Mediators and Drugs in Gastrointestinal Motility II

Endogenous and Exogenous Agents

Contributors

A. Bennett · G. Bertaccini · E. Corazziari · E. E. Daniel
M.A. Eastwood · G.J. Sanger · A.N. Smith · A. Torsoli

Editor

G. Bertaccini

Springer-Verlag Berlin Heidelberg New York 1982

Professor GIULIO BERTACCINI, M.D.
Head of the Department of Pharmacology,
School of Medicine, University of Parma
I-43100 Parma

With 74 Figures

ISBN-13:978-3-642-68476-0 e-ISBN-13:978-3-642-68474-6
DOI: 10.1007/978-3-642-68474-6

Library of Congress Cataloging in Publication Data. Main entry under title:
Mediators and drugs in gastrointestinal motility. (Handbook of experimental pharmacology; v. 59)
Contents: 1. Morphological basis and neurophysiological control – 2. Endogenous and exogenous agents.
Includes bibliographies and index. 1. Gastrointestinal system – Motility. 2. Gastrointestinal agents. 3. Neurotransmitters. 4. Gastrointestinal hormones. I. Baumgarten, H.G. II. Bertaccini, G. (Giulio), 1932–. III. Series.
[DNLM: 1. Gastrointestinal motility – Drug effects.
W1 HA51L v. 59 pt. 1/WI 102 M489] QP905.H3 vol. 59 [QP145] 615'.1s [612'.32] AACR2 81-21349
ISBN-13:978-3-642-68476-0

Softcover reprint of the hardcover 1st edition 1982

2122/3130-543210

Handbook of Experimental Pharmacology

Continuation of Handbuch der experimentellen Pharmakologie

Vol. 59/II

List of Contributors

Professor A. Bennett, Department of Surgery, King's College Hospital, Medical School, University of London, Denmark Hill, GB-London SE5 8RX

Professor G. Bertaccini, Head of the Department of Pharmacology, School of Medicine, University of Parma, I-43100 Parma

Professor E. Corazziari, Cattedra di Gastroenterologia, II Clinica Medica, Policlinico Umberto I, University of Rome, I-00100 Roma

Professor E. E. Daniel, Faculty of Health Sciences, Department of Neurosciences, McMaster University, 1200 Main Street West, Hamilton, Ontario, Canada L8S 4J9

Dr. M.A. Eastwood, Gastrointestinal Unit, University of Edinburgh, Western General Hospital, GB-Edinburgh EH4 2XU

Dr. G. J. Sanger, Beecham Pharmaceuticals, Medicinal Research Centre, GB-Harlow, Essex CM 19 5AD

A. N. Smith, Gastrointestinal Unit, University of Edinburgh, Western General Hospital, GB-Edinburgh EH4 2XU

Professor A. Torsoli, Cattedra di Gastroenterologia, II Clinica Medica, Policlinico Umberto I, University of Rome, I-00100 Roma

Preface

This volume places more emphasis on endogenous mediators of gut motility than on drugs used to treat patients with deranged motility. In this respect it resembles most other books on gastroenterology, for while only a relatively small number of drugs are really useful for a rational therapy, a tremendous amount of data is available on neural and hormonal factors regulating the motility of the alimentary canal. Moreover, it must be considered that some of the drugs which can routinely be employed to modify deranged motility of the digestive system are represented by pure or slightly modified endogenous compounds (e.g., cholecystokinin, its C-terminal octapeptide and caerulein), and it is easy to foresee that their number is destined to increase in the near future. Other drugs are simply antagonists of physiological substances acting on specific receptors (e.g., histamine H_2-blockers and opioid compounds).

The real explosion of research in this field and the extreme specialization often connected with the use of very sophisticated techniques and methodologies would probably have required a larger number of experts to cover some very specific fields from both an anatomical (lower esophageal sphincter, stomach, pylorus, small and large intestine) and a biochemical (hormones, candidate hormones, locally active substances, neurotransmitters etc.) point of view. However, in order to avoid involving too many collaborators (originally only one volume on gastrointestinal motility had been planned) and because many outstanding investigators were already engaged at the time when the work had to be organized. I decided to write about some topics myself although I had scarcely done sufficient work to justify authorship: I hope that this decision will at least result in greater homogeneity and perhaps objectivity. To avoid excessive length, the motility of the biliary system was not included in this volume, which nevertheless, attempts to provide the reader with the best of more than 2,000 papers. Our aim has been to interpret and clarify concepts derived from different disciplines and to provide not only an exhaustive compilation of data but also a synthesis, sometimes critical, of most pieces of information. Controversies were reported even though they sometimes represented a certain overlapping: however, in my opinion the diversity of views may be provocative and may act as a useful incentive for workers in the field.

As for exogenous agents, the book is not intended to be encyclopedic in its treatment of gastrointestinal pharmacology: the most important agents, such as the drugs acting on opioid receptors, some anticholinergics, and some laxatives, are extensively discussed, whereas others, like the new histamine H_2-receptor antagonists, which are mainly involved in secretory processes are barely mentioned. Finally a consistent number of figures and tables summarizes useful information and clarifies the most impressive data. The literature survey which formed the basis for the book was concluded in July 1981.

I wish to thank Professor H. HERKEN for selecting me as Editor of this volume and for giving me the opportunity of reporting in many chapters the results of my personal experience. I am very grateful to the authors for accepting the invitation to contribute, even though not all of them managed to meet the deadline for delivery of manuscripts. The delay in publication which this caused is offset by the excellent quality of this work. I should also like to thank Dr. GABRIELLA CORUZZI and Dr. CARMELO SCARPIGNATO of the Institute of Pharmacology, University of Parma Medical School, who helped me to overcome all the difficulties (and there were quite a lot) which I encountered during the drawing up of the manuscript and the collection of references.

GIULIO BERTACCINI

Contents

Motilin

Neurotensin

Bombesin

CHAPTER 2c

Peptides: Pancreatic Hormones. G. BERTACCINI. With 4 Figures

Glucagon

Insulin

Pancreatic Polypeptide

CHAPTER 2d

Peptides: Other Hormones. G. BERTACCINI. With 4 Figures

Vasopressin

Calcitonin

Coherin

Thyrotropin-Releasing Hormone

CHAPTER 2e

Peptides: Locally Active Peptides ("Vasoactive Peptides"). G. BERTACCINI
With 7 Figures

Angiotensin

Bradykinin

CHAPTER 3

Amines: Histamine. G. BERTACCINI. With 4 Figures

CHAPTER 4

Acidic Lipids: Prostaglandins. A. BENNETT and G. J. SANGER. With 1 Figure

CHAPTER 5

Pharmacology of Adrenergic, Cholinergic, and Drugs Acting on Other Receptors in Gastrointestinal Muscle. E. E. DANIEL

CHAPTER 7

Motility and Pressure Studies in Clinical Practice
A. TORSOLI and E. CORAZZIARI. With 15 Figures

Contents

Part I: Morphological Basis and Neurophysiological Control

CHAPTER 1

Endogenous Substances Which Can Affect Gastrointestinal Motility

G. BERTACCINI

General Introduction

All the compounds described in this chapter are "physiologic" in the sense that they occur in the organism under physiologic conditions. Of course, this does not imply that their action on the motility of the digestive system must necessarily be considered as "physiologic;" not all of these compounds participate directly in the physiologic regulation of peristalsis. However, the ability to modify motor activity of the digestive tract appears to be a common property of these substances.

The peptide compounds are represented by the true gastrointestinal hormones, gastrin, cholecystokinin, secretin, and gastric inhibitory polypeptide (GIP), by the pancreatic hormones, insulin and glucagon, and by the so-called candidate hormones (GROSSMAN 1974b), i.e., suspected but not yet proven to be hormonal agents since they do not possess as yet all the prerequisites to reach hormonal status. This is the case of vasoactive intestinal peptide (VIP), motilin, pancreatic polypeptide (PP), neurotensin, substance P, and other substances which were shown to be present in the gastrointestinal tract only by radioimmunoassay or immunohistochemistry: bombesin-like peptide, somatostatin-like peptide, enkephalins, etc. Other peptides which can affect gastrointestinal motility are represented by coherin, found in the posterior pituitary gland, thyrotropin-releasing hormone (TRH), first found in the hypothalamus, then in the gut and the pancreas, and calcitonin, the thyroid hormone whose primary effect is to lower the calcium concentration in the blood. Finally, peptides which have a primary role in the vascular muscle (so-called vasoactive peptides, like angiotensin, bradykinin, vasopressin) can also exert a remarkable effect on intestinal motility.

Besides the peptides, biogenic amines like histamine, 5-hydroxytryptamine, dopamine, and acidic lipids such as the prostaglandins will be considered in this chapter. For many years all of these compounds have been considered as "humoral" mediators and in a certain way they have been opposed to the "nervous" mediators. Now this distinction appears to be something of an artifact and can no longer be maintained. In fact, in the last few years it has been recognized that some gastrointestinal peptides like VIP, enkephalins, substance P, also occur in nerves (surprising localizations have been reported: not only gastrin in the vagus, but even gastrin-like immunoreactivity and insulin-like immunoreactivity were found after stimulation of sciatic and brachial nerves of the cat (UVNÄS-WALLENSTEN 1979a, b; UVNÄS-WALLENSTEN et al. 1979). Finally, some peptides are located in endocrine-like cells which, however, do not discharge their products into the blood and thus are presumed to exert a local, paracrine function (Fig. 1). If the situation is that de-

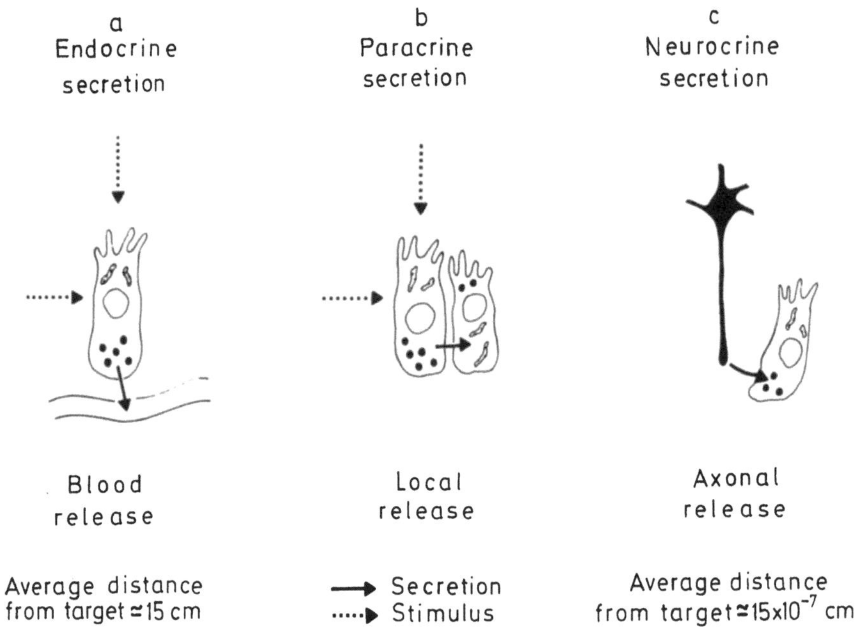

Fig. 1a–c. Diagrammatic representation of the mode of delivery of peptides acting as gut hormones **a**, paracrine messengers **b**, or neurotransmitters **c**. The possibility exists that the same molecule could function in each of these systems in the same organism

scribed in Fig. 1, the selectivity of the actions of the messengers at specific target levels appears to be a real problem. According to GROSSMAN (1979b), selectivity for products of neurocrine or paracrine secretions is achieved by the close proximity to those targets which are to be activated; for endocrine or mixed kinds of secretion several factors may intervene: the blood–brain barrier may exclude access to the central nervous system and a similar mechanism may also be hypothesized in some peripheral synaptosomes which could keep the messengers away from the receptors. In the case of peptides, the different molecular forms which have been. described may activate different targets. In other cases, different mechanisms may be envisaged, according to the quantity of secretions: small amounts being able to activate quite close targets and large amounts causing generalized effects. Of course, these represent speculations which must await adequate studies in order to be checked and accepted as true events.

Summing up, many chemical messengers can be delivered from the cell of origin ("regulator cells," according to GROSSMAN 1979b) to their specific target by neurocrine, endocrine, or paracrine secretion (Fig. 1); for this reason the term "hormone" may sometimes be inappropriate for such compounds and other new terms have been recently suggested to designate the products of these "policrine" secretions. WINGATE (1976) proposed the generic title for the gastrointestinal polypeptides of "eupeptides," constituting the "eupeptide system" and suggesting the idea of eupeptic, or good digestive function (which these peptides clearly promote). GROSSMAN (1979a, b), including also nonpeptidic compounds, proposed the terms "chemitters," (a contraction of "chemical transmitters") or "regulins" (as products

Table 1. In vivo interactions among secretions of endogenous peptides affecting gastrointestinal motility

Hormone	Species	Stimulation of release	Inhibition of release	References
Gastrin	Dog	Insulin		UNGER et al. (1967)
	Human	Insulin		REHFELD (1971)
	Dog	Insulin		KANETO et al. (1969)
	Dog	Glucagon		KANETO et al. (1970)
	Rat	Histamine		KAHLSON et al. (1964)
(Pentagastrin)	Human	HPP		FLOYD et al. (1977)
	Pig	Calcitonin		COOPER et al. (1972)
	Dog	PP		BLOOM and POLAK (1978)
	Rat	Histamine		HAKANSON et al. (1977)
Cholecystokinin	Dog	Insulin		UNGER et al. (1967)
	Rat	Insulin		RAPTIS et al. (1969)
	Monkey	Insulin		GLICK et al. (1970)
	Human	Insulin		DUPRÉ et al. (1969)
	Dog	Glucagon		UNGER et al. (1967)
	Pig	Calcitonin		CARE et al. (1971)
(Cerulein)	Rat	Insulin		AGOSTI (1969)
	Dog	Insulin		BERTACCINI et al. (1970)
	Human	Insulin		FALLUCCA et al. (1972)
	Dog	Glucagon		DE CARO et al. (1970)
	Human	HPP		ADRIAN et al. (1977)
	Human	Calcitonin		PASSERI et al. (1975)
	Pig	Calcitonin		CARE and BATES (1971)
Secretin	Rat	Insulin		RAPTIS et al. (1969)
	Dog	Insulin		UNGER et al. (1967)
	Monkey	Insulin		GLICK et al. (1970)
	Human	Insulin		DUPRÉ et al. (1966)
	Dog/human		Gastrin	BUNCHMAN et al. (1971)
	Human	HPP		ADRIAN et al. (1978)
Glucagon	Dog	Insulin		LEFEBVRE and LUYCKX (1966)
	Human	Insulin		YALOW and BERSON (1960)
	Cat		Gastrin	BECKER et al. (1973a, b)
	Human	Calcitonin		MELVIN et al. (1970)
GIP	Dog	Insulin		PEDERSON et al. (1975)
	Human	Insulin		DUPRÉ (1973)
	Rat	Glucagon		BROWN et al. (1975)
	Human	Glucagon		BROWN et al. (1975)
	Dog	PP		BLOOM and POLAK (1978)
	Dog		Gastrin	VILLAR et al. (1975)
VIP	Cat	Insulin		SCHEBALIN et al. (1977)
	Cat	Glucagon		SCHEBALIN et al. (1977)
	Dog	PP		BLOOM and POLAK (1978)
	Dog		Gastrin	VILLAR et al. (1975)
	Dog	Somatostatin		IPP et al. (1978)
Bombesin	Dog	Gastrin		BERTACCINI et al. (1974)
	Human	Gastrin		BASSO et al. (1977)

Table 1 (continued)

Hormone	Species	Stimulation of release	Inhibition of release	References
	Cat	Gastrin		G. BERTACCINI (unpublished)
	Dog	CCK		FENDER et al. (1976)
	Dog	PP		TAYLOR et al. (1978)
	Human	HPP		DE MAGISTRIS et al. (1979)
	Dog	GIP		BECKER et al. (1978)
	Rat	PG (F series)		M. IMPICCIATORE (unpublished work)
	Human	Enteroglucagon		BLOOM et al. (1979)
	Human	Motilin		BLOOM et al. (1979)
	Human	Neurotensin		BLOOM et al. (1979)
	Guinea pig	Catecholamines		E.S. VIZI (unpublished work 1971)
	Dog	ACH		KOWALEWSKI and KOLODEJ (1976)
	Dog		VIP	MELCHIORRI et al. (1975)
	Cat		VIP	MELCHIORRI et al. (1975)
	Human		VIP	MELCHIORRI et al. (1975)
	Human	Glucagon		FALLUCCA et al. (1978)
Somatostatin	Dog		Insulin	SAKURAI et al. (1974)
	Dog		Glucagon	SAKURAI et al. (1974)
	Human		Insulin	MORTIMER et al. (1974)
	Human		Glucagon	MORTIMER et al. (1974)
	Human		Gastrin	BLOOM et al. (1974b)
	Human		Enteroglucagon	LEROITH et al. (1975)
	Dog		PP	GYR et al. (1978)
	Human		HPP	ADRIAN (1978)
	Human		CCK	SCHLEGEL et al. (1977)
	Human		Secretin	SCHLEGEL et al. (1977)
	Rat		Gastrin	OBIE and COOPER (1979)
Calcitonin	Cat		Gastrin	BECKER et al. (1973a)
	Human		Gastrin	BECKER et al. (1974)
	Human		Insulin	D'ONOFRIO et al. (1978)
Bradykinin	Rat	ADH		HARRIS (1970)
	Cat	ADH		ROCHA e SILVA and HARRIS (1970)
Neurotensin	Dog	Insulin		BROWN and VALE (1976)
	Dog	Glucagon		BROWN and VALE (1976)
	Dog	Gastrin		ISHIDA (1977)
Oxitocin	Dog	VIP		EBEID et al. (1979)
Substance P	Rat	Glucagon		BROWN and VALE (1976)
	Rat	Histamine		JOHNSON and ERDÖS (1973)
	Dog		Insulin	SASAKI (1976)
	Dog	Glucagon		PATTON et al. (1976)
	Dog		Gastrin	SASAKI (1976)
Enkephalin	Dog		Secretin	CHEY et al. (1980)
Histamine	Rat	Vasopressin		DOGTEROM et al. (1976)

Table 1 (continued)

Hormone	Species	Stimulation of release	Inhibition of release	References
Insulin	Human	PP		SCHWARTZ (1978)
(Hypo-	Human	Gastrin		KORMAN et al. (1973)
glycemia)	Dog	Gastrin		CSENDES et al. (1972)
	Human	HPP		FLOYD et al. (1977)
	Human		Motilin	CHRISTOFIDES et al. (1978)
	Calf	Glucagon		BLOOM et al. (1974c)
	Human	Glucagon		BLOOM et al. (1974c)

of "regulator cells"). It is probable that other neologisms are going to be coined and only the future will say which will endure.

Since most of these substances have multiple actions, attempts have been made to establish rigorous criteria which could enable us to distinguish between "physiologic" and "pharmacologic" effects (GROSSMAN 1973, 1974a). Physiologic effects were considered those which could be seen after endogenous release by physiologic stimuli (like meals) and which, after mimicking endogenous release by exogenous infusions, determine blood levels of the corresponding hormone similar to those encountered after physiologic stimuli. Pharmacologic effects were considered those obtained with amounts higher than those required for the preceding condition. However, the situation is complicated by a number of very important factors which may represent a noticeable source of errors.

a) Ingestion of food represents a stimulus for the release of a series of endogenous substances which, besides acting as separate entities, may release in their turn (or prevent the release of) other substances (see Table 1) and in addition can interact with each other with consequent synergistic or antagonistic effects. Of course when speaking of interactions, not only humoral but also nervous interactions must be considered (see Table 2) again with a number of other possibilities of synergisms and antagonisms; the final biologic result thus represents the algebraic sum of all these different effects which multiply in close parallelism with the continuous discoveries of active principles. It is obvious that intravenous infusion of single compounds cannot be expected to reproduce the natural event exactly.

b) Reliable radioimmunoassays are very few up to now; they give different results according to the antibodies used in the various laboratories and they may or may not distinguish among the different molecular forms of the hormones. Very often data reported in the literature give such inadequate information on the radioimmunologic techniques that some specific guidelines have actually been offered for the preparation of manuscripts (WALSH 1978).

c) Last, but certainly not least, if we admit that the same compound may be simultaneously released by endocrine, paracrine, and neurocrine secretion, who could say whether an intravenous bolus injection or even a continuous infusion of 1–100 μg is detected by the target tissue any more easily or to any greater extent than a few picograms released in close proximity to the target cell itself?

The availability of specific inhibitors could play a crucial role in establishing physiologic tasks for the chemical messengers. Unfortunately, we have at our dis-

Table 2. Influence of vagal or splanchnic stimulation on the release of endogenous substances which can affect gastrointestinal motility

	Species	Stimulation of release	Inhibition of release	References
Vagal stimulation	Human	HPP		SCHWARTZ et al. (1976)
	Dog	Insulin		FROHMAN et al. (1967)
	Baboon	Insulin		DANIEL and HENDERSON (1967)
	Dog	Glucagon		KANETO et al. (1974)
	Cat	Insulin		UVNÄS et al. (1975)
	Cat	Gastrin		UVNÄS et al. (1975)
	Pig	VIP		SCHAFFALITZKY DE MUCKADELL (1977)
	Dog	Gastrin		LANCIAULT et al. (1973)
	Goose	Calcitonin		FRANCHIMONT and HEYNEN (1976)
	Cat	Somatostatin		UVNÄS-WALLENSTEN (1978)
Splanchnic stimulation	Cat	Glucagon	Insulin	BLOOM and EDWARDS (1975)
	Dog	Glucagon	Insulin	BLOOM and EDWARDS (1975)
	Calf	Glucagon	Insulin	BLOOM et al. (1973)
	Sheep	Glucagon	Insulin	BLOOM and EDWARDS (1975)
	Dog	Glucagon	Gastrin	BLOOM and EDWARDS (1975)
	Cat	Glucagon	Gastrin	BLOOM and EDWARDS (1975); BLAIR et al. (1975)

posal only specific inhibitors limited to amino compounds and we are still waiting to increase the number of the very few antagonists of peptide transmitters.

All these premises must be carefully considered when evaluating the effects of the compounds described in Chaps. 2–4 in which all the aforementioned substances will be reported. Conversely, substances which, under particular experimental or pathologic conditions, may produce besides their primary effects a moderate action on the motility of the digestive system (parathyroid hormone, female sex hormones, thyroxine etc.), will not be considered.

References

Adrian TE, Bloom SR, Besterman HS, Barnes AJ, Cooke TJ, Russel RC, Faber RG (1977) Mechanism of pancreatic polypeptide release in man. Lancet 1:161–163

Adrian TE, Bloom SR, Besterman HS, Bryant MG (1978) PP-physiology and pathology. In: Bloom SR (ed) Gut hormones. Churchill Livingstone, Edinburgh London, pp 254–260

Agosti A (1969) Hypoglycemic activity of caerulein in the rat. Pharmacol Res Commun 1:94–96

Basso N, Lezoche E, Giri S, Percocco M, Speranza V (1977) Acid and gastrin levels after bombesin and calcium infusion in patients with incomplete antrectomy. Am J Dig Dis 22:125–128

Becker HD, Konturek SJ, Reeder DD, Thompson JC (1973a) Effect of calcium and calcitonin on gastrin and gastric secretion in cats. Am J Physiol 225:277–280

Becker HD, Reeder DD, Thompson JC (1973b) Effect of glucagon on circulating gastrin. Gastroenterology 65:28–35

Becker HD, Reeder DD, Scurry MT (1974) Inhibition of gastrin release and gastric secretion by calcitonin in patients with peptic ulcer. Am J Surg 127:71–75

Becker HD, Börger HW, Scafmayer A, Werner M (1978) Bombesin releases GIP in dogs. Scand J Gastroenterol [Suppl 49] 13:14

Bertaccini G, De Caro G, Melchiorri P (1970) The effects of caerulein on insulin secretion in anaesthetized dogs. Br J Pharmacol 40:78–85

Bertaccini G, Erspamer V, Melchiorri P, Sopranzi N (1974) Gastrin release by bombesin in the dog. Br J Pharmacol 52:219–225

Blair EL, Grund ER, Reed JD, Sanders DJ, Sanger G, Shaw B (1975) The effect of sympathetic nerve stimulation on serum gastrin, gastric acid secretion, and mucosal blood flow responses to meat extract stimulation in anaesthetized cats. J Physiol (Lond) 253:493–504

Bloom SR, Edwards AV (1975) The release of pancreatic glucagon and inhibition of insulin in response to stimulation of the sympathetic innervation. J Physiol (Lond) 253:157–173

Bloom SR, Polak JM (1978) Enteropancreatic axis. In: Grossman MI, Speranza V, Basso N, Lezoche E (eds) Gastrointestinal hormones and pathology of the digestive system. Plenum, New York, pp 151–163

Bloom SR, Edwards AV, Vaughan NJA (1973) The role of the sympathetic innervation in the control of plasma glucagon concentration in the conscious calf. J Physiol (Lond) 233:457–466

Bloom SR, Edwards AV, Vaughan NJA (1974a) The role of the autonomic innervation in the control of plasma glucagon concentration in the calf. J Physiol (Lond) 236:611–623

Bloom SR, Mortimer CH, Thorner MO et al. (1974b) Inhibition of gastrin and gastric-acid secretion by growth-hormone release-inhibiting hormone. Lancet 2:1106–1109

Bloom SR, Vaughan NJA, Russel RCG (1974c) Vagal control of glucagon release in man. Lancet 2:546–549

Bloom SR, Chatei MA, Christofides ND et al. (1979) Bombesin infusion in man, pharmacokinetics and effect on gastrointestinal and pancreatic hormonal peptides. J Endocrinol 83:P51

Brown JC, Dryburgh JR, Ross SA, Dupré J (1975) Identification and actions of gastric inhibitory polypeptide. Rec Prog Horm Res 31:487–532

Brown M, Vale M (1976) Effects of neurotensin and substance P on plasma insulin, glucagon and glucose levels. Endocrinology 98:819–822

Bunchman HH, Reeder DD, Thompson JC (1971) Effect of secretin on the serum gastrin response to a meal in man and in dog. Surg Forum 22:303–305

Care AD, Bruce JB, Boelkinst J, Kenny AD, Conaway H, Anast CS (1971) Role of pancreozymin-cholecystokinin and structurally related compounds as calcitonin secretagogue. Endocrinology 89:262

Chey WY, Coy DM, Konturek SJ, Schally AV, Tasler J (1980) Enkephalin inhibits the release and action of secretin on pancreatic secretion in the dog. J Physiol (Lond) 298: 429–436

Christofides ND, Bloom SR, Besterman HS (1978) Physiology of motilin II. In: Bloom R (ed) Gut hormones. Churchill Livingstone, Edinburgh London, pp 343–350

Cooper CW, Schwesinger WH, Ontjes DA, Mahgoub AM, Munson PL (1972) Stimulation of secretion of pig thyrocalcitonin by gastrin and related peptides. Endocrinology 91:1079–1089

Csendes A, Walsh JH, Grossman MI (1972) Effects of atropine and of antral acidification on gastrin release and acid secretion in response to insulin and feeding in dogs. Gastroenterology 63:257–263

Daniel PM, Henderson JR (1967) The effect of vagal stimulation on plasma insulin and glucose levels in the baboon. J Physiol (Lond) 192:317–326

De Caro G, Improta G, Melchiorri P (1970) Effect of caerulein infusion on glucagon secretion in the dog. Experientia 26:1145–1146

De Magistris L, Delle Fave G, Khon A, Schwartz TW (1979) Stimulation of pancreatic-polypeptide and gastrin secretion by bombesin in man. Ital J Gastroenterol 11:139A

Dogterom J, Van Wimersma TB, De Wied D (1976) Histamine as an extremely potent releaser of vasopressin in the rat. Experientia 32:659–660

D'Onofrio F, Sgambato S, Carbone L, Giuliano D, Siniscalchi N, Varano R (1978) The effect of calcitonin on plasma insulin response to glucose in normal, obese and prediabetic subjects. Diabetologia 15:228P
Dupré J, Rojas L, White JJ, Unger RH, Beck JC (1966) Effects of secretin on insulin and glucagon in portal and periferal blood in man. Lancet 2:26–27
Dupré J, Curtis JD, Unger RH, Waddell RW, Beck, JC (1969) Effects of secretin, pancreozymin or gastrin on the response of the endocrine pancreas to administration of glucose or arginine in man. J Clin Invest 48:745–757
Dupré J, Ross SA, Watson D, Brown JC (1973) Stimulation of insulin secretion by gastric inhibitory polypeptide in man. J Clin Endocrinol Metab 37:826–828
Ebeid AM, Attia RR, Sundaram P, Fischer JE (1979) Release of vasoactive intestinal peptide in the central nervous system in man. Am J Surg 137:123–127
Fallucca F, Carratù R, Tamburrano G, Javicosi M, Menzinger G, Andreani D (1972) Effects of caerulein and pancreozymin on insulin secretion in normal subjects and in patients with insulinoma. Horm Metab Res 4:55
Fallucca F, Delle Fave GF, Gambardella S, Mirabella C, De Magistris L, Carratù R (1978) Glucagon secretion induced by bombesin in man. In: Grossman MI, Speranza V, Basso N, Lezoche E (eds) Gastrointestinal hormones and pathology of the digestive system. Plenum, New York, pp 259–261
Fender HR, Curtis PJ, Rayford PL, Thompson JC (1976) Effect of bombesin on serum gastrin and cholecystokinin in dogs. Surg Forum 37:414–416
Floyd JC Jr, Fajans SS, Pek S, Chance RE (1977) A newly recognised pancreatic polypeptide; plasma levels in health and disease. Rec Prog Horm Res 33:519–570
Franchimont P, Heynen GA (1976) Relationships between CT and other hormones. In: Franchimont P, Heynen G (eds) Parathormone and calcitonin radioimmunoassay in various medical and osteoarticular disorders. Masson, Paris, pp 73–78
Frohman LA, Ezdinli EZ, Javid R (1967) Effect of vagotomy and vagal stimulation on insulin secretion. Diabetes 16:443–448
Glick Z, Baile CA, Mayer J (1970) Insulinotropic and possible insulin-like effects of secretin and cholecystokinin-pancreozimin. Endocrinology 86:927–931
Grossman MI (1973) What is physiological? Gastroenterology 65:994
Grossman MI (1974a) What is physiological?: Round 2. Gastroenterology 67:766–767
Grossman MI (1974b) Candidate hormones of the gut. Gastroenterology 67:730–755
Grossman MI (1979a) Neural and hormonal regulation of gastrointestinal function: an overview. Annu Rev Physiol 41:27–33
Grossman MI (1979b) Chemical messengers: a view from the gut. Fed Proc 38:2341–2343
Gyr K, Kayasseh L, Haecki W, Girard J, Rittman WW, Stalder GA (1978) The release of pancreatic polypeptide (PP) by test meal and HCl and its response to somatostatin (SST) and atropine in dogs. Scand J Gastroenterol [Suppl 49] 13:71
Hakanson R, Rehfeld JF, Liedberg G, Sundler F (1977) Colchicine inhibits stimulated release of gastric histamine but not activation of histidine decarboxylase. Experientia 33:305–306
Harris NC (1970) Release of the antidiuretic hormone by bradykinin in rats. In: Sicuteri F, Rocha e Silva M, Back N (eds) Bradykinin and related kinins. Plenum, New York, pp 609–614
Ipp E, Dobbs RE, Unger RH (1978) Vasoactive intestinal peptide stimulates pancreatic somatostatin release. FEBS Lett 90:76–78
Ishida T (1977) Stimulatory effect of neurotensin on insulin and gastrin secretion in dogs. Endocrinol Jpn 24:335–342
Johnson AR, Erdös EG (1973) Release of histamine from mast cells by vasoactive peptides. Proc Soc Exp Biol Med 142:1252–1256
Kahlson G, Rosengren E, Svahn D, Thunberg G (1964) Mobilization and formation of histamine in the gastric mucosa as related to acid secretion. J Physiol (Lond) 174:400–416
Kaneto A, Tasaka Y, Kosaka K, Nakao K (1969) Stimulation of insulin secretion by the C-terminal tetrapeptide amide of gastrin. Endocrinology 84:1098–1106
Kaneto A, Mizuno Y, Tasaka V, Kosaka K (1970) Stimulation of glucagon secretion by tetragastrin. Endocrinology 86:1175–1180

Kaneto A, Miki E, Kosaka K (1974) Effects of vagal stimulation on glucagon and insulin secretion. Endocrinology 95:1005–1010
Korman MG, Hansky J, Coupland GAE, Cumberland VH (1973) Serum gastrin response to insulin hypoglycemia: studies after parietal cell vagotomy and after selective gastric vagotomy. Scand J Gastroenterol 8:235–239
Kowalewski K, Kolodej A (1976) Effect of bombesin a natural tetradecapeptide, on myoelectrical and mechanical activity of isolated ex vivo perfused, canine stomach. Pharmacology 14:8–19
Lanciault G, Bonoma C, Brooks FP (1973) Vagal stimulation, gastrin release and acid secretion in anesthetized dogs. Am J Physiol 225:546–552
Léfèbvre PJ, Luyckx A (1966) Glucagon stimulated insulin release. Lancet 2:248–250
Leroith D, Vinik AI, Epstein S, Baron P, Olkenitzky MN, Pimstone BL (1975) S Am Med J 49:1–60
Melchiorri P, Improta G, Sopranzi N (1975) Inibizione della secrezione di VIP da parte della bombesina nel cane, nel gatto e nell'uomo. Rend Gastroenterol [Suppl 1] 7:57
Melvin KEV, Voelkel EF, Tashjian AH Jr (1970) Medullary carcinoma of the thyroid: stimulation by calcium and glucagon of calcitonin secretion. In: Proceedings of the Second International Symposium on Calcitonin (Abstr). Heinemann, London, p 487P
Mortimer CH, Turnbridge WMG, Carr D et al. (1974) Effects of growth-hormone release-inhibiting hormone on circulating glucagon, insulin and growth hormone in normal, diabetic, acromegalic and hypopituitary patients. Lancet 1:697–701
Obie JF, Cooper CW (1979) Bombesin stimulates gastrin secretion in the rat without increasing serum calcitonin. Proc Soc Exp Biol Med 162:437–441
Passeri M, Carapezzi C, Ceccato S, Monica C, Strozzi D, Palummeri E (1975) Possible role of caerulein on calcitonin secretion in man. Experientia 31:1234–1235
Patton G, Brown M, Dobbs R, Vale W, Unger RH (1976) Effects of neurotensin and substance P on insulin and glucagon release by the perfused dog pancreas. Metabolism [Suppl 1] 25:1465
Pederson RA, Schubert HE, Brown JC (1975) Gastric inhibitory polypeptide. Its physiologic release and insulinotropic action in the dog. Diabetes 24:1050–1056
Raptis S, Goberna R, Schröder KE, Ditschuneit HH, Pfeiffer EF (1969) Die Wirkung der intestinalen Hormone Sekretin und Pankreozymin bei der totalpankreatektomierten Ratte. Verh Dtsch Ges Inn Med 75:650–653
Rehfeld FJ (1971) Effect of gastrin and its C-terminal tetrapeptide on insulin secretion in man. Acta Endocrinol 66:169–176
Rocha e Silva M, Harris MC (1970) The release of vasopressin by a direct central action of bradykinin. In: Sicuteri F, Rocha e Silva M, Back N (eds) Bradykinin and related kinins. Plenum, New York, pp 561–570
Sakurai H, Dobbs R, Unger RH (1974) Somatostatin-induced changes in insulin and glucagon secretion in normal and diabetic dogs. J Clin Invest 54:1395–1402
Sasaki H (1976) Effects of substance P. Metabolism [Suppl 1] 25:1463
Schaffalitzky de Muckadell OB, Fahrenkrug OB, Holst JJ (1977) Release of vasoactive intestinal peptide (VIP) by electric stimulation of vagal nerves. Gastroenterology 72:373–375
Schebalin M, Said SI, Makhlouf GM (1977) Stimulation of insulin and glucagon secretion by vasoactive intestinal peptide. Am J Physiol 232:E197–E200
Schlegel W, Raptis S, Dollinger HC, Pfeiffer EF (1977) Inhibition of secretin, pancreozymin and gastrin release and their biological activities by somatostatin. In: Bonfils S, Fromageot P, Rosselin G (eds) Hormonal receptors in digestive tract physiology. Elsevier, Amsterdam Oxford New York, pp 361–377
Schwartz TW (1978) Vagal regulation of PP secretion. In: Bloom SR (ed) Gut hormones. Churchill Livingstone, Edinburgh London, pp 261–264
Schwartz TW, Rehfeld JF, Stadil F, Larsson LI, Chance RE, Moon N (1976) Pancreatic polypeptide response to food in duodenal ulcer patients before and after vagotomy. Lancet 1:1102–1105
Taylor IL, Walsh JH, Carter DC, Wood J, Grossman MI (1978) Effect of atropine and bethanechol on release of pancreatic polypeptide and gastrin by bombesin in dogs. Scand J Gastroenterol [Suppl 49] 13:183

Unger RH, Ketterer H, Dupré J, Eisentraut AM (1967) The effect of secretin, pancreozymin and gastrin on insulin and glucagon secretion in anesthetized dogs. J Clin Invest 46:630–645
Uvnäs B, Uvnäs-Wallensten K, Nillson G (1975) Release of gastrin on vagal stimulation in the cat. Acta Physiol Scand 94:167–176
Uvnäs-Wallensten K (1978) Vagal release of antral hormones. In: Bloom SR (ed) Gut hormones. Churchill Livingstone, Edinburgh London, pp 389–393
Uvnäs-Wallensten K (1979a) Vagal, gastrinergic transmission. In: Rehfeld JF, Amdrup E (eds) Gastrins and the vagus. Academic Press, London New York San Francisco, pp 115–122
Uvnäs-Wallensten K (1979b) Release of gastrin and insulin by electrical vagal stimulation and sulphonuric drugs from endocrine cells and nerves in the cat. In: Rosselin G, Fromageot P, Bonfils S (eds) Hormone receptors in digestion and nutrition. Elsevier, Amsterdam Oxford New York, pp 493–500
Uvnäs-Wallensten K, Efendic S, Uvnäs B, Lundberg JM (1979) Release of gastrin from the skeletal muscle and from the antral mucosa in cats induced by sulfonuric drugs. Acta Physiol Scand 106:267–270
Villar HV, Fender HR, Rayford PL, Ramus NI, Thompson JC (1975) Inhibition of gastrin release and gastric secretion by GIP and VIP. In: Thompson JC (ed) Gastrointestinal hormones. University of Texas Press, Austin, pp 467–473
Walsh JH (1978) Radioimmunoassay methodology for articles published in gastroenterology. Gastroenterology 75:523–524
Wingate D (1976) The eupeptide system: a general theory of gastrointestinal hormones. Lancet 1:529–532
Yalow RS, Berson SA (1960) Immunoassay of plasma insulin concentrations in normal and diabetic man: insulin secretory response to glucose and other agents. J Clin Invest 39:1041–1052

CHAPTER 2a

Peptides: Gastrointestinal Hormones

G. BERTACCINI

Gastrin

A. Introduction

The history of hormones, which began as a physiologic era with the discovery of secretin by BAYLISS and STARLING in 1902, turned into a biochemical era with the isolation of gastrin by GREGORY and TRACY in 1964. From pig antral mucosa these authors isolated two heptadecapeptides that they named gastrin I and gastrin II, according to the absence (I) or presence (II) of a sulfated group on the tyrosyl residue in the sixth position (starting unconventionally from the COOH terminus). Since then, gastrin heptadecapeptides have been purified from the antral mucosa of several species (including human, dog, pig, cat, sheep, and cow) and found to differ in only one or two amino acid substitutions in the middle of the linear peptide chain (GREGORY 1974). The development of immunologic methods of study made it possible to measure gastrin in tissues and body fluids and established the heterogeneity of this peptide which can be present in several forms because of its biosynthetic pathways and enzymatic degradation: a "big gastrin" with 34 amino acid residues (this is referred to as G 34), the heptadecapeptide "little gastrin," (G 17), and a "minigastrin" isolated from gastrinoma tissue by GREGORY and TRACY (1974) and thought initially to be the COOH terminal tridecapeptide of G 17. It has since become apparent that there is an additional tryptophan at the NH_2 terminus, bringing the total of aminoacid residues to 14 (G 14) (GREGORY et al. 1979), in the same sequence as in the COOH terminal tetradecapeptide of G 17. According to REHFELD and LARSSON (1979) the predominant molecular form of gastrin in the gut is a small peptide corresponding to its COOH terminal tetrapeptide amide but this is still a matter of controversy (DOCKRAY and GREGORY 1980). The various forms of gastrin are presented in Table 1. The proportion of sulfated to nonsulfated gastrins varies, but usually they are present in about equal amounts. The table also shows the gastrin-like peptide most commonly used, pentagastrin, a commercially available synthetic pentapeptide consisting of the COOH terminal tetrapeptide amide of gastrin plus a β-alanyl residue and an NH_2 terminal blocking group (*t*-butyloxycarbonyl). Since its pharmacologic actions parallel those of natural gastrin it will be discussed in this chapter even though pentagastrin is a synthetic compound and not an endogenous substance. Finally, two immunoreactive components have been found in tissues and in the circulation which are probably larger peptides since they emerge with smaller elution volumes from Sephadex gel-filtration columns: the so called "big big gastrin" (YALOW and BERSON 1971, 1972) and

Table 1. The gastrins[a]

Big (G 34)		Little (G 17)					Mini-gastrin (G 14)	Tetra-gastrin	1-13-NTF of G 17
Human	Pig	Human	Pig	Cow, sheep	Dog	Cat	Human	Pig	Pig
pGlu	–								
Leu	–								
Gly	–								
Pro	Leu								
Gln	–								
Gly	–								
His	–								
Pro	–								
Ser	Pro								
Leu	–								
Val	–								
Ala	–								
Asp	–								
Pro	Leu								
Ser	Ala								
Lys	–								
Lys	–								
Gln	–	pGlu	–	–	–	–			–
Gly	–	–	–	–	–	–			–
Pro	–	–	–	–	–	–			–
Trp	–	–	–	–	–	–	–		–
Leu	Met	–	Met	Val	Met	–	–		Met
Glu	–	–	–	–	–	–	–		–
Glu	–	–	–	–	–	–	–		–
Glu	–	–	–	–	Ala	–	–		–
Glu	–	–	–	–	–	–	–		–
Glu	–	–	–	Ala	–	Ala	–		–
Ala	–	–	–	–	–	–	–		–
Tyr	–	–	–	–	–	–	–		–
Gly	–	–	–	–	–	–	–		–
Trp	–	–	–	–	–	–	–	–	
Met	–	–	–	–	–	–	–	–	
Asp	–	–	–	–	–	–	–	–	
Phe-NH_2	–	–	–	–	–	–	–	–	

[a] NTF = NH_2 terminal fragment; pGlu = pyroglutamic acid; – = same as human. All these gastrins (except tetragastrin) occur in two forms: unsulfated tyrosine = I, and sulfated tyrosine = II. For references see text

"component 1" (REHFELD and STADIL 1973). These have not been characterized chemically or biologically.

The COOH terminal portion of the gastrin molecule has all the biologic effects of the whole molecule and even the dipeptide amide shows traces of activity (BERTACCINI 1972). However, the potencies of the natural peptides or their synthetic partial sequences must be defined very carefully. Not only must the activity of a given amount of exogenously administered peptide be considered, but also their half-lives in the organism. For instance, the COOH terminal tetrapeptide, tetragas-

Table 2. Structure–activity relationship of gastrin-like and cholecystokinin-like polypeptides on longitudinal muscle strips of guinea pig ileum[a]

Acetylcholine		ED_{50} (*M*)	Relative potency	α
		2.7×10^{-8}	1.0	1.2
Lys-...-Ile-Ser-Asp-Arg-Asp-Tyr(SO_3H)-Met-Gly-Trp-Met-Asp-Phe-NH_2	CCK PZ	2.01×10^{-8}	1.3	1
pGlu-Asp-Tyr(SO_3H)-Thr-Gly-Trp-Met-Asp-Phe-NH_2	Cerulein	2.5×10^{-9}	10.8	1
pGlu-Tyr(SO_3H)-Thr-Gly-Trp-Met-Asp-Phe-NH_2	Phyllocerulein	2.7×10^{-9}	10.0	1
Asp-Tyr(SO_3H)-Met-Gly-Trp-Met-Asp-Phe-NH_2	CCK PZ octapeptide	4.8×10^{-9}	5.6	1
Tyr(SO_3H)-Met-Gly-Trp-Met-Asp-Phe-NH_2	CCK PZ heptapeptide	6×10^{-9}	4.5	1
Tyr(SO_3H)-Thr-Gly-Trp-Met-Asp-Phe-NH_2	Cerulein heptapeptide	4×10^{-9}	6.7	1
Z(NO_2)-Tyr(SO_3H)-Gly-Trp-Met-Asp-Phe-NH_2	Gastrin II hexapeptide	10^{-8}	2.7	1
p-...-Glu-Ala-Tyr-Gly-Trp-Met-Asp-Phe-NH_2	Gastrin I (human)	9.2×10^{-8}	0.29	0.9
pGlu-Asp-Tyr-Thr-Gly-Trp-Met-Asp-Phe-NH_2	Desulfated cerulein	10^{-7}	0.27	0.9
Ac-Thr-Gly-Trp-Met-Asp-Phe-NH_2	Cerulein hexapeptide	4×10^{-8}	0.67	0.7
H_2-Tyr-Gly-Trp-Met-Asp-Phe-NH_2	Gastrin I hexapeptide	10^{-7}	0.27	0.7
H-Gly-Trp-Met-Asp-Phe-NH_2	Cerulein pentapeptide	10^{-6}	0.027	0.8
BOC-Ala-Trp-Met-Asp-Phe-NH_2	Pentagastrin	9×10^{-7}	0.03	0.8
H-Trp-Met-Asp-Phe-NH_2	Tetragastrin	1.2×10^{-6}	0.02	0.6
BOC-Met-Asp-Phe-NH_2	Tripeptide	5.5×10^{-6}	0.0049	0.6
Met-Asp-Phe-NH_2	Tripeptide	6.6×10^{-6}	0.0041	0.6
Asp-Phe-NH_2	Dipeptide	7.2×10^{-6}	0.0037	0.6

[a] ED_{50} values represent the concentrations of different polypeptides required for half-maximal response. Since it has been shown that all these peptides act via acetylcholine release, the half-maximal contraction produced by acetylcholine was taken as a requirement for ED_{50} value of peptides. Relative potency of peptides relative to that of acetylcholine. α: maximal response produced by cholecystokinin was taken as unity. *t*-butyloxycarbonyl. Z(NO_2), *p*-nitrobenzyloxycarbonyl. CCK PZ, cholecystokinin pancreozymin. Each ED_{50} value has been calculated from response to 6–9 concentrations of the peptide in 2–4 preparations. (Vizi et al. 1974)

trin, is one-sixth as potent as G 17 in terms of acid secretory response and G 34 is actually more potent than G 17 when equimolar doses are infused into dogs (WALSH et al. 1974; CARTER et al. 1979). However, almost five times as great a molar increment in serum G 34 is needed to elicit the same degree of gastric secretion as a given increment of G 17. The bulk of the research on the effects of gastrin on the motility of the gastrointestinal tract was performed with G 17 (little gastrin) and, especially, with the synthetic derivative, pentagastrin. The structure–activity relationships of gastrin (G 17) and some natural and synthetic analogs on longitudinal muscle strips of the guinea pig is shown in Table 2 (VIZI et al. 1974). Exhaustive review articles concerning gastrin and its biologic functions as well as the structure–activity relationship problems have been published (HIATT and WELLS 1974; WALSH and GROSSMAN 1975a, b; GREGORY 1978; NILSSON 1980).

B. Effects on the Lower Esophageal Sphincter

One of the hottest controversies about the physiologic regulation of gut motility concerns the role of gastrin in the function of the lower esophageal sphincter (LES). The differences in the results obtained might be connected at least to a certain extent with profound differences in the techniques and in the animal species used. In vitro techniques, though they allow a more precise evaluation of the mechanism of action of the physiologic or pharmacologic compounds, cannot, because of obvious anatomic alterations, give results which can be transferred to the physiologic in vivo situation. In vivo studies, which were, of course, more important because of their clinical implications also varied when different procedures were followed. For example, the technique with unperfused manometric catheters yielded lower values for LES pressure (reflecting closure tension) than that with perfused catheters; anesthetized animals responded differently from conscious ones, etc. All these aspects have been carefully examined in recent exhaustive reviews (CHRISTENSEN 1975; GOYAL and RATTAN 1978, FISHER and COHEN 1980).

I. Excitation

1. In Vitro Studies

In the isolated LES from the opossum, gastrin I was shown (LIPSHUTZ and COHEN 1971, 1972; LIPSHUTZ et al. 1971) to provoke a dose-related contraction, with a lower threshold concentration (10^{-13} *M*) and a higher peak tension in muscle strips cut from the sphincter region than in strips cut from the midesophagus, gastric fundus, or antrum. The LES proved to be more sensitive to gastrin than to either acetylcholine or noradrenaline. The contractions were antagonized by tetrodotoxin and anticholinergics but not by ganglion-blocking agents and were potentiated by physostigmine. These results suggested that gastrin excites acetylcholine release at the cholinergic neuroeffector. A subsequent careful study by COHEN and GREEN (1973) showed that gastrin I increased both the maximum velocity of shortening and the peak force of the isolated LES of the opossum, the maximum effect being obtained with a concentration of 1 ng/ml. Recent data for rat and guinea pig LES were reported by TAKAYANAGI and KASUYA (1977). They used tetragastrin (5×10^{-6} g/ml) which, in the rat, induced a contraction unaffected by atropine or tetrodotoxin. The maximum response was only $13\% \pm 6\%$ that to acetylcholine. In the guinea pig, the effect was even less.

The first in vitro data for the activity of gastrin in the human lower esophagus muscle strip were those of BENNETT et al. (1967), who reported that gastrin (0.05–0.5 μg/ml) caused contraction of strips from both circular and longitudinal muscle layers. Pentagastrin behaved like gastrin, but was less active and more prone to tachyphylaxis. Apparently, the effect of gastrin or pentagastrin was independent of the cholinergic system, since it was not affected by neostigmine. The spasmogenic effect of pentagastrin (3.8–78 μ*M*) on human LES in vitro was confirmed quite recently by BURLEIGH (1979).

2. In Vivo Studies

a) Experimental Animals

Most of the studies have been performed in the opossum. This species was found to be the most suitable for the investigation of LES function and is anatomically similar to the human. In the opossum species, *Didelphis marsupialis virginiana*, gastrin I was found (COHEN and SNAPE 1975) to cause a dose-related increase in LES pressure with a peak effect at 1 μg kg^{-1} h^{-1}. Pentagastrin (6 μg kg^{-1} h^{-1} or 0.5–5 μg/kg by bolus injection) caused rises in LES pressure of 41%–92% in the bush-tailed phalanger, *Trichosurus vulpecula*, and 113%–197% in the pig-tailed macaque, *Macaca nemestrina*, (DE CARLE and GLOVER 1975). In the restrained conscious baboon (BROWN et al. 1976; BYBEE et al. 1977) bolus injections of pentagastrin (0.1–6.4 μg/kg) were also shown to cause dose-related contractions of the LES, with maximum effect at 1.6 μg/kg. This effect was not modified by cimetidine or by somatostatin, but was abolished by atropine. Recent studies (RATTAN et al. 1976; RYAN and DUFFY 1978) showed that in the anesthetized opossum, pentagastrin or gastrin I, given either as a bolus or by continuous infusion, produced a dose-dependent rise in LES pressure, the peak responses occurring at 1 μg/kg and 32 μg kg^{-1} h^{-1}, respectively. Unlike some of the in vitro studies, this action was unaffected by atropine or edrophonium in doses (100 μg/kg) which were able to abolish or potentiate, respectively, the contractile activity of acetylcholine, suggesting that the action is not mediated through excitatory cholinergic neurons. RATTAN and GOYAL (1978) found that the late component of the LES contration induced by gastrin I (1 μg/kg i.v.) in the anesthetized opossum utilizes the verapamil-sensitive influx of extracellular calcium, whereas the early phase of the LES contraction ($\leqq$ 1 min) may utilize the verapamil-insensitive intracellular calcium activation system.

The ability of endogenous gastrin to affect sphincter closure tension was also tested immunologically in the opossum, with variable results. According to LIPSHUTZ et al. (1972), injection of increasing amounts of a rabbit gastrin antiserum progressively lowered resting LES pressure, with a maximal inhibition of 80% $\pm 3.1\%$. Gastrin antiserum also inhibited the LES response to endogenous gastrin (gastric deacidification) and to exogenous intravenous administration of gastrin I, while leaving unaffected the spasmogenic action of acetylcholine. According to a double-blind study of GOYAL and MCGUIGAN (1976), administration of gastrin antiserum resulted in the binding of 85%–90% of circulating gastrin but did not reduce sphincter pressure. The authors drew the conclusion that circulating gastrin may not be an important determinant of basal sphincter pressure. Although there were some differences in the techniques used in the two studies, these differences do not appear to explain the variability in the results obtained, which remain largely puzzling.

In the conscious dog, ZWICK et al. (1976) found that pentagastrin (0.5–3 μg/kg by i.v. bolus injection) contracts the LES, mainly through direct activity on the smooth muscle and to a lesser extent through an effect on preganglionic cholinergic neurons. In anesthetized dogs, a slight increase in LES pressure was obtained with i.v. infusion of human G 17 I in doses (5 $\mu g\ kg^{-1}\ h^{-1}$) which produced unphysiologically high gastrin blood levels. The levels of gastrin measured were physiologic only with an infusion dose of 0.5 $\mu g\ kg^{-1}\ h^{-1}$, which was below the threshold for increasing LES pressure (JENNEWEIN et al. 1976). ITOH et al. (1978a) showed that pentagastrin (1.8 $\mu g\ kg^{-1}\ h^{-1}$) had an inhibitory effect on the naturally occurring interdigestive contractions in both the LES and the stomach body and antrum. This emphasizes the importance of the physiologic situation, digestive or interdigestive phase, in altering the LES response to gastrin.

Apparently there is a developmental mutation of the baseline and the contraction of LES from birth through 5 weeks. In the first days, pentagastrin causes a decrease in pressure, then is ineffective for about 2 weeks and, finally, begins to contract the LES, by 3 weeks (SPEDALE et al. 1978).

b) Humans

An enormous amount of data have been published in the last decade about both healthy subjects and patients, and evidence, both for and against a physiologic role of gastrin in the regulation of LES function has been presented, with the latter being more convincing. In one of the early studies in humans (CASTELL and HARRIS 1970), it was found that pentagastrin (1 μg/kg s.c.) raised pressure, recorded manometrically from the sphincter, in parallel with the increase in gastric acid secretion. Acid itself lowered sphincter pressure and alkalinization of the stomach increased it. Since peptone broth also increased pressure, CASTELL and HARRIS suggested that both exogenous and endogenous gastrins increase closure tension in the LES region. Several subsequent observations suggested that LES pressure changes that occurred in response to altered gastric pH might be mediated by changes in serum gastrin levels, indeed, LES pressure was shown to decrease, with some exceptions (KLINE et al. 1974, 1975) during gastric acidification (CASTELL and HARRIS 1970; CASTELL and LEVINE 1971; BAILES et al. 1972; LIPSHUTZ et al. 1973; HIGGS et al. 1974; MCCALLUM and WALSH 1979) and to increase during gastric alkalinization. However, the newer techniques for quantitative evaluation of serum gastrin have provided data suggesting that LES pressure changes are indeed pH related but not gastrin mediated (HIGGS et al. 1974). LES pressure was found to increase after a protein meal and some parallelism between LES pressure and serum gastrin concentrations was observed in some investigations (NEBEL and CASTELL 1972; MORRIS et al. 1974; DODDS et al. 1975). Moreover, continuous infusions of synthetic human gastrin I (HEIL et al. 1977; DOMSCHKE et al. 1978) or of pentagastrin (CORAZZIARI et al. 1978) were found to increase LES pressure at serum gastrin levels which did not exceed those normally found in response to a meal (FREELAND et al. 1975). However, the LES pressure responses were quantitatively smaller than those that occur concomitantly with similar total immunoreactive gastrin levels evoked by administration of a protein meal to the same subjects (FREELAND et al. 1976). It is most probable that, although increases in serum gastrin concentrations may contribute to the increase in LES pressure observed after feeding, it cannot be explained exclusively on the basis of endogenous gastrin release. Decreased basal gastrin concentrations and decreased integrated gastrin release have been demonstrated (LIPSHUTZ et al. 1974; FARRELL et al. 1974), thus it was suggested that hypogastrinemia may contribute to pathogenesis of LES incompetence.

After distal gastric resection, symptomatic gastroesophageal reflux and more-or-less severe esophagitis have been reported (BINGHAM 1958; HELSINGER 1960; COX 1961; WINDSOR 1964) and this could indicate that the abnormal sphincter function was due to a decreased release of gastrin. However, neither decreased serum gastrin levels nor lower resting LES pressure have been demonstrated convincingly in these patients (SIEWERT et al. 1977). In addition, in patients with different degrees of gastroesophageal symptoms (WRIGHT et al. 1975; HIGGS et al. 1976) or with diseases characterized by hypergastrinemia (COHEN and HARRIS 1972; SIEWERT et al. 1973; FARRELL et al. 1973), no correlation was found between LES pressure and serum gastrin levels.

Other pieces of information which were against rather than for a physiologic role of gastrin are the following observations. Pentagastrin was found to cause a dose-related increase in LES pressure but only when given as a bolus i.v. injection (0.5–1 μg/kg; with very high and short-lasting peak blood levels) and not when given by the much more physiologic continuous i.v. infusion (0.1–2.5 $\mu g\ kg^{-1}\ h^{-1}$; with blood levels more like those that are found under physiologic conditions and are capable of inducing a good acid secretory response; CALVERT et al. 1975; WALKER et al. 1975; ITOH et al. 1978b). A similar lack of LES contraction was observed after stimulation of endogenous gastrin release by protein instillation (CSENDES et al. 1978a, b), or by ingestion of cimetidine (WALLIN et al. 1979), even in subjects who did respond to bolus injection of pentagastrin (DENT and HANSKY 1976; HENDERSON et al. 1978).

Another important contribution, which supports a growing theory that there may be little relationship between endogenous gastrin levels and the basal sphincter tone, came from the work of ECKARDT et al. (1978), who showed that in 15 patients who had undergone a very carefully mapped antrectomy, in spite of a substantial decrease in their fasting serum gastrin values there was no proportional decrease in resting LES pressure. Other investigators (JENSEN et al. 1978b) concluded that gastrin by itself is not likely to be a physiologic regulator of LES tone in humans, since they observed that the serum concentrations of G 34 required to produce half-maximal stimulation of LES (300–400 fmol/ml) were well above the physiologic range of G 34 responses to a protein meal (20–25 fmol/ml). The same authors observed that the peak increases of LES pressure after equimolar doses of G 34 and G 17 were similar, but the responses to G 34 were more prolonged, consistent with the longer half-life of G 34.

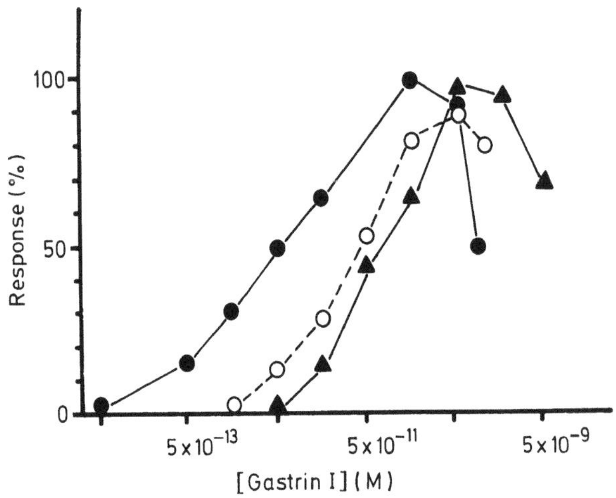

Fig. 1. Dose–response curve of human gastrin I alone *(solid circles)* and in combination with secretin (3×10^{-19} *M*) *(open circles)* or with cholecystokinin (7.5×10^{-13} *M triangles*) on LES circular muscle. Active tension is expressed as a percentage of maximum response to gastrin I when given alone. (Adapted from LIPSHUTZ and COHEN 1972; FISHER et al. 1975)

Both cholecystokinin and secretin were found to inhibit gastrin-induced contractions of the LES (Fig. 1; LIPSHUTZ and COHEN 1972; FISHER et al. 1975). Contrasting findings were also obtained about the role of gastrin in the pathophysiology of disorders of LES function. The LES response to an intravenous bolus of pentagastrin was found to be increased in patients suffering from diffuse esophageal spasm (ECKARDT and KRUEGER 1974; ORLANDO and BOZYMSKI 1979), who were, however, unresponsive to infusion with gastrin (G 17, 25 pmol kg^{-1} h^{-1}; LANE et al. 1977, 1979). Other authors (MORRIS et al. 1978) obtained different results (no differences in sensitivity to pentagastrin between controls and patients with symptomatic diffuse esophageal spasms) and claimed that the pentagastrin test cannot be relied upon to provoke the spasms in these patients.

In patients with achalasia, opposite findings were also reported: COHEN et al. (1971) and COHEN (1975) demonstrated an exaggerated pressure response of the LES to gastrin, with maximal LES pressure at low serum gastrin levels, whereas CORAZZIARI et al. (1977, 1978) found that in achalasic patients, infusion of pentagastrin in doses (0.012 μg kg^{-1} min^{-1}) which produced statistically significant increases of LES pressure in normal and in antrectomized subjects was absolutely ineffective. Apparently consistent results were reported for patients with hiatus hernia (SIEWERT et al. 1974; SCHEURER and HALTER 1976), in whom the LES response to pentagastrin was found to be reduced; a good correlation between the degree of this reduction and the severity of symptoms actually suggested that a LES pentagastrin test can be used to diagnose their condition.

II. Inhibition

Along with all these observations suggesting the existence of gastrin receptors that cause LES excitation and are located in the LES muscle and/or in excitatory neurons, there are other data which suggest that there are also gastrin receptors that mediate LES inhibition. In the opossum and the dog, it has been reported that increasing the dose of gastrin above the dose which produces maximal contraction of the LES leads to a diminution of the effect of gastrin (COHEN and SNAPE 1975). This sort of autoinhibition was thought to be due to simultaneous stimulation of the inhibitory receptors for gastrin in the LES with the supramaximal dose of the peptide.

At present, the existence of inhibitory receptors for gastrin in the LES is controversial. Some authors suggest that these receptors may be the H_2-receptors, since they found that the autoinhibition of gastrin was abolished by pretreatment with metiamide (COHEN and SNAPE 1975), which was also able to block in vitro the inhibitory effect of gastrin on KCl-induced contractions. However, other authors (RATTAN et al. 1976) were unable to confirm these findings in the anesthetized opossum and suggested a simple, direct contractile effect of gastrin. Finally, other investigators (ZWICK et al. 1976) found that in the unanesthetized dog the inhibitory effect of pentagastrin at supramaximal doses of the hormone was antagonized by atropine. They found that hexamethonium (2 mg/kg i.v.) depressed the response to 3 μg/kg pentagastrin and increased the response to 6 μg/kg. Propranolol (2 mg/kg i.v.) also prolonged the effect of pentagastrin. They concluded that the stimulatory effect of pentagastrin is mainly due to a direct effect, but that it also has a less prominent action on preganglionic cholinergic neurons. The autoinhibition of pentagastrin seems to be mediated, at least in part, via the preganglionic neurons, acting through adrenergic receptors. Pentagastrin-induced LES contraction in humans was found to be potentiated by truncal vagotomy (HIGGS and CASTELL 1975) and by somatostatin (250 μg/kg i.v.; RÖSCH et al. 1976). However, it was not established whether somatostatin acts by blocking gastrin-sensitive inhibitory receptors or by reducing endogenous plasma glucagon levels or, finally, by decreasing cyclic AMP activity within the smooth muscle. Vasoactive intestinal peptide (VIP; 0.8–32 μg kg^{-1} h^{-1}) also inhibited the response of LES to pentagastrin (1.6 μg kg^{-1} h^{-1}) without decreasing basal pressure; however, even the smallest doses induced plasma levels of radioimmunoassayable VIP higher than those encountered normally (DOMSCHKE et al. 1978). Apparently, atropine infusion (12 μg kg^{-1} h^{-1}) or single injection (1 mg) did not inhibit LES stimulation by submaximal or maximal doses of G 17 in humans (JENSEN et al. 1978a). It is obvious that further studies are needed to clarify all these important points.

To conclude, at this time the evidence regarding the physiologic role of gastrin in the regulation of LES pressure and the precise mechanism of action of the peptide is incomplete and it is probably advisable to consider this problem as JOHNSON (1977) suggested in his beautiful review on gastrointestinal hormones: "the best view is on open-minded one." On the other hand it appears to have been unequivocally demonstrated that gastrin in high (pharmacologic) doses can affect the lower esophageal sphincter, with a predominant contractile action.

C. Effects on the Stomach

The effects of gastrin on the electrical and mechanical activity of the fundus and the body of the stomach differ from those on the antrum, in keeping with the different physiologic roles of the two regions. The effects observed by various investigators have also differed according to the experimental conditions, the animal species, and the techniques used to evaluate the motor responses to gastrin.

I. In Vitro Studies

1. Experimental Animals

The early in vitro studies showed that gastrin caused small contractions of the rat fundus strip preparation, rat antrum and body of the stomach, guinea pig sacculus rotundus, hamster stomach strip, and cat stomach fundus (BENNETT 1965; MIKOS and VANE 1967). Threshold stimulant doses varied, for the different preparations, between 0.01 and 1 μg/ml. Tachyphylaxis appeared to be a rather common feature and the action of gastrin appeared in some cases (hamster stomach) to be a direct one and in other cases to be, at least partially nerve mediated. In the opossum, gastrin I (10^{-10}–10^{-9} *M*) was found to stimulate antral muscle and to have no effect on the pyloric circular muscle or even to inhibit the contraction of this muscle induced by secretin (LIPSHUTZ and COHEN 1972). In a recent study (YATES et al. 1978), performed with isolated preparations from young ferrets and kittens, with simultaneous recording of motility and secretion of the gastric fundus, pentagastrin (6.5×10^{-8} and 6.5×10^{-7} *M*) was found to increase the spontaneous contractions and the basal tone of the muscle, the kitten being less sensitive than the ferret. Small doses of atropine (10^{-6} *M*) inhibited the motility but not the secretion induced by pentagastrin; higher doses (10^{-3} *M*) also reduced secretion but did not abolish it. The authors suggested that gastrin acted on motility, but not on secretion, through excitation of the cholinergic nerves (ROTH et al. 1979).

In the guinea pig stomach, gastrin (0.05 μg/ml) stimulated antral rhythmic activity and raised the fundal basal pressure. However, the mechanisms of action seemed to be different, since the antral motor effects were significantly blocked by atropine and tetrodotoxin whereas the fundal effects were not (GERNER and HAFFNER 1977). Apparently, in the fundus the action of gastrin was inhibited specifically by mepyramine, suggesting that there is either a local release of histamine induced by gastrin or a direct effect of gastrin on the H_1-receptors (GERNER et al. 1979). Pretreatment with gastrin tended to reduce the maximal contracting response to CCK in the guinea pig antrum, simulating a noncompetitive interaction between the two hormones (GERNER and HAFFNER 1978). Conversely, in the cat the increase in the frequency of the slow wave component and in the amplitude of phasic contraction induced in a preparation of the antrum by pentagastrin (1.25–2.5×10^{7} g/ml) were completely unaffected by atropine (2.5×10^{-6} g/ml) or tetrodotoxin (1.6×10^{-7} g/ml; (OHKAWA and WATANABE 1977a).

In strips of circular muscle of the dog antrum, gastrin increased both the frequency and the amplitude of spontaneous contractions, with maximal amplitude changes observed at 3.5×10^{-9} *M*. The response to gastrin was reduced (−35%) by atropine (1×10^{-6} *M*) and unaffected by tripelennamine (1×10^{-3} *M*) or cimetidine (1×10^{-3} *M*) Secretin (1.5×10^{-8} *M*) reduced the maximal response but did not change the median effective dose (ED_{50}) of gastrin (FARA and BERKOWITZ 1978; FARA et al. 1979). Again in canine antral circular muscle, pentagastrin was shown (EL-SHARKAWY and SZURSZEWSKI 1978) to increase the size of the plateau potential and the frequency of the action potential complex and also to produce a marked diastolic depolarization between action potentials. The effects of pentagastrin were apparently due to a direct action on the smooth muscle cell, but it is of interest that a previous work by SZURSZEWSKI (1975) had shown that in the longitudinal muscle of canine antrum pentagastrin could exert at least part of its stimulant action through a release of acetylcholine from intramural cholinergic nerves. A sophisticated microelectrode technique, with recording of the electrical activity of single cells in the corporal circular muscle, enabled it to be established that the pentagastrin-induced increase in the plateau potential causes the increase in phasic activity through electromechanical coupling, but it is not likely that the depolarization alone causes the increase in tone. Thus, pentagastrin probably acts through some direct form of "hormonomechanical coupling" to affect tone (MORGAN and SZURSZEWSKI 1978). The same technique, with simultaneous recording of mechanical activity was used to evaluate the potency of G 34 which was slightly greater than those of G 17 and pentagastrin. The effects on the size of the action potential plateau occurred at a lower range of concentrations than the effect on frequency (5×10^{-12} compared with 5.5×10^{-10} M; MORGAN et al. 1978). According to MORGAN and SZURSZEWSKI (1980), pentagastrin caused an increase in conductance of antral preparations during the plateau of the action potential but not between action potentials, as was the case in corporal preparations. It was suggested that pentagastrin increases the force of contractions by a voltage-dependent process involving the opening of voltage-dependent calcium channels whereas the peptide increases the tone by a voltage- independent process, possibly involving a nonregenerative increase in calcium movements through voltage-independent channels.

2. Humans

Gastrin (0.05–0.6 μg/ml) and pentagastrin (1–5 μg/ml) caused contraction in 42 of 88 strips from the body and the antrum (the same percentage of positive responses was obtained with the circular and the longitudinal muscle) of human stomachs removed during surgery. After washing, a slow recovery was noted and tachyphylaxis was present, usually after pentagastrin but not after gastrin I or II (BENNETT et al. 1967). The authors did not offer any explanation for the relatively low percentage of strips that responded to gastrin and stated that the gastrin stimulated receptors are on or in the smooth muscle cell, since its action was not affected by hexamethonium (20 μg/ml), local anesthetics (40 μg/ml), neostigmine (0.1–0.5 μg/ml), or hyoscine (0.2–0.4 μg/ml). In subsequent studies (CAMERON et al. 1970), the number of strips which did not contract after gastrin administration (0.01 μg/ml for antral strips and 0.1 μg/ml for body strips) was not statistically significant. In this study, gastrin was found to increase the amplitude (but not the frequency) of the spontaneous rhythmic contractions, with little effect on the tone of the muscle. Contractions of human stomach (both body and antrum, with recording of longitudinal and circular muscle contractions) were observed after addition of gastrin COOH terminal hexapeptide (0.1–0.3 μg/ml; VIZI et al. 1973; G. BERTACCINI unpublished work 1974). Apparently, the circular muscle layer was more sensitive to the peptide than is the longitudinal layer.

According to a recent study (HARA 1980) the circular muscle of the human stomach responded to concentrations of tetragastrin as low as 10^{-14}–10^{-12} g/ml, the maximum contraction being obtained with 10^{-8} g/ml. The increase in the amplitude of spontaneous contractions induced by tetragastrin was partly suppressed by atropine (10^{-6} g/ml) and by tetrodotoxin (10^{-7} g/ml) while it was enhanced by neostigmine (10^{-6} g/ml). The effect of tetragastrin was also partly reduced by secretin.

II. In Vivo Studies

1. Experimental Animals

The first experiments with the denervated fundic pouch of the conscious dog (GREGORY and TRACY 1964) showed that gastrin I or II (10–50 µg i.v.) increased tone and frequency of spontaneous contractions and this effect was reduced but not blocked by atropine (1 mg). Subsequent studies (ISENBERG and GROSSMAN 1969) showed that gastrin stimulated rhythmic antral contractions in the intact stomach of the dog as well as in the innervated antral pouch. Gastrin I had the same effect as crude gastrin and gastrin II. All the peptides were given by i.v. infusion. Further investigations (SCHUURKES and CHARBON 1979) confirmed the antral effects of gastrin and showed that pentagastrin could increase the mean frequency of slow waves in the antrum from 4.6–5.8 cycles/min and the amplitude of contractions in the antrum more than in the corpus. Moreover pentagastrin increased dose-dependently (128–2,048 ng/kg i.v.) also the tone of the corpus. In other studies, together with the increase of frequency, a parallel decrease in the amplitude of antral contractions was noted (SUGAWARA et al. 1969). Paradoxically, a simultaneous delay in gastric emptying was noted (DOZOIS and KELLY 1971) and it was suggested that pentagastrin might act on sites other than the antrum (COOKE et al. 1972). Gastric emptying was also slowed in the calf (BELL et al. 1975) after infusion of pentagastrin (0.01–0.03 µg kg^{-1} min^{-1}) which in this species was shown to act predominantly by inhibiting gastric muscle in both the body and the antrum. Indeed, intravenous administration of pentagastrin (0.025–0.2 µg/kg) caused also a dose-dependent inhibition of electromyogram registered in the abomasum of the calf (BELL et al. 1977). Human gastrin I (0.5–2 µg kg^{-1} h^{-1} i.v.) caused a marked decrease in emptying from the omasum of the sheep (ONAPITO et al. 1978).

Parallel studies on canine myoelectric and motor activities (KELLY 1975) showed that pentagastrin (0.1 µg kg^{-1} min^{-1} i.v.), inhibits the phasic contractions of the proximal part of the stomach, thus enhancing gastric accomodation to distension and slowing gastric emptying of liquids. At the same time, pentagastrin increases the frequency of the gastric pacemaker, abolishes the interdigestive migrating myoelectric complex and induces a regular sequence of peristaltic contractions in the antrum, which enhances gastric mixing and grinding of solids. In the isolated perfused stomach preparation from dogs pentagastrin and endogenously released gastrin had the same effects as in in vivo experiments (KOWALEWSKI et al. 1975a). Similar results were obtained with pig stomach (KOWALEWSKI et al. 1975b).

All these different factors in the inhibition of contractility in the fundus and in the increase in frequency associated with decrease of amplitude of antral contractions are likely to be the major factors responsible for the slowed gastric emptying. The "acid–secretin–neural" pathways were much less important (the effect of gastrin was unaffected by neutralization with $NaHCO_3$), as was the alteration of duodenal motility (the effect of gastrin was present even when the cycles of the duodenal pacemaker potential were not increased).

Contractions that appear during the interdigestive state in both the Heidenhain pouch and the main stomach of the dog were inhibited by administration of pentagastrin exactly as they were by the ingestion of food (ITOH et al. 1978b) or by antral irrigation with acetylcholine (THOMAS et al. 1979). Pentagastrin (unlike administration of food) caused a dose-dependent (0.125–4 $\mu g\ kg^{-1}\ h^{-1}$) increase in gastric basic electrical rhythm (BER) in the conscious dog (PEARCE et al. 1978). The studies of STRUNZ and GROSSMAN (1977) showed that canine antrum is extremely sensitive to G 17 I (threshold dose = 12.5 $pmol\ kg^{-1}\ h^{-1}$) and that the stimulatory action of gastrin may be considered to be physiologic, since the ED_{50} for this action is no greater than that for acid secretion. Moreover, this action has a strong cholinergic component, since it is strongly inhibited by atropine (0.1 mg/kg) and by vagotomy.

In the anesthetized dog and in the anesthetized rat, pentagastrin and gastrin I were found to cause a small but constant contraction of the gastroduodenal junction (MANTOVANI and BERTACCINI 1971; BERTACCINI et al. 1973). In the rat, both pentagastrin and gastrin were recently shown to cause a dose-dependent delay of gastric emptying (BERTACCINI and SCARPIGNATO 1981; Figs. 2, 3). In the cat, an erratic contraction of the gastroduodenal junction was also observed after administration of pentagastrin (0.5–4 µg/kg; BEHAR et al. 1979). Very small, graded "physiologic" doses of G 17 I produced, in both the stomach and the duodenum, graded increases in frequency of pacemaker potentials and in the incidence of pacemaker potentials with action potentials (STRUNZ et al. 1979). When intragastric pressure was measured (WILBUR and KELLY 1974; VALENZUELA and GROSSMAN 1975), pentagastrin in very low doses (1 $\mu g\ kg^{-1}\ h^{-1}$) was shown to decrease it, when gastric acid was not neutralized and in much higher doses after gastric neutralization (up to 8 $\mu g\ kg^{-1}\ h^{-1}$). However, in the intact dog (STRUNZ and GROSSMAN 1978), infusion of gastrin (G 17 II) at the dose which produced maximal acid secretion (400 $pmol\ kg^{-1}\ h^{-1}$) had no effect on emptying or gastric volume.

The neonatal development of gastric motility and responses to pentagastrin were studied in dogs (MALLOY et al. 1979). Gastric contraction rates increased progressively during the first two weeks of life: pentagastrin (8 µg/kg s.c.) decreased contraction after the ninth day but had no effect during the first week. Apparently the response to pentagastrin was dose dependent and was not altered by gastric perfusion with sodium bicarbonate.

2. Humans

In humans, the activity of gastrin on the stomach has been investigated by means of different techniques for evaluation of the motor and electrical activity, as well as of gastric emptying in healthy subjects and in patients. The early experiments in humans, which gave contrasting results for the action of gastrin on the intestine, showed unequivocally a stimulatory effect of the hormone or of pentagastrin on gastric antrum muscle (MISIEWICZ et al. 1967). Pentagastrin was apparently more

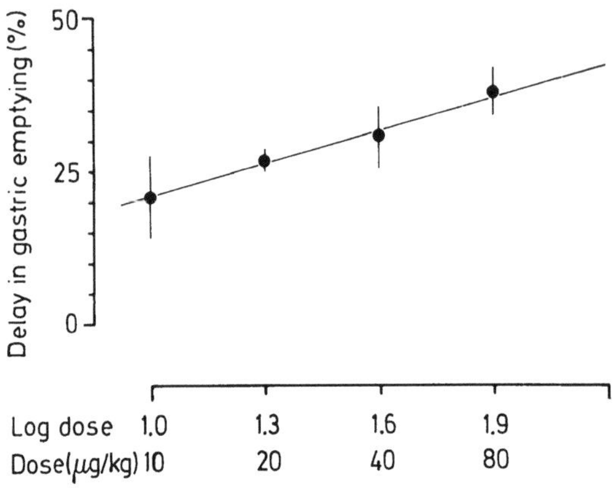

Fig. 2. Gastric emptying in conscious rats. Delay in gastric emptying induced by pentagastrin calculated as a percentage difference in comparison with controls taken as 100%. Dose–response relationship of pentagastrin (administered intraperitoneally 5 min before the test meal). (C. SCARPIGNATO and G. BERTACCINI, unpublished work 1981)

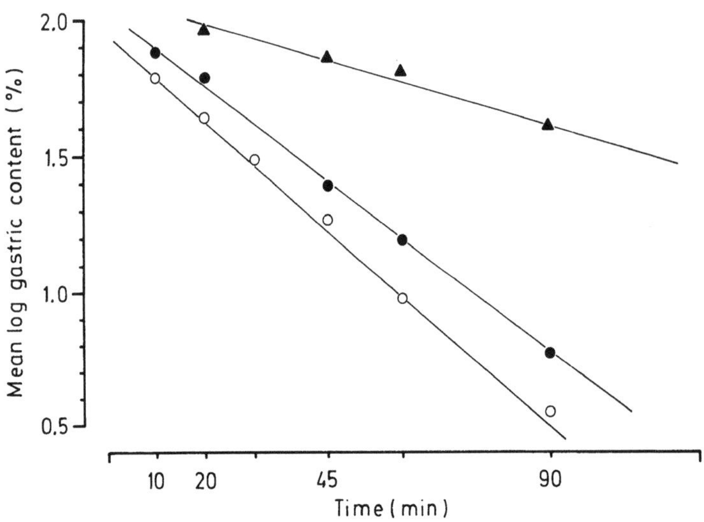

Fig. 3. Gastric emptying in conscious rats. Semilogarithmic plot of gastric content versus time. *Open circles*, controls; *solid circles*, pentagastrin 80 μg/kg, 5 min before the test meal; *triangles*, human gastrin I 80 μg/kg 5 min before the meal. (C. SCARPIGNATO and G. BERTACCINI, unpublished work 1981)

active than gastrin in stimulating antral motility, increasing both intraluminal pressures and mean height of the waves (which was not affected by gastrin). Other investigators (SZÉKELY et al. 1969) demonstrated roentgenologically an increase in frequency and amplitude of antral peristalsis, with a corresponding decrease in periodicity, after administration of 0.5 mg pentagastrin intramuscularly. Electrical activity was modified in the same way by pentagastrin (0.5 mg s.c. or 0.1 μg kg^{-1} min^{-1}) and by gastrin I (1 μg kg^{-1} h^{-1}; MONGES and SALDUCCI 1972; KWONG et al. 1972). Both compounds increased the frequency of the pacemaker potentials (by about 35%) and increased the occurrence of bursts of action potentials superimposed on cycles of the pacemaker potential. Both exogenous pentagastrin (2 μg kg^{-1} h^{-1}) and endogenous gastrin (released by infusion of glycine and NaOH) were found to have no effect on resting pyloric pressure but to inhibit pyloric contraction to different stimuli (FISHER et al. 1973; FISHER and BODEN 1976). Reflux of duodenal contents, which may be an important etiologic factor in several gastroesophageal disorders, could be facilitated by elevating the serum gastrin concentrations (HARVEY 1975).

HUNT and RAMSBOTTOM (1967) first observed a delay in gastric emptying after administration of gastrin II (0.125–3 μg/min). Subsequent studies with different techniques (MEVES et al. 1975; HAMILTON et al. 1976; MACGREGOR et al. 1978) confirmed that intravenous pentagastrin (1.2–6 μg kg^{-1} h^{-1}) slowed the gastric emptying rates for both liquid and solid foods. Pentagastrin (6 μg/kg s.c.) was found to stimulate rhythmic discontinuous contractions, with pressures significantly higher in the pylorus and lower in the antrum: this could probably account for the delay in emptying (WHITE and KEIGHLEY 1978). Other studies confirmed the contraction of the pylorus after i.v. administration of pentagastrin (0.6 μg/kg), together with an increase in antral motility and in the linkage of antral to duodenal contractions (MUNK et al. 1978). However, there is still no good evidence of correlation between pentagastrin-induced changes in myoelectric activity patterns in the stomach and the observed pentagastrin-induced slowing of gastric emptying. Quite recently it was observed that pentagastrin (6 μg kg^{-1} h^{-1}) increased gastric emptying in patients with duodenal and gastric ulcer, probably because of an abnormal sensitivity of the patients to the peptide or of pyloric dysfunction (GAMBLIN et al. 1977; DUBOIS and CASTELL 1978). Surprisingly, a significant increase in gastric emptying rate was also observed in healthy subjects after intragastric administration of G 17, while maintaining the intraluminal pH at 7 (PITTINGER et al. 1978; FIDDIAN-GREEN and QUINN 1978).

D. Effects on the Small and Large Intestine

I. In Vitro Studies

Because of the easy availability of rather homogenous material and of a completely standardized technique, the guinea pig ileum, either as whole intestine preparation or as a pure longitudinal muscle preparation, was used in most classical investigations of the mechanism of action of gastrin and its analogs. In one of the early papers on this topic, BENNETT (1965) reported that gastrin II caused a rapid contraction of the guinea pig ileum which sometimes declined spontaneously before washing. Tachyphylaxis could be prevented if there was an interval of at least 15 min between two consecutive administrations of the peptide. Mepyramine, methysergide, and hexamethonium did not significantly modify the effects of gastrin, which were, on the contrary, inhibited by hyoscine (4 ng/ml) and potentiated by eserine (20–100 ng/ml). In addition, other indirect evidence that gastrin acted predominantly by stimulation of postganglionic cholinergic nerves was provided by the inhibitory effects of cooling and of anoxia (which blocked nerve conduction) and of morphine (which blocked the release of acetylcholine).

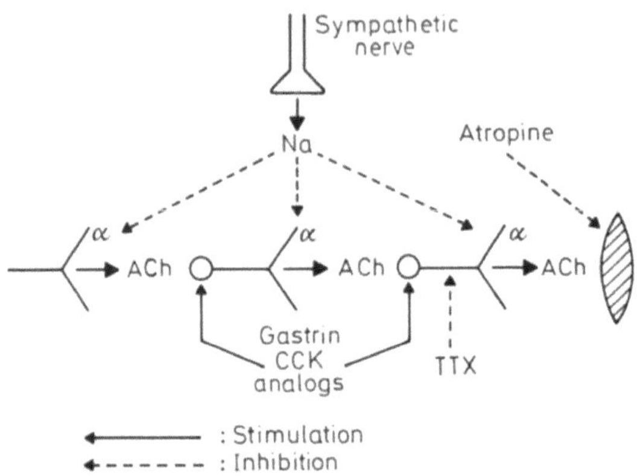

Fig. 4. Scheme of the mode of action of the peptides of the gastrin–CCK family. It is likely that they can stimulate the cell bodies of both "interneuronal" and "preeffector" fibers producing acetylcholine release from these nerve terminals ("interneuronal") which synapse with other ganglion cells and also from those ("preeffector") which come directly into relation with smooth muscle

However, definite and direct proof that gastrin I and other peptides of the same family act predominantly through release of acetylcholine from the myenteric (Auerbach) plexus was obtained by VIZI et al. (1973) as shown in Fig. 4. They were able to confirm all the previous indirect proofs and also to measure the quantity of acetylcholine released by gastrin I (5×10^{-7} g/ml) and found this value to be 134.5 ng g^{-1} min^{-1}, compared with a value of 65 ng g^{-1} min^{-1} in control tissues (without treatment with gastrin). The acetylcholine release by gastrin and some related peptides from the longitudinal muscle strip of guinea pig ileum is shown in Table 3. The same authors (VIZI et al. 1974) demonstrated that gastrin and related peptides elicited reciprocal responses from the two muscle layers of guinea pig ileum, similar to their responses to electrical stimulation (Fig. 5). The dose-dependent contractions of the longitudinal muscle and the relaxation of the circular muscle layer in response to peptides were followed by a contraction of the circular muscle and a relaxation of the longitudinal muscle. These alternating contractions of the two coats were inhibited by tetrodotoxin (TTX, 10^{-6} *M*). In these experiments cross-tachyphylaxis between peptides of the gastrin and of the cholecystokinin (CCK) series was also observed and this suggested a common receptor for both types of peptides. However, recent very accurate experiments (ZETLER 1979) have shown some interesting qualitative differences between pentagastrin, on the one hand and CCK OP and cerulein on the other which suggest different receptor sites. Unlike CCK-like peptides, pentagastrin was antagonized by TTX, in a purely noncompetitive way, and it showed a surprisingly high sensitivity to morphine and to β-endorphin, the pA_2 values for the opioid peptides against CCK OP and pentagastrin being significantly different. The simultaneous recording of contractions of longitudinal and circular muscle layers showed that pentagastrin (as well as CCK), in doses which were just on the threshold for motor-stimulating effects by themselves, were highly effective in increasing the frequency of peristaltic contractions evoked by distension of isolated ileal segments.

Table 3. Acetylcholine release by gastrin-related polypeptides (octapeptide amide of cholecystokinin, gastrin I, cerulein, pentagastrin) from longitudinal muscle strips of guinea pig ileum

	Acetylcholine release[a]							
	Control	Peptide	Control	Noradrenaline (10^{-6} g/ml) + peptide	Control	Tetrodotoxin (5×10^{-7} g/ml) + peptide	Control	Hexa-methonium[b] (3 ± 10^{-4} g/ml)
	($ng\ g^{-1}\ min^{-1}$)							
Octapeptide amide of cholecystokinin	76.4 ± 18.1	209.5 ± 83.5[c]	68.5 ± 9.1	51.0 ± 10.5	68.6	31.4	53.5 ± 8.1	181.4 ± 15.2[c]
(5×10^{-8} g/ml)	(3)	(3)	(3)	(3)	60.9	20.8	(3)	(3)
Gastrin I (5×10^{-7} g/ml)[d]	65.1 ± 9.6	134.5 ± 13.4[c]	70.2	31.4	55.6	48.5	54.3	106.5
	(5)	(5)			60.2	40.1		
Cerulein (5×10^{-8} g/ml)	54.2 ± 10.6	117.3 ± 27.6[c]	64.7 ± 6.8	47.5 ± 6.3	60.3 ± 4.1	38.1 ± 7.1[c]	51.8 ± 8.4	136.4 ± 14.2[c]
	(6)	(6)	(5)	(5)	(3)	(3)	(4)	(4)
Pentagastrin (5×10^{-7} g/ml)[d]	63.5 ± 8.3	120.4 ± 16.1[c]	58.4 ± 6.2	41.2 ± 4.2			61.4	103.6
	(3)	(3)	(3)	(3)			69.5	127.1

[a] Values represent the mean ± standard errors of the acetylcholine release from the nerve terminals of the myenteric plexus. The number of experiments is given in parentheses. 1-min collection periods

[b] Hexamethonium was added to the bath 5 min before administration of peptides. The concentrations of peptide used caused the maximum effect on acetylcholine output. Additional increase in concentration failed to produce any higher increase of acetylcholine release. These concentrations also produced a maximal effect on contraction of longitudinal muscle of guinea pig ileum. This statement is based on a dose–response curve study

[c] The change is significant, $P < 0.01$

[d] In order to avoid tachyphylaxis that was otherwise observed to the effect of gastrin (pentagastrin), 15 min were allowed to elapse before the next dose of gastrin (pentagastrin) was administered. (Vizi et al. 1973)

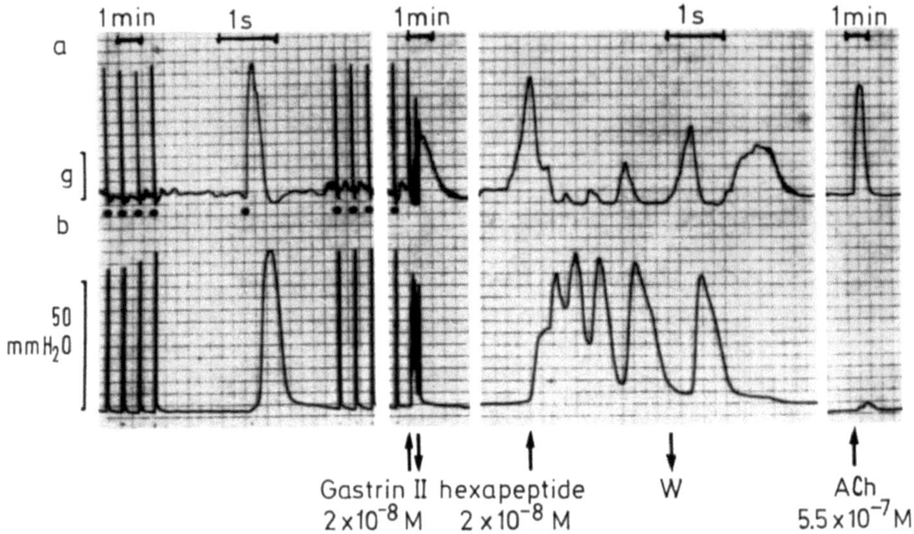

Fig. 5 a, b. Responses of the longitudinal **a** and circular muscle **b** layer of guinea pig ileum to gastrin II hexapeptide and stimulation. Supramaximal field stimulation as indicated by *dots* (20 Hz for 2 s, 1 ms, 6 V/cm) Krebs solution. Organ bath, 5 ml. Note the alternating contractions of the two muscle layers in response to peptide and stimulation. Acetylcholine added to the bath contracted only the longitudinal muscle. *W* washout. In the middle of each tracing, the paper speed was increased as indicated by the time marks. (VIZI et al. 1974)

The potentiating effect of pentagastrin was blocked by atropine and tetrodotoxin, confirming previous findings. Hexamethonium decreased but did not abolish the response to pentagastrin, suggesting that sites of action of the peptide were both preganglionic and postganglionic (CHIJIKAWA and DAVISON 1974). Small contractions were observed in rat duodenum and rat and cat colon with relatively high concentrations of gastrin II (0.2–2 μg/ml). While duodenum, ileum, and rectum from the rabbit, the mouse, and the chick appeared to be insensitive to gastrin (BENNETT 1965; MIKOS and VANE 1967), more recent techniques have shown that gastrin, as well as cholecystokinin and cerulein, is able to increase the smooth muscle tone in rabbit small intestine and to cause the appearance of action potentials while leaving the slow waves virtually unaltered. All these changes were completely blocked by tetrodotoxin (10^{-5} *M*) (YAU 1974). The effect of the COOH terminal hexapeptide of gastrin and the interference of the sympathetic system on the motor activity of rabbit jejunum is shown in Fig. 6. Different data were obtained for cat small intestine (OHKAWA and WATANABE 1977 b), in which both the electrical and the mechanical activity of the smooth muscle was examined. Tetragastrin (7.5×10^{-7}–1.5×10^{-6} g/ml) and pentagastrin (5×10^{-7}–2.5×10^{-6} g/ml) inhibited the spike activity and the phasic contractions and did not affect the slow waves. The tone of the smooth muscle was decreased. All these changes were probably due to direct effects on smooth muscle since they were completely unaffected by tetrodotoxin, atropine, or sympatholytic compounds. In the isolated cat colon, very low concentrations of gastrin I (10^{-13}–10^{-11} *M*) were found to in-

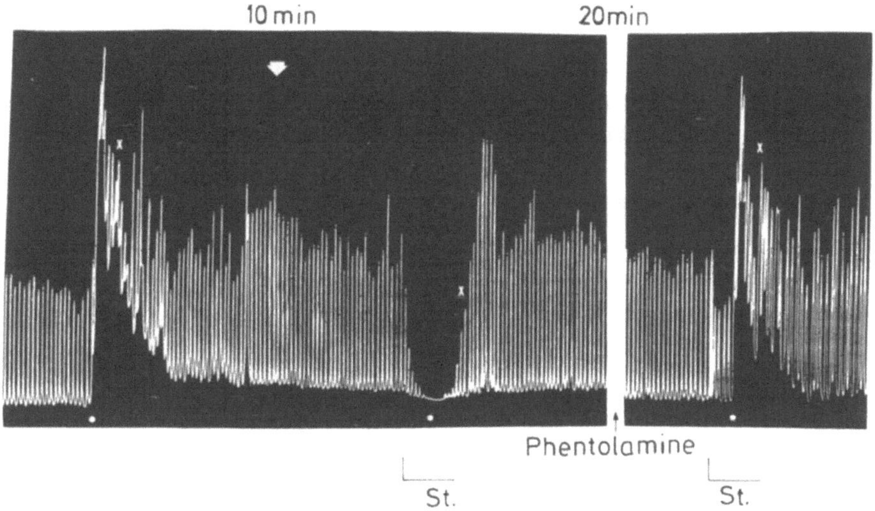

Fig. 6. Inhibitory effect of sympathetic nerve stimulation on the response to gastrin II hexapeptide of rabbit jejunum (Finkleman preparation). Sympathetic nerve stimulation (St.) for 30 s as indicated (20 Hz, 0.5 ms, 10 V). Propanolol, (2×10^{-6} g/ml) was present throughout the experiment. It only slightly reduced the inhibitory effect of exogenous (10^{-6} g/ml) and endogenous (sympathetic nerve stimulation) noradrenaline on pendular movement. The contractions are recorded on a smoked drum by an isotonic writing lever. The smoked drum was stopped for 20 min at the time indicated by the *arrow*. More than 10 min elapsed between two consecutive administrations of gastrin II hexapeptide to avoid tachyphylaxis. *Dots* indicate drug added to the bath, and *crosses* indicate washout of drugs. Krebs solution (20 ml) bubbled with a gas mixture of 95% O_2 + 5% CO_2. Note that the failure of sympathetic stimulation to reduce the effect of gastrin II hexapeptide in the presence of phentolamine (2×10^{-6} g/ml) indicates the importance of receptors in the presynaptic inhibitory effect of noradrenaline. (Vizi et al. 1973)

crease spike activity, the slow waves remaining tightly coupled. Higher concentrations of gastrin (10^{-9}–10^{-8} *M*) disturbed the congruence of the slow wave frequencies and completely uncoupled slow wave activity, abolishing all slow wave propagation. This suggested that smooth muscle cells may have two receptors for motor activity, a high affinity receptor controlling spike genesis and a lower affinity receptor controlling membrane coupling between cells (Snape and Cohen 1979). Gastrin and CCK (which behaves in the same way) could thus play a modulating role in colonic motor function and high hormone concentrations might disrupt the normal myogenic control, leading to deranged motility.

In studies conducted with human bowel, gastrin I or II and pentagastrin were found (Bennett and Whitney 1966; Bennett et al. 1967; G. Bertaccini unpublished work 1974) to have no stimulant effects on the duodenum or the ileum and to contract the colon and the sigmoid weakly. In this case, threshold doses were 0.5–2 μg/ml for gastrin and 2–10 μg/ml for pentagastrin or COOH terminal gastrin hexapeptide. In one other study with human colonic circular muscle, gastrin I (10^{-12}–10^{-8} *M*) was found to be inactive (Weiss et al. 1976).

II. In Vivo Studies

On the whole, the different areas of the gut examined in vivo were much less sensitive to gastrin than the antrum, though the hormone was shown to induce more-or-less unmistakable changes in different animal species and also in humans.

1. Experimental Animals

Both pentagastrin (0.125–4 μg kg^{-1} h^{-1}; PEARCE et al. 1978) and human gastrin I (50–200 pmol kg^{-1} h^{-1}; STRUNZ et al. 1979) were found to increase the rate of duodenal BER in the dog dose-dependently. Very large doses of gastrin (400 pmol/kg given i. v. over 1 min) strongly inhibited electrical activity and neither pacemaker potentials nor action potentials could be identified. This strong inhibition usually ceased within 10 min. In other studies (CHEY et al. 1974), pentagastrin (1 μg kg^{-1} h^{-1}) was shown to increase motor activity of dog duodenum to approximately the same extent as CCK OP. As for the jejunum and the ileum, the early experiments of TRACY and GREGORY (1964) showed that gastrin (50 μg i.v.) caused a prompt, sustained spasm or a rapid series of contractions, followed by inhibition, chiefly of tone but often of motility as well.

Subsequent studies (WEISBRODT et al. 1974) concerned the effects of pentagastrin on the myoelectric activity of the small intestine in conscious dogs. The peptide, when infused into fasted animals, was shown to change the pattern of myoelectric activity from that of a fasted condition to that of a fed condition and the authors suggested that the change in myoelectric activity caused by the ingestion of food may in part be due to the release of gastrin. The opposite conclusion was drawn by EECKHOUT et al. (1978), on the basis of results obtained in probably more "physiologic" experiments, i.e., when serum gastrin levels were changed by giving specific test meals. Other investigators (WINGATE et al. 1977, 1978) reported that pentagastrin (0.1–4 μg kg^{-1} h^{-1}) abolished duodenal and jejunal migrating myoelectric complexes (MMC), substituting irregular spiking activity, but had little effect on ileal MMC. The "obliterative" effect of pentagastrin on the interdigestive myoelectric complex was not altered by vagotomy; very often the cessation of pentagastrin infusion was followed by an activity front in the duodenum (MARIK and CODE 1975). Moreover, a dose-related acceleration of the duodenal pacemaker was observed. In the dog, pentagastrin (25 μg i.v.) was found to produce rapid, tonic contraction of isolated perfused vascular segments along the circular axis and a simultaneous relaxation along the longitudinal axis. These responses were followed by long periods of tachyphylaxis. However, during these periods CCK OP was able to stimulate motility, suggesting different receptor sites for the two peptides (STEWART and BURKS 1976).

In contrast, a complete failure of pentagastrin (0.001–8 μg/kg i.v.) to change intestinal motility from the duodenum to the ileum in fasted anesthetized dogs was reported quite recently (SCHUURKES et al. 1978). Futhermore, the colon was remarkably stimulated by pentagastrin (1 μg kg^{-1} h^{-1}).

In the intestine of the cat, an inhibitory effect of pentagastrin on the electrical and mechanical activities, which seemed either directly on the smooth muscle or mediated through a mechanism independent of β-receptors, was observed (OHKAWA 1978).

In the rat, the total small bowel transit time was significantly prolonged during gastrin infusion secondary to a retarded propagation velocity in the distal small bowel. The slower transport rate during gastrin infusion was coupled to an increase of the mixing of gut contents. Pretreatment with cimetidine did not abolish these changes, suggesting that they were not correlated with gastric hypersecretion (GUSTAVSSON et al. 1978).

2. Humans

In a preliminary study, SMITH and HOGG (1966) found stimulation of motility by single i.v. injections of 25 or 50 μg gastrin II widespread throughout the gastrointestinal tract, except in the sigmoid colon, which was inhibited. These effects were notably decreased by administration of atropine (0.6 mg). At the same time, LOGAN and CONNELL (1966) reported stimulation of rectal and colonic motor activity and an occasional inhibition of the sigmoid after intravenous (0.25–0.5 μg/kg) but not after subcutaneous (1–4 μg/kg) pentagastrin administration. The effect on the ileum, when present, was always very slight. However, in exhaustive studies by MISIEWICZ et al. (1967), it was found that pentagastrin (0.01 μg kg^{-1} min^{-1}) increased antral activity only, leaving those in the gastric fundus, the right colon, sigmoid, and rectum unaffected, provided that the gastric secretion was aspirated. The authors suggested that gastrin is not directly concerned in the mediation of the gastrocolic reflex; of course, the different doses of gastrin or pentagastrin employed and the different kinds of administration (bolus injections or continuous infusions) may be responsible for these discrepancies.

In a study carried out in patients with permanent ileostomy, gastrin I (1 g kg^{-1} h^{-1}) significantly increased the frequency of action potentials in the terminal ileum concomitantly with the motor activity (WATERFALL et al. 1972). Pentagastrin (0.5 μg/kg i.v.) and gastrin I (0.1–0.2 μg kg^{-1} h^{-1}) were shown to affect colonic myoelectric activity by increasing the number of spike potentials but to leave the slow wave activity or frequency unaffected. They were approximately as effective as CCK OP (SNAPE et al. 1977, 1978). The effect of gastrin and related compounds on motor activity of the gastrointestinal tract in different species is summarized in Table 4. Recent experiments in which the intraluminal pressures in the rectum and the sigmoid in healthy volunteers and in patients with Chagas' disease were recorded showed that pentagastrin (0.1 μg/kg i.v.) stimulated motility in normal subjects and was much less effective, if at all, in the patients, probably because of the denervation of the myenteric plexus peculiar to the Chagas megacolon (MENGHELLI et al. 1978). In patients with irritable colon syndrome, fasting and poststimulation serum gastrin levels were the same as those of age- and sex-matched controls (GEOGHEGAN and FIELDING 1978).

E. Conclusions

Gastrin, being the first gastrointestinal hormone to be synthesized and available for experimental studies, had the privilege of being the subject of an enormous number of investigations. It is obvious that the effects of gastrin in regulating motor activity of the gastrointestinal tract cannot be considered of the same impor-

Table 4. Effect of gastrin and related compounds on motor activity of gastrointestinal tract

Target	Compounds[a]	Effect[b] In vitro	Effect[b] In vivo	Species
Lower esophageal sphincter	Gastrin I; pentagastrin	++ I	++ D	Opossum
	Tetragastrin	+D		Rat
	Pentagastrin		++	Monkey
	Pentagastrin; gastrin I		+ D, I	Dog
	Gastrin I; pentagastrin	+ D	++	Human
Stomach (body and fundus)	Gastrin I and II	+ I	+	Dog
	Gastrin I	+ I		Rat
	Gastrin I	+ D		Hamster
	Gastrin I	++		Opossum
	Pentagastrin	+ D		Ferret and cat
	Pentagastrin	++ D		Guinea pig
	Pentagastrin		−	Calf
	Gastrin I and II; pentagastrin hexagastrin	+		Human
Stomach (antrum)	Gastrin I	++		Opossum
	Gastrin I	++ I		Guinea pig
	Gastrin I and II; pentagastrin	++ I	++ I	Dog
	Pentagastrin		−	Calf
	Gastrin I; pentagastrin Gastrin II; hexagastrin	++ D	++	Human
Pylorus	Gastrin I		−	Human
	Gastrin I; pentagastrin		+ D	Rat
	Gastrin I		−	Opossum
Small intestine	Gastrin I and II; pentagastrin; hexagastrin	++ I		Guinea pig
	Gastrin I	+		Rat
	Gastrin I	+		Rabbit
	Tetragastrin; pentagastrin	+D	−	Cat
	Gastrin I; pentagastrin		++; −	Dog
Large intestine	Pentagastrin; gastrin I		++	Dog
	Gastrin I; pentagastrin; hexagastrin	+	+; −; O	Human

[a] Gastrin = human G 17

[b] ++ and + strong or moderate stimulatory effect; − inhibitory effect. D, I direct or indirect effect on the smooth muscle. For references see text

tance as those regulating gastric secretion. However, at least from a pharmacologic viewpoint they appear to be of considerable interest in both in vitro and in vivo studies which were performed with sophisticated techniques for the evaluation of mechanical and electrical activity and which were often correlated with studies on plasma gastrin levels. The recent recognition, however, of the various molecular forms of gastrin, each of which displays a different degree of potency and a different half-life, represents an important source of error, since radioimmunoassay techniques are unable to discriminate between them. It is possible that some investigators were not sufficiently conscious of the hazards connected with extrapolations of data and generalization of conclusions drawn from results obtained under particular experimental conditions. The logical consequence is that many data reported in the literature should be carefully reconsidered in the light of these new aquisitions and checked in the light of new methodological improvements.

Physiologic problems are tremendously complex; the possible release of gastrin from the nerves, the type of response to the different molecular forms of gastrin occurring in the gut wall or reaching the muscle through the bloodstream and the numberless possibilities of interactions between the gastrins, and all the other nervous and/or humoral mediators occurring in the gastrointestinal tract represent problems which cannot as yet be solved. Of course all the doubts regarding physiologic problems, are reflected, and magnified, in pathologic conditions involving modest or remarkable changes in plasma gastrin levels.

References

Bailes R, Picker S, Bremmer CG (1972) The effect of intragastric aluminum hydroxide on lower esophageal sphincter pressure. S Afr Med J 46:1387–1389

Bayliss WM, Starling EH (1902) On the causation of the so-called "peripheral reflex secretion" of the pancreas. Proc R Soc Lond [Biol] 69:352–353

Behar J, Biancani P, Zabinski MP (1979) Characterization of feline gastroduodenal junction by neural and hormonal stimulation. Am J Physiol 236:E45–E51

Bell FR, Titchen DA, Watson DJ (1975) The effects of pentagastrin on gastric (abomasal) motility in the unweaned calf. J Physiol (Lond) 251:12P–13P

Bell FR, Titchen DA, Watson DJ (1977) The effects of the gastrin analogue, pentagastrin, on the gastric electromyogram and abomasal emptying in the calf. Res Vet Sci 23:165–170

Bennett A (1965) Effect of gastrin on isolated smooth muscle preparations. Nature 208:170–173

Bennett A, Whitney B (1966) A pharmacological study of the motility of the human gastrointestinal tract. Gut 7:307–316

Bennett A, Misiewicz JJ, Waller SL (1967) Analysis of the motor effects of gastrin and pentagastrin on the human alimentary tract *in vitro*. Gut 8:470–474

Bertaccini G (1972) Pharmacological actions of kinins occurring in amphibian skin. *In:* Pharmacology and the future of man. Proceedings of the 5th International Congress of Pharmacology, San Francisco. Karger, Basel, pp 336–346

Bertaccini G, Scarpignato C (1981) Effects of some cholecystokinin (CCK)-like peptides on gastric emptying of a liquid meal in the rat. Br J Pharmacol 72:103P–104P

Bertaccini G, Impicciatore M, De Caro G (1973) Action of caerulein and related substances on the pyloric sphincter of the anaesthetized rat. Eur J Pharmacol 22:320–324

Bingham J (1958) Oesophageal structures after gastric surgery and nasogastric intubation. Br Med J 2:817–819

Brown FC, Dubois A, Castell DO (1976) Failure of H_2-receptor blockade with cimetidine to affect resting lower esophageal sphincter pressure and response to pentagastrin. Gastroenterology 70:A867

Burleigh DE (1979) The effects of drugs and electrical field stimulation on the human lower oesophageal sphincter. Arch Int Pharmacodyn Ther 240:169–176

Bybee DE, Brown FC, Georges LP, Castell DO, McGuigan JE (1977) Somatostatin (GHRIH) inhibition of hormonally induced increases in lower esophageal sphincter pressure (LESP). Clin Res 25:A570

Calvert CH, Parks TG, Buchanan KD (1975) The relationship of lower oesophageal sphincter pressure to plasma gastrin concentration. Gut 16:A403

Cameron AJ, Phillips SF, Summerskill WHJ (1970) Comparison of effects of gastrin, cholecystokinin-pancreozymin, secretin, and glucagon on human stomach muscle in vitro. Gastroenterology 59:539–545

Carter DC, Taylor IL, Elashoff J, Grossman MI (1979) Reappraisal of the secretory potency and disappearance rate of pure human minigastrin. Gut 20:705–708
Castell DO, Harris LD (1970) Hormonal control of gastro-esophageal sphincter strength. N Engl J Med 282:886–889
Castell DO, Levine SM (1971) A new mechanism for treatment of heartburn with antacids: lower esophageal sphincter response to gastric alkalinization. Ann Intern Med 74:223–227
Chey WY, Gutiérrez J, Yoshimori M, Hendricks J (1974) Gut hormones on gastrointestinal motor function. In: Chey WY, Brooks FP (eds) Endocrinology of the gut. Slack, Thorofare, NJ, pp 192–211
Chijikwa JB, Davison JS (1974) The action of gastrin-like polypeptides on the peristaltic reflex in guinea-pig intestine. J Physiol (Lond) 238:68P–70P
Christensen J (1975) Pharmacology of the esophageal motor function. Annu Rev Pharmacol Toxicol 15:243–258
Cohen S (1975) Symptomatic diffuse esophageal spasm and its relation to gastrin supersensitivity. Ann Intern Med 82:714–715
Cohen S, Green FE (1973) The mechanics of esophageal muscle contraction. Evidence of an inotropic effect of gastrin. J Clin Invest 52:2029–2040
Cohen S, Harris LD (1972) The lower esophageal sphincter. Gastroenterology 63:1066–1073
Cohen S, Snape WJ (1975) Action of metiamide on the lower esophageal sphincter. Gastroenterology 69:911–919
Cohen S, Lipshutz W, Hughes W (1971) Role of gastrin supersensitivity in the pathogenesis of lower esophageal sphincter hypertension in achalasia. J Clin Invest 50:1241–1247
Cooke AR, Chvasta TE, Weisbrodt NW (1972) Effect of pentagastrin on emptying and electrical and motor activity of the dog stomach. Am J Physiol 223:934–938
Corazziari E, Pozzessere C, Dani S, Delle Fave GF, De Magistris L, Anzini F (1977) Lower esophageal sphincter pressure (LESP) response to intravenous infusions of pentagastrin (PG). Gastroenterology 72:A1041
Corazziari E, Pozzessere C, Dani S, Anzini F, Torsoli A (1978) Lower oesophageal sphincter response to intravenous infusions of pentagastrin in normal subjects, antrectomized and achalasic patients. Gut 19:1121–1124
Cox KR (1961) Oesophageal structure after gastrectomy. Br J Surg 49:307–313
Csendes A, Öster M, Brandsborg O, Möller J, Brandsborg M, Amdrup E (1978a) Gastroesophageal sphincter pressure and serum gastrin studies following food intake before and after vagotomy for duodenal ulcer. Scand J Gastroenterol 13:437–441
Csendes A, Öster M, Brandsborg O, Möller J, Brandsborg M, Amdrup E (1978b) Gastroesophageal sphincter pressure and serum gastrin: reaction to food stimulation in normal subjects and in patients with gastric or duodenal ulcer. Scand J Gastroenterol 13:879–884
De Carle DJ, Glover WE (1975) Independence of gastrin and histamine receptors in the lower oesophageal sphincter of the monkey and possum. J Physiol (Lond) 245:78P–79P
Dent J, Hansky J (1976) Relationship of serum gastrin response to lower oesophageal sphincter pressure. Gut 17:144–146
Dockray GJ, Gregory RA (1980) Does the C-terminal tetrapeptide of gastrin and CCK exist as an entity? Nature 286:742
Dodds WJ, Hogan WJ, Miller WN, Barrera RF, Arndofer RC, Stef JJ (1975) Relationship between serum gastrin concentration and lower esophageal sphincter pressure. Dig Dis Sci 20:201–207
Domschke W, Lux G, Domschke S, Strunz U, Bloom SR, Wünsch E (1978) Effect of vasoactive intestinal peptide on resting and pentagastrin-stimulated lower esophageal sphincter pressure. Gastroenterology 75:9–12
Dozois RR, Kelly KA (1971) Gastrin pentapeptide and delayed gastric emptying. Am J Physiol 221:113–117
Dubois A, Castell DO (1978) Abnormal gastric emptying response to pentagastrin in duodenal ulcer. Scand J Gastroenterol [Suppl 49] 13:50
Eckardt VF, Kruger A (1974) The effect of pentagastrin on esophageal peristalsis in diffuse esophageal spasm. Clin Res 22:A693

Eckardt VF, Grace ND, Osborne MP, Fischer JE (1978) Lower esophageal sphincter pressure and serum gastrin levels after mapped antrectomy. Arch Intern Med 138:243–245

Eeckhout C, De Wever I, Peeters T, Hellemans J, Vantrappen G (1978) Role of gastrin and insulin in postprandial disruption of migrating complex in dogs. Am J Physiol 235:E666–E669

El-Sharkawy TY, Szurszewski JH (1978) Modulation of canine antral circular smooth muscle by acetylcholine, noradrenaline, and pentagastrin. J Physiol (Lond) 279:309–320

Fara JW, Berkowitz JM (1978) Effects of histamine and gastrointestinal hormones on dog antral smooth muscle in vitro. Scand J Gastroenterol [Suppl 49] 13:60

Fara JW, Praissman M, Berkowitz JM (1979) Interaction between gastrin, CCK, and secretin on canine antral smooth muscle in vitro. Am J Physiol 236:E39–E44

Farrell RL, Nebel OT, McGuire AT, Castell DO (1973) The abnormal lower esophageal sphincter in pernicious anaemia. Gut 14:767–772

Farrell RL, Castell DO, McGuigan JE (1974) Measurements and comparisons of lower esophageal sphincter pressure and serum gastrin levels in patients with gastroesophageal reflux. Gastroenterology 67:415–422

Fiddian-Green RG, Quinn TS (1978) Physiological actions of luminal gastrin in human gastric juice. Gut 19:A435

Fisher RS, Boden G (1976) Gastrin inhibition of the pyloric sphincter. Am J Dig Dis 21:468–472

Fisher RS, Cohen S (1980) Effects of gut hormones on gastrointestinal sphincters. In: Jerzy Glass G (ed) Gastrointestinal hormones. Raven, New York, pp 613–638

Fisher RS, Lipshutz W, Cohen S (1973) The hormonal regulation of pyloric sphincter function. J Clin Invest 52:1289–1296

Fisher RS, Di Marino AJ, Cohen S (1975) Mechanism of cholecystokinin-inhibition of lower esophageal sphincter pressure. Am J Physiol 228:1469–1473

Freeland GR, Higgs RH, Castell DO, McGuigan JE (1975) Lower esophageal sphincter (LES) and gastric acid (GA) response to intravenous infusion of synthetic human gastrin heptadecapeptide I (HGH). Gastroenterology 68:A894

Freeland GR, Higgs RH, Castell DO, McGuigan JE (1976) Lower esophageal sphincter and gastric acid responses to intravenous infusions of synthetic human gastrin I heptadecapeptide. Gastroenterology 71:570–574

Gamblin GT, Dubois A, Castell DO (1977) Contrasting, effect of pentagastrin on gastric emptying in normals and patients with gastric ulcer. Clin Res 25:A17

Geoghegan J, Fielding JF (1978) Brief report serum gastrin and the irritable bowel syndrome. Ir J Med Sci 147:156

Gerner T, Haffner JFW, (1977) The role of local cholinergic pathways in the motor response to cholecystokinin and gastrin in isolated guinea-pig fundus and antrum. Scand J Gastroenterol 12:751–757

Gerner T, Haffner JFW (1978) Interactions of cholecystokinin (CCK-PZ) and gastrin on motor activity of isolated guinea-pig antrum and fundus. Scand J Gastroenterol 13:789–794

Gerner T, Haffner JFW, Norstein J (1979) The effects of mepyramine and cimetidine on the motor responses to histamine, cholecystokinin, and gastrin in the fundus and antrum of isolated guinea-pig stomachs. Scand J Gastroenterol 14:65–72

Goyal RK, McGuigan JE (1976) Is gastrin a major determinant of basal lower esophageal sphincter pressure? A double-blind controlled study using high titer gastrin antiserum. J Clin Invest 57:291–300

Goyal RK, Rattan S (1978) Neurohumoral, hormonal, and drug receptors for the lower esophageal sphincter. Gastroenterology 74:598–619

Gregory RA (1974) The Bayliss-Starling lecture 1973. The gastrointestinal hormones: a review of recent advance. J Physiol (Lond) 241:1–32

Gregory RA (1978) The gastrins: structure and heterogeneity. In: Grossman M, Speranza V, Basso N, Lezoche E (eds) Gastrointestinal hormones and pathology of the digestive system. Plenum, New York London, pp 75–83

Gregory RA, Tracy HJ (1964) The constitution and properties of two gastrins extracted from hog antral mucosa. Gut 5:103–117

Gregory RA, Tracy HJ (1974) Isolation of two minigastrins from Zollinger-Ellison tumour tissue. Gut 15:683–685

Gregory RA, Tracy HJ, Harris JI, Runswick MJ, Moore S, Kenner GW, Ramage R (1979) Minigastrin: corrected structure and synthesis. Hoppe Seylers Z Physiol Chem 360:73–80

Gustavsson S, Jung B, Lundqvist G, Nilsson F (1978) Propulsion and mixing of small bowel contents during exogenous gastrin infusion. An experimental study in rats. Acta Chir Scand 144:103–108

Hamilton SG, Sheiner HJ, Quinlan MF (1976) Continuous monitoring of the effect of pentagastrin on gastric emptying of solid food in man. Gut 17:273–279

Hara Y (1980) Actions of tetragastrin on smooth muscles of human stomach. Eur J Physiol 386:127–134

Harvey RF (1975) Hormonal control of gastrointestinal motility. Dig Dis Sci 20:523–539

Heil T, Mattes P, Raptis S (1977) Effects of somatostatin and human gastrin I on the lower esophageal sphincter in man. Digestion 15:461–468

Helsinger N (1960) Oesophagitis following total gastrectomy. Acta Clin Scand 118:190–201

Henderson JM, Lidgard G, Osborne DH, Carter DC, Heading RC (1978) Lower oesophageal sphincter response to gastrin pharmacological or physiological? Gut 19:99–102

Hiatt GA, Wells RF (1974) Clinical physiology review: gastrin. Am J Gastroenterol 62:59–66

Higgs RH, Castell DO (1975) Increased response of the lower esophageal sphincter after truncal vagotomy. Clin Res 23:A16

Higgs RH, Smyth RD, Castell DO (1974) Gastric alkalinization; effect on lower esophageal sphincter pressure and serum gastrin. N Engl J Med 291:486–490

Higgs RH, Humphries TJ, Castell CO, McGuigan JE (1976) Lower esophageal sphincter pressure and serum gastrin levels after cholinergic stimulation. Am J Physiol 231:1250–1253

Hunt JN, Ramsbottom N (1967) Effect of gastrin II on gastric emptying and secretion during a test meal. Br Med J 4:386–387

Isenberg JI, Grossman MI (1969) Effect of gastrin and SC 15396 on gastric motility in dogs. Gastroenterology 56:450–455

Itoh Z, Honda R, Hiwatashi K (1978a) Hormonal control of the lower oesophageal sphincter in man and dog: reevaluation of the present manometric methods for diagnosis of gastro-oesophageal reflux. In: Grossman M, Speranza V, Basso N, Lezoche E (eds) Gastrointestinal hormones and pathology of the digestive system. Plenum, New York London, pp 121–131

Itoh Z, Takayanagi R, Takeuchi S, Issgiki S (1978b) Interdigestive motor activity of Heidenhain pouches in relation to main stomach in conscious dogs. Am J Physiol 234:E333–E338

Jennewein HM, Hummelt H, Siewert R, Waldeck F (1976) The effect of intravenous infusion of synthetic human gastrin-I on lower esophageal sphincter (LES) pressure in the dog and its relation to gastrin level. Digestion 14:376–380

Jensen DM, McCallum RW, Walsh JH (1978a) Failure of atropine to inhibit gastrin-17 stimulation of the lower esophageal sphincter in man. Gastroenterology 75:825–827

Jensen DM, McCallum RW, Walsh JH (1978b) Human lower oesophageal sphincter (LES) response to submaximal and maximal effective doses of synthetic human big gastrin (G-34) and gastrin I (G-17). In: Duthie HL (ed) Gastrointestinal motility in health and disease. MTP Press, Lancaster, pp 337–338

Johnson LR (1977) Gastrointestinal hormones and their functions. Annu Rev Physiol 39:135–158

Kelly KA (1975) The effect of pentagastrin on canine gastric myoelectric and motor activity. In: Thompson G (ed) Gastrointestinal hormones. University of Texas Press, Austin London, pp 381–389

Kline MM, Curry N, Sturdevant RAL, McCallum RW (1974) Effect of gastric alkalinization on lower esophageal sphincter pressure and serum gastrin. Gastroenterology 66:A724

Kline MM, McCallum RW, Curry N, Sturdevant RAL (1975) Effect of gastric alkalinization on lower esophageal sphincter pressure and serum gastrin. Gastroenterology 68:1137–1139
Kowalewski K, Zajac S, Kolodej A (1975a) Effect of release of endogenous gastrin on myoelectrical and mechanical activity of isolated canine stomach. Pharmacology 13:56–64
Kowalewski K, Zajac S, Kolodej A (1975b) The effect of drugs on the electrical and mechanical activity of the isolated porcine stomach. Pharmacology 13:86–95
Kwong NK, Brown BH, Whittakez GE, Duthie HL (1972) Effect of gastrin I, secretin and cholecystokinin-pancreozymin on the electrical activity, motor activity, and acid output of the stomach in man. Scand J Gastroenterol 7:161–170
Lane W, McCallum R, Ippoliti A (1977) The effect of gastrin heptadecapeptide on esophageal contractions in patients with diffuse esophageal spasm. Clin Res 25:A111
Lane WH, Ippoliti AF, McCallum RW (1979) Effect of gastrin heptadecapeptide (G17) on oesophageal contractions in patients with diffuse oesophageal spasm. Gut 20:756–759
Lipshutz W, Cohen S (1971) Physiological determinants of lower esophageal sphincter function. Gastroenterology 61:16–24
Lipshutz W, Cohen S (1972) Interaction of gastrin I and secretin on gastrointestinal circular muscle. Am J Physiol 222:775–781
Lipshutz W, Tuch AF, Cohen S (1971) A comparison of the site of action of gastrin I on lower esophageal sphincter and antral circular smooth muscle. Gastroenterology 61:454–460
Lipshutz W, Hughes W, Cohen S (1972) The genesis of lower esophageal sphincter pressure: its identification through the use of gastrin antiserum. J Clin Invest 51:522–529
Lipshutz W, Gaskins RD, Lukash WM, Sode J (1973) Pathogenesis of lower esophageal sphincter incompetence. N Engl J Med 289:182–184
Lipshutz W, Gaskins RD, Lukash WM, Sode J (1974) Hypogastrinemia in patients with lower esophageal sphincter incompetence. Gastroenterology 67:423–427
Logan CJH, Connell AM (1966) The effect of a synthetic gastrin-like pentapeptide (I.C.I. 50,123) on intestinal motility in man. Gastroenterology 1:996–999
MacGregor IL, Wiley ZD, Martin PM (1978) Effect of pentagastrin infusion on gastric emptying rate of solid food in man. Am J Dig Dis 23:72–75
Malloy MH, Morriss FH, Denson SE, Weisbrodt NW, Lichtenberger LM, Adcock EW (1979) Neonatal gastric motility in dogs: maturation and response to pentagastrin. Am J Physiol 236:E562–E566
Mantovani P, Bertaccini G (1971) Action of caerulein and related substances on gastrointestinal motility of the anaesthetized dog. Arch Int Pharmacodyn Ther 193:362–371
Marik F, Code CF (1975) Control of the interdigestive myoelectric activity in dogs by the vagus nerves and pentagastrin. Gastroenterology 69:387–395
McCallum RW, Walsh JH (1979) Relationship between lower esophageal sphincter pressure and serum gastrin concentration in Zollinger-Ellison syndrome and other clinical settings. Gastroenterology 76:65–81
Menghelli UG, Godoy RA, Padovan W, Santos JCM, Dantas RO, Oliveira RB (1978) L'action de la pentagastrine sur la motilité du sigmoide et du rectum normaux et sur le megacolon chagasique. VI th World Congr Gastroenterol, Madrid, June 5–9, 1978, p 205
Meves M, Beger HG, Hüthwohl BB (1975) The effect of some gastrointestinal hormones on gasric evacuation in man. In: Vantrappen G (ed) Fifth International Symposium on Gastrointestinal Motility. Typoff, Herentals, pp 327–332
Mikos E, Vane JR (1967) Effects of gastrin and its analogues on isolated smooth muscles. Nature 214:105–107
Misiewicz JJ, Holdstock DJ, Waller SL (1967) Motor responses of the human alimentary tract to near-maximal infusions of pentagastrin. Gut 8:463–469
Monges H, Salducci J (1972) Variations of the gastric electrical activity in man produced by administration of pentagastrin and by introduction of water or liquid nutritive substance into the stomach. Am J Dig Dis 17:333–338
Morgan KG, Szurszewski JH (1978) Effects of pentagastrin on intracellular electrical activity of canine corpus. Gastroenterology 74:A1069

Morgan KG, Szurszewski JH (1980) Mechanisms of phasic and tonic actions of pentagastrin on canine gastric smooth muscle. J Physiol (Lond) 301:229–242
Morgan KG, Schmalz PF, Go VLW, Szurzewski JH (1978) Effects of pentagastrin G_{17} and G_{34} on the electrical and mechanical activities of canine antral smooth muscle. Gastroenterology 75:405–412
Morris SJ, Perez C, Rogers AI (1978) Sensitivity of esophageal peristalsis to pentagastrin in patients with symptomatic diffuse esophageal spasm. Gastroenterology 74:A1137
Morris DW, Shoen H, Brooks FP, Cohen S (1974) Relationship of serum gastrin and lower esophageal sphincter pressure in normals and patients with antrectomy. Gastroenterology 66:75
Munk JF, Hoare M, Johnson AG (1978) Hormonal influence of pyloric diameter and antral motility in man: Gut 19:A435
Nebel OT, Castell DO (1972) Lower esophageal sphincter pressure changes after food ingestion. Gastroenterology 66:778–783
Nilsson G(1980) Gastrin: isolation, characterization, and functions. In: Jerzy Glass GB (ed) Gastrointestinal hormones (comprehensive endocrinology). Raven, New York
Ohkawa H (1978) Inhibition of the electrical and mechanical activities of the intestinal smooth muscle by pentagastrin. Tohoku J Exp Med 125:271–279
Ohkawa H, Watanabe M (1977a) Effects of gastrointestinal hormones on the electrical and mechanical activity of the cat stomach. Tohoku J Exp Med 122:287–298
Ohkawa H, Watanabe M (1977b) Effects of gastrointestinal hormones on the electrical and mechanical activities of the cat small intestine. Jpn J Physiol 27:71–79
Onapito SJ, Donawick WJ, Merritt AM (1978) Effects of gastrin on emptying and composition of digesta of the omasum of sheep. Am J Vet Res 39:1455–1458
Orlando RC, Bozymski EM (1979) The effects of pentagastrin in achalasia and diffuse esophageal spasm. Gastroenterology 77:472–477
Pearce EAN, Wingate DL, Wünsch E (1978) The effects of gastrointestinal hormones and feeding on the basic electric rhythm of the stomach and duodenum of the conscious dog. J Physiol (Lond) 276:41P–42P
Pittinger G, Kothary P, Fiddian-Green RG (1978) The effect of luminal gastrin on the rate of gastric emptying. Clin Res 26:A665
Rattan S, Goyal RK (1978) Influence of verapamil on the stimulated lower esophageal sphincter pressure. Gastroenterology 74:A1082
Rattan S, Coln D, Goyal RK (1976) The mechanism of action of gastrin on the lower esophageal sphincter. Gastroenterology 70:828–831
Rehfeld JF, Larsson LI (1979) The predominanting molecular form of gastrin and cholecystokinin in the gut is a small peptide corresponding to their COOH-terminal tetrapeptide amide. Acta Physiol Scand 105:177–119
Rehfeld JF, Stadil F (1973) Gel-filtration studies on immunoreactive gastrin in serum from Zollinger-Ellison patients. Gut 14:369–373
Rösch W, Lux G, Schittenhelm W, Demling L (1976) Interaction of somatostatin and pentagastrin on lower oesophageal sphincter pressure (LESP) in man. Acta Hepatogastroenterol (Stuttg) 23:209–212
Roth SH, Schofield B, Yates JC (1979) Effects of atropine on secretion and motility in isolated gastric mucosa and attached muscularis externa from ferret and cat. J Physiol (Lond) 292:351–361
Ryan JP, Duffy KR (1978) LES pressure response to pentagastrin: effect of cholinergic augmentation and inhibition. Am J Physiol 234:E301–E305
Scheurer U, Halter F (1976) Lower esophageal sphincter in reflux esophagitis. Scand J Gastroenterol 11:629–634
Schuurkes JAJ, Charbon GA (1979) Pentagastrin stimulates tonic and phasic contractile activity of the canine stomach. Arch Int Pharmacodyn Ther 239:128–137
Schuurkes JAJ, Beijer HJM, Brouwer FAS, Charbon GA (1978) Motor effects of graded doses of pentagastrin on the gut of the anesthetized dog. Arch Int Pharmacodyn Ther 234:97–106
Siewert R, Jennewein HM, Arnold R, Creutzfeldt W (1973) The lower oesophageal sphincter in the Zollinger-Ellison-Syndrome. Ger Med Man 3:101–102

Siewert R, Weiser F, Jennewein HM, Waldeck F (1974) Clinical and manometric investigations of the lower esophageal sphincter and its reactivity to pentagastrin in patients with hiatus hernia. LES-pentagastrin-test. Digestion 10:287–297

Siewert R, Weiser HF, Lepsien G, Jennewein H, Waldeck F, Arnold R, Creutzfeldt W (1977) The relationship between serum IRG levels and LES pressure under various conditions. Digestion 15:162–174

Smith AN, Hogg D (1966) Effect of gastrin II on the motility of the gastrointestinal tract. Lancet 1:403–404

Snape WJ Jr, Cohen S (1979) Effect of bethanecol, gastrin I, or cholecystokinin on myoelectrical activity. Am J Physiol 236:E458–E463

Snape WJ Jr, Carlson GM, Cohen S (1977) Human colonic myoelectric activity in response to prostigmine and the gastrointestinal hormones. Am J Dig Dis 22:881–887

Snape WJ Jr Matarazzo SA, Cohen S (1978) Effect of eating and gastrointestinal hormones on human colonic myoelectrical and motor activity. Gastroenterology 75:373–378

Spedale SB, Morriss FH, Denson SE, Adcock EW (1978) Neonatal lower esophageal sphincter pressure in dogs: maturation and response to pentagastrin. Clin Res 26:A827

Stewart JJ, Burks TF (1976) Investigation of the intestinal smooth muscle response to pentagastrin. Pharmacologist 18:181

Strunz UT, Grossman MI (1977) Antral motility stimulated by gastrin: a physiological action affected by cholinergic activity. In: Chey WY, Brooks FP (eds) Endocrinology of the gut. Slack, Thorofare, NJ, pp 233–243

Strunz UT, Grossman MI (1978) Effect of intragastric pressure on gastric emptying and secretion. Am J Physiol 235:E552–E555

Strunz UT, Code CF, Grossman MI (1979) Effect of gastrin on electrical activity of antrum and duodenum of dogs. Proc Soc Exp Biol Med 161:25–27

Sugawara K, Isaza J, Woodward ER (1969) Effect of gastrin on gastric motor activity. Gastroenterology 57:649–658

Székely A, Major T, Romvári H (1969) Über die Wirkung von Pentagastrin auf die Magenmotilität. Fortsch Geb Roentgenstr Ver Roentgenprax 111:841–846

Szurszewski JH (1975) Mechanism of action of pentagastrin and acetylcholine on the longitudinal muscle of the canine antrum. J Physiol (Lond) 252:335–361

Takayanagi I, Kasuya Y (1977) Effects of some drugs on the circular muscle of the isolated lower esophagus. J Pharm Pharmacol 29:559–560

Thomas PA, Schang JC, Kelly KA, Go VLW (1979) Inhibition of interdigestive proximal gastric motor cycles by endogenously – released gastrin. Gastroenterology 76:A1262

Tracy HJ, Gregory RA (1964) Physiological properties of a series of synthetic peptides structurally related to gastrin I. Nature 204:935–938

Valenzuela JE, Grossman MI (1975) Effect of pentagastrin and caerulein on intragastric pressure in the dog. Gastroenterology 69:1383–1384

Vizi SE, Bertaccini G, Impicciatore M, Knoll J (1973) Evidence that acetylcholine released by gastrin and related polypeptides contributes to their effect on gastrointestinal motility. Gastroenterology 64:268–277

Vizi SE, Bertaccini G, Impicciatore M, Mantovani P, Zséli J, Knoll J (1974) Structure-activity relationship of some analogues of gastrin and cholecystokinin on intestinal smooth muscle of the guinea pig. Naunyn Schmiedebergs Arch Pharmacol 284:233–243

Walker CO, Frank SA, Manton J, Fordtran JS (1975) Effect of continuous infusion of pentagastrin on lower esophageal sphincter pressure and gastric acid secretion in normal subjects. J Clin Invest 56:218–225

Wallin L, Madsen T, Brandsborg M, Brandsborg O, Larsen NE (1979) The influence of cimetidine on basal gastroesophageal sphincter pressure, intragastric pH, and serum gastrin concentration in normal subjects. Scand J Gastroenterol 14:349–353

Walsh JH, Grossman MI (1975a) Gastrin (first of two parts). N Engl J Med 292:1324–1334

Walsh JH, Grossman MI (1975b) Gastrin (second of two parts). N Engl J Med 292:1377–1384

Walsh JH, Debas HT, Grossman MI, (1974) Pure human big gastrin: immunochemical properties, disappearance half-time and acid stimulating action in dogs. J Clin Invest 54:477–485

Waterfall WE, Brown BH, Duthie HL, Whittaker GE (1972) The effects of humoral agents on the myoelectrical activity of the terminal ileum. Gut 13:528–534
Weisbrodt NW, Copeland EM, Kearley RW, Moore EP, Johnson LR (1974) Effects of pentagastrin on electrical activity of small intestine of the dog. Am J Physiol 227:425–429
Weiss SM, Hughes SR, Paskin DL, Lipshutz WH (1976) Effects of drugs and hormones on human colon muscle. Clin Res 24:A293
White CM, Keighley MRB (1978) An explanation of the paradoxical effect of pentagastrin on gastric motility. Gut 19:A434–A435
Wilbur BG, Kelly KA (1974) Gastrin pentapeptide decreases canine gastric transmural pressure. Gastroenterology 67:1139–1142
Windsor C (1964) Gastro-oesophageal reflux after partial gastrectomy Br Med J 2:1233–1234
Wingate D, Thompson H, Pearce E, Dand A (1977) Similar-but different: the myoelectric response to cholecystokinin and pentagastrin in the conscious dog. Gut 18:A966
Wingate DL, Pearce EA, Hutton M, Dand A, Thompson HH, Wünsch E (1978) Quantitative comparison of the effects of cholecystokinin, secretin, and pentagastrin on gastrointestinal myoelectric activity in the conscious fasted dog. Gut 19:593–601
Wright LF, Slaughter RL, Gibson RG, Hirschowitz BI (1975) Correlation of lower esophageal sphincter pressure and serum gastrin level in man. Am J Dig Dis 20:603–606
Yalow RS, Berson SA (1971) Further studies on the nature of immunoreactive gastrin in human plasma. Gastroenterology 60:203–214
Yalow RS, Berson SA (1972) And now, "big, big" gastrin. Biochem Biophys Res Commun 48:391–395
Yates JC, Schofield B, Roth SH (1978) Acid secretion and motility of isolated mammalian gastric mucosa and attached muscularis externa. Am J Physiol 234:E319–E326
Yau WM (1974) The actions of cholecystokinin and related peptides on the small intestinal muscle. In: Chey WY, Brooks FP (eds) Endocrinology of the gut. Slack, Thorofare, NJ, pp 212–219
Zetler G (1979) Antagonism of cholecystokinin-like peptides by opioid peptides, morphine or tetrodotoxin. Eur J Pharmacol 60:67–77
Zwick R, Bowes KL, Daniel EE, Sarna SK (1976) Mechanism of action of pentagastrin on the lower esophageal sphincter. J Clin Invest 57:1644–1651

Cholecystokinin

A. Introduction

The history of cholecystokinin (CCK) starts with its discovery by Ivy and Oldberg (1928), continues with the discovery of pancreozymin by Harper and Raper (1943) and then proceeds by slow, successive steps in the research that led to the important conclusion that contraction of the gallbladder (cholecystokinin) and stimulation of pancreatic enzyme secretion (pancreozymin) were effects of a single peptide, which was isolated in 1964 by Jorpes et al. (for a complete review see Jorpes and Mutt 1973). However, in view of the first activity attributed to it, Grossman (1970) suggested that it be called cholecystokinin, with the understanding that it also has the action of pancreozymin. Mutt and Jorpes (1968), when describing the partial sequence of cholecystokinin, described another form of the hormone, known as cholecystokinin variant, which has the same amino acid composition as cholecystokinin but has six additional amino acids at the NH_2 terminus. Quite recently several molecular forms of CCK have been demonstrated by bioassay and/

or radioimmunoassay to be present in intestinal and in cerebral tissue (for review see MUTT 1979). It is possible that the larger molecular forms represent precursors of the more active CCK octapeptide (CCK OP) which seems to be present (or predominant) in both the brain and the gut in which also a small peptide, corresponding to the COOH terminal tetrapeptide amide is present (REHFELD and LARSSON 1979). Apparently CCK OP is the predominant immunoreactive form found in the dog vagus (DOCKRAY et al. 1980). All the different forms of CCK are listed in Table 1, together with a series of peptides in amphibian skin discovered by ERSPAMER and co-workers (ANASTASI et al. 1967, 1969; ERSPAMER 1970; MONTECUCCHI et al. 1977) and found to be quite similar to CCK from both the chemical and pharmacologic points of view.

B. Structure–Activity Relationships

As we have already said (see Chap. 2a, Gastrin), CCK and gastrin belong to the same family of peptides: the smallest fragment which still retains the spectrum of activity of gastrin is the COOH terminal tetrapeptide, which is the same as that of CCK (Gly-Trp-Met-Asp-Phe-NH_2).

We will not discuss here the complex problem of structure-activity relationships in the entire gastrin–cholecystokinin group, which includes those with action on gastric and pancreatic secretions, on the biliary system, etc. Here we will deal especially with problems connected with gastrointestinal motility. Comparative bioassays of a large number of analogs and derivatives of CCK OP and cerulein, and of shorter COOH terminal fragments have given considerable amounts of information about the structural requirements for the activities of CCK (for review see MUTT 1979). It has been found that:

1) CCK OP is, even on a molar basis, several times more potent than CCK 33.

2) The sulfated tyrosyl residue in position 7 from the COOH terminus is of decisive importance for the maintenance of the biologic activity and this phenomenon was seen more strongly in vitro than in vivo (possibly because of a certain degree of metabolism of the injected material in vivo) in the studies of FARA and ERDE (1978) with cerulein. The striking difference in activity between sulfated and nonsulfated forms suggests that sulfation and desulfation may be an efficient regulatory mechanism.

3) The position of the tyrosine-*O*-sulfate residue is also of importance; moving it to the left by insertion of an amino acid residue or to the right by elimination of a threonyl or the threonyl and glycyl residues yielded compounds with no activity on smooth muscle.

4) The changes observed after substitution of the methionyl residue at position 6 from the COOH terminus were largely dependent on the kind of substituent: tryptophan, phenylalanine, glycine, and tyrosine gave compounds with lower activity, whereas threonine did not change the activity and the more stable norleucyl residue actually enhanced the potency of the octapeptide molecule.

5) Shortening the heptapeptide molecule caused a strong decline in potency, however, there was still some degree of activity of the COOH terminal tripeptide and even of the dipeptide Asp-Phe-NH_2 (LIN 1972; BERTACCINI 1972; VIZI et al. 1974).

Table 1. Structure of cholecystokinin (porcine CCK 33) and its natural analogs[a]

CCK variant (39)[b]	CCK (33)	CCK (27)	CCK (12)	CCK OP (8)	Tetrapeptide (4)	Cerulein (Ceruletide) (10)	Asn^2, Leu^5-Cerulein (10)	Phyllocerulein (9)
Tyr								
Ile								
Gln								
Gln								
Ala								
Arg								
Lys	–							
Ala	–							
Pro	–							
Ser	–							
Gly	–							
Arg	–							
Val	–	–						
Ser	–	–						
Met	–	–						
Ile	–	–						
Lys	–	–						
Asn	–	–						
Leu	–	–						
Gln	–	–						
Ser	–	–						
Leu	–	–						
Asp	–	–						
Pro	–	–						
Ser	–	–						
His	–	–						

Arg	–	–						
Ile	–	–	–					
Ser	–	–	–					
Asp	–	–	–			pGlu	–	
Arg	–	–	–			Gln	Asn	pGlu
Asp	–	–	–	–		–	–	Glu
Tyr–HSO_3	–	–	–	–		–	–	–
Met	–	–	–	–		Thr	Leu	–
Gly	–	–	–	–		–	–	–
Trp	–	–	–	–	–	–	–	–
Met	–	–	–	–	–	–	–	–
Asp	–	–	–	–	–	–	–	–
Phe–NH_2	–	–	–	–	–	–	–	–

[a] The dashes (–) indicate the same amino acid residue as that in the column to the left
[b] Figures in parentheses indicate the number of residues in each peptide

C. Effects on the Lower Esophageal Sphincter

Most of the data for intact animals (opossum and cats) and for humans have shown that cholecystokinin and CCK OP cause a dose- dependent decrease in lower esophageal sphincter (LES) pressure, the maximum decrease being between 70% and 80%. Bolus injections were generally employed (RESIN et al. 1973; STURDEVANT and KUN 1974; FISHER et al. 1975) because intravenous infusion apparently does not modify basal LES pressure though it is able to inhibit the response to pentagastrin partially (STURDEVANT and KUN 1974). The fat-induced inhibition of LES pressure (NEBEL and CASTELL 1973) was probably related to CCK release from the duodenum, but this should be confirmed by reliable radioimmunoassay of CCK, which has not been done so far.

A recent study in the anesthetized cat (BEHAR and BIANCANI 1977) showed that the inhibitory effect of CCK OP (maximal relaxation obtained with 300–400 μg/kg), was unaffected by atropine or by adrenergic blocking agents, but was antagonized by tetrodotoxin (TTX). The authors suggested that CCK OP acts at two receptor sites: one on postganglionic inhibitory (nonadrenergic, noncholinergic) neurons responsible for sphincter relaxation and one on smooth muscle, causing contraction. The sum of the effects is LES relaxation, and contraction becomes apparent only when the innervation of the LES is abolished by tetrodotoxin. Recent experiments DENT et al. 1978 a) in the opossum, gave data at variance with previous data, suggesting remarkable species differences. They showed that CCK OP (10–800 μg/kg) caused a dose-related increase in LES pressure and phasic contractions of the esophageal body. CCK OP was apparently acting directly on smooth muscle, since its effect was unaffected by the common inhibitors. In contrast to data obtained in the cat, there was no demonstrable effect on inhibitory esophageal nerves in the opossum. Studies performed on in vitro strips from opossum LES showed that both CCK and CCK OP contract the sphincter, acting as partial agonists of gastrin (lower threshold dose and smaller maximum response). This stimulatory effect was blocked by tetrodotoxin and atropine, suggesting that the action is mediated through a release of acetylcholine (FISHER et al. 1975). It may be thought that not only the action on inhibitory neurons but also the competitive inhibition of the gastrin effect may play a role in the inhibitory action of CCK observed in vivo.

Cerulein was also found to cause contraction of the opossum LES, an effect which was apparently potentiated by tetrodotoxin, thus suggesting a neural inhibitory component in the action of the peptide (GOYAL and RATTAN 1978). It was hypothesized that the effect of cerulein, unlike that of CCK, may be more marked on the muscle receptor (causing contraction) than on the neural receptor (causing relaxation). This difference between the actions of cerulein and CCK needs to be confirmed.

The first study performed in humans (RESIN et al. 1973) showed that CCK OP (2.5–40 ng/kg i.v.) produced a dose-related decrease in LES pressure (down to 60% of basal pressure). The effect was rapid in onset, reached a peak within 4 min, and lasted about 10 min. Results similar to those with CCK were obtained by giving continuous infusion of cerulein (1–8 ng kg^{-1} min^{-1} for 15 min) to 16 normal subjects (PANDOLFO et al. 1977). Surprisingly, CCK OP (5–80 ng/kg i.v.) was shown in other studies to cause a slight, dose-independent decrease in LES pressure in achalasia patients (DENT et al. 1978b). Atropine, which by itself reduced LES pressure, did not inhibit the effect of CCK OP. The significance of this phenomenon is still obscure.

The general conclusions which can be drawn, in accordance with those of FISHER and COHEN (1980), are as follows: (a) CCK and its analogs have a predominantly inhibitory effect on LES pressure in vivo, though some exceptions are possible in the different species; (b) the effect in vitro is usually a stimulatory one and probably depends on the release of acetylcholine; (c) CCK may antagonize the effect of gastrin, probably by a competitive mechanism.

D. Effects on the Stomach

I. In Vivo Studies

Most of the studies reported in the literature were done in the dog because of the easy availability of animals prepared with gastric fistulas, denervated Heidenhain pouches, or antral pouches. Motility was studied by recording intraluminal pressure or by transducers applied directly to the serosal surface. The first observations of the effects of a pure, synthetic analog of CCK on gastrointestinal motility were made with the decapeptide cerulein (ceruletide), which preceded those made with CCK OP or with highly purified CCK. The early results with extracts containing variable amounts of CCK were not completely reliable because it has been recognized, that they were contaminated with secretin and GIP, which could noticeably affect the action of CCK. As with gastrin, the effects of cholecystokinin and its analogs, also differed in the proximal and the distal stomach.

The early experiments with cerulein showed that the peptide caused a dose-related increase in motor activity of the denervated gastric pouch of both anesthetized and conscious dogs when administered either subcutaneously (0.2–1 μg/kg) or intravenously (5–50 ng/kg; BERTACCINI et al. 1968). Cerulein (10–100 ng/kg i.v.) was also able to induce a potent dose-dependent stimulation of the pyloric antrum, affecting the amplitude and the frequency of the antral waves more than the tonus (MANTOVANI and BERTACCINI 1971; Fig. 1). The stimulatory effect of cerulein on the innervated stomach of conscious dogs was also observed, though much higher doses had to be used (0.1–0.5 μg/kg i.v.) (BERTACCINI and IMPICCIATORE 1975). While stimulation of both antrum and pyloric sphincter was also observed with CCK OP (0.1–1.6 $\mu g\ kg^{-1}\ h^{-1}$; CHEY et al. 1972; ISENBERG and CSENDES 1972) and with CCK (128–4,096 mU/kg i.v.; SCHUURKES and CHARBON 1978), all the recent studies performed with different techniques indicate a predominantly inhibitory effect of CCK and analogs on the proximal stomach. In the presence of gastric neutralization, a dose of cerulein as low as 63 $ng\ kg^{-1}\ h^{-1}$, which is the ED_{50} for pancreatic protein secretion, produced significant inhibition of gastric motility as measured by the decrease in intragastric pressure (VALENZUELA and GROSSMAN 1975). This confirmed the inhibitory effect of CCK OP (0.5 μg/kg or 0.4 $\mu g\ kg^{-1}\ h^{-1}$) observed in the dog's antrum stimulated by balloon distension (CHEY et al. 1974). Other studies of the effect of CCK OP on antral mechanical and myoelectric activ-

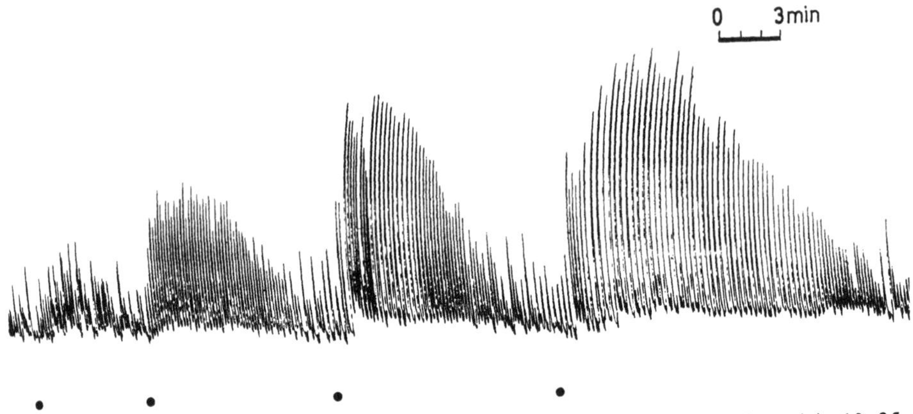

Fig. 1. Motility in the canine pyloric antrum. *Dots* indicate i.v. injection of cerulein 10, 25, 50, and 100 ng/kg. (MANTOVANI and BERTACCINI 1971)

ity showed that the peptide caused a significant increase in mechanical activity and in the mean percentage frequency of spike potentials on slow waves without changing the frequency of slow waves (LEE et al. 1974; CASTRESANA et al. 1978).

According to SCHANG and KELLY (1980), CCK OP (15–250 ng kg^{-1} h^{-1}) inhibited the interdigestive cycles in both proximal gastric pouch and duodenum. After the infusion was stopped, cyclic activity and intrapouch pressure returned promptly to control values. The authors suggested that CCK mimicks the effect of feeding and may have a role in inducing the fed pattern of motility in the proximal stomach after meals.

In the conscious cat CCK (0.25–16 Ivy dog units kg^{-1} h^{-1}) or CCK OP (0.5–2 μg kg^{-1} h^{-1}) caused dose-dependent changes of antral motility. The peptides increased the frequency of low amplitude contractions and decreased the force of contractions (DESVIGNE et al. 1980). These effects, which were similar to those elicited by pentagastrin (0.5–8 μg kg^{-1} h^{-1}) could be interpreted as an action on the mixing function of the stomach.

A remarkable spasmogenic effect was observed in the in situ pylorus of the rat (BERTACCINI et al. 1973, 1974). In this preparation, cerulein caused a spasmogenic contraction, lasting 1–20 min according to the dose (2–160 ng/kg i.v.), which was unaffected by the common inhibitors and was probably due to a direct activity of the peptide on the pylorus. The potency of cerulein (apart from that of bombesin which was approximately equiactive) exceeded by 3–1,000 times those of all the other peptide and nonpeptide spasmogenic compounds. Only adrenaline and other sympathomimetic compounds or PGE_1 were able to inhibit or sometimes to prevent the spasmogenic effect of cerulein on the rat pylorus. In the gastroduodenal junction of the cat, CCK OP (50–800 ng/kg) had an erratic effect, sometimes causing relaxation, sometimes contractions, and only rarely a biphasic effect. However, the most common feature was a fall in baseline intraluminal pressure (BEHAR et al. 1979).

Different data were obtained for the forestomach of the sheep, probably because of differing experimental conditions. FAUSTINI et al. (1973, 1979) observed a potent relaxant effect of cerulein on the reticulum and the omasum (0.1–1 ng/kg, by bolus i.v. injection) and a complete block of rhythmic motility with a continuous infusion of the peptide (0.1 ng kg^{-1} min^{-1}). WILSON (1975), using CCK (2.5 U/kg i.v.), found a reduction of frequency of contractions in the rumen to 80% of the control values, but an increase in the amplitude of the contractions to 144% of the control values. This effect was not modified by pretreatment with α- or β-sympathetic blocking agents or tripelennamine. The proventriculus and duodenum of the chicken were stimulated by intravenous infusion of cerulein (0.25 ng kg^{-1} min^{-1}; ANGELUCCI et al. 1969).

Contrasting findings were obtained for the activity of cholecystokinin in the human pylorus FISHER and COHEN (1973), administering CCK 2 U kg^{-1} h^{-1} i.v., reported a complete lack of response whereas MUNK et al. (1978) observed a strong contraction of the pylorus and an antral inhibition following 1 U/kg CCK given by i.v. injection. The response was decidedly higher in patients with gastric or duodenal ulcer than in controls. As for cerulein, a constant relaxant effect on the stomach corpus, together with an increase in the tone of the gastroduodenal junction, was observed in healthy subjects (GROSSI et al. 1970; BORTOLOTTI et al. 1970; ORLANDINI et al. 1972). The early data have been confirmed by studies of gastric myoelectric and mechanical activity after administration of cerulein (0.5–12.5 ng kg^{-1} min^{-1} i.v.) and some gastrointestinal hormones. The peptide decreased both the motility index and the basal frequency of electric rhythm. The molar potency for inhibiting gastric motor activity decreased in the order: secretin > glucagon > cerulein > cholecystokinin (BORTOLOTTI et al. 1975). Conversely, a noticeable increase in antral peristalsis, similar to, but more pronounced than that elicited by serotonin and cholecystokinin, was observed following i.v. administration of cerulein (10–40 ng/kg) by X-ray examination (SZEKELI et al. 1975). Probably, different doses and different techniques are responsible for some of the aforementioned discrepancies.

1. Gastric Emptying

The early experiments in both dogs and humans showed that cholecystokinin inhibited gastric motor activity (JOHNSON et al. 1966; DINOSO et al. 1969). In these studies 10% pure CCK was given by bolus i.v. injection. However, subsequent studies showed that this activity seen with impure CCK preparations could not be ascribed solely to such contaminants as GIP or secretin. In fact it was demonstrated (CHEY et al. 1970; STERZ et al. 1974; DEBAS et al. 1975; YAMAGISHI and DEBAS 1978) that 20% pure CCK or the synthetic CCK OP, as well as endogenous CCK released by L-tryptophan administration, could dose-dependently inhibit gastric emptying in both dogs and humans. This action is probably a physiologic effect of CCK, since it was obtained with doses which were approximately the same as those necessary for the cholecystokinin and pancreozymin effects (3 U kg^{-1} h^{-1} for CCK and 125 ng kg^{-1} h^{-1} for CCK OP). Cerulein was also found to delay gastric emptying when given by i.v. infusion (3 ng kg^{-1} min^{-1}), intramuscularly (0.25–0.75 μg/kg), or even by nasal insufflation (1 μg/kg; ORLANDINI et al. 1972). This was confirmed quite recently by means of a labeled meal by SCARPIGNATO et al. (1980).

The mechanism through which CCK regulates gastric emptying in humans and dogs probably involves a drop in intragastric pressure due to relaxation of the

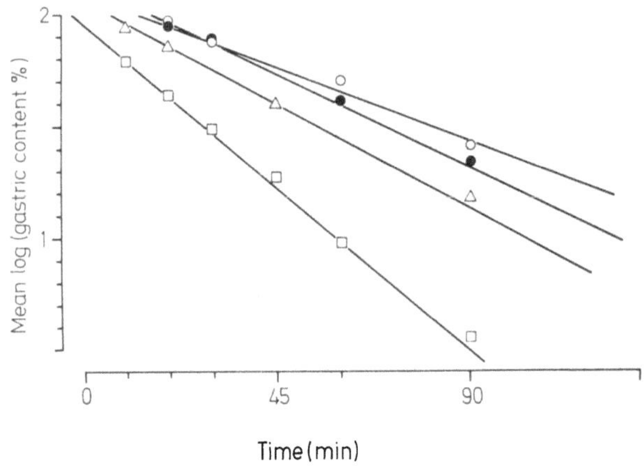

Fig. 2. Semilogarithmic plot of gastric content as a function of time. *Open circles* CCK; *solid circles*, cerulein 1 μg/kg; *triangles*, cerulein 0.25 μg/kg; *squares*, controls

proximal gastric wall plus other more distal mechanisms, since CCK was shown to delay gastric emptying even when intragastric pressure was kept constant by means of a barostat (STRUNZ and GROSSMAN 1978). Contraction of the pylorus, inhibition of motor activity in the first portion of the duodenum, and increased motility, starting from the distal duodenum may all be factors contributing to the delay in gastric emptying. The contraction of the pyloric sphincter was probably the most important factor in the dose-dependent delay in gastric emptying in the rat observed quite recently by C. SCARPIGNATO and G. BERTACCINI (unpublished work 1981) after intraperitoneal administration of cerulein (0.25–5 μg/kg) or the COOH terminal heptapeptide of CCK (1 μg/kg; Fig. 2). This effect was shown to be completely independent of gastric hypersecretion induced by cerulein (BERTACCINI et al. 1968) since it was completely unchanged by pretreatment with cimetidine in doses able to produce a complete block of gastric secretion (50 mg/kg; BERTACCINI and SCARPIGNATO 1981).

II. In Vitro Studies

CCK (0.1 U/ml) was found to contract both antral and body strips from human stomach. The effect was seen on the amplitude more than on the frequency of spontaneous contractions (CAMERON et al. 1967). Cerulein had a similar effect in very low threshold doses (1–5 ng/ml; BERTACCINI et al. 1971) and its effect was prevented by tetrodotoxin, indicating a nerve-mediated action (VIZI et al. 1973). Cerulein, which has been shown to be a rather weak stimulant of hamster and toad stomach (BERTACCINI et al. 1968), was shown to be a very potent stimulant of the isolated guinea pig stomach (DEL TACCA et al. 1972), the threshold concentration being between 2 and 5×10^{-10} g/ml. The effect was largely nerve mediated, as it was considerably decreased but not completely abolished by pretreatment with tetrodotoxin or atropine.

More detailed studies with 25% pure CCK (GERNER et al. 1975, 1976) showed that the peptide (0.02–0.75 U/ml) dose-dependently increased the basal pressure in the fundus, with variable effects on the rhythmic activity. In the antrum, it increased the amplitude of the rhythmic contractions, leaving their frequency and the basal pressure unaltered. Again in the isolated guinea pig stomach GERNER and HAFFNER (1977) and GERNER et al. (1979) found that antral activity stimulated by CCK (0.38 U/ml) was inhibited by atropine or tetrodotoxin, whereas the CCK-induced increase in fundus pressure was only slightly decreased by the two inhibitors. Mepyramine also inhibited CCK-induced contractions. These data were completely confirmed with synthetic CCK OP, which apparently is 3–6 times more potent than CCK (20% pure) (GERNER 1979).

After preexposure to gastrin, the antral dose–response curve to CCK was flattened, the lower maximal response suggesting that gastrin acted as a partial agonist with CCK (GERNER and HAFFNER 1978). CCK was also found to increase the frequency of the slow wave component and the amplitude of phasic contractions in the cat's stomach, apparently through a completely atropine-resistant direct effect on the smooth muscle (OHKAWA and WATANABE 1977).

A dose-related contractile effect of CCK OP (10^{-12}–10^{-9} *M*) on isolated smooth muscle cells from amphibian and guinea pig stomach was observed. Atropine, at concentrations (5×10^{-8} *M*) which completely abolished the contractile effect of acetylcholine (ACh), only partially inhibited the response to CCK OP, suggesting the possibility of separate receptor sites for the two substances. Some interaction between CCK OP and ACh was suggested, however, since a combination of the two compounds at doses less than the ED_{50} caused a marked potentiation in the guinea pig cells which was not seen when the two compounds were given at the maximal doses (BITAR et al. 1977, 1979). A remarkable effect on the isolated proventriculus and duodenum of the chicken was reported (ANGELUCCI et al. 1969). However, the mechanism of action was not investigated.

CCK and CCK OP caused dose-dependent (4.8×10^{-11}–3.5×10^{-9} *M*) increases in the amplitude and frequency of isometric tension in circular and longitudinal antral muscle of the dog. These effects were not blocked by tetrodotoxin and were decreased but not abolished by atropine. CCK OP was able to shift to the left the dose–response curve to gastrin but not to change the calculated maximal response. The reverse was also true, and gastrin had a similar effect on the dose–response curve of CCK OP (FARA et al. 1979). These findings indicate additive kinetics and support the hypothesis that CCK and gastrin share a common receptor site. However, CCK OP significantly increased adenyl cyclase activity in the antral muscle in concentrations as low as 10^{-13}–10^{-11} *M*, whereas gastrin was inactive even at 10^{-8} *M*. (BAUR et al. 1978).

A striking spasmogenic effect on isolated pylorus from the opossum was reported after administration of CCK (FISHER et al. 1973). The maximum response was obtained with concentrations of 10^{-10}–10^{-12} *M*. Secretin acted synergistically with CCK whereas gastrin I acted as a competitive antagonist of cholecystokinin.

CCK OP and the variant form CCK 39 were both more potent than CCK 33 in increasing the force and the frequency of spontaneous contractions of the dog antrum. They also increased the frequency and the amplitude of gastric action potential. All these effects were atropine-resistant (MORGAN et al. 1978).

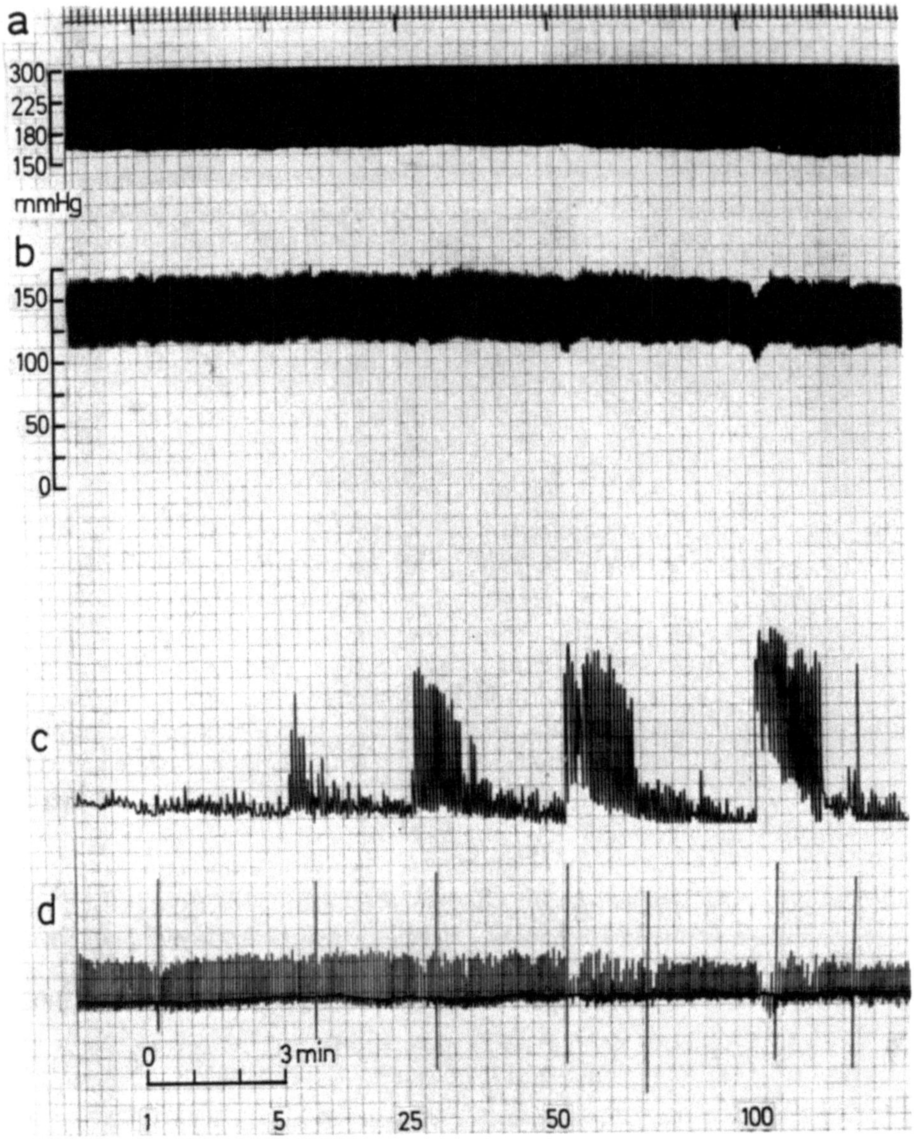

Fig. 3 a–d. Ileal motility in the dog. **a** tachogram; **b** arterial pressure; **c** intestinal motility; **d** pneumogram. Doses of cerulein in ng/kg i.v.

E. Effects on Small and Large Intestine

I. In Vivo Studies

1. Experimental Animals

Cholecystokinin and its analogs had a mixture of stimulatory and inhibitory effects on gut motility though the stimulatory effects were largely predominant. The early studies with very impure extracts of CCK (for review see JORPES and MUTT 1973)

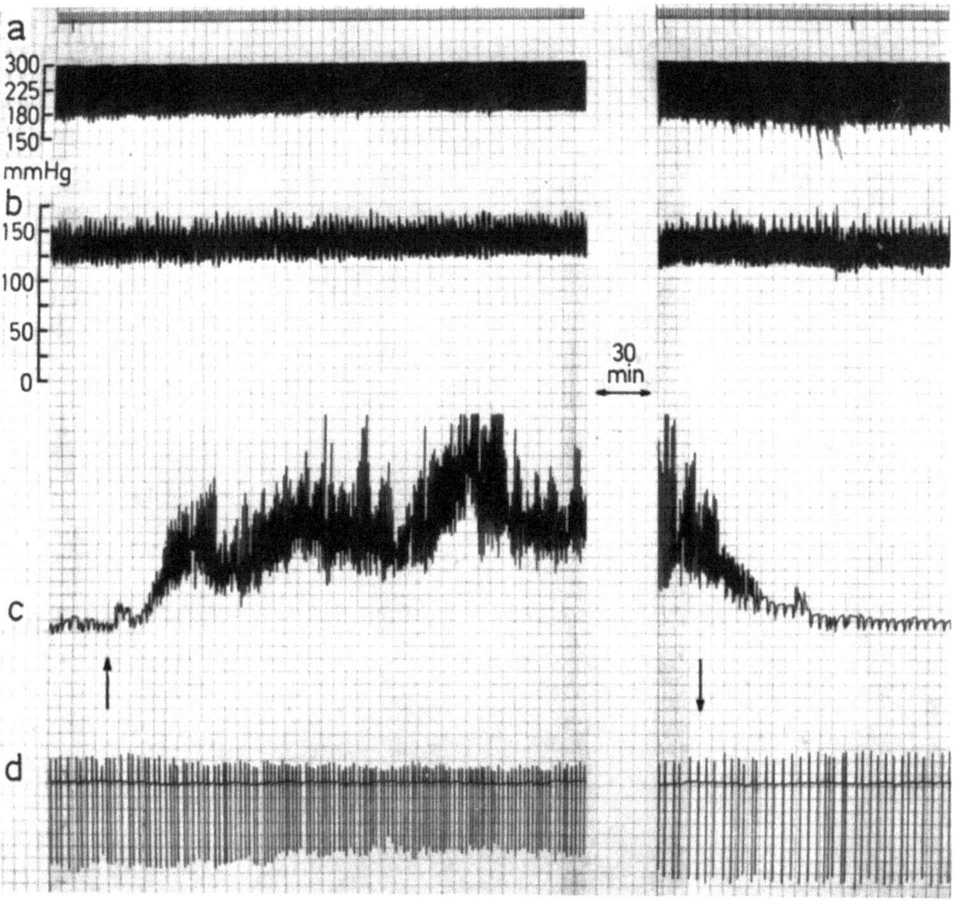

Fig. 4a–d. Ileal motility in the dog. The *upward arrow* indicates the start of the cerulein infusion (10 ng kg^{-1} min^{-1}); the *downward arrow* indicates the end of the infusion

were less reliable than those with pure synthetic cerulein, which were then followed by those with CCK OP or with highly purified CCK preparations. In the intact conscious dog, cerulein caused diarrhea after i.v. (0.1–0.5 µg/kg) or s.c. (1–4 µg/kg) administration. In the anesthetized dog, manometric recording of gut motility showed a dose-dependent stimulatory effect of the peptide after i.v. administration of between 1–5 and 100–500 ng/kg. The small intestine appeared to be more sensitive than the large intestine and the effect was partially atropine resistant (Figs. 3–5). The molar potency of cerulein exceeded by 3–1,000 times those of other spasmogenic peptide and nonpeptide compounds and could be detected with doses 0.2–0.5% of those needed to induce cardiovascular or respiratory changes (BERTACCINI et al. 1968, 1970; MANTOVANI and BERTACCINI 1971). Similar stimulatory activity with increase in amplitude of pressure waves was observed in the dog (DAHLGREN 1966, 1967; RAMIREZ and FARRAR 1970; NAKAYAMA 1973; STEWART and BASS 1976; G. BERTACCINI unpublished work 1981) after i.v. injection of CCK (0.1–1 U/kg) or CCK OP (50–500 ng/kg).

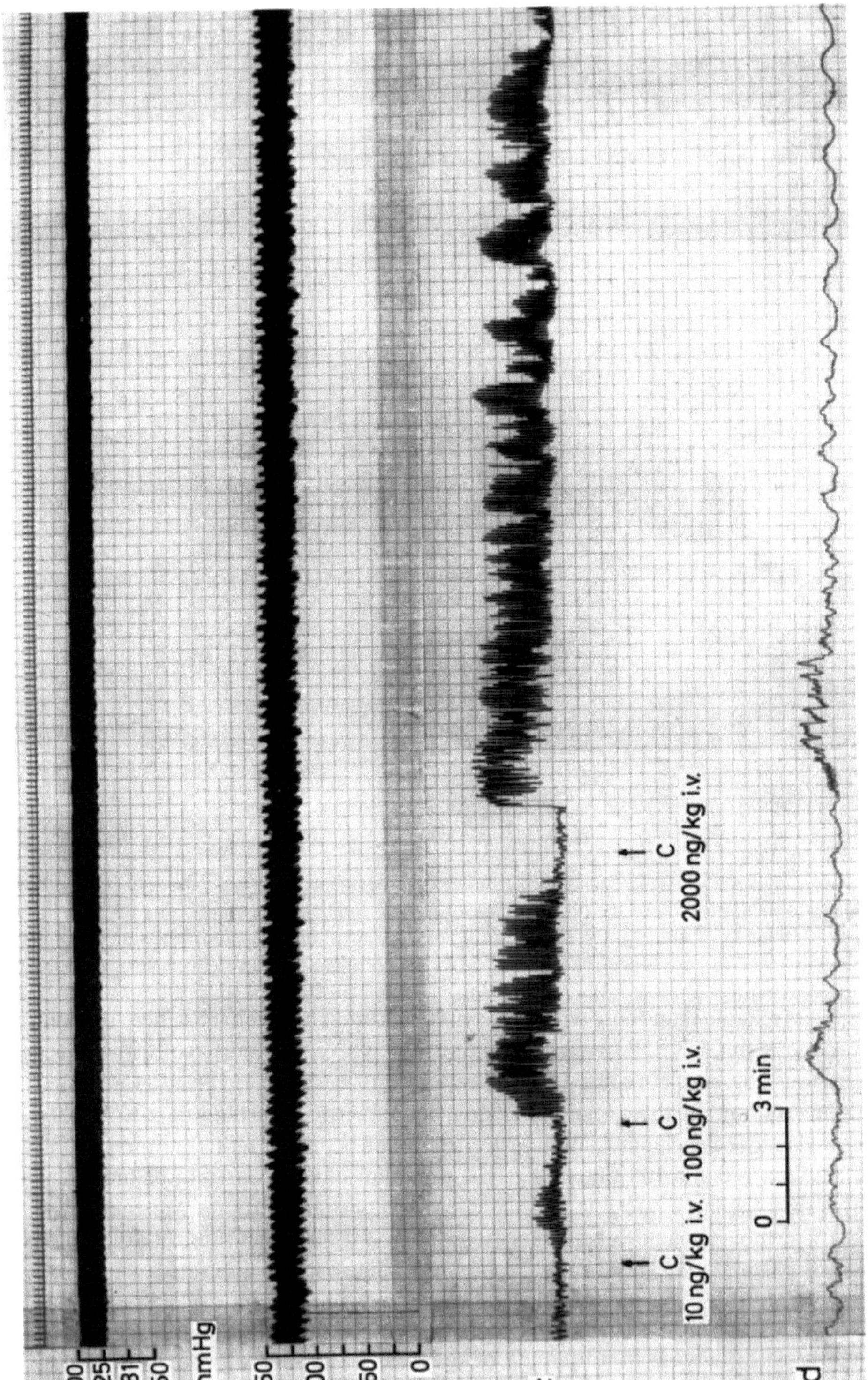
a
300
225
181
150
mmHg
b
150
100
50
0
c
d
C
10 ng/kg i.v.
C
100 ng/kg i.v.
C
2000 ng/kg i.v.
0
3 min

Duodenal and jejunal but not colonic motor activities were found to increase dose-dependently after i.v. injection of CCK (500–4,000 mU/kg; SCHUURKES and CHARBON 1978). CCK (1 Ivy dog unit/kg i.v.) was also able to promote peristalsis in dogs and in rabbits in which a mechanical ileus had been produced (DAHLGREN and THORÉN 1967).

As to changes on myoelectric activity, CCK OP (125–1,000 ng kg^{-1} h^{-1} i.v.) increased dose-dependently the number of slow waves with superimposed spike potentials in the small bowel of fasted dogs and hence stimulated small bowel contractions (MUKHOPADHYAY et al. 1977). Since the doses used were similar to those able to stimulate pancreatic secretion, the authors concluded that stimulation of bowel motility is a physiologic action of CCK. WINGATE et al. (1978) also found a significant relation between increasing spike activity in the dog jejunum and highly purified CCK dosage but in their experiments there was no relationship between CCK and spike activity in the duodenum or ileum. CCK (0.5–2 U kg^{-1} h^{-1}) diminished or abolished migrating complexes in the duodenum and jejunum but not in the ileum. CCK, whose action was similar in some respects to that of pentagastrin but different in others (CCK had no consistent effect on gastric or duodenal pacemakers), was considered to cause a "partial" disconnection of the intestinal smooth muscle from the extraenteric center. According to a recent study (PEARCE et al. 1978), CCK had no dose-dependent effect, but low doses (0.125 and 0.25 μg kg^{-1} h^{-1}) slowed the duodenal basic electrical rhythm (BER) in conscious dogs, exactly as did secretin. The above observations are consistent with the idea that the motor response to food is probably mediated by additional neural or humoral mediators besides CCK and gastrin.

Rabbits and cats were less sensitive than dogs (threshold stimulant dose for duodenal motility in the cat was 2 U CCK; LIEDBERG 1969). In the rabbit, threshold doses of cerulein were 10 ng/kg i.v. and 0.5 μg/kg s.c. (NAKAMURA et al. 1973). In the rabbit, both CCK (4–8 U/kg every 3 min) and cerulein (300 ng/kg every 3 min) were found to accelerate the movement of papillary region. Lower doses of CCK (0.5–2 U kg^{-1} h^{-1}) caused a depression in the same area. These effects were inhibited by secretin but not by atropine (KOBAYASHI et al. 1978).

In the cat, CCK relaxed the duodenum in the part surrounding the sphincter of Oddi but tended to contract more distal parts (PERSSON and EKMAN 1972). The stimulant action on cat jejunum was inhibited by pretreatment with atropine (2 mg/kg; HEDNER et al. 1967). Cerulein (0.3–1 μg/kg i.v.) increased motility in the guinea pig colon and greatly enhanced the response to pelvic nerve stimulation (DEL TACCA et al. 1970).

In a very accurate study in the rat (SCOTT and SUMMERS 1976), cerulein was shown to increase motility and to induce uniform distribution of contractions with time, in doses of 1 and 10 ng kg^{-1} min^{-1}. Larger doses (1 μg kg^{-1} min^{-1}) strongly inhibited contractions. The two smaller doses accelerated transit and the highest dose slowed it. The change in transit was specifically connected to the effect on contractions, since no significant change in water movement occurred. Accelera-

◀ **Fig. 5 a–d.** Tachogram **a**; arterial pressure **b**; ileal motility **c** and colonic motility **d** in the dog. *C*, Cerulein by intravenous (i.v.) or intramuscular (i.m.) injection

Table 2. Effect of cerulein on human gastrointestinal tract (radiologic technique)

Dose (ng/kg)	Route of administration	Subjects	Transit time[a] (min)	Range
0		35	280 ± 56	180–420
125	i.m.	6	170 ± 28	145–210
250	i.m.	8	115 ± 15	88–130
500	i.m.	8	36 ± 12	20– 55
750	i.m.	5	35 ± 9	20– 45
1 500	nasal	5	45 ± 14	25– 60
1 ng kg^{-1} min^{-1}	i.v.	5	120 ± 10	90–135

[a] From the stomach to the cecum; ± standard error

tion of intestinal transit was also observed in the mouse (NAKAMURA et al. 1973; PICCINELLI et al. 1973; HORN 1977) after intravenous, subcutaneous, or intraperitoneal administration of doses ranging between 0.1 and 50 µg/kg.

Finally, striking atropine-resistant villokinetic activity was shown after intravenous infusion of cerulein (0.2–2 ng kg^{-1} min^{-1}), which stimulated the pump-like movements of the duodenojejunal villi of chicken, pigeon, and cat (ANGELUCCI et al. 1972). Moreover, cerulein antagonized the glucagon-induced and PGE_1-induced depression of villous motility in the dog (IHÁSZ et al. 1976).

2. Humans

Studies performed in humans by several investigators, using manometric techniques or fluorography and cinematography or simultaneous recording of myoelectric and mechanical activity have largely confirmed the results obtained in animals. The early studies (MONOD 1964; MORIN et al. 1966) which showed an accelerated passage of X-ray contrast medium through the intestine under the influence of extracts containing CCK were confirmed by DAHLGREN (1967) who used a sample of pure cholecystokinin and proved that the peristalsis-promoting effect was elicited by the hormone itself and not by contaminating peptides. Another attempt was made by PARKER and BENEVENTANO (1970) to evaluate the utility of CCK (50–100 Ivy dog units) for accelerating and refining contrast studies of the small bowel. In the first portion of the duodenum, cerulein (1–5 ng $kg^{-1}min^{-1}$; BERTACCINI et al. 1971; BERTACCINI and AGOSTI 1971; LABÒ et al. 1972) and cholecystokinin (1 U kg^{-1} h^{-1}; ADLERCREUTZ et al. 1960; TORSOLI et al. 1961; ÖIGAARD et al. 1975; OSNES 1975; LABÒ and BORTOLOTTI 1976) both had an inhibitory effect on both the motility index (abolition of rhythmic contractions with no change in the tone) and the BER frequency. The inhibitory effect on the proximal duodenum resembles the relaxant effect of CCK and cerulein on the sphincters of Oddi of several species including humans and confirms the early observations of ALBOT and KAPANDJI (1958), who demonstrated similar behavior of the distal part of the bile tract and the duodenum. In any case, it is not unusual for a substance to act at the same time as a stimulant in some intestinal segments and a relaxant in others. Indeed, this has been shown to occur with pentagastrin, with 5-hydroxytryptamine, and even with some natural substance P analogs, such as physalemin (BERTACCINI et al. 1965; NISTICÒ and CALIFANO 1969).

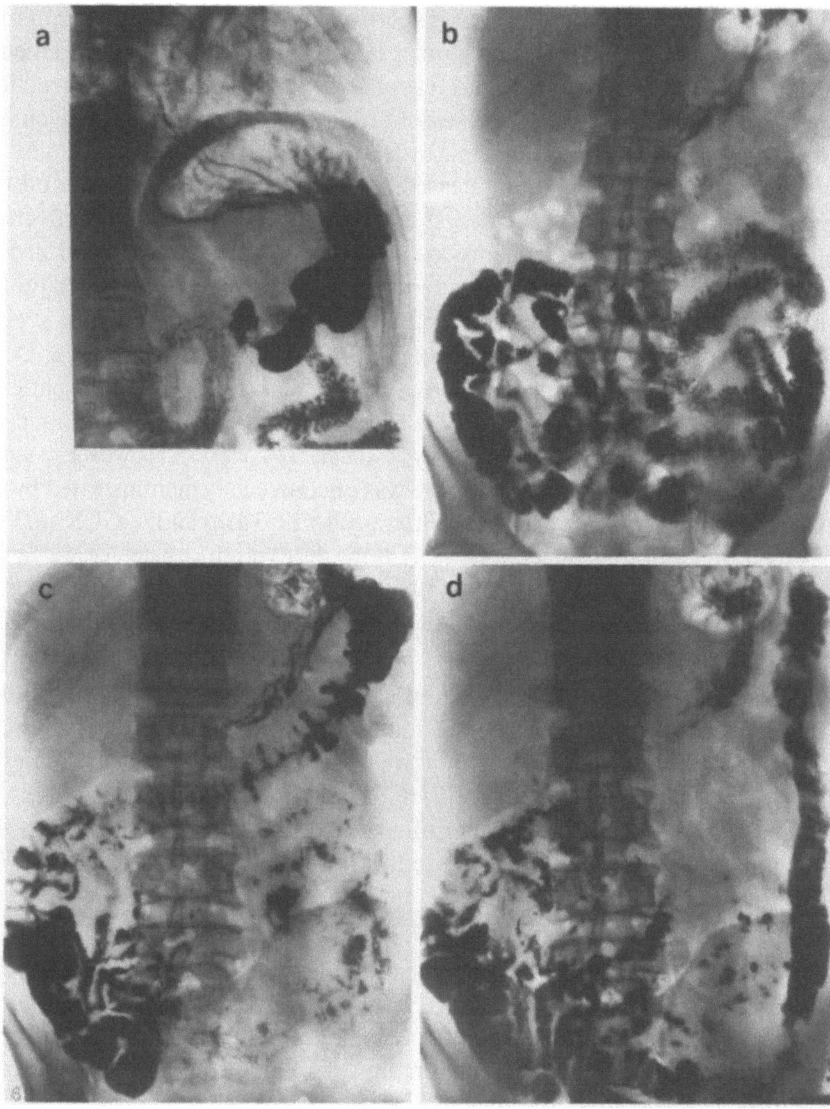

Fig. 6a–d. X-ray examination of the gastrointestinal tract. Basal radiogram; **a** 20, **b** 40, **c** and **d** 60 min after administration of cerulein (1 μg/kg i.m.)

From the distal portion of the duodenum down to the rectum, the effect of CCK and its analogs was always a stimulatory one (BERTACCINI and AGOSTI 1971; FLECKENSTEIN and ÖIGAARD 1977). The consequence was an increased propulsion in the gut and decreased transit time from the stomach to the cecum (Table 2). An example of the tremendous acceleration of transit that can be obtained in humans with cerulein is shown in Fig. 6. The decrease in mean transit time along the jejunum observed after CCK treatment was primarily related to hypermotility induced by the peptide, however, the increase in net water, sodium, and chloride secretion into the lumen observed in some experiments could also play a certain role (MATUCHANSKY et al. 1972). Recent studies (CORAZZIARI et al. 1976) in patients submitted to total gastrectomy and esophagojejunoduodenal reconstruction showed that cerulein induced dose-related motor activity in the transposed jejunal loops. Doses of cerulein were of the same order of magnitude (0.25 ng kg^{-1} min^{-1}) as the amounts of cholecystokinin released by a conventional fatty meal and for this reason the authors state that colecystokinin has a physiologic motor effect on the human jejunum; the same conclusions were drawn from studies performed in healthy subjects, who showed a marked increase in motor activity of distal duodenum, jejunum and sigmoid colon after intravenous infusion of CCK (1–4 U kg^{-1} h^{-1}; DINOSO et al. 1973; GUTIERREZ et al. 1974; ÖIGAARD et al. 1975; DOLLINGER et al. 1975). The stimulatory activity of CCK in the colon of 20 patients with irritable colon syndrome observed by HARVEY and READ (1973) was not confirmed in patients with the same disease by WALLER et al. (1973). However, a stimulant effect of cerulein on the human colon was unequivocally demonstrated by X-ray examination (RAMORINO et al. 1970; BERTACCINI 1973a, b) and of CCK (0.5 U/kg i.v.) with pressure transducer systems (CHOWDHURY and LORBER 1975). Quite recently also EBERHARDT and DYRSZKA (1980) found that patients with irritable colon syndrome and control subjects did not differ with regard to CCK-induced slow cycle pressure waves in the colon.

Apparently the response of the rectum was minimal or absent (CHOWDHURY and LORBER 1975). Cerulein (2 ng kg^{-1} min^{-1} every 30 min) was shown to enhance sigmoid motility in subjects with normal and prolonged total gastrointestinal transit times (POZZESSERE et al. 1979). CCK did not affect slow wave activity or frequency but increased the number of spike potentials in the rectum and the rectosigmoid, with a consequent increase in motor activity (SNAPE et al. 1977). CCK OP (20 ng kg^{-1} h^{-1}) also caused a maximum increase in spike activity and a significant increase in the motility index in the colon.

Atropine (1 mg bolus) did not significantly alter the spike potential activity stimulated by CCK OP (LONDON et al. 1980). Since atropine, ineffective against CCK OP, was found to inhibit the gastrocolonic response to eating, the authors suggested that CCK which is a direct stimulus of colonic contractions, yet plays no role in the gastrocolonic response.

It is likely that endogenous CCK plays an important role in the increased segmental motor activity of the colon observed after meals, at least through an interaction with other gastrointestinal peptides, the importance of gastrin being surely less, since the motor response to food was also observed in patients after antrectomy or total gastrectomy (HOLDSTOCK and MISIEWICZ 1970). In addition, intraduodenal administration of essential amino acids and sodium oleate was shown to increase significantly motor activity of the sigmoid colon of normal subjects in which pentagastrin (0.6 μg kg^{-1} h^{-1}) had no effect (MESHKINPOUR et al. 1974).

With roentgenographic techniques, an acceleration of peristalsis and a striking decrease in transit time in the small intestine of normal and pathologic subjects after administration of CCK (75 Ivy dog units i.v.), CCK OP (5–20 ng/kg i.v.) or cerulein (250–750 ng/kg i.m.; 1 ng kg^{-1} min^{-1} i.v.; 1,500 ng/kg nasal administration) could be shown (MORIN et al. 1966; RAMORINO et al. 1970; HEDNER and RORS-

Table 3. Therapeutic effect of cerulein in some pathologic conditions concerning gut motility

Syndrome	Patients Reference	Dose of cerulein and route of administration	No effect
Paralytic ileus	45 [1], [2], [3], [4]	0.75 μg/kg i.m. (× 1–4)	5
	55 [5]	0.75 μg/kg i.m.	5
	24 [6]	0.5 μg/kg i.m.	2
	20 [7]	0.5 μg/kg i.m.	1
	20 [8]	0.75 μg/kg i.m.	
	25 [9]	0.5–1.5 μg/kg (i.m. or i.v. infusion)	
	25 [10]	0.5 μg/kg i.m. (× 1–4)	7
	51 [11]	0.3 μg/kg i.m. or 1.25 ng $kg^{-1}min^{-1}$	4
	178 [12]	0.5 μg/kg i.m.	8
	16 [13]	0.25 μg kg^{-1} h^{-1} (× 2 h)	4
	[a] [14]	0.3 μg/kg i.m.	[a]
	40 [15]	[a]	[a]
	30 [21]	2 ng $kg^{-1}min^{-1}$ (× 45 min)	2
	10 [22]	0.3 μg/kg i.m. (× 2)	
	10 [22]	0.5 μg/kg i.m. (× 2)	
	3 [23]	1.2–25 ng kg^{-1} min^{-1} i.v.	
Chronic fecal stasis	54 [16]	3 ng kg^{-1} min^{-1} (× 6 h)	5
	30 [3]	0.75 μg/kg i.m. (× 1–2)	7
	6 [17]	2–4 ng kg^{-1} min^{-1} (× 20 min)	
Megacolon	14 [3], [4], [18]	3 ng kg^{-1} min^{-1} (× 30 min)	4
Hirschsprung's disease	1 [19]	0.5 μg/kg i.m. (1 per day)	
	2 [20]	0.25 μg/kg i.m. (1 per day)	

[a] Quantitative data were not reported

[1] Agosti et al. (1971); [2] Agosti et al. (1972); [3] Bertaccini (1973a); [4] G. Bertaccini (unpublished work 1980); [5] Bonomo et al. (1972); [6] Fumoto and Watanuki (1975); [7] Horn et al. (1976); [8] Aloisio et al. (1976); [9] Carpino and Di Negro (1976); [10] Pandolfo et al. (1978); [11] Uggeri and Santamaria (1977); [12] Haas and Rueff (1978); [13] Hartung and Waldmann (1978); [14] Horn et al. (1978); [15] Naveiro (1978); [16] E. Bonomo (unpublished work 1971); [17] Lanfranchi et al. (1973); [18] Bertaccini (1973a); [19] Kapila et al. (1975); [20] Bertaccini et al. (1971); [21] Montero et al. (1980); [22] Sommoggy et al. (1980); [23] Neidhardt et al. (1980)

man 1972; Levant et al. 1974; Bertaccini and Agosti 1971; Novak 1975; Rapela et al. 1976; Robbins et al. 1980; Sargent 1980; Sargent et al. 1980).

The use of small doses of cerulein (0.25 μg/kg i.m. or 1 ng kg^{-1} min^{-1}) was recommended by radiologists to obtain a faster transit time with an intact column of barium and a consequently excellent delineation of the distal small bowel (Orlandini et al. 1972; Bertaccini 1973; Lorber 1980). Of course, owing to the delay in gastric emptying induced by the peptide (Scarpignato et al. 1981), the radiologist should allow for sufficient filling of the upper jejunum before administration of cerulein.

When different doses were used, excellent dose–response curves were obtained. These data suggested that CCK or its analogs may be useful for treatment of paralytic ileus and other diseases connected with alterations in motility (see Table 3), as pointed out at recent international meetings (International Symposium on Gastrointestinal Hormones and Pathology of the Digestive System, Rome, June 1977;

2nd International Symposium on Gastrointestinal Hormones, Valdres, Norway, August–September 1978; XI Internationaler Kongress für Gastroenterologie, Hamburg, June 1980).

In human studies with CCK, CCK OP or cerulein the harmful side effects were always modest and short-lasting. They consisted of dry mouth, nausea, flushing, mild tachycardia, and sweating. The most common complaints, however, were abdominal pain, cramps, and, occasionally, vomiting or diarrhea. Of course these symptoms cannot be considered to be true side effects, since they are strictly connected with the stimulant effect of the peptides on the motility of the bowel. In any case, all the possible discomforts caused by the peptides lasted only a few minutes after single administrations; in the case of continuous infusions they disappeared as soon as the infusion was discontinued.

II. In Vitro Studies

The effects of CCK and its analogs were different, both quantitatively and qualitatively in the different areas of the gut. However, a predominantly stimulant effect was observed. As we have already said, the early data obtained with CCK extracts were not entirely reliable because of the presence of contaminating stimulatory and/or inhibitory substances in the very impure CCK preparations. Those carried out with synthetic cerulein on isolated bowel preparations from different species were rather disappointing, probably because the experimental conditions, in which cerulein was compared with the tremendously active kinins (both bradykinins and tachykinins), were not the best for cerulein (BERTACCINI et al. 1968). Subsequently, more accurate experiments revealed that the peptide was indeed a very good stimulant of the gastrointestinal tract in vitro too and this was also true for synthetic CCK OP.

Inhibition of motility following cerulein administration in the proximal part of the human duodenum with a complete disappearance of phasic movements, was noted but there was no effect on the tone. This inhibitory effect was followed by complete recovery after washing and was not affected by administration of tetrodotoxin and was thus considered to be myogenic in origin (BERTACCINI et al. 1971, 1979).

The duodenum from the opossum was employed by ANURAS and COOKE (1978), in an interesting investigation. They found CCK (5×10^{-9}– 5×10^{-7} *M*) and cerulein (10^{-9}–2×10^{-7} *M*) to stimulate phasic contractions of the circular, but not the longitudinal muscle layer, dose-dependently. This stimulatory activity was not blocked by tetrodotoxin, indicating direct muscle stimulation. The cat duodenum surrounding the sphincter of Oddi, but not the more distal portion, was relaxed by cholecystokinin (PERSSON and EKMAN 1972) whereas rabbit duodenum was contracted by cerulein. These different situations found their counterparts in the choledocoduodenal junction, which was relaxed in the cat but contracted in the rabbit, after either exposure to cerulein (SARLES et al. 1976) or Boots pancreozymin (0.01–0.2 U/ml; NAKAYAMA 1973). Duodena from rats, hamsters, dogs, and guinea pigs were found to contract in response to cerulein, the threshold stimulant doses varying between 0.1 and 1.5 μg/ml (BERTACCINI et al. 1979). CCK OP (0.1–0.5 ng/ml) and cholecystokinin (0.003 Ivy dog units/ml) were found to stimulate dose-dependently both the longitudinal and the circular muscle layers of the guinea pig ileum. The contractile effect was completely inhibited by atropine (0.08 μg/ml) and by tetrodotoxin (0.4 μg/ml; HEDNER and RORSMAN 1968; HEDNER 1970). Rabbit duodenum, jejunum, and colon were also strongly contracted by Boots pancreozymin (0.01–0.1 U/ml) and by cerulein (10^{-10}–10^{-8} g/ml; NAKAYAMA 1973, NAKAYAMA et al. 1972). Surprisingly, cat small intestine was inhibited by CCK (0.01–0.05 U/ml), as evidenced in both electrical and mechanical activity, which were remarkably inhibited, even in the presence of tetrodotoxin or atropine (OHKAWA and WATANABE 1977).

In vitro studies gave a classical demonstration that cerulein, in concentrations as low as 10^{-12} *M*, caused marked augmentation of the peristalsis of both the small and the large intestine of the guinea pig (FRIGO et al. 1971). It also caused a coordinated motor response in both muscle layers of the guinea pig and the rabbit ileum, with alternating contractions of the longitudinal and the circular muscle (LECCHINI and GONELLA 1973; VIZI et al. 1974). The remarkable activity on the circular muscle, which exceeded by far those of a number of spasmogenic peptides (G. BERTACCINI unpublished work 1981), was completely abolished by tetrodotoxin (LECCHINI et al. 1976). The striking effect of cerulein on the peristaltic reflex in the guinea pig ileum was recently confirmed by HOLZER and LEMBECK (1979), who found that the peptide (0.2 pmol/min) was able to initiate peristalsis when intraluminal pressure was not raised and to increase the efficiency of the peristaltic reflex under conditions of isometric longitudinal contraction. Moreover cerulein (2 pmol/min) was able to counteract the inhibition of peristalsis induced by FK 33-824 (a synthetic enkephalin). In the guinea pig ileum and colon, cerulein was shown to act predominantly by releasing acetylcholine from the myenteric plexus. Only a very small percentage of the contractile activity was due to a direct effect on the smooth muscle (DEL TACCA et al. 1970). Concentrations of cerulein and other CCK-like peptides as low as 5×10^{-8} *M* were able to increase the release of acetylcholine to two or three times above control levels.

Both exogenous and endogenous noradrenaline decreased the acetylcholine release and the contraction of the smooth muscle induced by CCK-like peptides, suggesting that the tonic activity of the sympathetic nervous system exerts a continuous control on the stimulating action of the peptides (VIZI et al. 1973). In the isolated guinea pig ileum, it was also shown that doses of CCK which were by themselves just at the threshold for motor stimulating effects were highly effective in increasing the frequency of peristaltic contractions evoked by distension of the segments (CHIJIKWA and DAVISON 1974). Acetylcholine did not elicit the same effect and it was thought that the lowering of the threshold of the peristaltic reflex is due to the action of CCK on the intramural cholinergic nerves.

That CCK OP acts via stimulation of myenteric plexus neurons was recently confirmed by DOCKRAY and HUTCHISON (1980). They showed that preparations of the guinea pig ileum longitudinal muscle without adherent plexuses failed to respond to CCK OP in concentrations up to 320 pmol/ml (in normal preparations the stimulatory effect of the peptide was present even with 1–2 pmol/ml). Innervated preparations treated with tetrodotoxin or incubated at 15 °C also failed to respond to CCK OP. Not only morphine (which blocks the release of acetylcholine) but also Met-enkephalin and Leu-enkephalin were shown to shift the dose–

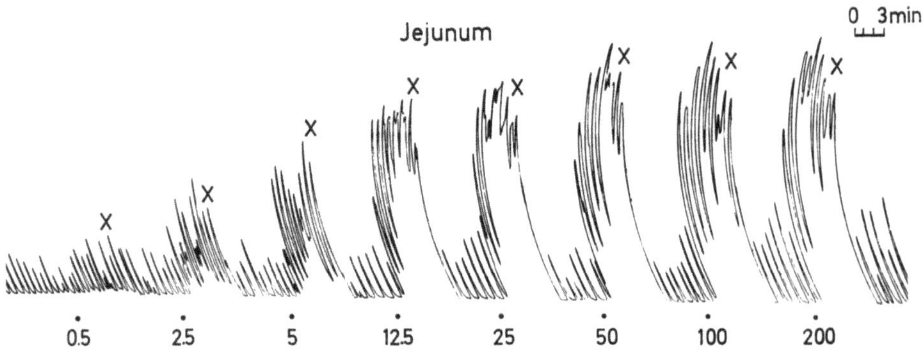

Fig. 7. Dose–response relationship of CCK OP on human isolated jejunum. Doses are in ng/ml

response curves of CCK OP and cerulein to the right in parallel fashion. Naloxone abolished the effect of enkephalins against CCK OP (ZETLER 1979a, b). Quite recently it has been shown (FONTAINE et al. 1978) that cerulein in low concentrations (4.7×10^{-10} *M*) which had no stimulatory effects, sensitized the guinea pig ileum to the effects of various cholinergic and noncholinergic agonists. In the presence of tetrodotoxin, higher concentrations (3.7×10^{-9} *M*) were inactive by themselves, but were able to potentiate the effects of different agonists, probably because of a nonspecific effect at the muscle level. According to very recent data (ZSÉLI et al. 1979), PGE_1 (2.8–28 n*M*) consistently and dose-dependently increased contractions evoked by CCK in the guinea pig ileum as well as those induced by endogenous or exogenous acetylcholine. On the contrary, indomethacine (2.7 μ*M*) decreased the contractions induced by both compounds, an effect which was reversed by PGE_1. The authors suggested that PGE_1 potentiates CCK-induced contractions by increasing the response to released ACh. The effect of indomethacine suggests that endogenous PGE_1 may modulate the effect of CCK and related peptides. In the isolated cat colon, CCK OP (exactly like gastrin) was found to exert different effects on the myoelectric activity according to the concentrations used. At 10^{-11} *M*, it increased spike activity with an increase in the percent of slow waves with spike potentials: at 10^{-9} and 10^{-8} *M*, it provoked slow wave uncoupling and abolished slow wave propagation (SNAPE and COHEN 1978, 1979). The increase in spike potential activity was not blocked by atropine (10^{-7} *M*), suggesting a direct effect of CCK on the smooth muscle (LONDON et al. 1980).

In human colonic circular muscle, CCK (10^{-12}–10^{-8} *M*) was found to be inactive (WEISS et al. 1976). This finding, which could be due to the experimental conditions, is in contrast with many observations made with cerulein in which it was found to stimulate human colonic muscle both in vitro and in vivo (RAMORINO et al. 1970; BERTACCINI et al. 1971, 1972; ORLANDINI et al. 1972). Cholecystokinin (Boots) and synthetic CCK OP were also found to stimulate human taenia coli, apparently through a direct effect on the smooth muscle (EGBERTS and JOHNSON 1977). In human isolated preparations, from the small and large intestine, the stimulatory effects of cerulein and CCK were found to be dose dependent (Figs. 7, 8) and strongly inhibited, but not completely prevented, by pretreatment with ei-

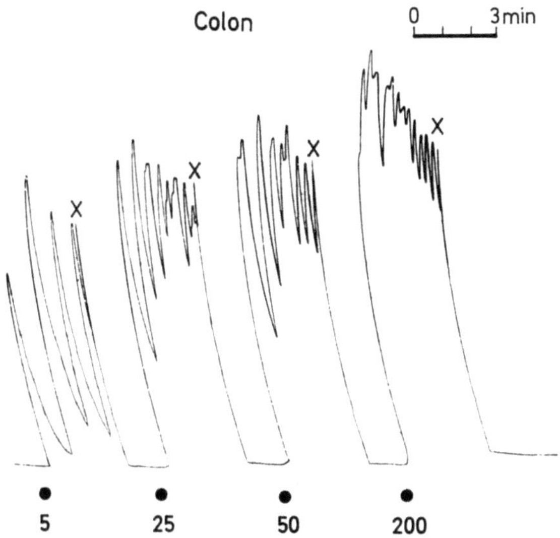

Fig. 8. Dose–response relationship of CCK OP in human isolated colon. Doses are in ng/ml

ther atropine or tetrodotoxin, suggesting that a small part of the effect of the peptide could be related to a direct action on the smooth muscle (BERTACCINI et al. 1971; DEL TACCA et al. 1974). The effects of CCK on colonic muscle are consistent with the idea that the hormone may be one of the substances involved in the gastrocolic responses. It is probable that CCK acts synergistically with nerve stimuli and/or other humoral agents.

The complex effects of CCK and its analogs on different in vitro and in vivo preparations from the gastrointestinal tracts of various species are shown schematically in Table 4. The data reported were mainly obtained with cerulein and CCK OP.

F. Conclusions

From a physiologic viewpoint, cholecystokinin (in its various molecular forms) is probably one of the most important hormones involved in the regulation of physiologic peristalsis. The fact that such minute amounts of CCK are sufficient to affect intestinal motility under all the possible in vivo and in vitro experimental conditions is consistent with the idea that its action in the gut is one of the physiologic actions of the peptide which, of course, may be important not only when acting by itself but also when interacting with other mediators. From a pharmacologic viewpoint, the results obtained with CCK OP and with cerulein suggest that these two peptides represent good alternatives to the intact CCK molecule. They have very similar activities both from a quantitative and a qualitative point of view, and they are pure, synthetic compounds and commercially available. In addition, they are useful tools for the study of gastrointestinal motility in vitro and in vivo, and they also have useful clinical applications in both diagnosis and therapy, especially

Table 4. Effects of CCK-like peptides on different segments of the gastrointestinal tract from experimental animals and humans

Target	Effect[a]	Species; technique	Mechanism of action[b]
Lower esophageal sphincter	–	Human; in vivo	NT
	∓	Opossum; in vivo	NT
	–	Cat; in vivo	M–D
	+	Opossum; in vitro	M–D
	+	Rat; in vitro	NT
Stomach (body and fundus)	–	Dog; in vivo	NT
	–	Human; in vivo	NT
	+ +	Human; in vitro	M*
	+	Hamster, toad; in vitro	NT
	+ +	Guinea pig; in vitro	M*
	+	Cat; in vitro	D
Stomach (antrum)	–	Human; in vivo	NT
	+ +	Human; in vitro	M*
	+ +	Dog; in vivo	NT
	+	Dog; in vitro	D
Pylorus	+ +	Rat; in vivo and in vitro	D
	+ +	Human; in vivo	NT
	+ +	Dog; in vivo	NT
	±	Cat; in vivo	NT
Duodenum	– –	Human; in vivo	NT
	– –	Human; in vitro	D
	–	Cat; in vivo and in vitro	NT
	+ +	Dog; in vivo	NT
	+	Dog, rat, hamster; in vitro	NT
	+	Rabbit; in vivo and in vitro	M
	+ +	Guinea pig; in vitro	NT
	+ +	Opossum; in vitro	D
	+	Chicken; in vitro and in vivo	NT
Small intestine	+ +	Human; in vivo	NT
	+ +	Human; in vitro	M*
	+ +	Dog; in vivo	M*
	+	Dog; in vitro	NT
	+ +	Guinea pig; in vitro	M*
	+ +	Rabbit; in vitro	M
	+	Rabbit; in vivo	M
	+	Mouse, rat; in vivo	NT
	+	Cat; in vivo	NT
	–	Cat; in vitro	D
Large intestine	+	Human; in vivo and in vitro	NT/D–M
	+	Dog; in vivo and in vitro	NT/M
	+ +	Cat; in vitro	NT
	+ +	Guinea pig; in vivo and in vitro	M*
	+	Rabbit; in vitro and in vivo	M
Villi	+	Pigeon, chicken, goose, cat; in vivo	D

[a] + or + + = moderate or strong stimulatory effect; – or – – = moderate or strong inhibitory effect
[b] D = direct activity; M or M* = totally or partially* nerve-mediated effect; NT = not tested

since the clinical studies performed so far have appeared to indicate that these peptides are relatively harmless. Leaving aside their usefulness for examination of the biliary system, first predicted by IVY in 1947, and of exocrine pancreatic function, their importance in the examination of the gastrointestinal tract and as therapeutic agents for the treatment of syndromes characterized by reduced motility seems to be well established, as a growing number of publications testifies clearly. From this point of view, cholecystokinin (like its analogs) surely represents, among the gastrointestinal hormones, a really very important "drug."

References

Adlercreutz E, Pettersson T, Adlercreutz H, Gribbe P, Wegelius C (1960) Effect of cholecystokinin on duodenal tonus and motility. Acta Med Scand 167:339–342

Agosti A, Bertaccini G, Paolucci R, Zanella E (1971) Cerulein treatment for paralytic ileus. Lancet 1:395

Agosti A, Paolucci R, Zanella E, Bertaccini G (1972) Preliminary studies on the effects of cerulein in paralytic ileus. Chir Gastroenterol 6:122–128

Albot G, Kapandji M (1958) Troubles fonctionnels synergiques biliaires et duodénaux. In: Vittel (ed) Congres international de la fonction biliaire. Masson, Paris, pp 255–277

Aloisio F, Giannoni MF, Montesani C, Pizzirani F (1976) Effetti del ceruletide nel trattamento dell'ileo paralitico postoperatorio. Chir Ital 28:846–853

Anastasi A, Erspamer V, Endean R (1967) Isolation and structure of caerulein an active decapeptide from the skin of *Hyla caerulea*. Experientia 23:699–700

Anastasi A, Bertaccini G, Cei JM, De Caro G, Erspamer V, Impicciatore M (1969) Structure and pharmacological actions of phyllocaerulein, a caerulein-like nonapeptide. Its occurrence in extracts of the skin of *Phyllomedusa sauvagei* and related Phyllomedusa species. Br J Pharmacol 37:198–206

Angelucci L, Baldieri M, Linari G (1969) Actions of caerulein on secretions and motility of the digestive tract in the chicken. In: Mantegazza P, Horton EW (eds) Prostaglandins, peptides, and amines. Academic Press, London, pp 147–156

Angelucci L, Micossi L, Cantalamessa F (1972) The action of caerulein on the motility of intestinal villi of avians. Arch Int Pharmacodyn Ther [Suppl] 196:89–91

Anuras S, Cooke R (1978) Effects of some gastrointestinal hormones on two muscle layers of duodenum. Am J Physiol 234:60–63

Baur S, Grant B, Spaulding RS (1978) Adenylate cyclase of antral muscle: hormonal and neural regulation. Gastroenterology 74:A1006

Behar J, Biancani P (1977) Effect of cholecystokinin-octapeptide on lower esophageal sphincter. Gastroenterology 73:57–61

Behar J, Biancani P, Zabinski MP (1979) Characterization of feline gastroduodenal junction by neural and hormonal stimulation. Am J Physiol 236:E45–E51

Bertaccini G (1972) Pharmacological actions of kinins occurring in amphibian skin. In: Pharmacology and the future of man. Proc 5th Int Congr Pharmacol, 5, San Francisco. Karger, Basel, pp 336–346

Bertaccini G (1973a) Pharmacology and clinical use of caerulein. In: Bory J, Mozsik G (eds) Symposium on gastrin and its antagonists: Akadémiai Kiadò, Budapest, pp 47–66

Bertaccini G (1973b) Action of caerulein on the motility of the biliary system and the gastrointestinal tract in man. Med Chir Dig 2:133–138

Bertaccini G, Agosti A (1971) Action of caerulein on intestinal motility in man. Gastroenterology 60:55–63

Bertaccini G, Impicciatore M (1975) Action of bombesin on the motility of the stomach. Naunyn Schmiedebergs Arch Pharmacol 289:149–156

Bertaccini G, Scarpignato C (1981) Effects of some cholecystokinin (CCK) – like peptides on gastric emptying of a liquid meal in the rat. Br J Pharmacol 72:103P–104P

Bertaccini G, Cei JM, Erspamer V (1965) Occurrence of physalaemin in extracts of the skin of *Physalaemus fuscumaculatus* and its pharmacological actions on extravascular smooth muscle. Br J Pharmacol 25:363–379
Bertaccini G, De Caro G, Endean R, Erspamer V, Impicciatore M (1968) The actions of caerulein on the smooth muscle of the gastrointestinal tract and the gall bladder. Br J Pharmacol 34:291–310
Bertaccini G, Mantovani P, Piccinin GL (1970) Activity ratio between intestinal and cardiovascular actions of caerulein and related substances in the anaesthetized dog. In: Sicuteri F, Rocha e Silva M, Back N (eds) Bradykinin and related kinins. Plenum, New York London, pp 213–220
Bertaccini G, Agosti A, Impicciatore M (1971) Caerulein and gastrointestinal motility in man. Rend Gastroenterol 3:23–27
Bertaccini G, Agosti A, Mantovani P, Impicciatore M, Romano A (1972) Azione della caeruleina sul tubo gastroenterico umano in vitro. Boll Soc Ital Biol Sper 48:322–325
Bertaccini G, Impicciatore M, De Caro G (1973) Action of caerulein and related substances on the pyloric sphincter of the anaesthetized rat. Eur J Pharmacol 22:320–324
Bertaccini G, Impicciatore M, De Caro G, Chiavarini M, Burani A (1974) Further observations on the spasmogenic activity of caerulein on the rat pylorus. Pharmacol Res Commun 6:23–34
Bertaccini G, Zappia L, Molina E (1979) "In vitro" duodenal muscle in the pharmacological study of natural compounds. Scand J Gastroenterol [Suppl 54] 14:25
Bitar KN, Zfass AM, Farrar JI, Makhlouf GM (1977) Isolated gastric muscle cells: demonstration of the direct myogenic effect of cholecystokinin. Gastroenterology 72:A1030
Bitar KN, Zfass AM, Makhlouf GM (1979) Isolated guinea pig gastric smooth muscle cells: interaction of acetylcholine (ACh) and the octapeptide of cholecystokinin (CCK-OP). Gastroenterology 76:A1100
Bonomo E, Calabi W, Fantoni A, Seveso M (1972) Risultati preliminari sull'impiego della caeruleina nel trattamento dell'ileo paralitico post-operatorio e della stasi fecale cronica. Ann Med 16:171
Bortolotti M, Miglioli M, Lanfranchi GA, Barbara L (1970) L'azione della caeruleine sull' attività elettrica e meccanica dello stomaco nell'uomo. Gastroenterologia 22:147–179
Bortolotti M, Sansone G, Sanavio C (1975) Effects of some gut hormones on gastric myoelectric and mechanical activity in man. Rend Gastroenterol 7:135
Cameron AJ, Phillips SF, Summerskill WHJ (1967) Effect of cholecystokinin on motility of human stomach and gallbladder muscle "in vitro." Clin Res 15:416–420
Carpino Boeri A, Di Negro G (1976) Studio dell'attività terapeutica del ceruletide nell'ileo paralitico conclamato. Atti Accad Med Lomb 31:1–5
Castresana M, Lee KY, Chey WY, Yajima H (1978) Effects of motilin and octapeptide of cholecystokinin on antral and duodenal myoelectric activity in the interdigestive state and during inhibition by secretin and gastric inhibitory polypeptide. Digestion 17:300–308
Chey WY, Hitanant S, Hendricks J, Lorber SH (1970) Effect of secretin and cholecystokinin on gastric emptying and gastric secretion in man. Gastroenterology 58:820–827
Chey WY, Yoshimori M, Hendricks J, Kimani S (1972) Effects of C-terminal octapeptide of cholecystokinin (CCK) on the motor activities of the antrum and pyloric sphincter in dogs. Gastroenterology 62:733
Chey WY, Gutierrez J, Yoshimori M, Hendricks J (1974) Gut hormones on gastrointestinal motor function. In: Chey WJ, Brooks FP (eds) Endocrinology of the gut. Slack, Thorofare, NJ; pp 194–211
Chijikwa JB, Davison JS (1974) The action of gastrin-like polypeptides in the peristaltic reflex in guinea-pig intestine. J Physiol (Lond) 238:68P–70P
Chowdhury AR, Lorber SH (1975) Effect of glucagon on cholecystokinin and prostigmin-induced motor activity of the distal colon and rectum in humans. Gastroenterology 68:875
Corazziari E, Tonelli F, Pozzessere C, Dani S, Anzini F, Torsoli A (1976) The effects of graded doses of caerulein on human jejunal motor activity. Rend Gastroenterol 8:190–193

Dahlgren S (1966) Cholecystokinin: pharmacology and clinical use. Acta Chir Scand [Suppl] 357:256–260

Dahlgren S (1967) The effect of cholecystokinin on duodenal motility. Acta Chir Scand 133:403–405

Dahlgren S, Thorén L (1967) Intestinal motility in low small bowel obstruction. Acta Chir Scand 133:417–421

Debas HT, Farooq O, Grossman MI (1975) Inhibition of gastric emptying is a physiological action of cholecystokinin. Gastroenterology 68:1211–1217

Del Tacca M, Soldani G, Crema A (1970) Experiments on the mechanism of action of caerulein at the level of the guinea-pig ileum and colon. Agents Actions 1:176–182

Del Tacca M, Pacini S, Amato G, Falaschi C, Crema A (1972) Action of caerulein on the isolated guinea pig stomach. Eur J Pharmacol 17:171–174

Del Tacca M, Soldani G, Crema A (1974) Effects of caerulein on the isolated human ileum. Rend Gastroenterol 6:165–167

Dent J, Dodds WJ, Hogan WJ, Arndorfer RC (1978a) Pressor effect of cholecystokinin-octapeptide on the opossum lower esophageal sphincter. Gastroenterology 74:A1025

Dent J, Dodds WJ, Hogan WJ, Arndorfer RC (1978b) CCK-OP: a useful agent for evaluating lower esophageal sphincter (LES) denervation in human. Gastroenterology 74:A1025

Desvigne C, Gelin ML, Vagne M, Roche M (1980) Effect of cholecystokinin and pentagastrin on motility and gastric secretion in the cat. Digestion 20:265–276

Dinoso V, Chey WY, Hendricks J, Lorber SH (1969) Intestinal mucosal hormones and motor function of the stomach in man. J Appl Physiol 26:326–329

Dinoso VP, Meshkinpour H, Lorber SH, Gutiérrez JG, Chey WY (1973) Motor responses of the sigmoid colon and rectum to exogenous cholecystokinin and secretin. Gastroenterology 65:438–444

Dockray GJ, Hutchison JB (1980) Cholecystokinin octapeptide in guinea-pig ileum myenteric plexus: localization and biological action. J Physiol (Lond) 300:28–29

Dockray GJ, Gregory RA, Tracy HJ (1980) Cholecystokinin octapeptide in dog vagus nerve: identification and accumulation on the cranial side of ligatures. J Physiol (Lond) 301:50P

Dollinger HC, Berz R, Raptis S, Von Uexküll TH, Goebell H (1975) Effects of secretin and cholecystokinin on motor activity of human jejunum. Digestion 12:9–16

Eberhardt G, Dyrszka H (1980) The effect of cholecystokinin (CCK) on symptoms and motility in the irritable colon syndrome. Abstr XIth Int Congr Gastroenterol. Thieme, Stuttgart p 191

Egberts E-H, Johnson AG (1977) The effect of cholecystokinin on human *taenia coli*. Digestion 15:217–222

Erspamer V (1970) Progress report: caerulein. Gut 11:79–87

Fara JW, Erde SM (1978) Comparison of in vivo and in vitro responses to sulfated and non-sulfated ceruletide. Eur J Pharmacol 47:359–363

Fara JW, Praissman M, Berkowitz M (1979) Interaction between gastrin, CCK, and secretin on canine antral smooth muscle in vitro. Am J Physiol 236:39–44

Faustini R, Beretta C, Cheli R, De Gresti A (1973) Some effects of caerulein on the motility of sheep forestomach and gall bladder. Pharmacol Res Commun 5:383–387

Faustini R, Ormas P, Galbiati A, Beretta C (1979) Tachykinins and forestomachs. 1st Congr Eur Assoc Vet Pharmacol and Toxicol (EAVPT), Utrecht 25–28 Sept

Fisher RS, Cohen S (1973) Phyloric sphincter dysfunction in patients with gastric ulcer. N Engl J Med 288:273–276

Fisher RS, Cohen S (1980) Effect of gut hormones on gastrointestinal sphincters. In: Jerzy Glass GB (ed) Gastrointestinal hormones. Raven, New York, pp 613–638

Fisher RS, Lipshutz W, Cohen S (1973) The hormonal regulation of pyloric sphincter function. J Clin Invest 52:1289–1296

Fisher RS, Di Marino AJ, Cohen S (1975) Mechanism of cholecystokinin inhibition of lower esophageal sphincter pressure. Am J Physiol 228:1469–1473

Fleckenstein P, Öigaard A (1977) Effects of cholecystokinin on the motility of the distal duodenum and the proximal jejunum in man. Scand J Gastroenterol 12:375–378

Fontaine J, Famaey JP, Seaman I, Reuse J (1978) Inhibition of caerulein and physalaemin-induced contractions of guinea-pig isolated ileum by non-steroidal antiinflammatory drugs and various steroids and their reversal by prostaglandin E_1. Prostaglandins Med 1:351–357
Frigo GM, Lecchini S, Falaschi C, Del Tacca M, Crema A (1971) On the ability of caerulein to increase propulsive activity in the isolated small and large intestine. Naunyn Schmiedebergs Arch Pharmakol Exp Pathol 268:44–58
Fumoto T, Watanuki T (1975) Effect of ceruletide on post-operative intestinal peristalsis. Farmaco [Prat] 30:579–584
Gerner T (1979) Pressure responses to OP-CCK compared to CCK-PZ in the antrum and fundus of isolated guinea-pig stomachs. Scand J Gastroenterol 14:73–77
Gerner T, Haffner JFW (1977) The influence of graded distension and carbachol on the motor response to cholecystokinin in isolated guinea pig antrum and fundus. Scand J Gastroenterol 12:745–757
Gerner T, Haffner JFW (1978) Interactions of cholecystokinin (CCK-PZ) and gastrin on motor activity of isolated guinea-pig antrum and fundus. Scand J Gastroenterol 13:789–794
Gerner T, Maehlumshagen P, Haffner JFW (1975) The effect of cholecystokinin on the in vitro motility of the guinea-pig stomach. Scand J Gastroenterol [Suppl 35] 10:48–50
Gerner T, Maehlumshagen P, Haffner JFW (1976) Pressure-responses to cholecystokinin in the fundus and antrum of isolated guinea-pig stomachs. Scand J Gastroenterol 11:823–827
Gerner T, Haffner JFW, Norstein J (1979) The effects of mepyramine and cimetidine on the motor responses to histamine, cholecystokinin, and gastrin in the fundus and antrum of isolated guinea-pig stomachs. Scand J Gastroenterol 14:65–72
Goyal RK, Rattan S (1978) Neurohumoral, hormonal, and drug receptors for the lower esophageal sphincter. Gastroenterology 74:598–619
Grossi F, Del Duca T, Spada S, Grassi M (1970) Influenze della caeruleina sulla motilità gastrointestinale nell'uomo. Clin Ter 54:321–327
Grossman MI (1970) Proposal: use the term cholecystokinin in place of cholecystokinin-pancreozymin. Gastroenterology 58:128
Gutiérrez JG, Chey WY, Dinoso VP (1974) Actions of cholecystokinin and secretin on the motor activity of the small intestine in man. Gastroenterology 67:35–41
Haas W, Rueff FL (1978) Caerulein in der Therapie der postoperativen Darmatonie und des Ileus. Therapiewoche 28:8939–8944
Harper AA, Raper HS (1943) Pancreozymin, a stimulant of the secretion of pancreatic enzymes in extracts of the small intestine. J Physiol (Lond) 102:115–125
Hartung H, Waldmann D (1978) Clinical experiences with ceruletide-continuous intravenous drip in the treatment of the paralytic ileus. Scand J Gastroenterol [Suppl 49] 13:81
Harvey RF, Read AE (1973) Effect of cholecystokinin on colonic motility and symptoms in patients with the irritable-bowel syndrome. Lancet 1:1–3
Hedner P (1970) Effect of the C-terminal octapeptide of cholecystokinin on guinea-pig ileum and gall-bladder *in vitro*. Acta Physiol Scand 78:232–235
Hedner P, Rorsman G (1968) Structure essential for the effect of cholecystokinin on the guinea pig small intestine. Acta Physiol Scand 74:58–68
Hedner P, Rorsman G (1972) Acceleration of the barium meal through the small intestine by the C-terminal octapeptide of cholecystokinin. Am J Roentgenol 116:245–248
Hedner P, Persson H, Rorsman G (1967) Effect of cholecystokinin on small intestine. Acta Physiol Scand 70:250–254
Holdstock DJ, Misiewicz JJ (1970) Factors controlling colonic motility: colonic pressures and transit after meals in patients with total gastrectomy, pernicious anemia or duodenal ulcer. Gut 11:100–110
Holzer P, Lembeck F (1979) Effect of neuropeptides on the efficiency of the peristaltic reflex. Naunyn Schmiedebergs Arch Pharmacol 307:257–264
Horn JM (1977) The effect of caerulein on the postoperative intestinal atony (Abstr). In: Speranza V, Basso N, Lezoche E (eds) Int symp gastrointestinal horm and pathol of the dig system, Rome, June 13–15. Arti Grafiche Tris, Rome, pp 69–70

Horn J, Merkle P, Hümpfner K (1976) Die Beeinflussung der postoperativen Darmatonie durch Caerulein. Chirurg 47:233–235

Horn J, Altunbay S, Herfarth C (1978) Ceruletide in the treatment of postoperative intestinal atonia. Scand J Gastroenterol [Suppl 49]13:91

Ihász M, Koiss I, Németh EP, Folly G, Papp M (1976) Action of caerulein, glucagon or prostaglandin E_1 on the motility of intestinal villi. Pfluegers Arch 364:301–304

Isenberg JI, Csendes A (1972) Effect of octapeptide of cholecystokinin on canine pyloric pressure. Am J Physiol 222:428–431

Ivy AC (1947) Motor disfunction of biliary tract. Am J Roentgenol 57:1–11

Ivy AC, Oldberg E (1928) A hormone mechanism for gall bladder contraction and evacuation. Am J Physiol 86:599–613

Johnson LP, Brown JC, Magee DF (1966) Effect of secretin and cholecystokinin-pancreozymin extracts on gastric motility in man. Gut 7:52–57

Jorpes JE, Mutt V (eds) (1973) Secretin, cholecystokinin, pancreozymin, and gastrin. In: Handbook of experimental pharmacology, vol XXXIV. Springer, Berlin Heidelberg New York

Jorpes E, Mutt V, Toczko K (1964) Further purification of cholecystokinin and pancreozymin. Acta Chem Scand 18:2408–2410

Kapila L, Haberkorn S, Nixon HH (1975) Chronic adynamic bowel simulating Hirschsprung's disease. J Pediatr Surg 10:885–892

Kobayashi K, Mitani E, Yamada H (1978) The effects of cholecystokinin caerulein and endogenous cholecystokinin on the movement of the papillary region. Jpn J Gastroenterol 75:481–491

Labò G, Bortolotti M (1976) Effect of gut hormones on myoelectric and manometric activity of the duodenum in man. Rend Gastroenterol 8:64

Labò G, Barbara L, Lanfranchi GA, Bortolotti M, Miglioli M (1972) Modification of the electrical activity of the human intestine after serotonin and caerulein. Dig Dis Sci 17:363–373

Lanfranchi GA, Bortolotti M, Miglioli M, Baldi F (1973) Azione della caeruleina sulla motilità del colon. Minerva Dietol Gastroenterol 19:78–86

Lecchini S, Gonella J (1973) Modification by caerulein of action potential activity in circular smooth muscle of isolated small intestine. J Pharm Pharmacol 25:261–262

Lecchini S, D'Angelo L, Tonini M, Perucca E, Gatti G, Teggia Droghi M (1976) Effects of some autonomic drugs on the electrical activity of intestinal circular muscle. Boll Soc Ital Biol Sper 52:1158–1161

Lee KY, Hendricks J, Chey WY (1974) Effects of gut hormones on motility of the antrum and duodenum in dogs. Gastroenterology 66:A729

Levant JA, Kun L, Jachna J, Sturdevant RAL, Isenberg JI (1974) The effects of graded doses of C-terminal octapeptide of cholecystokinin on small intestinal transit time in man. Am J Dig Dis 19:207–209

Liedberg G (1969) The effect of vagotomy on gall bladder and duodenal pressures during rest and stimulation with cholecystokinin. Acta Chir Scand 135:695–700

Lin TM (1972) Gastrointestinal actions of the C-terminal tripeptide of gastrin. Gastroenterology 63:922–923

London R, Cohen S, Snape W Jr (1980) The action and role of cholecystokinin on distal colonic function. Gastroenterology 78:1210

Lorber SH (1980) Small bowel transit time. Am J Roentgenol 135:648–649

Mantovani P, Bertaccini G (1971) Action of caerulein and related substances on gastro-intestinal motility of the anaesthetized dog. Arch Int Pharmacodyn Ther 193:362–371

Matuchansky C, Huet PM, Mary JY, Rambaud JC, Bernier JJ (1972) Effects of cholecystokinin and metoclopramide on jejunal movements of water and electrolytes and on transit time of luminal fluid in man. Eur J Clin Invest 2:169–175

Meshkinpour H, Dinoso VP, Lorber SH (1974) Effect of intraduodenal administration of essential amino acids and sodium oleate on motor activity of the sigmoid colon. Gastroenterology 66:373–377

Monod E (1964) Action entéro-kinétique de la cécékine. Arch Mal Appar Dig 53:607–608

Montecucchi P, Falconieri Erspamer G, Visser J (1977) Occurrence of Asn^2, Leu^5-cerulein in the skin of the African frog *Hylambates maculatus*. Experientia 33:1138–1139
Montero VF, Laganga AM, Garcia EA (1980) Usefulness of caerulein in the treatment of post-operative intestinal atony. J Intern Med Res 8:98–104
Morgan KG, Schmalz PF, GoVLW, Szerszewski JH (1978) Electrical and mechanical effects of molecular variants of CCK on antral smooth muscle. Am J Physiol 235:E324–E329
Morin G, Besançon F, Grall A, Jouve R, Garat JP, Debray C (1966) La cholécystokinine appliquée au radiodiagnostique de l'intestine grêle: nouvelle technique de radiocinématographie complète en quelques minutes, avec 62 observations. Entret Bichat Radiol 247–250
Mukhopadhyay AK, Thor PJ, Copeland EM, Johnson LR, Weisbrodt NW (1977) Effect of cholecystokinin on myoelectric activity of small bowel of the dog. Am J Physiol 232:E44–E47
Munk JF, Hoare M, Johnson AG (1978) Hormonal influence of pyloric diameter and antral motility in man. Gut 19:A435
Mutt V (1979) Chemistry of the cholecystokinins. In: Rehefeld JF, Amdrup E (eds) Gastrins and the vagus. Academic Press, London New York San Francisco, pp 57–71
Mutt V, Jorpes JE (1968) Structure of porcine cholecystokinin-pancreozymin. 1. Cleavage with thrombin and with trypsin. Eur J Biochem 6:156–162
Nakamura N, Koyama Y, Kojima T, Takahira H (1973) Effects of caerulein on intestinal tract and gall-bladder. Jpn J Pharmacol 23:107–120
Nakayama S (1973) The effects of secretin and cholecystokinin on the sphincter muscles. In: Fujita T (ed) Gastro-entero-pancreatic endocrine system – a cell-biological approach. Igaku Shoin, Tokyo, pp 145–154
Nakayama S, Neya T, Tsuchiya K, Takeda M, Yamasato T, Watanabe K (1972) Effects of caerulein on the movements of the gastrointestinal tract and the biliary system. Pharmacometrics 6:1163–1173
Naveiro MC (1978) Efectos de la ceruleina sobre la motilidad intestinal y el ileo paralítico (Abstr). In: 6th World Congr Gastroenterol, Madrid, June 5–9, p 200
Nebel OT, Castell DO (1973) Inhibition of the lower esophageal sphincter by fat; a mechanism for fatty food intolerance. Gut 14:270–274
Neidhardt B, Hartwich G, Schneider MU, König HI (1980) Ceruletid (caerulein) treatment in cytostatic atonic gut and paralytic ileus. Dtsch Med Wochenschr 105:1220–1221
Nisticò G, Califano G (1969) Inhibitory activity of physalaemin on rat oesophageal motility in vivo. Arch Int Pharmacodyn Ther 181:414–423
Novak D (1975) Beschleunigung der Dünndarmpassage mit Caerulein. Dtsch Med Wochenschr 100:2488–2491
Novak D (1977) Significance of caerulein in the roentgenology of small intestine. In: Speranza V, Basso N, Lezoche E (eds) Int Symp Gastrointestinal Horm and Pathol of the Dig System, Rome, June 13–15. Arti Grafiche Tris, Rome, p A66
Öigäard A, Dorph S, Christensen KC, Christiansen L (1975) The effect of cholecystokinin on electrical spike potentials and intraluminal pressure variations in the human small intestine. Scand J Gastroenterol 10:257–262
Ohkawa H, Watanabe M (1977) Effects of gastrointestinal hormones on the electrical and mechanical activities of the cat small intestine. Jpn J Physiol 27:71–79
Orlandini I, Impicciatore M, Bertaccini G (1972) Diagnostica radiologica dell'apparato digerente sotto controllo farmacologico. In: Abstracts of the 25th Congr S.I.R.M.N., Montecatini Terme. Soc Ital Radiol Med, Acquapendente, pp 1–101
Osnes M (1975) The effect of secretin and cholecystokinin on the duodenal motility in man. Scand J Gastroenterol [Suppl 35] 10:22–26
Pandolfo N, Bortolotti M, Nebiacolombo G, Sansone G, Mattioli F (1977) Action of caerulein on lower oesophageal sphincter pressure. In: Speranza V, Basso N, Lezoche E (eds) Symp Gastrointestinal Horm and Pathol of the Dig System. Rome, June 13–15. Arti Grafiche Tris, Rome
Pandolfo N, Mortola GP, Parodi E, Moresco L (1978) L'impiego della ceruleina nel trattamento dell'ileo paralitico post-operatorio. Riforma Med 93:149–152

Parker JG, Beneventano TC (1970) Acceleration of small bowel contrast study by cholecystokinin. Gastroenterology 58:679–684
Pearce EAN, Wingate DL, Wünsch E (1978) The effects of gastrointestinal hormones and feeding on the basic electric rhythm of the stomach and duodenum of the conscious dog. J Physiol (Lond) 276:41P–42P
Persson GGA, Ekman M (1972) Effect of morphine, cholecystokinin, and sympathomimetics on the sphincter of Oddi and intraluminal pressure in cat duodenum. Scand J Gastroenterol 7:345–351
Piccinelli D, Ricciotti F, Catalani A, Sale P (1973) The action of caerulein on gastro-intestinal propulsion in mice. Naunyn Schmiedebergs Arch Pharmakol Exp Pathol 279:75–82
Pozzessere C, Corazziari E, Dani S, Anzini F, Torsoli A (1979) Basal and caerulein stimulated motor activity of sigmoid colon in chronic constipation. Ital J Gastroenterol 11:107–109
Ramirez M, Farrar JT (1970) The effect of secretin and colecystokinin-pancreozymin on the intraluminal pressure of the jejunum in the unanesthetized dog. Am J Dig Dis 15:539–544
Ramorino ML, Ammaturo MV, Anzini F (1970) Effects of caerulein on small and large bowel motility in man. Rend Gastroenterol 2:172–175
Rapela RO, Gutstein D, Naveiro JJ, Morel J (1976) Acción de la ceruleina sobre la motilidad intestinal. Rev Argent Chir 30:14–16
Rehfeldt JF, Larsson LI (1979) The predominating molecular form of gastrin and cholecystokinin in the gut is a small peptide corresponding to their COOH-terminal tetrapeptide amide. Acta Physiol Scand 105:117–119
Resin H, Stern DH, Sturdevant RAL, Isenberg JI (1973) Effect of the C-terminal octapeptide of cholecystokinin on lower esophageal sphincter pressure in man. Gastroenterology 64:946–949
Robbins AH, Wetzner SM, Landy MD (1980) Ceruletide-assisted examination of the small bowel. Am J Roentgenol 134:343–347
Sargent EN (1980) Efficacy and tolerance study of ceruletide for roentgenography of the gastrointestinal tract (Abstr) XI th Int Congr Gastroenterol. Thieme, Stuttgart, p 376
Sargent EN, Halls JM, Colletti P, Wieler M (1980) Efficacy and tolerance of ceruletide in radiography of the small intestine. Radiology 136:57–60
Sarles JC, Bidart JM, Devaux MA, Echinard C, Castagnini A (1976) Action of cholecystokinin and caerulein on the rabbit sphincter of Oddi. Digestion 14:415–423
Scarpignato C, Zimbaro G, Vitulo F, Bertaccini G (1980) Caerulein delays gastric emptying of solids in man. Arch Int Pharmacodyn Ther 249:98–105
Schang JC, Kelly KA (1980) Inhibition of canine interdigestive proximal gastric motility by cholecystokinin-octapeptide (CCK-OP). Gastroenterology 78:1253
Schuurkes JAJ, Charbon GA (1978) Motility and hemodynamics of the canine gastrointestinal tract. Stimulation by pentagastrin, cholecystokinin, and vasopressin. Arch Int Pharmacodyn Ther 236:214–227
Scott LD, Summers RW (1976) Correlation of contractions and transit in rat small intestine. Am J Physiol 230:132–137
Sommoggy St v, Theisinger W, Fraunhofer B (1980) Medikamentöse Beeinflussung der postoperativen Darmatonie (Abstr). XI th Int Congr Gastroent, Hamburg, June 8–13. Thieme, Stuttgart, pH 5.8
Snape WJ Jr, Cohen S (1978) Stimulation of the isolated cat colon with gastrin or octapeptide of cholecystokinin. Scand J Gastroenterol [Suppl 49] 13:169
Snape WJ, Cohen S (1976) Effect of bethanechol, gastrin I or cholecystokinin on myoelectrical activity. Am J Physiol 236:E458–E463
Snape WJ Jr, Carlson GM, Cohen S (1977) Human colonic myoelectric activity in response to prostigmin and the gastrointestinal hormones. Am J Dig Dis 22:881–887
Sterz P, Guth P, Sturdevant R (1974) Gastric emptying in man: delay by octapeptide of cholecystokinin and L-tryptophan. Clin Res 22:A174
Stewart JJ, Bass P (1976) Effect of intravenous C-terminal octapeptide of cholecystokinin and intraduodenal ricinoleic acid on contractile activity of the dog intestine. Proc Soc Exp Biol Med 152:213–217

Strunz UT, Grossman MI (1978) Effect of intragastric pressure on gastric emptying and secretion. Am J Physiol 235:E552–E555
Sturdevant RAL, Kun T (1974) Interaction of pentagastrin and the octapeptide of cholecystokinin on the human lower oesophageal sphincter. Gut 15:700–702
Szekely A, Major T, Romvari H (1975) Röntgenkymographische Untersuchung der die Magenperistaltik steigernden Wirkung von intravenös gegebenem Caerulein. Fortschr Roentgenstr 122:167–169
Thoren L (1967) Intestinal motility in low small bowel obstruction. Acta Chir Scand 133:417–421
Torsoli A, Ramorino ML, Colagrande C, Demaio G (1961) Experiments with cholecystokinin. Acta Radiol (Stockh) 55:193–206
Uggeri F, Santamaria A (1977) Ceruletide and intestinal atony: preliminary results. In: Speranza V, Basso N, Lezoche E (eds) Int Symp Gastrointestinal Horm and Pathol of the Dig System, Rome, June 13–15. Arti Grafiche Tris, Rome, p A176
Valenzuela JE, Grossman MI (1975) Effect of pentagastrin and caerulein on intragastric pressure in the dog. Gastroenterology 69:1383–1384
Vizi SE, Bertaccini G, Impicciatore M, Knoll J (1973) Evidence that acetylcholine released by gastrin and related polypeptides contributes to their effect on gastrointestinal motility. Gastroenterology 64:268–277
Vizi ES, Bertaccini G, Impicciatore M, Mantovani P, Zsèli J, Knoll J (1974) Structure-activity relationship of some analogues of gastrin and cholecystokinin on intestinal smooth muscle of the guinea-pig. Naunyn Schmiedebergs Arch Pharmakol Exp Pathol 284:233–243
Waller SL, Carvalhinhos A, Misiewicz JJ, Russell RI (1973) Effect of cholecystokinin on colonic motility. Lancet 1:264
Weiss SM, Hughes SR, Paskin DL, Lipshutz WH (1976) Effects of drugs and hormones on human colon muscle. Clin Res 24:A293
Wilson RC (1975) Mechanism of secretin inhibition of rumen motility. Dissertation Abstr Int B35 4081
Wingate DL, Pearce EA, Hutton M, Dand A, Thompson HH, Wünsch E (1978) Quantitative comparison of the effects of cholecystokinin, secretin, and pentagastrin on gastrointestinal myoelectric activity in the conscious fasted dog. Gut 19:593–601
Yamagishi T, Debas HT (1978) Cholecystokinin inhibits gastric emptying by acting on both proximal stomach and pylorus. Am J Physiol 234:E375–E378
Zetler G (1979a) Enkephalins as antagonists of cholecystokinin-like peptides. Naunyn Schmiedebergs Arch Pharmakol Exp Pathol [Suppl] 307:R51
Zetler G (1979b) Antagonism of cholecystokinin-like peptides by opioid peptides, morphine or tetrodotoxin. Eur J Pharmacol 60:67–77
Zséli J, Török TL, Vizi ES, Knoll J (1979) Effect of prostaglandin E_1 and indomethacin on responses of longitudinal muscle of guinea-pig ileum to cholecystokinin. Eur J Pharmacol 56:139–144

Secretin

A. Introduction

Secretin was discovered in 1902 by BAYLISS and STARLING and is the first member of the big family of gastrointestinal hormones. It was also the first polypeptide to be called a hormone. Although the importance of this discovery was soon recognized, six decades elapsed before JORPES and MUTT (1961) were able to purify and subsequently identify the amino acid sequence of secretin. The peptide was then synthesized by BODANSZKY et al. (1966). Secretin is composed of 27 amino acid res-

Table 1. The secretin family[a]

GIP	Glucagon	Secretin	VIP
(43)[b]	(29)	(27)	(28)
Tyr	His	–	–
Ala	Ser	–	–
Glu	Gln	Asp	–
Gly	–	–	Ala
Thr	–	–	Val
Phe	–	–	–
Ile	Thr	–	–
Ser	–	–	Asp
Asp	–	Glu	Asn
Tyr	–	Leu	Tyr
Ser	–	–	Thr
Ile	Lys	Arg	–
Ala	Tyr	Leu	–
Met	Leu	Arg	–
Asp	–	–	Lys
Lys	Ser	–	Gln
Ile	Arg	Ala	Met
Arg	–	–	Ala
Gln	Ala	Leu	Val
Gln	–	–	Lys
Asp	–	Arg	Lys
Phe	–	Leu	Tyr
Val	–	Leu	–
Asn	Gln	–	Asn
Trp	–	Gly	Ser
Leu	–	–	Ile
Leu	Met	Val–NH_2	Leu
Ala	Asp		Asn–NH_2
Gln	Thr		
Gln			
Lys			
Gly			
Lys			
Lys			
Ser			
Asp			
Trp			
Lys			
His			
Asn			
Ile			
Thr			
Gln			

[a] The dashes (–) indicate the same amino acid residue as that in the column to the left

[b] Figures in parentheses indicate the number of residues in each peptide

idues (molecular weight 3,055 daltons), 14 of which are in the same positions as in porcine glucagon. The structure of secretin and those of the other members of the secretin family are shown in Table 1.

The amino acids between position 5 and position 13 form a helix (BODANSZKY et al. 1969) and it has been suggested that the intact secretin molecule is necessary for complete biologic activity (GROSSMAN 1969). A certain degree of stimulation of pancreatic secretion observed with COOH terminal fragments of the secretin molecule (23, 21, 19, 15, 13, and 6 amino acid fragments) has, in fact, been attributed not to the intrinsic activity of the fragments but to their competition with secretin and the displacement of tightly bound secretin from acceptor sites on pancreatic cells (BITAR et al. 1977). In contrast, it was recently found (KÖNIG et al. 1979) that NH_2 terminal fragments may have a little intrinsic activity: secretin-(1-14), S-(1-15)-NH_2, and S-(1-21)NH_2 exerted slight activity on pancreatic secretion. Some inhibition of duodenal motility has also been observed with analogs of native secretin: (DSer^2)-S had weak activity, whereas (DAla^4 Val^5)-S, (Glu^3)-S, and (DAla^4)-S seemed to be more active, but precise quantitative data were not reported.

B. Action on the Lower Esophageal Sphincter

Secretin, administered intravenously (1–2.3 U kg^{-1} h^{-1}) or released endogenously after duodenal acidification, was shown to be ineffective in changing resting lower esophageal sphincter (LES) pressure in humans (COHEN and LIPSHUTZ 1971). Only larger "pharmacologic" doses were reported to decrease resting LES pressure (LIPSHUTZ 1976; ITOH et al. 1978). In contrast, the peptide (0.65 U kg^{-1} h^{-1}) did inhibit the LES pressure response to an intravenous bolus injection of gastrin I significantly and shifted the gastrin dose–response curve to higher doses, while the maximal sphincter response was still attained. The selective competitive antagonism with secretin and the low doses required to decrease the effect of gastrin appear to suggest that secretin is one of the factors interacting with gastrin in the physiologic regulation of human LES competence.

No interaction between the effects of glucagon (which is another strong inhibitor of the action of gastrin on the LES) and secretin, on pentagastrin-stimulated LES has been found (CHRISTIANSEN and BORGESKOV 1974).

In the dog, secretin had little effect on LES contractile activity during the interdigestive state and slightly decreased the contractile force of the LES during the digestive state but only when given in large doses. The peptide did not influence motilin-induced contractions (ITOH et al. 1978). In the conscious baboon, secretin was very weak in modifying resting LES pressure and antagonized the LES pressure response to pentagastrin only when very high doses (512 μg kg^{-1} h^{-1}) were employed (BROWN et al. 1978). In these experiments, secretin appeared to be twice as active as glucagon. The potency ratio of VIP to secretin was 16:1 for reduction of basal LES pressure by 50%, but was 32:1 for inhibition of pentagastrin-stimulated LES pressure (SIEGEL et al. 1979). In the anesthetized cat, secretin was shown to have a weak relaxant effect with LES pressure falling only by 25% (doses of 4–8 U/kg i.v. had to be employed). Secretin appeared to inhibit LES muscle by direct action since its effect was not antagonized by the common antagonists and tetrodotoxin (BEHAR et al. 1979). In the isolated LES from the opossum, secretin was virtually ineffective when given alone but was able to inhibit the contractions induced by gastrin I competitively, even in very low doses (3×10^{-19} M; LIPSHUTZ and COHEN 1972).

C. In Vivo Effects on the Stomach

Secretin is endowed with a remarkable inhibitory effect on the gastric fundus and especially on the antrum. In the dog, both the amplitude and the frequency of the spontaneous contractions have been shown to be inhibited by natural or synthetic secretin (VAGNE et al. 1968; SUGAWARA et al. 1969; CHEY et al. 1969; CHVASTA and COOKE 1973). The motor inhibition, which was also observed in denervated pouches, was dose dependent (0.5–4 U/kg) (VALENZUELA 1976), had an immediate onset and lasted 5–20 min. Food-induced motor activity has also been found to be inhibited by secretin (WALKER et al. 1972), as is motility stimulated by balloon distension or by administration of gastrin or CCK OP (CHEY et al. 1974). The antral action potentials, the electrical correlate of smooth muscle contractions, were found to diminish after secretin administration to dogs (0.1 U kg^{-1} min^{-1}) or humans (0.5–6 U kg^{-1} h^{-1}; KELLY et al. 1969; KWONG et al. 1972; BORTOLOTTI et al. 1975). When the infusion was discontinued, recovery was obtained within 3–5 min. In the isolated canine stomach perfused ex vivo, only high doses of secretin (16–32 U) were able to inhibit the electrical response activity to vagal stimulation. They also produced a decrease in mechanical activity in the antrum and antagonized the stimulant effect of pentagastrin (KOWALEWSKI and KOLODEJ 1977).

In the rat, secretin (0.1–0.5 U/kg) has been shown (BERTACCINI et al. 1973) to have a remarkable spasmogenic effect on the pyloric sphincter. The response was of the all-or-nothing type, so that no dose–response curve could be demonstrated (Fig. 1). This effect might be a physiologic action protecting against possible regurgitation into the stomach of alkaline pancreatic juice stimulated by secretin.

Secretin (3.4 U/kg i.v.) was also able to decrease the amplitude and frequency of rumen contraction in the sheep. This effect was accompanied by increased intracellular levels of cyclic AMP (WILSON 1975). Secretin (1 U/kg) was found to inhibit gastric motility in humans also, both under basal conditions and after administration of cholinomimetic agents (JOHNSON et al. 1966; CHEY et al. 1967, 1974; DINOSO et al. 1969), and again in humans, secretin (2–3 U kg^{-1} h^{-1}) was shown to contract the pyloric sphincter (PHAOSAWASDI et al. to be published). However, the serum concentration of secretin necessary to stimulate the pylorus (1 U kg^{-1} h^{-1}) far exceeds that found after duodenal acidification (FISHER et al. 1973; FISHER and COHEN 1980). Maximum pyloric contraction was obtained in normal subjects with a combination of secretin (1 U kg^{-1} h^{-1}) plus CCK (2 U kg^{-1} h^{-1}); this combination, however, was found to be ineffective in gastric ulcer patients (FISHER and COHEN 1973).

D. Gastric Emptying

As a consequence of the inhibitory activity in the stomach combined with the possible stimulation of the pyloric sphincter, the obvious effect of secretin was to lower

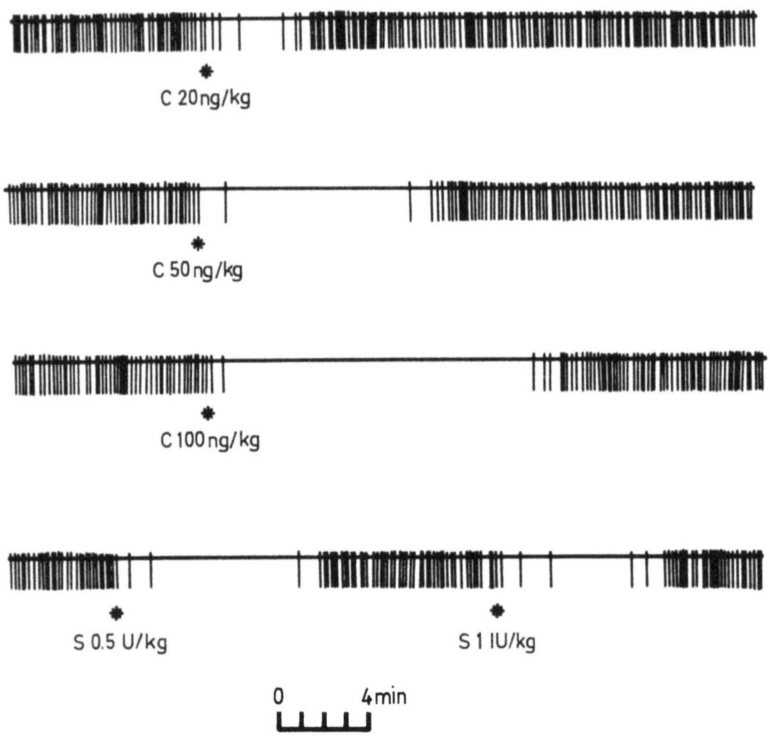

Fig. 1. Gastric emptying in the anesthetized rat. Each stroke of the drop counter represents one drop of duodenal effluent during continuous infusion of physiologic saline through the esophagus. *C*, COOH terminal octapeptide of CCK; *S*, secretin. *Asterisks* indicate injections. Note the good dose–response relation with CCK OP and the lack of correlation with secretin. (G. BERTACCINI unpublished work 1980)

the rate of gastric emptying in the rat (0.1–0.5 U/kg; G. BERTACCINI unpublished work 1980), in the dog (4 and 8 U kg^{-1} h^{-1}; CHVASTA and COOKE 1973) and in humans (1 U/kg; DINOSO et al. 1969; VAGNE and ANDRE 1971; CHEY et al. 1970; MEVES et al. 1975.

The doses needed to delay gastric emptying were usually larger than those required for inhibition of gastric acid secretion, but in some experiments were similar to those that induced pancreatic HCO_3^- secretion (VALENZUELA 1976). However, if we accept that in humans, the postprandial secretin blood levels correspond to an exogenous hormone dose of approximately 0.03 U kg^{-1} h^{-1} (STRUNZ 1979), it is evident that all the studies on gastric motility have been performed with doses which far exceed this physiologic dose and may be considered as truly pharmacologic doses.

E. In Vitro Effects on the Stomach

One of the early in vitro studies of the human stomach is that of CAMERON et al. (1970), who observed that secretin (both natural and synthetic) caused a decrease in amplitude of rhythmic contractions in both antral and body strips, as well as a true relaxation, as shown by an increase in resting strip length between contractions. However, no attempt was made to obtain a dose–response curve and only one dose (1 U/ml) was used in that study.

In one of the most recent in vitro studies, the interaction of secretin with gastrin and CCK on canine antrum was investigated. Secretin, which was found to be inactive by itself (2.5×10^{-8} *M*), was shown to shift to the right the dose–response curve to gastrin, and also to decrease the calculated maximal response but not to change the ED_{50}. Secretin had a similar effect on the responses to CCK OP (FARA et al. 1979). Therefore, secretin inhibits gastrin and CCK in a noncompetitive way and it does not affect the affinity of these peptides for their receptors.

In the isolated guinea pig stomach, secretin by itself was usually ineffective and only occasionally produced a slight transient decrease in basal tension. In the antrum, but not in the fundus, the hormone (13×10^{-8} *M*) markedly inhibited the motor response to CCK noncompetitively, whereas it was ineffective against acetylcholine-induced contractions (GERNER and HAFFNER 1978).

Surprisingly, unlike its effect in other stomach preparations, secretin (0.05–0.25 U/ml) apparently increased the frequency of the slow wave component and the amplitude of phasic contraction in the cat stomach. This effect, which was atropine resistant and tetrodotoxin resistant, was blocked only by verapamil and potentiated by imidazole, suggesting that cyclic AMP plays a role in the antral region stimulated by secretin (OHKAWA and WATANABE 1977a). The hormone was indeed shown to activate the adenylate cyclase of a membrane preparation from canine gastric antrum in concentrations as low as 1×10^{-11} *M* (BAUR et al. 1979), being much more potent than glucagon, CCK, or gastrin.

In the antral muscle of the opossum, secretin had little effect over a wide dose range but it inhibited the stimulant action of gastrin. Conversely, in the pyloric muscle, secretin caused a dose-dependent increase (3×10^{-15}–3×10^{-13} *M*) in the active tension. This effect was antagonized noncompetitively by gastrin (10^{-16} *M*). The reciprocal gastrin–secretin antagonism was found to be selective and not to alter the response of the antrum or the pylorus to other agonists (LIPSHUTZ and COHEN 1972; FISHER et al. 1973).

F. Effects on the Intestine

On the intestine of experimental animals and humans, secretin has a predominantly inhibitory effect, as it does on the LES and the stomach. Both mechanical and electrical activity were shown to be decreased, the effects being more striking in the proximal than in the distal regions.

Studies of mechanical activity showed that secretin induced a dose-dependent (0.2–1 U/kg i.v.) inhibitory effect on duodenal motor activity in the dog (WALKER et al. 1972), an effect which had already been seen on the hypermotility induced by the bethanechol chloride preparation, Urecholine (CHEY et al. 1967). Interestingly, in experiments in which the adrenal glands were excluded from the circulation, secretin apparently showed no inhibitory effect on dog small intestine, while it increased considerably the regional blood flow in the superior mesenteric region (FASTH et al. 1972).

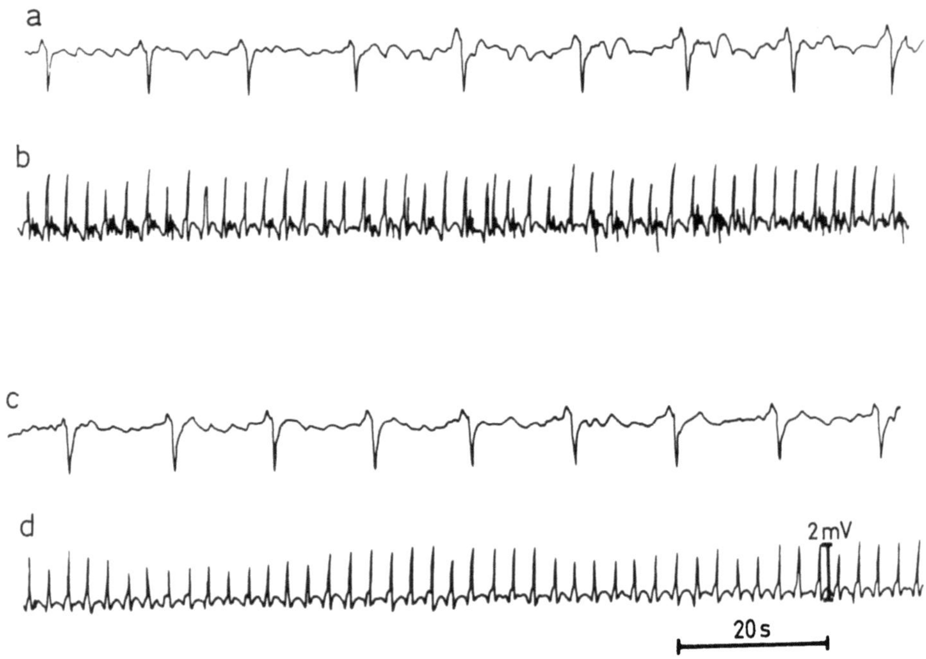

Fig. 2a–d. Electrical activity recorded from the stomach **a, c** and the duodenum **b, d** in an unanesthetized dog. The intense spike activity observed in duodenum under basal conditions **b** disappears during infusion with secretin (0.1 U $kg^{-1}min^{-1}$, **d**. (R. CAPRILLI unpublished work 1979)

In the duodenum of the conscious dog (Fig. 2), secretin in very low doses (0.5 U kg^{-1} h^{-1}) slowed the basic electrical rhythm (BER), which was not affected by food (PEARCE et al. 1978). In higher doses (1.5 U kg^{-1} h^{-1}) it also markedly decreased duodenal pressure and actually abolished motor activity fronts (DI MAGNO et al. 1978). In the small bowel of the dog, both endogenous (following intraduodenal acidification) and exogenous (0.5–6 U kg^{-1} h^{-1}) secretin caused delays in the onset of the interdigestive myoelectric complex and decreases in the total percentage of slow waves, with superimposed spike potentials. However, low or medium doses of secretin did not produce any marked alteration in the pattern of fed activity, slow wave frequency, or the caudal migration of the interdigestive migrating myoelectric complex (MUKHOPADHYAY et al. 1975; WINGATE et al. 1978). These results confirmed the early data of HERMON-TAYLOR and CODE (1970). Secretin (0.25 and 0.5 U/kg) was able to decrease the mean percentage incidence of spike potentials stimulated by motilin in the duodenum and the antrum. It had the same effect against CCK OP in the stomach but not in the duodenum (CASTRESANA et al. 1978). In the dog ileum, only very high doses (1–5 U/kg i.v.) were able to inhibit cerulein-induced stimulation (MANTOVANI and BERTACCINI 1971). The motility of the canine intestinal villi was also inhibited by secretin (NEMETH et al. 1973).

In the rabbit, secretin was shown to inhibit the spontaneous contraction of the jejunum both in vivo (0.5–5 U/ml) and in vitro (0.05–1 U/ml; NAKAYAMA 1973). Surprisingly, both the cat stomach and the cat small intestine responded to secretin with stimulation instead of inhibition. In the cat isolated ileum, secretin (0.01–

0.05 U/ml) increased dose-dependently the tone of the preparation without altering the frequency of the phasic contractions. Spikes on the slow waves disappeared after administration of secretin, probably because of the depolarization of the membrane potential of the smooth muscle cells. These changes were not influenced by tetrodotoxin (1.6×10^{-7} g/ml) or atropine (2.5×10^{-6} g/ml), suggesting that the secretin effect is not mediated via an excitatory cholinergic nerve pathway. Reciprocal secretin–pentagastrin and secretin–CCK antagonisms were also observed, though the nature of the antagonisms was not established (OHKAWA and WATANABE 1977b). In isolated duodenum from cat and opossums, secretin did not have any appreciable effect on either circular or longitudinal muscle strips (ANURAS and COOKE 1978).

In humans, secretin (1 U/kg or 1 U kg^{-1} h^{-1}) inhibited duodenal motor activity both under basal conditions (OSNES 1975) and after stimulation with metacholine (CHEY et al. 1967) exactly as it did in the stomach. Its efficacy and potency on both mechanical and electrical activity were slightly lower than those of glucagon (CORAZZIARI 1976; LABÒ and BORTOLOTTI 1976) and it was therefore suggested that secretin may be used for hypotonic duodenography (GUTIÉRREZ et al. 1974b). The peptide (1–2 U kg^{-1} h^{-1}) was also shown to decrease the amplitude and the duration of the arrhythmic phase I and phase III waves in the duodenum and the jejunum, an effect quite opposite to that of CCK (DOLLINGER et al. 1975). Indeed, secretin was able to antagonize the stimulant effect of CCK, which in turn was able to antagonize the effect of secretin (GUTIÉRREZ et al. 1974).

In patients with terminal ileostomy, secretin (1 U kg^{-1} h^{-1}) caused a significant decrease in motility of the terminal ileum plus a decrease in the frequency of action potentials, while it left unaffected the configuration and the frequency of the pacemaker potential (WATERFALL et al. 1972). These changes are consistent with the idea that small bowel digestion is aided by a decrease in the rate of advance of the intraluminal contents after the release of secretin when the gastrin meal has reached the duodenum. In healthy subjects, secretin (0.25–1 U/kg) caused a dose-related increase in plasma secretin and a simultaneous dose-related inhibition of food-stimulated motor activity of the distal colon (DINOSO et al. 1976).

The motor activity of the sigmoid colon was also decreased by secretin, which showed reciprocal antagonism with CCK (DINOSO et al. 1973). Moreover, secretin (2 U kg^{-1} h^{-1}) caused marked inhibition of food-stimulated motor wave activity in the distal colon and decreased the motility index from 45.6 to 17.5. An inhibitory effect on the rectum was present but not statistically significant. No effect was noted on the internal anal sphincter pressure. Unlike glucagon, secretin did not suppress morphine-induced motor activity (CHOWDHURY and LORBER 1977). Myoelectric and motor activity in the rectum and rectosigmoid did not appear to be affected by secretin (1 U/kg; SNAPE et al. 1977).

G. Conclusions

The inhibitory effect of secretin on gastrointestinal motility, is very seldom observed under basal conditions but is remarkable when motility is increased by mechanical distension or by pretreatment with gastrin or cholecystokinin. The only segment which appears to be stimulated, at least in some species, is the pylorus. On the whole, secretin appears to be one of the most important endogenous inhibitory substances and it is likely that it plays an inhibitory role in the physiologic control of the intricate networks modulating the humoral (or neurohumoral) regulation of gut motility.

References

Anuras S, Cooke AR (1978) Effects of some gastrointestinal hormones on two muscle layers of duodenum. Am J Physiol 234:E60–E63

Baur S, Grant B, Spaulding RK (1979) Effect of hormonal and neuronal agents on adenylate cyclase from smooth muscle of the gastric antrum. Biochem Biophys Acta 584:365–374

Bayliss WM, Starling EH (1902) The mechanism of pancreatic secretion. J Physiol (Lond) 28:325–353

Behar J, Field S, Marin C (1979) Effect of glucagon, secretin, and vasoactive intestinal polypeptide on the feline lower esophageal sphincter: mechanism of action. Gastroenterology 77:1001–1007

Bertaccini G, Impicciatore M, De Caro G (1973) Action of caerulein and related substances on the pyloric sphincter of the anaesthetized rat. Eur J Pharmacol 22:320–324

Bitar KN, Zfass AM, Bodanszky M, Mackhlouf GM (1977) Activity of C-terminal partial sequences of secretin. Clin Res 25:307A

Bodanszky M, Ondetti MA, Levine SD et al. (1966) Synthesis of a heptacosapeptide amide with the hormonal activity of secretin. Chem Ind (Lond) 42:1757–1758

Bodanszky A, Ondetti MA, Mutt V, Bodanszky M (1969) Synthesis of secretin. IV. Secondary structure in a miniature protein. J Am Chem Soc 91:944–949

Bortolotti M, Sanavio C, Sansone G, Labò G (1975) Modifications in human gastric motility induced by secretin and by glucagon. Rend Gastroenterol 7:240

Brown FC, Siegel SR, Castell DO, Johnson LF, Said SI (1978) Effects of vasoactive intestinal polypeptide (VIP) on the lower esophageal sphincter in awake baboons: comparison with glucagon and secretin. Scand J Gastroenterol [Suppl 49] 13:32

Cameron AJ, Phillips SF, Summerskill WHJ (1970) Comparison of effects of gastrin, cholecystokinin-pancreozymin, secretin, and glucagon on human stomach muscle in vitro. Gastroenterology 59:539–545

Castresana M, Lee KY, Chey WY, Yajima H (1978) Effects of motilin and octapeptide of cholecystokinin on antral and duodenal myoelectric activity in the interdigestive state and during inhibition by secretin and gastric inhibitory polypeptide. Digestion 17:300–308

Chey WY, Lorber SH, Kusakcioglu O, Hendricks J (1967) Effect of secretin and pancreozymin-cholecystokinin on motor function of stomach and duodenum. Fed Proc 26:383, A710

Chey WY, Kosay S, Hendricks J, Lorber SH (1969) Effect of secretin on the motor activity of the stomach and Heidenhain pouch in dogs. Am J Physiol 217:848–852

Chey WY, Hitanant S, Hendricks J, Lorber SH (1970) Effect of secretin and cholecystokinin on gastric emptying and gastric secretion in man. Gastroenterology 58:820–827

Chey WY, Gutiérrez J, Yoshimori M, Hendricks J (1974) Gut hormones on gastrointestinal motor function. In: Chey WY, Brooks FP (eds) Endocrinology of the gut. Slack, Thorofare NJ, pp 194–211

Chowdhury AR, Lorber SH (1977) Effects of glucagon and secretin on food- or morphine-induced motor activity of the distal colon, rectum, and anal sphincter. Am J Dig Dis 22:775–780

Christiansen J, Borgeskov S (1974) The effect of glucagon and the combined effect of glucagon and secretin on lower esophageal sphincter pressure in man. Scand J Gastroenterol 9:615–618

Chvasta TE, Cooke AR (1973) Secretin-gastric emptying and motor activity: natural versus synthetic secretin. Proc Soc Exp Biol Med 142:137–142

Cohen S, Lipshutz WH (1971) Hormonal regulation of human lower esophageal sphincter competence: interaction of gastrin and secretin. J Clin Invest 50:449–454

Corazziari E (1976) Mechanical activity of the second portion of human duodenum. Rend Gastroenterol 8:64

Di Magno EP, Hendricks JC, Dozois RR, Go VLW (1978) Effects of secretin on the canine duodenal (D) pancreatic duct (PD) and pancreatic sphincter yield (SY) pressures (P) and duodenal motor activity fronts (AF). Gastroenterology 74:A1026

Dinoso V Jr, Chey WY, Hendricks J, Lorber SH (1969) Intestinal mucosal hormones and motor function of the stomach in man. J Appl Physiol 26:326–329

Dinoso VP, Meshkinpour H, Lorber SH, Gutiérrez JG, Chey WY (1973) Motor responses of the sigmoid colon and rectum to exogenous cholecystokinin and secretin. Gastroenterology 65:438–444

Dinoso VP, Murthy SNS, Clearfield HR, Chey WY (1976) The effects of exogenous secretin on food-stimulated motor activity of the distal colon-correlation with plasma gastrin and secretin. Gastroenterology 70:A878

Dollinger HC, Berz R, Raptis S, Uexküll T Von, Goebell H (1975) Effects of secretin and cholecystokinin on motor activity of human jejunum. Digestion 12:9–16

Fara JW, Praissman M, Berkowitz JM (1979) Interaction between gastrin, CCK, and secretin on canine antral smooth muscle in vitro. Am J Physiol 236:E39–E44

Fasth S, Filipsson S, Hultén L, Martinson J (1972) The effect of the gastrointestinal hormones on small intestinal motility and blood flow. Experientia 29:982–984

Fisher RS, Cohen S (1973) Pyloric-sphincter dysfunction in patients with gastric ulcer. N Engl J Med 288:273–276

Fisher RS, Cohen S (1980) Effect of gut hormones on gastrointestinal sphincters. In: Jerzy Glass GB (ed) Comprehensive endocrinology. Gastrointestinal hormones. Raven, New York, pp 613–638

Fisher RS, Lipshutz W, Cohen S (1973) The hormonal regulation of pyloric sphincter function. J Clin Invest 52:1289–1296

Gerner T, Haffner JFW (1978) The inhibitory effect of secretin and glucagon on pressure response to cholecystokinin-pancreozymin in isolated guinea-pig stomach. Scand J Gastroenterol 13:537–544

Grossman MI (1969) Structure of secretin. Gastroenterology 57:610–611

Gutiérrez JG, Chey WY, Dinoso VP (1974a) Actions of cholecystokinin and secretin on the motor activity of the small intestine in man. Gastroenterology 67:35–41

Gutiérrez JG, Chey WY, Shah A, Holzwasser G (1974b) Use of secretin in hypotonic duodenography. Radiology 113:563–566

Hermon-Taylor JH, Code CF (1970) Effect of secretin on small bowel myoelectric activity of conscious healthy dogs. Am J Dig Dis 15:545–550

Itoh Z, Honda R, Hiwatashi K, Takahashi I (1978) Hormonal control of the lower esophageal sphincter in man and dog: reevaluation of the present manometric method for diagnosis of GE reflux. In: Grossman M, Speranza V, Basso N, Lezoche E (eds) Gastrointestinal hormones and pathology of the digestive system. Plenum, New York London, pp 121–131

Johnson LP, Brown JC, Magee DF (1966) Effect of secretin and cholecystokinin-pancreozymin extracts on gastric motility in man. Gut 7:52–57

Jorpes E, Mutt V (1961) On the biological activity and amino acid composition of secretin. Acta Chem Scand 15:1790–1791

Kelly KA, Woodward ER, Code CF (1969) Effect of secretin and cholecystokinin on canine gastric electrical activity. Proc Soc Exp Biol Med 130:1060–1063

König W, Bickel M, Wissmann H, Uhmann R, Geiger R (1979) Secretin analogues. In: Rosselin G, Fromageot P, Bonfils S (eds) Hormone receptors in digestion and nutrition. Elsevier/North Holland, Amsterdam Oxford New York, pp 137–143

Kowalewski K, Kolodej A (1977) Effect of secretin on myoelectrical and mechanical activity of the isolated canine stomach perfused ex vivo. Pharmacology 15:73–83

Kwong NK, Brown BH, Whittaker GE, Duthie HL (1972) Effect of gastrin I, secretin and cholecystokinin-pancreozymin on the electrical activity, motor activity, and acid output of the stomach in man. Scand J Gastroenterol 7:161–170
Labò G, Bortolotti M (1976) Effect of gut hormones on myoelectric and manometric activity of the duodenum in man. Rend Gastroenterol 8:64
Lipshutz WH (1976) Physiology of the gastro-oesophageal junction and hiatus hernia. In: Bouchier ID (ed) Recent advances in gastroenterology, vol 3. Churchill Livingstone, Edinburgh London, pp 1–26
Lipshutz W, Cohen S (1972) Interaction of gastrin I and secretin on gastrointestinal circular muscle. Am J Physiol 222:775–781
Mantovani P, Bertaccini G (1971) Action of caerulein and related substances on gastrointestinal motility of the anaesthetized dog. Arch Int Pharmacodyn Ther 193:363–371
Meves M, Beger HG, Hüthwohl B (1975) The effect of some gastrointestinal hormones on gastric evacuation in man. In: Vantrappen G (ed) Fifth International Symposium on Gastrointestinal Motility. Typoff, Herentals, pp 327–332
Mukhopadhyay AK, Johnson LR, Copeland EM, Weisbrodt NW (1975) Effect of secretin on electrical activity of small intestine. Am J Physiol 229:484–488
Nakayama S (1973) The effects of secretin and cholecystokinin on the sphincter muscles. In: Fujita T (ed) Gastro-entero-pancreatic endocrine system – a cell-biological approach. Igaku Shoin, Tokyo, pp 145–154
Nemeth EP, Ihász M, Folly G, Papp M (1973) The action of secretin, trypsin, and histamine on the motility of canine intestinal villi. Am J Gastroenterol 60:607–615
Ohkawa H, Watanabe M (1977a) Effects of gastrointestinal hormones on the electrical and mechanical activity of the cat stomach. Tohoku J Exp Med 122:287–298
Ohkawa H, Watanabe M (1977b) Effects of gastrointestinal hormones on the electrical and mechanical activities of the cat small intestine. Jpn J Physiol 27:71–79
Osnes M (1975) The effect of secretin and cholecystokinin on the duodenal motility in man. Scand J Gastroenterol [Suppl 35] 10:22–26
Pearce EAN, Wingate DL, Wünsch E (1978) The effects of gastrointestinal hormones and feeding in the basic electric rhythm of the stomach and duodenum of the conscious dog. J Physiol (Lond) 276:41P–42P
Phaosawasdi K, Boden G, Kolts B, Fisher RS (to be published) Hormonal effects on pyloric sphincter pressure: are they of physiological importance? Clin Res
Siegel SR, Brown FC, Castell DO, Johnson LF, Said SI (1979) Effects of vasoactive intestinal polypeptide (VIP) on lower esophageal sphincter in awake baboons. Dig Dis Sci 24:345–349
Snape WJ Jr, Carlson GM, Cohen S (1977) Human colonic myoelectric activity in response to prostigmin and the gastrointestinal hormones. Am J Dig Dis 22:881–887
Strunz U (1979) Hormonal control of gastric emptying. Acta Hepatogastroenterol (Stuttg) 26:334–341
Sugawara K, Isaza J, Curt J, Woodward ER (1969) Effect of secretin and cholecystokinin on gastric motility. Am J Physiol 217:1633–1638
Vagne M, André C (1971) The effect of secretin on gastric emptying in man. Gastroenterology 60:421–424
Vagne M, Stening GF, Brooks FP, Grossman MI (1968) Synthetic secretin: comparison with natural secretin for potency and spectrum of physiological actions. Gastroenterology 55:260–267
Valenzuela JE (1976) Effect of intestinal hormones and peptides on intragastric pressure in dogs. Gastroenterology 71:766–769
Walker DG, Stewart JJ, Bass P (1972) The effect of secretin on the fed pattern of gastric and duodenal contractile activity. Surg Gynecol Obstet 134:807–809
Waterfall WE, Brown BH, Duthie HL, Whittaker GE (1972) The effects of humoral agents on the myoelectrical activity of the terminal ileum. Gut 13:528–534
Wilson RC (1975) Mechanism of secretin inhibition of rumen motility. PhD dissertation Abstr Int B 35, Nr. 8, 4081
Wingate DL, Pearce EA, Hutton M, Dand A, Thompson HH, Wünsch E (1978) Quantitative comparison of the effects of cholecystokinin, secretin, and pentagastrin on gastrointestinal myoelectric activity in the conscious fasted dog. Gut 19:593–601

Gastric Inhibitory Polypeptide

A. Introduction

Gastric inhibitory polypeptide (GIP) was isolated during the purification of cholecystokinin (BROWN et al. 1969, 1970). In 1971 BROWN and DRYBURGH published the complete amino acid sequence and in 1975 YAJIMA et al. synthesized the entire molecule. GIP is a 43 amino acid polypeptide with a molecular weight of 5,105 daltons. Of the first 26 amino acids 15 are in the same positions as in porcine glucagon and 9 of the first 26 are in the same positions as in secretin (see Table 1 in Chap. 2a, Secretin). The 17 COOH terminal amino acids are not common to any other known intestinal peptide. Since the discovery that in addition to having an inhibitory effect on gastric secretion GIP is also a powerful insulin-releasing hormone (BROWN 1977), GIP has been renamed glucose-dependent insulin-releasing peptide, which term recognizes both its insulinotropic effects and its dependence on the ambient glucose concentration, since it is ineffective when glucose is low.

B. Effects on Gastrointestinal Motility

Besides these two most important effects and a stimulatory effect on intestinal secretion (BARBEZAT and GROSSMAN 1971), GIP also has some effects on the motility of the gastrointestinal tract.

I. Lower Esophageal Sphincter

The effect of GIP on lower esophageal sphincter (LES) pressure in the cat was studied by manometric techniques. Both exogenous (0.2 µg kg^{-1} min^{-1} i.v.) and endogenous (released by intraduodenal administration of 20% glucose) peptides were shown to induce significant decrements in LES pressure both under basal conditions and when increased by pentagastrin (SINAR et al. 1978).

II. Intragastric Pressure

GIP was shown to decrease intragastric pressure significantly in dogs (VALENZUELA 1976). The maximal decrease in intragastric pressure produced by GIP was small in comparison with those produced by other peptides like VIP, secretin, or cholecystokinin. However, the threshold dose for GIP was 500 ng kg^{-1} h^{-1}, that is to say the same dose that is the ED_{50} for the inhibition of pentagastrin-induced acid secretion. If inhibition of gastric secretion is a physiologic effect of GIP, it may be suggested that inhibition of gastric motility is also a physiologic effect of the peptide. Indeed, one suggested method for investigating whether or not an effect is physiologic is to show that the ED_{50} for that effect is not significantly different from the ED_{50} for the action of the hormone on its primary target (DEBAS and GROSSMAN 1975). These recent results are in accord with previous studies by PEDERSON (1971), who showed that GIP (1 µg kg^{-1} h^{-1}) was able to suppress pentagastrin-stimulated or acetylcholine-stimulated antral motor activity.

III. Intraluminal Pressure

In the conscious dog, LIN (1980) observed that GIP increased the intraluminal pressure of the gastroduodenal junction, but decreased that of the antrum, descending duodenum, gallbladder, and choledochal sphincter, thus exerting a predominant inhibitory effect; however no quantitative data were reported.

C. Interactions

The demonstration that oral administration of glucose with a consequent increase in serum GIP concentration, delayed gastric emptying in humans (MAYLE et al. 1978) is consistent with the idea that GIP may play a role in the regulation of gastric motility. Of course, other substances (like insulin) may intervene in such a situation and may interact in a negative or positive sense with the action of GIP.

In the stump-tailed macaque, *Macaca arctoides*, it has been shown that feeding increased electromechanical activity in the right colon, cecum, and transverse colon. This was accompanied by a significant increase in serum GIP, whereas no changes in serum gastrin or cholecystokinin were observed (SILLIN et al. 1978). The authors suggested that GIP was responsible for the increase in colon contractions, which they called the "gastrocolic response." However, no data are available on a possible relationship between exogenous GIP and this type of colonic response which might be species specific or might be due to interactions with other humoral mediators.

As to possible interactions with other gastrointestinal peptides, GIP (0.25–0.5 μg/kg) was found to reduce significantly the mean percentage incidence of spike potentials in the dog antrum and duodenum stimulated by motilin. Although the percentage incidence of spike potentials produced by cholecystokinin COOH terminal octapeptide also appeared to be lowered in both antrum and duodenum by GIP, the changes were not statistically significant (CASTRESANA et al. 1978). Further studies are needed to clarify whether or not this inhibitory effect of GIP is one of its physiologic properties.

References

Barbezat GO, Grossman MI (1971) Intestinal secretion: stimulation by peptides. Science 174:422–424

Brown JC (1977) GIP: gastric inhibitory polypeptide or glucose-dependent insulinotropic polypeptide? Metab Ther 6:1–2

Brown JC, Dryburgh JR (1971) A gastric inhibitory polypeptide. II. The complete amino-acid sequence. Can J Biochem 49:867–872

Brown JC, Pederson RA, Jorpes JE, Mutt V (1969) Preparation of highly active enterogastrone. Can J Physiol Pharmacol 47:113–114

Brown JC, Mutt V, Pederson RA (1970) Further purification of a polipeptide demonstrating enterogastrone activity. J Physiol (Lond) 209:57–64

Castresana M, Lee KY, Chey WY, Yajima H (1978) Effect of motilin and octapeptide of cholecystokinin on antral and duodenal myoelectric activity in the interdigestive state and during inhibition by secretin and gastric inhibitory polypeptide. Digestion 17:300–308

Debas HT, Grossman MI (1975) Inhibition of gastric emptying is a physiological action of cholecystokinin. Gastroenterology 68:1211–1217

Lin TS (1980) Effects of insulin and glucagon on secretory and motor function of the gastrointestinal tract. In: Jerzy Glass GB (ed) Gastrointestinal hormones. Raven, New York, pp. 639–691

Mayle JE, Wolfe MM, Caldwell JH, O'Dorisio TM, Cataland S, Thomas FB (1978) Gastric emptying and serum inhibitory polypeptide (GIP) after oral glucose. Gastroenterology 74:1063

Pederson RA (1971) The isolation and physiological actions of gastric inhibitory polypeptide. PhD dissertation, University of British Columbia, Vancouver

Sillin LF, Condon RE, Schulte WJ, Woods JH, Bass P, Go VWL (1978) The relationship between gastric inhibitory peptide and right colon electromechanical activity after feding (Abstr). In: Duthie HL (ed) Gastrointestinal motility in health and disease. MTP Press, Lancaster, pp 361–362

Sinar DR, D'Dorisio TM, Mazzaferri EL, Mekhjian HS, Caldwell JH, Thomas FB (1978) Effect of gastric inhibitory polypeptide on lower esophageal sphincter pressure in cats. Gastroenterology 75:263–267

Valenzuela JE (1976) Effect of intestinal hormones and peptides on intragastric pressure in dogs. Gastroenterology 71:766–769

Yajima H, Ogawa H, Kubota M et al. (1975) Synthesis of the tritracontapeptide corresponding to entire aminoacid sequence of gastric inhibitory polypeptide. J Am Chem Soc 97:5593–5594

CHAPTER 2b

Peptides: Candidate Hormones

G. BERTACCINI

Substance P

A. Introduction

About 50 years ago (VON EULER and GADDUM 1931) substance P (SP) was obtained from extracts of equine brain and intestine which were able to stimulate contraction of rabbit bowel which had been pretreated with atropine. The active moiety found in the dried extracts was given the provisional name "preparation P" and was shown to differ from all the other stimulants known at that time. Many years later its structure was identified as a peptide with 11 amino acid residues (CHANG et al. 1971) and it was synthesized. MEINARDI and CRAIG (1966) found several peptides with SP-like activity in the brain and gut of different mammalian species and suggested that this activity may be possessed by a family of related peptides rather than by a single substance. ZETLER (1970) came to a similar conclusion. This heterogeneity, which is both biologic and immunologic (NILSSON and BRODIN 1977), finds its counterpart in the heterogeneity of several gastrointestinal hormones and "candidate" hormones. Only recently have we come to recognize that substance P is the prototype of a long and still growing list of peptides present both in brain and gut.

By means of immunofluorescence, substance P was found to be present in several areas of the central nervous system and the spinal cord in many species including humans. Fluorescence microscopy enabled PEARSE and POLAK (1975) to show this peptide to be present in the nerve plexuses of the intestine and also in endocrine cells of intestinal mucosa. With radioimmunoassay techniques, NILSSON et al. (1975) have made new and important findings about the presence of SP-like immunoradioactivity in human and canine plasma. Little is known about the mechanisms of the synthesis of SP or its destruction in tissues. Unlike angiotensin or bradykinin, SP does not appear to be split from a precursor protein. The peptide is thought to be stored in its active form. Moreover, the fact that activity exhibited by the entire SP amino acid sequence is retained down to the COOH terminal hexapeptide suggests that enzymes which inactivate SP in the tissues must be capable of lysing peptide bonds present in the COOH terminal pentapeptide sequence.

Substance P was first studied, from a pharmacologic point of view, as a hypotensive compound and as a smooth muscle stimulant. Its effects are numerous, including stimulation of all the extravascular smooth muscle and stimulation of lacrimal and salivary secretion. SP also inhibits insulin release from the pancreas.

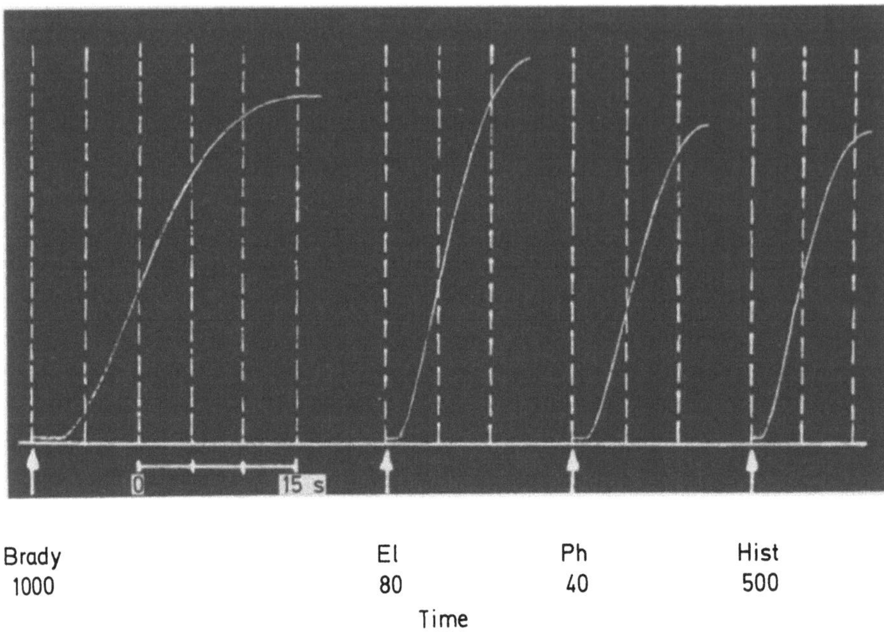

Fig. 1. Guinea pig ileum preparation. Contractions produced by bradykinin *Brady*, eledoisin *El*, physalemin *Ph*, and histamine *Hist*. All doses in ng/bath (10 ml). (BERTACCINI et al. 1965a)

Table 1. Structure of SP and its natural analogs

Structure[a]	Trivial name	Source
Arg-Pro-Lys-Pro-Gln-Gln-*Phe*-Phe-*Gly-Leu-Met-*NH_2	Substance P	Mammals
pGlu-Pro-Ser-Lys-Asp-Ala-*Phe*-Ile-*Gly-Leu-Met-*NH_2	Eledoisin	Octopods
pGlu-Ala-Asp-Pro-Asn-Lys-*Phe*-Tyr-*Gly-Leu-Met-*NH_2	Physalemin	Frogs
pGlu-Ala-Asp-Pro-Lys-Thr-*Phe*-Tyr-*Gly-Leu-Met-*NH_2	(Lys^5 Thr^6)-physalemin	Frogs
pGlu-Pro-Asp-Pro-Asn-Ala-*Phe*-Tyr-*Gly-Leu-Met-*NH_2	Uperolein	Frogs
pGlu-Asn-Pro-Asn-Arg-*Phe*-Ile-*Gly-Leu-Met-*NH_2	Phyllomedusin	Frogs
Asp-Val-Pro-Lys-Ser-Asp-Gln-*Phe*-Val-*Gly-Leu-Met-*NH_2	Kassinin	Frogs

[a] The amino acid residues which are common to the different peptides are *italicized*. (For references, see BERTACCINI 1980)

Apparently, this peptide can play two roles in the pain pathway: in the spinal cord it may be involved in the transmission of pain, while in the brain it may act as a modulator of pain sensitivity. SP is the prototype of a series of naturally occurring peptides that are characterized by the promptness of their stimulant effects on smooth muscle, which suggested the name tachykinins (fast-acting kinins, from the Greek *tachus* fast) as opposed to the group of bradykinins (slow-acting kinins, from the Greek *bradus* slow; Fig. 1).

B. Structure–Activity Relationships

The tachykinins whose structures have been elucidated and confirmed by synthesis are listed in Table 1 and both the structure, and the origin are indicated. The peptides discovered more recently are kassinin, found in the skin of the African frog *Kassina senegalensis* (ANASTASI et al. 1977) and synthesized by YAJIMA et al. (1978) and (Lys^5 Thr^6)-physalemin found in the skin of the Australian frog *Uperoleia rugosa* (T. NAKAJIMA and V. ERSPAMER unpublished work 1980). Another kassinin-like peptide namely (Glu^2 Pro^5)-kassinin was found quite recently to occur in the skin of the East African tree frog *Hylambates maculatus* (T. NAKAJIMA unpublished work 1980).

The study of tachykinins, which at first appeared to be of only academic interest, has proved to be of definite importance in the elucidation of the structure of SP and for studying the relationship of structure to activity. Moreover, results obtained with the natural tachykinins in different animal species may have the same importance as those achieved with pure synthetic SP because it is quite possible that rat, guinea pig, or dog SP may be more closely related structurally and biologically to one of the aforementioned tachykinins than to the *bovine* SP used as the reference test compound so far, as the only synthetic SP available. In this connection LAZARUS et al. (1980) discovered in mammalian tissues, a substance with an immunoreactivity resembling that of physalemin. In the gastrointestinal tract and in other tissues, physalemin-like immunoreactivity contained an amino acid sequence common to the NH_2 terminal region of both physalemin and uperolein (-Asp-Pro-Asn-). Without entering into the details of the important and complex problem of structure–activity relationships, in systematic research that included natural and synthetic SP-like substances, it was found (BERTACCINI 1976) that the typical biologic activity is related to the presence of a COOH terminal pentapeptide with a phenylalanyl residue at position 5 from the COOH terminus and the sequence Gly-Leu-Met-NH_2 in the COOH terminal tripeptide. These findings were recently confirmed in a study of a series of synthetic SP analogs (YANAIHARA et al. 1977) and a series of eledoisin and physalemin analogs (DE CASTIGLIONE 1978), tested for their contractile activity on guinea pig ileum and on rabbit large intestine.

The COOH terminal pentapeptide sequence is therefore considered to contain the *basic information*. Attachment of additional amino acids can lead to a "reinforcement effect" (OEHME et al. 1972). The COOH terminal heptapeptide is actually three times as active as the whole SP molecule (KITAGAWA et al. 1979). (Ile^8)-SP was found to be almost twice as active as SP on the guinea pig ileum, whereas (Ile^7 Ile^8)-SP had a very low activity, confirming the importance of the phenylalanyl residue at position 5 from the COOH terminus (RACKUR et al. 1979), which was further emphasized in other studies in which Ala- residue was substituted in different positions in the SP molecule (COUTURE et al. 1979).

C. Action on Gut Motility

Mainly, results obtained with the pure, synthetic peptide will be quoted in this review since those referring to crude preparations might be invalid because of possible interference with other active substances. Results obtained with the other natural tachykinins will be also be cited. The data available in this field of research are mainly concerned with experimental animals since SP cannot be given to humans because of the strong hypotensive effect which parallels the effect on the bowel, or even predominates. For the same reason, in experimental animals most of the results available were obtained by means of in vitro techniques. However, some in vivo experiments have been reported.

I. In Vitro Studies

The action of SP on the gastrointestinal smooth muscle of several animal species is generally a spasmogenic one. Only in freshwater crayfish *(Astacus astacus* and *Astacus torrentium)* did SP inhibit contractions of the terminal intestine (UMRATH and GRALLERT 1967). Isolated intestinal preparations from other fishes, such as the flapper skate *Raja batis*, the plaice *Pleuronectes platessa*, and the ballan wrasse *Labrus bergylta*, have been reported to contract in the presence of SP preparations (SKRABANEK and POWELL 1977; BURY and MASHFORD 1977b). Because of the good dose-related contractions elicited by the peptide, the usual lack of tachyphylaxis (if repeated administrations are followed by adequate rest periods), and the minute amounts needed to induce contractions in the smooth muscle of the bowel, the bioassay of SP has generally been performed in isolated gut preparations, the most common being the guinea pig ileum, the rabbit jejunum, the chicken rectal cecum, and the goldfish *(Carassius auratus)* intestine. Appropriate use of different inhibitors and prior removal of interfering substances allowed good evaluation of SP in extracts of various tissues before the development of radioimmunologic techniques.

The smooth muscle stimulant effect is very potent. The most sensitive gastrointestinal preparations have been found to be, besides those already mentioned as used in the bioassay, the golden hamster jejunum and the isolated human jejunum and ileum. The rabbit duodenum is about one-half as sensitive, the human duodenum one-quarter to one-fifth, and the rat duodenum and colon one-tenth to one-twentieth as sensitive. These results concern only the longitudinal muscle. In the human sigmoid colon, BENNETT (1975) observed contraction of the circular muscle layers with SP, while in the guinea pig ileum, SP was said to be ineffective on the circular muscle. A remarkable difference in sensitivity was found in the two muscle layers of the opossum duodenum (FAULK et al. 1977); the longitudinal muscle responded to SP with a tonic contraction at 5×10^{-13} *M*, whereas the circular muscle responded with a tonic followed by a phasic contraction only to 5×10^{-5} *M*.

According to MILENOV et al. (1978a) SP (10^{-8}–10^{-7} *M*) was able to stimulate the tone of the fundus and the body of guinea pig isolated stomach and to decrease the phasic contractions, but it did not affect the motility of the antrum. The peptide was also shown to increase simultaneously the number and the amplitude of spike discharges and to decrease the amplitude of slow potentials in the stomach body. Methoxyverapamil and sodium nitroprussiate, in concentrations (10^{-6} *M*) which blocked the spontaneous phasic contractions, did not inhibit the tonic activation induced by SP.

The bulk of the data about the spasmogenic effect of SP (and a tempting explanation of its mechanism of action) were obtained with guinea pig ileum. The early exhaustive experiments performed with purified SP extracts were those reported by PERNOW (1963). This investigator obtained spasmogenic activity of SP in a series of isolated gut preparations with very low concentrations of the peptide (0.05 U/ml, which corresponded to 0.002 μg pure SP preparation). Moreover, he observed not only a stimulant action of the peptide but a true effect on peristaltic activity, with an increase in amplitude and frequency of the intestinal contractions. Apparently the mode of action differed in longitudinal muscle, whose contraction was not altered by hexamethonium, and in circular muscle, whose contraction was completely blocked by hexamethonium.

Most of these early findings were confirmed with the guinea pig whole ileum preparation and synthetic SP, which proved to be much more potent than acetylcholine, histamine and, 5-hydroxytryptamine (5-HT; ROSELL et al. 1977). The ED_{50} value for SP was 2.5×10^{-9} *M*, for acetylcholine 1×10^{-7} *M*, and for histamine 4.2×10^{-7} *M*. The action of SP was unaffected by drugs which block the action of acetylcholine, histamine, and 5-hydroxytryptamine. It was similarly unaffected by tetrodotoxin, ganglion-blocking agents and indomethacin. Thus, the effect of the peptide was assumed to be mainly a direct one. According to early studies however (KOSTERLITZ and ROBINSON 1956), SP-induced contractions can be depressed by lowering the bath temperature more than can contractions due to any other compound acting directly on plain muscle and this suggested that SP may act, at least partially, through the nervous structures, since these are more thermosensitive than smooth muscle. Of course it cannot be excluded that the SP preparations used at that time could have been contamined by other indirectly acting spasmogenic compounds. On the other hand, PATON and ZAR (1968) compared the responses to SP in guinea pig ileum preparations with and without the myenteric (Auerbach's) plexus and obtained similar results. They concluded from this that SP acts primarily on the smooth muscle. Evidence for a partial indirect activity of SP, mediated through activation of cholinergic neurons, was recently provided by HOLZER and LEMBECK (1980) using the longitudinal muscle of the guinea pig ileum.

Direct activity of SP in eliciting both mechanical contraction and bursts of spike potentials in the guinea pig ileum has been observed also by YAU (1978), who reported that SP-induced changes were unaffected even by Lioresal, a compound which has been shown to antagonize both SP and acetylcholine by blocking the excitatory mono- and polysynaptic transmission at the primary afferent synapses in the spinal cord. The ED_{50} for the direct activity of SP on the intestine was 1×10^{-9} g/ml, a value which falls within the limits of the reported values of circulating levels of SP in several species (5×10^{-11}–2×10^{-9} g/ml) and this is support for the contention that SP is of physiologic importance. On the basis of results obtained with a number of synthetic analogs of SP, a model for the interaction of SP with lyotropic receptors on intestinal muscle was hypothesized (CHIPKIN et al. 1979). This interaction appears to involve three areas of the peptide molecule

1) The COOH terminal methionine amide residue, which was of crucial importance for activity;
2) The aromatic residues at positions 7 and 8 (Phe-Phe), and
3) The hydrophobic residues at positions 4–6 (Pro-Gln-Gln).

In the longitudinal muscle layer of guinea pig ileum, SP showed a dose-dependent (1.5–7.5×10^{-10} *M*) enhancement of the contractile response to transmural nerve stimulation and often increased the basal tone of the preparation (HEDQVIST and VON EULER 1975). At the same concentrations, the peptide failed to enhance the contractions to exogenous acetylcholine and this suggests a prejunctional effect of SP on cholinergic transmission, in addition to its direct stimulatory effect on the smooth muscle cell. Different results were obtained by COSTA et al. (1978), who found that SP did not significantly affect the cholinergic twitch contraction elicited by transmural electrical stimulation of the ileum (supramaximal voltage, 0.5 ms pulse duration, 0.1 Hz), while the nerve-mediated noncholinergic contraction of the ileum elicited by transmural stimulation at 20–50 Hz was markedly reduced by the peptide.

In recent experiments, HOLZER and LEMBECK (1979) found that SP initiated peristalsis in the guinea pig ileum and increased the efficiency of the peristaltic reflex in very low doses (2.4 pmol/min). Moreover the peptide was able to reduce the efficiency of pressure-induced peristalsis and to antagonize the inhibition of peristalsis induced by FK 33-824 (a synthetic enkephalin).

On ileal strips, a subthreshold dose of SP (5.7×10^{-9} *M*) did not antagonize the action of morphine or enkephalins (CHIPKIN and STEWART 1978). Different techniques could be responsible for this discrepancy, however, it is likely that receptors for SP and opiate receptors are separate entities. In recent experiments (ZETLER 1979), neither morphine (4.8×10^{-7} *M*) nor Met-enkephalin (6×10^{-7} *M*) were able to modify the concentration–response curves to SP. The effect of SP on the neurons of the myenteric plexus of the guinea pig has been investigated quite recently (KATAYAMA and NORTH 1978). Intracellular recordings were made from neurons within isolated ganglia adherent to longitudinal muscle and maintained in Krebs solution at 37 °C, to which SP and other drugs were added from time to time. In low concentrations (3–100 n*M*) the peptide caused a dose-related depolarization of the soma membrane, with rapid onset and easy reversibility. Iontophoretic application of SP directly onto the soma membrane also caused pronounced depolarizations which were unaffected by hexamethonium (100–200 μ*M*), atropine (1–2 μ*M*), naloxone (1 μ*M*), or enkephalin (1 μ*M*). The depolarization caused by SP was associated with an increase in neuronal input resistance. The low concentration of SP used and the fact that it both depolarizes and increases input resistance seem to indicate that SP is a powerful modulator of neuronal activity. Although there is no conclusive evidence that SP is an excitatory transmitter within the myenteric plexus, the mechanisms of action of SP and of a substance released by nerve stimulation do seem to be very similar.

1. Natural Analogs

Results obtained by FONTAINE et al. (1977) with guinea pig ileum and physalemin were at variance with those obtained with SP, inasmuch as they showed that physalemin significantly potentiated the contractions to exogenous acetylcholine (+65.1%), to nicotine (+57%), to 5-hydroxytryptamine (+25.9%), and to electrical stimulation (+19.3%) in concentrations (1.3×10^{-10} *M*) which had only a very slight effect on the basal intestinal tone. Only histamine was not potentiated by physalemin. In a preparation of the guinea pig whole ileum which allowed the simultaneous evaluation of the contraction of longitudinal and circular muscle, physalemin (1×10^{-10} M) was found (FONTAINE et al. 1978) to be active only on the longitudinal response of the peristaltic reflex: it enhanced the slow phase of the longitudinal reflex and increased the longitudinal tension while leaving unchanged the relaxation of the longitudinal muscle. The circular muscle responses were slightly decreased and this did not modify the expulsion wave. At higher concentrations (5×10^{-10} M), physalemin had a marked influence on the basal longitudinal tone, and interfered nonspecifically with the peristaltic waves in the same way as high doses of acetylcholine. In a "fatigued" preparation, the peptide increased the slow peristaltic activity.

The opposite was true when eledoisin was used instead of physalemin (BELESLIN 1969). When the passive intraluminal pressure was too low to induce peristaltic activity, physalemin was not able to trigger cyclic peristaltic waves, but only increased the longitudinal tone. Even doses of the peptide as high as 20 ng/ml were unable to restore normal peristaltic activity previously inhibited by hexamethonium, procaine, morphine, or atropine. FONTAINE et al. (1978) showed also that administration of both steroidal and nonsteroidal anti-inflammatory drugs (10–40 μg/ml) significantly inhibited contractions of the guinea pig ileum induced by physalemin whereas it inhibited to a lesser extent contractions induced by histamine or acetylcholine. The inhibition was reversed by addition of the prostaglandin, PGE_1 (2.5 ng/ml) to the bath. These data suggested that muscular receptors to physalemin would be more sensitive to the endogenous prostaglandin production or synthesis than cholinergic or histaminergic receptors.

Eledoisin, but not other vasoactive peptides (angiotensin and bradykinin), was able to antagonize the block of the peristaltic reflex induced by calcium chloride (BELESLIN and SAMARDZIC 1976). In the longitudinal muscle of the guinea pig ileum, other interesting information about the structure–activity relationships of the natural tachykinins was obtained (ZSÉLI et al. 1977). The good dose–response relationship, starting from very low threshold doses (10^{-10} M), and the direct activity on the smooth muscle were confirmed. The only substance capable of inhibiting the contractions induced by SP and its analogs was verapamil, indicating that these peptides may cause contractions of the guinea pig ileum by interfering with the transport of calcium ions. The order of potency in the group of tachykinins was: eledoisin > phyllomedusin > physalemin > uperolein > SP (kassinin was not tested).

Surprisingly, when contractions of the circular muscle layer were considered (recording the intraluminal pressure by the method described previously or by connecting several rings obtained by cutting the ileum in the direction of the circular muscle), not only were the peptides less active (doses 2–10 times higher were required to cause a marked spasmogenic effect), as could have been expected from the early experiments performed with SP (BROWNLEE and HARRY 1963), but the order of potency also changed noticeably, being as follows: kassinin = uperolein > eledoisin > phyllomedusin > physalemin > SP (BERTACCINI 1977; G. BERTACCINI and L. ZAPPIA unpublished work 1980). In this connection, ERSPAMER et al. (1975), ZAPPIA et al. (1978), and BERTACCINI and CORUZZI (1980) found completely different ratios of potencies among the different tachykinins when they examined various segments of the gastrointestinal tracts from rabbits, guinea pigs, rats, and humans, as reported in Table 2. Among all the tachykinins examined, kassinin, which

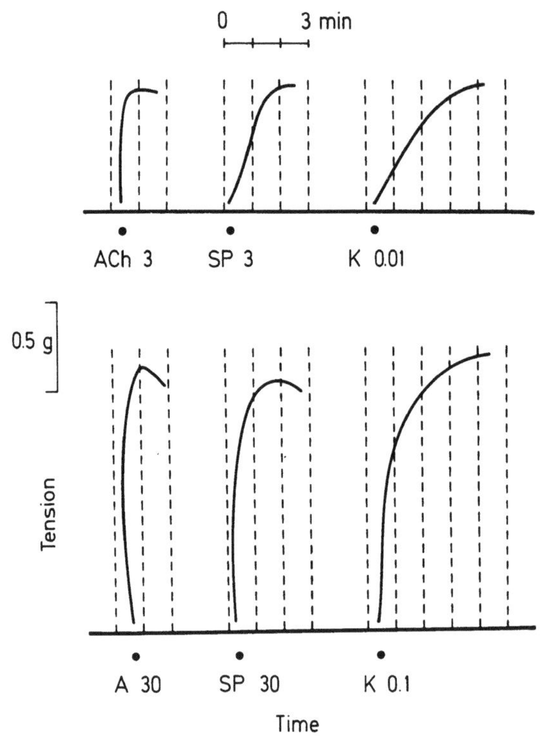

Fig. 2. Isolated lower esophageal sphincter *LES* of the rat, suspended in Krebs solution at 37 °C. Contractions produced by acetylcholine *ACh*, substance P *SP*, and kassinin *K*. All doses in μg/ml. Note the slow contractions induced by kassinin compared with the fast responses to acetylcholine and also to SP

in most preparation was the most potent peptide of the family, showed the last rapid onset of response and the slowest relaxation upon washing. This was clearly demonstrated in the rat duodenum (FALCONIERI ERSPAMER et al. 1980) and in the isolated lower esophageal sphincter of the rat (BERTACCINI and CORUZZI 1980; Fig. 2.

All the different segments of the alimentary canal were extremely sensitive to the tachykinins and threshold doses varied from 0.1 to 5 ng/ml according to the different preparations and the different compounds. It is clear from Table 2 that SP is, in almost all preparations, less potent than the other tachykinins and it is worth mentioning that the opposite is true when one examines the activity ratio with respect to the blood pressure in different species, SP being the most potent hypotensive peptide (ERSPAMER et al. 1975). Of course, this does not necessarily signify that SP is more important in the regulation of vessel tone than in that of intestinal motility. Moreover, in only a few investigations have other important parameters, besides "potency," been considered: the duration of the effect was evaluated in the in situ stomach of the rat and found to be independent of the potency of the peptides (BERTACCINI and CORUZZI 1977, see Sect. C. II); when the "efficacy," (that is maximum response) was considered, again some remarkable differences were found (see Table 3). In addition, the occurrence of tachyphylaxis was absolutely irregular, both for the peptides involved and for the preparations in

Table 2. Relative potencies of SP-like natural peptides (tachykinins) in different preparations from the gastrointestinal tract

Rat						
LES	Kassinin[c]	> Eledoisin	> Phyllomedusin	> Physalemin[c]	= Uperolein[c]	> SP[c]
Stomach	Eledoisin	> Physalemin	> Uperolein	> Phyllomedusin	> SP	
Pylorus	Eledoisin	> Phyllomedusin	> Physalemin	> Uperolein	> SP	
Gastric emptying	Phyllomedusin	> Physalemin	> Uperolein	= Eledoisin	> Kassinin	= SP
Duodenum	Eledoisin	> Physalemin	> SP			
Colon	Eledoisin	> Phyllomedusin	> Physalemin	> Uperolein	> SP	
Guinea pig						
Duodenum	Physalemin	> Eledoisin	= Phyllomedusin	= Uperolein	> SP	
Ileum LM[a]	Eledoisin	> Uperolein	> SP	> Phyllomedusin	> Physalemin	
Ileum CM[b]	Kassinin	= Uperolein	> Eledoisin	> Phyllomedusin	> Physalemin	> SP
Colon	Physalemin	> Eledoisin	> Uperolein	> SP	> Phyllomedusin	
Rabbit						
Duodenum	Eledoisin	= Physalemin	> Phyllomedusin	> SP		
Colon	Eledoisin	> Kassinin	> Phyllomedusin	> Physalemin	> Uperolein	> SP
Cat						
Duodenum	Physalemin	> Eledoisin	> SP			
Human						
Stomach	Phyllomedusin	> Eledoisin	= Uperolein	> Physalemin[c]	> SP[c]	
Duodenum	Uperolein	> Eledoisin	= Phyllomedusin[c]	> Physalemin	= Kassinin	> SP
Ileum	Eledoisin	= Kassinin	> Phyllomedusin	> Uperolein[c]		
Taenia coli	Eledoisin	= Kassinin	> Phyllomedusin	> Physalemin	> Uperolein[c]	> SP

[a] Longitudinal muscle
[b] Circular muscle
[c] tachyphylaxis (Only the "potency" in terms of lower threshold doses was considered)

Table 3. Efficacy of the natural tachykinins on different isolated preparations. Maximal response (that produced by SP taken as unity). Mean of the values obtained from 4–10 preparations

	Guinea pig ileum		Rat LES
	Longitudinal muscle	Circular muscle	
SP	1.00	1.00	1.00
Eledoisin	2.10	1.42	1.47
Physalemin	0.90	1.31	1.01
Phyllomedusin	0.92	1.18	1.71
Uperolein	1.39	1.40	0.75
Kassinin	NT	1.44	1.84

NT = not tested

which the phenomenon was observed (see Table 2). Also, the sensitivity of the tachykinins to atropine was erratic with respect to both the different peptides and the different preparations (BERTACCINI 1979).

Another important difference was pointed out by JOHNSON and ERDÖS (1973) who found that SP, but not eledoisin, is a very effective releaser of histamine. All these observations of quantitative and qualitative differences in this peptide family suggested that the so-far neglected NH_2 terminal part of these peptides may be of crucial importance for biologic activity, a situation apparently peculiar to the tachykinins. Summing up, early experiments apparently pointed out only the analogies among the different natural tachykinins and suggested that results obtained with one peptide could be extended to the other members of the same peptide family; recent data and the discovery of the importance of the NH_2 terminal part of the tachykinin sequences, support the idea that results obtained with one compound (SP, eledoisin, or physalemin) are valid only for that specific compound and under the particular experimental conditions of the investigation, unless they have been confirmed with all the available tachykinins. Contrasting findings obtained even when using the same peptide may be connected with the different experimental conditions, which may be of fundamental importance for the results obtained, since even slight differences may, in extreme cases, lead to opposite results.

2. Antagonists

A specific antagonist to SP has not yet been found, despite much research in this field. Most of the data available, however, refer to impure preparations of the peptide. Also, among the synthetic analogs of eledoisin and physalemin, no peptide endowed with specific antagonistic properties has been found, even among compounds completely devoid of stimulant activity. Therefore, it is at present virtually impossible to predict modifications which might lead to an antagonist. Apparently the only means of antagonizing SP is by repeated exposure of guinea pig ileum to large concentrations of SP, producing tachyphylaxis. In this connection it was found that, while SP (7.5×10^{-8} *M*) inhibited its own response, it had no effect on other muscle and neuronal receptors and did not change the responses to carbachol (10^{-7} *M*), dimethylpiperazinium (2×10^{-6} *M*), and 5-hydroxytryptamine

(10^{-6} *M*; COSTA et al. 1978; FRANCO et al. 1979). Moreover, "crossed tachyphylaxis" was observed among some tachykinins but not between SP and bradykinin or kallidin (LEMBECK and FISCHER 1967). BURY and MASHFORD (1976a) reported that the spasmogenic effect of SP on the guinea pig ileum was less susceptible to attenuation in the presence of tertiary amine local anesthetics than were the responses to acetylcholine, histamine, or barium chloride. The investigators suggested that different and more efficient channels for calcium entry into the smooth muscle cells are involved in the mechanism of contraction elicited by SP. The same authors (BURY and MASHFORD 1976b) reported nonspecific inhibition of SP-induced contractions by both 5-HT and some 5-HT antagonists. Phenoxybenzamine also inhibited SP nonspecifically (BURY and MASHFORD 1977a).

As for the opiate receptors which might be involved in some actions of SP according to DAVIES and DRAY (1977), it was shown that both naloxone ($\leqq 15$ µ*M*) and the opiate receptor agonists (morphine, codeine, and pethidine, $\leqq 20$ µ*M*) were absolutely ineffective in altering SP-induced contraction of the guinea pig ileum (ELLIOTT and GLEN 1978). CHIPKIN and STEWART (1978) also demonstrated that the action of SP on the guinea pig ileum is unaffected by stimulation (with morphine or enkephalins, in amounts of 3,000 and 1,500 n*M* respectively) or inhibition (with naloxone 5×10^{-9} *M*) of opiate receptors, and suggested that the receptors for SP and the opiate receptors are separate entities.

Presumably, earlier studies showing interaction of SP and morphine in the gut were biased by both impure SP extracts and the lack of such specific antagonists as naloxone. Of course, the possibility of a certain interaction, based on opposite presynaptic inhibitory effects of opiates, which decrease acetylcholine release, and a postsynaptic stimulant action of SP on intestinal muscle, cannot be totally excluded. Tetrodotoxin (1 µmol/l) and indomethacine (11 µmol/l) also had no effect on SP-induced contractions, thus excluding a participation of neural pathways and prostaglandins in the mode of action of SP. Potentiation of responses to SP in the guinea pig ileum were observed in the presence of lysergide and also of metoclopramide (6×10^{-6} *M*), but they both were found to be nonspecific in nature (BURY and MASHFORD 1976b). The same was true for potentiation by hexamethonium (BURY and MASHFORD 1977a, b). In a recent study dealing with the "affinity" and "intrinsic efficacy" of SP, OEHME et al. (1977) reported that the sequence–activity relationship for SP sequences is different in the normal guinea pig ileum compared with a desensitized preparation; this latter condition appears to be similar to the situation in the rat colon. The authors claim that the so-called spare receptors for SP are available only in the guinea pig ileum and are eliminated after desensitization. In the same study, the differences in the response to SP of guinea pig ileum and rat colon were emphasized by using verapamil (a Ca^{2+} antagonist), which apparently had a much stronger inhibitory effect on the SP-induced contraction in the guinea pig.

II. In Vivo Studies

The early experiments performed in vivo were described by PERNOW (1963) and concern rabbits and humans treated with purified SP extracts (30–50 U/min, i.v., in humans). Studies performed with a cineroentgenographic technique confirmed

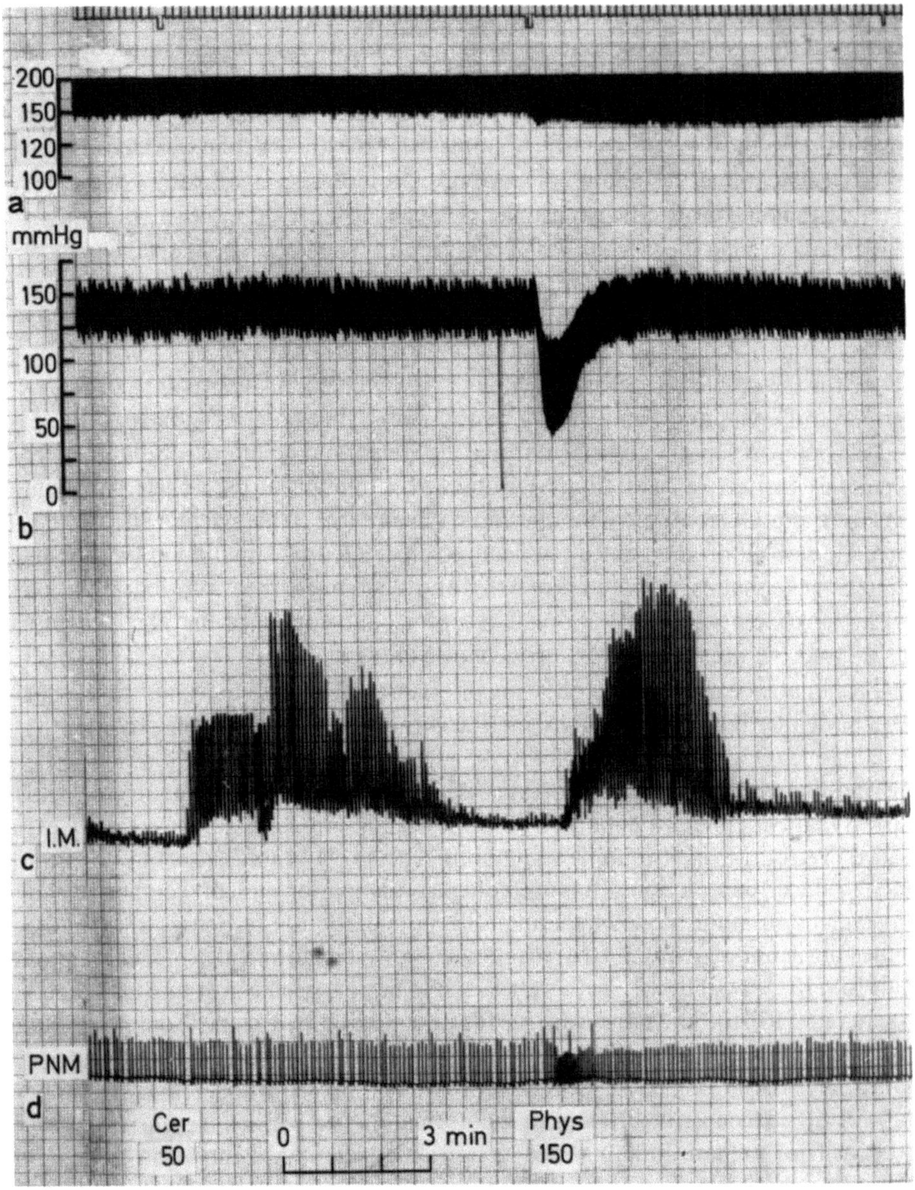

Fig. 3 a–d. Effect of physalemin on canine intestinal motility. Traces show tachogram **a**; arterial pressure **b**; ileal motility **c**; pneumogram **d**. *Cer*, cerulein; *Phys*, physalemin. Doses in ng/kg i.v. (BERTACCINI et al. 1970)

the in vitro data about the effects of SP on peristalsis. In patients with paralytic ileus, SP (total i.v. amounts of 1,000 U) induced both segmental movements and peristaltic activity, which ceased at the end of the infusion.

Later studies were performed with synthetic SP and synthetic tachykinins. In anesthetized cats and rabbits, eledoisin was found to exert a remarkable stimulant

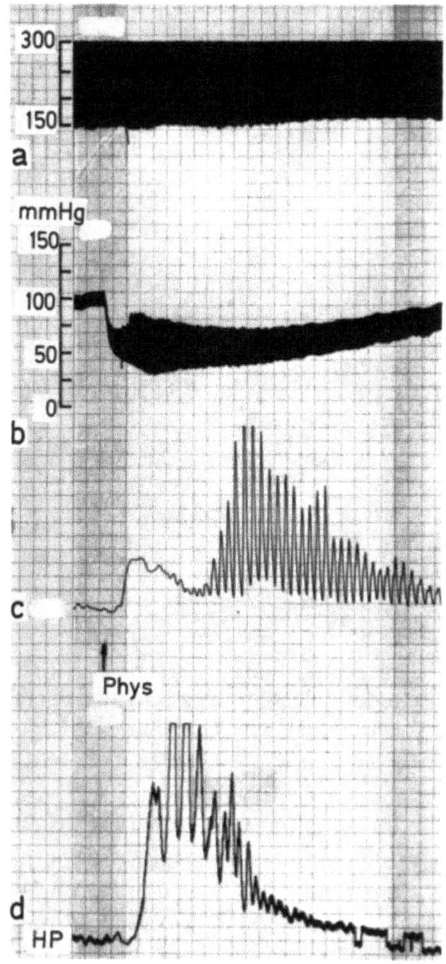

Fig. 4 a–d. Effect of physalemin on canine gastric and intestinal motility. Order of traces is the same as in Fig. 3. *HP*, Heidenhain pouch, *Phys*, physalemin in µg/kg i.v. Note the striking response on the tonus of the denervated gastric fundic pouch and the more prolonged ileal response. (G. BERTACCINI unpublished work 1973)

activity in the ileum which was not preceded (in contrast to bradykinin and kallidin) by an inhibitory phase (WINKLER et al. 1965). In conscious dogs, eledoisin (10–100 µg/kg s.c.) and physalemin (0.5–3 µg/kg i.v. or 30–300 µg/kg s.c.) caused a dose-related stimulation of the gastrointestinal tract with vomiting and evacuation of formed or watery stools. Recovery was relatively rapid and symptoms disappeared within 20–120 min, according to the dose and the route of administration (ERSPAMER and FALCONIERI ERSPAMER 1962; BERTACCINI et al. 1965 a). An example of the intestinal and gastric stimulation caused by physalemin in an anesthetized dog is shown in Figs. 3, 4. In experiments in conscious dogs (MILENOV et al. 1978 b), synthetic SP, in doses of 5–20 ng/kg, i.v., stimulated tonic activity of the stomach, decreasing or suppressing at the same time the "starvational peristaltic contrac-

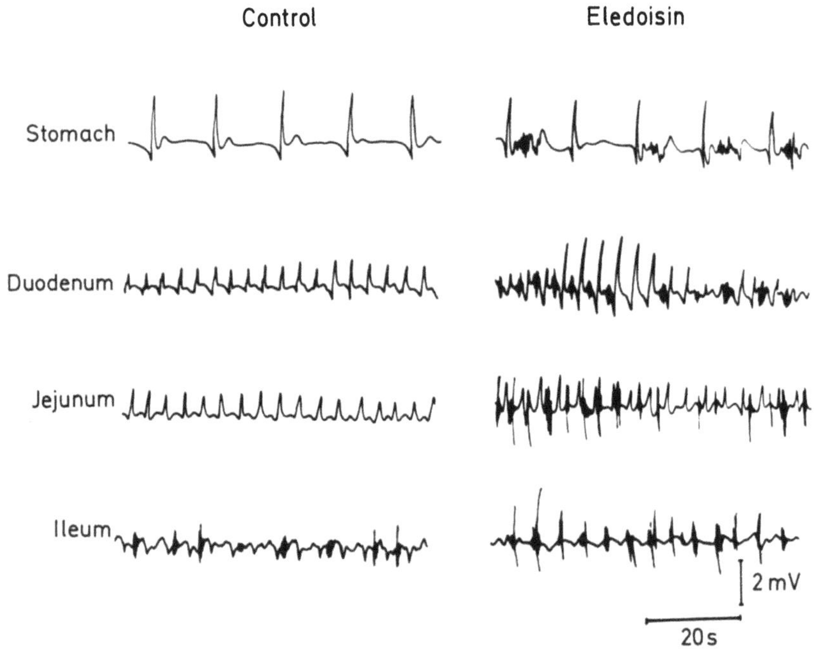

Fig. 5. Effect of eledoisin on electrical activity recorded in an unanesthesized dog with chronically implanted electrodes. Intense spiking activity occurs from the stomach to the ileum during the infusion of eledoisin (10 ng kg^{-1} min^{-1}). (R. CAPRILLI unpublished work 1975)

tion." In the ileum, the doses required to elicit obvious effects were higher (15–100 ng/kg i.v.). Again, mechanograms revealed tonic contractions followed by an increase in basal tonus. Apparently, the lower doses (15 ng/kg) triggered peristaltic contractions and the higher doses (100 ng/kg) reduced both their amplitude and their frequency.

Interesting results were also obtained with eledoisin and physalemin (CAPRILLI et al. 1976) which in low doses behaved like SP, but in high doses caused the appearance of diffuse spike activity, accompanied by intense local motor activity (Fig. 5). Pacemaker potentials were never affected. Atropine (0.1 mg/kg) left these mechanical effects of SP virtually unaffected. In the same experiments, SP also modified in a dose-dependent manner the myoelectric activity of the stomach and the ileum; spike discharges were markedly stimulated by SP, which also stimulated the propagation velocity of the basic electrical rhythm (BER), both in the stomach and in the small intestine. Mechanical and electrical changes appeared soon after administration of the peptide and vanished within 5 min. The authors suggested that the main effect of SP is a reinforcement of muscle wall contractions and that the peptide is a physiologic modulator of smooth muscle activity.

In the anesthetized cat, intra-arterial administration of SP (0.5, 1, 2, and 4 µg) caused prompt, powerful contractions of the stomach and the pylorus of about 5 min duration. Surprisingly these motor effects of SP were blocked by atropine (0.5 mg/kg i.v.) in contrast to most in vitro studies (EDIN et al. 1980). It is possible that effects of SP observed in these experimental conditions involve the activation of excitatory cholinergic neurons, presumably located in the intramural plexuses.

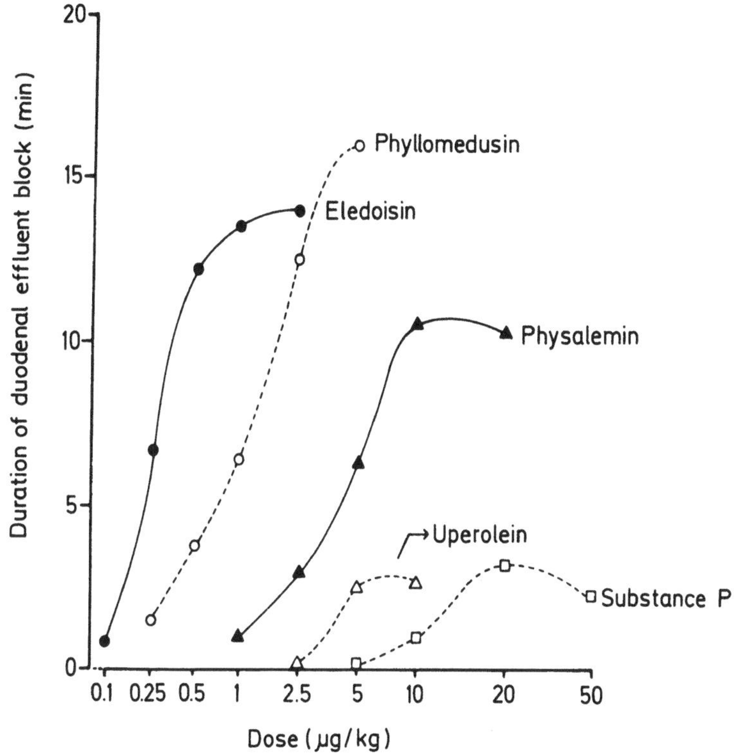

Fig. 6. Spasmogenic effect of substance P and its natural analogs on the pylorus of the anesthesized rat. Mean values from 4–8 experiments. (BERTACCINI and CORUZZI 1977)

In experiments performed with the in situ stomach of the anesthetized rat, BERTACCINI and CORUZZI (1977) found that SP and its natural analogs are endowed with a potent dose-related spasmogenic effect directly on the smooth muscle; not even the Ca^{2+}-antagonizing coumpound, verapamil, at the maximum doses tolerated, modified the action of the peptides. SP and related compounds acted on both the gastric body and the gastroduodenal junction (Fig. 6) and in this respect behaved like bombesin (BERTACCINI and IMPICCIATORE 1975) and not like cerulein and its analogs (BERTACCINI et al. 1973), which have been shown to affect only pyloric motility. Eledoisin appeared to be the most potent peptide in terms of threshold spasmogenic dose (0.1–1 μg/kg), SP was the least potent (threshold dose 5–10 μg/kg) and phyllomedusin appeared to be the most effective peptide in duration of the spasmogenic effect (20 min compared with a maximum of 18 min obtained with eledoisin and physalemin). We could not state, on the basis of our experiments, whether this parameter reflected a stronger binding capacity of phyllomedusin to the receptor sites or only a slower degree of metabolism. As a consequence of the contraction of the pylorus, the tachykinins delayed gastric emptying in the conscious rat. Phyllomedusin and physalemin were the most effective peptides, followed by uperolein and eledoisin; kassinin and SP were virtually inactive, suggesting that pylorus contraction was the main factor regulating gastric emptying in the rat (BERTACCINI et al. 1981).

Other interesting in vivo experiments have been reported quite recently on the action of SP on the lower esophageal sphincter (LES) of the opossum (MUKHOPADHYAY 1978). SP, administered intravenously (5–100 ng/kg) stimulated LES contraction from 16% to 169% above control values. No inhibitor affected the SP-induced LES contraction except atropine (40–500 μg/kg), which significantly but partially inhibited this contracting effect. Thus, the potent stimulant action on the LES seems to involve both cholinergic muscarinic and noncholinergic mechanisms. It is conceivable that SP may be a modulator of LES pressure, although the precise physiologic significance is not clear at present.

In the veterinary field, interesting experiments have been performed, by FAUSTINI's group, with cattle bowel strips in vitro, and on the anesthetized sheep (ORMAS et al. 1975, 1977; FAUSTINI et al. 1979). The authors obtained interesting results by using eledoisin and SP for their stimulatory activities on the forestomachs and the abomasum as well as on the intestine of ruminants. In the in vitro preparations, eledoisin exerted a stimulant action on all the different segments examined (reticulum–omasal sphincter, reticulum, omasum, rumen, abomasum, duodenum, jejunum, ileum, and colon). Maximum sensitivity was shown by abomasum, reticulum, and rumen (threshold stimulatory doses 2–20 ng/ml). The action of eledoisin was qualitatively identical to that of SP but it was 3–20 times as effective in the stomachs. It consisted of reinforcement of the tonic contractions and increase of the amplitude of phasic movements. In the segments which did not show spontaneous activity, both peptides caused the appearance of contractions, with a satisfactory dose–response relationship.

The action of the peptides appeared to be a direct one. In the in vivo experiments, eledoisin administered intravenously (25–100 ng/kg) stimulated the motility of all the segments examined, from the reticulum to the ileum; by contrast the large intestine was not affected by the peptide. In the reticulum, eledoisin was able to excite the rhythmic motility when it was naturally absent in response to fasting of the animals or previous pharmacologic blockade. A similar effect with SP was evident only with doses 20–30 times greater and was not consistently obtained. The effect of eledoisin appeared promptly and lasted for 5–10 min, then a complete return to basal levels of motility was noted. Among all the various antagonists tested, only dihydroergotamine (0.2 mg/kg) caused a considerable reduction in the stimulating effect of eledoisin on the duodenum and ileum, while propranolol (2.5 mg/kg) produced a potentiation in the duodenum. The authors, taking into account that in the ruminants eledoisin is devoid of any effect on the cardiovascular system, claim that the peptide may prove to be a valuable new therapeutic agent for the treatment of forestomach atonia, a frequent occurrence in ruminants.

D. Conclusions

All the findings reported raise the fundamental question of whether or not SP is involved in the regulation of peristalsis. The lack of direct action in vitro on the isolated circular muscle layer observed in some experiments is not necessarily inconsistent with a stimulatory effect of SP on peristalsis in the more complex situation in intact animals, where coordinated activity of the longitudinal and circular muscle layers is achieved through the nerve plexuses. Moreover, subsequent studies showed that by changing experimental conditions SP and its natural analogs are indeed capable of contracting the circular muscle layer. Also, in vitro studies often suggested contrasting effects; atropine, morphine, or neostigmine, in doses which had an obvious effect on peristalsis, were shown to have no effect on the SP content of the rat small intestine (LEMBECK and ZETLER 1962; FISCHER and GUTTMANN 1967). Similar results were obtained in the rabbit when atropine, reserpine, nicotine, and chlorpromazine were applied (RADMANOVIC 1964). Also in the rabbit, some cholinesterase inhibitors have been found to reduce intestinal SP concentrations, while hemicolinium apparently increased them (RADMANOVIC and RAKIC 1969). Evacuation of formed or watery stools, accompanied by more-or-less pronounced salivation and vomiting (depending on the dose employed) were observed in the dog after administration of SP or eledoisin or physalemin (ERSPAMER and FALCONIERI-ERSPAMER 1962; BERTACCINI et al. 1965a).

More recently, CUNHA MELO et al. (1973) suggested that the increased peristalsis induced in the rat by a purified scorpion toxin may be mediated partially by SP, since its effect was only partially inhibited by atropine. Other evidence in support of the theory that SP may be an essential stimulating factor for gut motility came from experiments in humans, showing for instance, that the amount of SP in intestinal segments was increased when motility was stimulated by the administration of hypertonic glucose. In addition, in patients with Hirschsprung's disease, the proximal hyperactive intestinal segments were shown to contain more SP than the controls, whereas the aganglionic, inactive colonic segments contained much less (TAFURI et al. 1974). In Chagas' disease, contrasting findings have been reported. Despite the reduction of the ganglion cells and nerve plexuses in the colonic and esophageal wall, HIAL et al. (1973) found no decrease of SP content in nine megaesophagus and five megacolon specimens. In subsequent very recent studies, LONG et al. (1980) found in rectal biopsy specimens from patients with Chagas' disease that the content of SP (together with that of vasoactive intestinal peptide and somatostatin) was considerably reduced (about 50%) in comparison with that of normal subjects. SP is also one of the substances which can be added to the list of possible mediators of the carcinoid syndrome.

In conclusion, though there are many data which apparently suggest a physiologic role for SP in the regulation of intestinal movements, these pieces of evidence are at present far from conclusive as to the definite function of the peptide in normal peristalsis.

References

Anastasi A, Montecucchi P, Erspamer V, Visser J (1977) Amino acid composition and sequence of kassinin, a tachykinin dodecapeptide from the skin of the African frog *Kassina senegalensis*. Experientia 33:857–858

Beleslin DB (1969) The action of eledoisin on the peristaltic reflex of guinea-pig isolated ileum. Br J Pharmacol 37:234–244

Beleslin DB, Samardzic R (1976) Observations on the ganglionic and neuromuscular blocking action of calcium in the guinea pig isolated ileum. Neuropharmacology 15:565–569

Bennett A (1975) Pharmacology of colonic muscle. Gut 16:307–311

Bertaccini G (1976) Active polypeptides of nonmammalian origin. Pharmacol Rev 28:127–177
Bertaccini G (1977) Action of substance P and some natural analogues on gastro-intestinal motility. In: Abstracts Joint Meeting of German and Italian Pharmacologists, Venezia, p 95
Bertaccini G (1979) Peptides from amphibian skin: mechanism of action on gastrointestinal motility. In: Rosselin G, Fromageot P, Bonfils S (eds) Hormone receptors in digestion and nutrition. Elsevier/North Holland, Amsterdam Oxford New York, pp 431–436
Bertaccini G (1980) Peptides of the amphibian skin active on the gut. I. Tachykinins (substance P-like peptides) and ceruleins. Isolation, structure, and basic functions. In: Jerzy Glass GB (ed) Gastrointestinal hormones. Raven, New York, pp 315–341
Bertaccini G, Coruzzi G (1977) Action of some natural peptides on the stomach of the anaesthetized rat. Naunyn Schmiedebergs Arch Pharmacol 298:163–166
Bertaccini G, Coruzzi G (1980) Action of substance P and its natural analogs on rat LES "in vitro." Ital J Gastroenterol 12:189–192
Bertaccini G, Impicciatore M (1975) Action of bombesin on the motility of the stomach. Naunyn Schmiedebergs Arch Pharmacol 289:149–156
Bertaccini G, Zappia L (to be published) Action of substance P and its natural analogs on the circular muscle of the guinea pig ileum Peptides 2 (Suppl. 2) 1981
Bertaccini G, Cei JM, Erspamer V (1965a) Occurrence of physalaemin in extracts of the skin of *Physalaemus Fuscumaculatus* and its pharmacological actions on extravascular smooth muscle. Br J Pharmacol 25:363–379
Bertaccini G, Cei JM, Erspamer V (1965b) The action of physalaemin on the systemic arterial blood pressure of some experimental animals. Br J Pharmacol 25:380–391
Bertaccini G, Mantovani P, Piccinin GL (1970) Activity ratio between intestinal and cardiovascular actions of caerulein and related substances in the anaesthetized dog. In: Sicuteri F, Rocha e Silva M, Back N (eds) Bradykinin and related kinins. Plenum, New York London, pp 213–220
Bertaccini G, Impicciatore M, De Caro G (1973) Action of caerulein and related substances on the pyloric sphincter of the anaesthetized rat. Eur J Pharmacol 22:320–324
Bertaccini G, De Castiglione R, Scarpignato C (1981) Effects of substance P and its natural analogues on gastric emptying in the conscious rat. Br J Pharmacol 12:221–223
Brownlee G, Harry J (1963) Some pharmacological properties of the circular and longitudinal muscle strips from the guinea-pig isolated ileum. Br J Pharmacol 21:544–554
Bury RW, Mashford ML (1976a) Interactions between local anesthetics and spasmogens on the guinea-pig ileum. J Pharmacol Exp Ther 197:633–640
Bury RW, Mashford ML (1976b) The effects of metoclopramide in modifying the response of isolated guinea-pig ileum to various agonists. J Pharmacol Exp Ter 197:641–646
Bury RW, Mashford ML (1977a) A pharmacological investigation of synthetic substance P on the isolated guinea-pig ileum. Clin Exp Pharmacol Physiol 4:453–461
Bury RW, Mashford ML (1977b) Substance P: its pharmacology and physiologic roles. Aust J Exp Biol Med Sci 55:671–735
Caprilli R, Frieri G, Palla R, Broccardo M (1976) Effects of eledoisin on gastrointestinal electrical activity. In: Smooth muscle. Abstr Int Symp on Physiol Pharmacol, Varna, p 12
Chang MM, Leeman SE, Niall HD (1971) Amino-acid sequence of substance P. Nature New Biol 232:86–87
Chipkin RE, Stewart JM (1978) Substance P and opioid interaction on stimulated and nonstimulated guinea pig ileum. Eur J Pharmacol 53:21–27
Chipkin RE, Stewart JM, Sweeney VE, Harris K, Williams R (1979) *In vitro* activities of some synthetic substance P analogs. Arch Int Pharmacodyn Ther 240:193–202
Costa M, Franco R, Furness JB (1978) The effect of substance P on intestinal nerves and muscle (Abstr 310). 7th Int Congr Pharmacol Paris, July 16–21, p 129
Couture R, Furnier A, Magnan J, St Pierre S, Regoli D (1979) Structure-activity studies on substance P. Can J Physiol Pharmacol 57:1427–1436
Cunha Melo JR, Freire-Maia L, Tafuri WL, Maria TA (1973) Mechanism of action of purified scorpion toxin on the isolated rat intestine. Toxicon 11:81–84

Davies J, Dray A (1977) Substance P and opiate receptors. Nature 268:351–352
De Castiglione R (1978) Tachichinine: rapporto struttura-attività. In: Abstr 19th Congr Ital Pharmacol Soc, Sept 24–27, Ancona, pp 168–169
Edin R, Lundberg JM, Lidberg P, Dahlström A, Ahlman H (1980) Atropine sensitive contractile motor effects of substance P on the feline pylorus and stomach in vivo. Acta Physiol Scand 110:207–209
Elliott JM, Glen JB (1978) The effects of some analgesic and neuroleptic drugs on the spasmogenic actions of substance P on guinea-pig ileum. J Pharm Pharmacol 30:578–579
Erspamer V, Falconieri Erspamer G (1962) Pharmacological actions of eledoisin on extravascular smooth muscle. Br J Pharmacol 19:337–354
Erspamer V, Negri L, Falconieri Erspamer G, Endean R (1975) Uperolein and other active peptides in the skin of the Australian leptodactylid frogs *Uperoleia* and *Taudactylus*. Naunyn Schmiedebergs Arch Pharmacol 289:41–54
Falconieri Erspamer G, Erspamer V, Piccinelli D (1980) Parallel bioassay of physalaemin and kassinin, a tachykinin dodecapeptide from the skin of the African frog *Kassina senegalensis*. Naunyn Schmiedebergs Arch Pharmacol 311:61–65
Faulk D, Anuras S, Christensen J (1977) The two muscle layers in duodenum differ in response to parasympathomimetic drugs, histamine, and substance P. Gastroenterology 72:A1057
Faustini R, Ormas P, Galbiati A, Beretta C (1979) Tachykinins and forestomachs. 1st Congr Eur Assoc Vet Pharmacol and Toxicol (E.A.V.P.T.), Utrecht, Sept 25–28
Fischer G, Guttmann B (1967) Beeinflussung des Substanz-P-Gehaltes des Darmes unter verschiedenen experimentellen Bedingungen. Z Biol 115:452–457
Fontaine J, Famaey JP, Reuse J (1977) Enhancement by physalaemin of the contractions induced by cholinomimetics in the guinea-pig ileum. J Pharm Pharmacol 29:449–450
Fontaine J, Van Nueten JM, Reuse J (1978) The action of physalaemin on the peristaltic reflex of guinea-pig isolated ileum. J Pharm Pharmacol 30:183–185
Franco R, Costa M, Furness JB (1979) Evidence that axons containing substance P in the guinea-pig ileum are of intrinsic origin. Naunyn Schmiedebergs Arch Pharmacol 307:57–63
Hedqvist P, Von Euler US (1975) Influence of substance P on the response of guinea pig ileum to transmural nerve stimulation. Acta Physiol Scand 95:341–343
Hial W, Diniz CR, Pittella JEH, Tafuri NL (1973) Quantitative study of P substance in the megaesophagus and megacolon of human *Trypanosoma cruzi* infections. J Trop Med Hyg 76:175–179
Holzer P, Lembeck F (1979) Effect of neuropeptides on the efficiency of the peristaltic reflex. Naunyn Schmiedebergs Arch Pharmacol 307:257–264
Holzer P, Lembeck F (1980) Neurally mediated contraction of ileal longitudinal muscle by substance P. Neurosci Lett 17:101–105
Johnson AR, Erdös EG (1973) Release of histamine from mast cells by vasoactive peptides. Proc Soc Exp Biol Med 142:1252–1256
Katayama Y, North RA (1978) Does substance P mediate slow synaptic excitation within the myenteric plexus? Nature 274:387–388
Kitagawa K, Ujita K, Kiso Y et al. (1979) Synthesis and activity of C-terminal heptapeptides of tachykinins and bombesin-like peptides. Chem Pharm Bull (Tokyo) 27:48–57
Kosterlitz HW, Robinson JA (1956) The effects of lowering the bath temperature on the responses of the isolated guinea-pig ileum. J Physiol (Lond) 131:7P–8P
Lazarus LH, Linnoila RI, Hernandez O, Di Augustine RP (1980) A neuropeptide in mammalian tissues with physalaemin-like immunoreactivity. Nature 287:555–558
Lembeck F, Fischer G (1967) Gekreuzte Tachyphylaxie von Peptiden. Naunyn Schmiedebergs Arch Pharmakol Exp Pathol 258:452–456
Lembeck F, Zetler G (1962) Substance P: a polypeptide of possible physiological significance, especially within the nervous system. Int Rev Neurobiol 4:159–215
Long RG, Bishop AE, Barnes AJ et al. (1980) Neural and hormonal peptides in rectal biopsy specimens from patients with Chagas' disease and chronic autonomic failure. Lancet 1:559–562

Meinardi H, Craig LC (1966) Studies of substance P. In: Erdös EG, Back N, Sicuteri F, Wilde AF (eds) Hypotensive peptides. Springer, Berlin Heidelberg New York, pp 594–606
Milenov K, Nieber K, Oehme P (1978a) A selective tonic activation of gastrointestinal smooth muscle by substance P. Arch Int Pharmacodyn Ther 235:219–229
Milenov K, Oehme P, Bienert M, Bergmann J (1978b) Effect of substance P on mechanical and myoelectrical activities of stomach and small intestines in conscious dog. Arch Int Pharmacodyn Ther 233:251–260
Mukhopadhyay AK (1978) Effect of substance P on the lower esophageal sphincter of the opossum. Gastroenterology 75:278–282
Nilsson G, Brodin E (1977) Tissue distribution of substance P-like immunoreactivity in dog, cat, rat, and mouse. In: Von Euler US, Pernow B (eds) Substance P. Raven, New York, pp 49–54
Nilsson G, Pernow B, Fisher GH, Folkers K (1975) Presence of substance P-like immunoreactivity in plasma from man and dog. Acta Physiol Scand 94:542–544
Oehme P, Bergmann J, Müller HG, Grupe R, Niedrich H, Vogt WE, Jung F (1972) Zur Pharmakologie von Hydrazinokarbonsäuren, Hydrazinopeptiden und andern Hydrazinderivaten. 9. Mitteilung: Untersuchungen zu Beziehungen zwischen biologischer Wirksamkeit und Struktur an heterologen Eledoisin- Penta- Hexa- und Oktapeptid-Sequenzen. Acta Biol Med Ger 28:121–131
Oehme P, Bergmann J, Bienert M, Hilse H, Piesche L, Minh Thu P, Scheer E (1977) Biological action of substance P: its differentiation by affinity and intrinsic efficacy. In: Von Euler US; Pernow B (eds) Substance P. Raven, New York, pp 327–335
Ormas P, Beretta C, Villalobos SJ, Pompa G, Andreini GC, Beretta C Jr, Faustini R (1975) Some effects of eledoisin on ruminant's reticular, omasal, ruminal and abomasal smooth muscles *in vitro* and *in vivo*. Pharmacol Res Commun 7:527–534
Ormas P, Castelli S, Beretta CM, Nilsson I, Galbiati A, Beretta C, Faustini R (1977) The effects of eledoisin on intestinal smooth muscle of ruminants. Folia Vet Lat 7:252–257
Paton WDM, Zar MA (1968) The origin of acetylcholine released from guinea-pig intestine and longitudinal muscle strips. J Physiol (Lond) 194:13–33
Pearse AGE, Polak JM (1975) Immunocytochemical localization of substance P in mammalian intestine. Histochemistry 41:373–375
Pernow B (1963) Pharmacology of substance P. Ann NY Acad Sci 104:393–402
Rackur G, Yamaguchi I, Leban JJ, Bjorkroth U, Rosell S (1979) Synthesis of peptides related to substance P and their activities as agonists and antagonists. Acta Chem Scand [B] 33:375–378
Radmanovic B (1964) Effects of vagotomy, vagus stimulation and various drugs on the substance P content in the small intestine of the rabbit. Acta Physiol Scand 61:272–278
Radmanovic B, Rakic M (1969) The effect of some anticholinesterase agents and of hemicholinium on the amount of substance P in rabbit brain and gut. Experientia 25:623–624
Rosell S, Björkroth U, Chang D et al. (1977) Effects of substance P and analogs on isolated guinea pig ileum. In: Von Euler US, Pernow W (eds) Substance P. Raven, New York, pp 83–88
Skrabanek P, Powell D (1977) Substance P. Annu Res Rev 1:1–181
Tafuri WL, Maria TA, Pittella JEH, Bogliolo L (1974) An electron microscopic study of the Auerbach's plexus and determination of substance P on the colon in Hirschsprung's disease. Virchows Arch [Pathol Anat] 362:41–50
Umrath K, Grallert M (1967) Über nervöse Hemmungssubstanzen der Wirbeltiere und über Wirkungsmechanismen von Psychopharmaka. Z Biol 115:322–364
Von Euler US, Gaddum JH (1931) An unidentified depressor substance in certain tissue extracts. J Physiol (Lond) 72:74–87
Winkler H, Bauer G, Gmeiner R (1965) Zur Wirkung von Bradykinin, Kallidin und Eledoisin auf den Katzen- und Kaninchen-Darm in situ. Naunyn Schmiedebergs Arch Exp Pharmakol Pathol 250:459–468
Yajima H, Sasaki T, Ogawa H, Fujii N, Segawa T, Nakata Y (1978) Studies on peptides, LXXVI[1,2]. Synthesis of kassinin, a new frog skin peptide. Chem Pharm Bull (Tokyo) 26:1231–1235

Yanaihara N, Yanaihara C, Horihashi M, Sato H, Iizuka Y, Hashimoto T, Sakagami M (1977) Substance P analogs: synthesis, biological, and immunological properties. In: Von Euler US; Pernow B (eds) Substance P. Raven, New York, pp 27–33
Yau WM (1978) Effect of Substance P on intestinal muscle. Gastroenterology 74:228–231
Zappia L, Molina E, Sianesi M, Bertaccini G (1978) Effects of natural analogues of substance P on the motility of human gastrointestinal tract *in vitro*. J Pharm Pharmacol 30:593–594
Zetler G (1970) Biologically active peptides (substance P). In: Lajtha A (ed) Handbook of neurochemistry. Plenum, New York, pp 135–148
Zetler G (1979) Antagonism of cholecystokinin-like peptides by opioid peptides, morphine or tetrodotoxin. Eur J Pharmacol 60:67–77
Zséli J, Molina E, Zappia L, Bertaccini G (1977) Action of some natural polypeptides on the longitudinal muscle of the guinea pig ileum. Eur J Pharmacol 43:285–287

Motilin

A. Introduction

Motilin is one of the newest gastrointestinal peptides. It was isolated by BROWN et al. (1971) from extracts of duodenal and jejunal mucosa. Its structure, established by SCHUBERT and BROWN (1974), is as follows:

1 2 3 4 5 6 7 8 9 10 11 12 13 14 15 16
Phe-Val-Pro-Ile-Phe-Thr-Tyr-Gly-Glu-Leu-Gln-Arg-Met-Gln-Glu-Lys-

17 18 19 20 21 22
Glu-Arg-Asn-Lys-Gly-Gln .

The decosapeptide corresponding to natural motilin was synthesized by YAJIMA et al. (1975).

Studies of the structure–activity relationship (WÜNSCH 1976; SEGAWA et al. 1976; ITOH et al. 1978c) revealed that the whole molecule is essential for biologic activity. However, some substitutions in the amino acid sequence can be made without loss of activity (13-Nle-14-desamidomotilin, or 13-Leu-Ldesamidomotilin have the same biologic activity as the natural peptide) or actually with an increase in activity (15-Gln-motilin is about 50% more potent than the natural peptide). As for some synthetic preparations of motilin fragments, motilin 1–6 and motilin 12–22 were found to be completely inactive. A very feeble activity (about $^{1}/_{200}$ of the potency of the entire molecule) was retained by the fragment motilin 7–22.

Motilin is very slightly inactivated by a single passage through the liver, suggesting that there are major sites of motilin metabolism other than in the liver. Motilin release by human duodenal mucosa is stimulated by acid or by bile salts both in vivo and in vitro. This release can be prevented by somatostatin, but not atropine (STRUNZ et al. 1979). It is deemed of interest that a pharmacologic compound, namely metoclopramide, which is known to accelerate gastric emptying (thus increasing acid in the duodenum) was described as a potent releaser of motilin. However the effect of metoclopramide on duodenal motility is apparently independent of motilin release (BORODY et al. 1980a).

B. Effects on Gastrointestinal Motility

I. In Vitro Studies

Extensive investigations concerning the in vitro effects of motilin on gastrointestinal motility (STRUNZ et al. 1975, 1976a, b, 1978; G. BERTACCINI unpublished work 1978) showed that the peptide has different activities in different species: guinea pig and rat preparations proved refractory to 13-Nle-motilin (concentrations up to 10×10^{-6} g/ml were tested), whereas preparations from rabbits and humans were highly sensitive to the peptide. In the rabbit, the order of sensitivity was: duodenum = jejunum > antrum (circular muscle) > colon (circular muscle). Contractile responses occurred in the most sensitive tissues, with threshold doses of 5×10^{-9} g/ml. Strips of stomach corpus and taenia coli were insensitive to motilin (up to 10×10^{-6} g/ml).

The action of motilin seemed to be a direct one on the smooth muscle, since it was unaffected by hexamethonium, tetrodotoxin, atropine, or pheniramine. Only verapamil blocked the spasmogenic effect of the peptide, suggesting a role for 13-Nle-motilin in the transport of Ca^{2+} into the cytosol of intestinal smooth muscle.

Vasoactive intestinal peptide (VIP; 3×10^{-8} *M*), but not secretin (10^{-7} *M*), was able to abolish motilin-induced contractions in rabbit antral muscle. This inhibition was unaffected by the common antagonists but it was counteracted by additional Ca^{+} ions (5.4×10^{-3} *M*). Surprisingly, VIP failed to influence contractions induced by motilin in the duodenum (Fig. 1). 13-Nle-motilin significantly potentiated the effect of acetylcholine on rabbit pyloric muscle. Motilin does not affect synthesis or degradation of acetylcholine from presynaptic sites, and therefore the cholinergic system may be sensitized by an allosteric effect of motilin. This could be the reason for the much greater effect of motilin observed in vivo, in which even subthreshold doses of the peptide may affect cholinergic-driven pyloric motor activity. 13-Nle-motilin was also shown to have no effect on the cyclic AMP content of antral and duodenal muscle from rabbits (SCHUBERT et al. 1975). As already pointed out, the effect of natural porcine motilin was found to be identical to that of the synthetic analog 13-Nle-motilin (STRUNZ et al. 1976b).

Isolated muscle strips taken from the lower esophageal sphincter (LES), fundus, antrum, and duodenum of dogs or pigs were reported to show no effects upon addition of motilin in concentrations of 10^{-15}–10^{-6} g/ml (JENNEWEIN et al. 1976; SEGAWA et al. 1976). However, in a very recent study (FOX et al. 1979) motilin was found to increase tone in the LES circular muscle strips from the opossum in doses as low as about 5 pg/ml. This effect was atropine sensitive. In the same study, motilin was also shown to be released in the LES by field stimulation of nerves as well as muscle and by K^{+} depolarization. Quite recently it was reported that motilin exerts a considerable spasmogenic effect on the isolated LES from rats (threshold

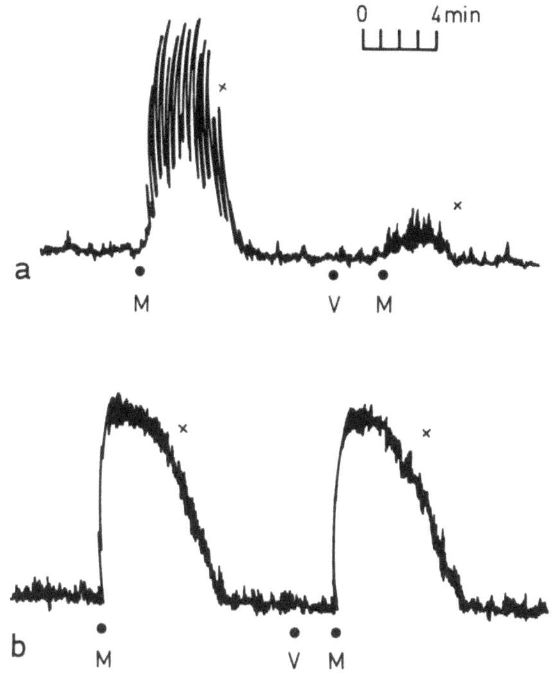

Fig. 1. a Inhibitory effect of VIP (V, 2×10^{-8} *M*) on the contraction induced by motilin (M, 3×10^{-8} *M*) in rabbit circular antral muscle. **b** Lack of inhibitory effect of VIP (V, 2×10^{-7} *M*) on the contraction induced by motilin (M, 2×10^{-7} *M*) on the isolated rabbit duodenum. *Crosses* indicate washout

dose 1.1×10^{-8} *M*) and guinea pigs (threshold dose 3.7×10^{-7} *M*). Tachyphylaxis was a common feature in both preparations, however no attempt was made to investigate the mechanism of action of the peptide (BERTACCINI et al. 1980).

In canine gastric muscle strips, when transmural nerve stimulation (200 μs duration) was used to "activate" the myenteric plexus, motilin markedly increased the excitatory response of the muscle to the nerve stimulation (MORGAN et al. 1979). The effect of motilin was greatest at lower frequencies and when submaximal current intensities were used. Thus motilin is likely to release acetylcholine from myenteric nerve terminals. Of course, this effect is more easily observed in vivo because the myenteric plexus is in an "activated state." These data once again emphasize the importance of the experimental conditions to evaluate correctly the action of an active substance in experiments in vitro.

13-Nle-motilin (10^{-7} g/ml) was found to affect electrical activity of rabbit circular duodenal muscle. The peptide reduced or abolished the typical specific slow waves, stimulated slow fluctuations of membrane potential typical of a minute rhythm and induced the appearance of trains of spikes associated with muscle contractions (RIEMER et al. 1977). Sodium depletion, as well as low temperature reduced the response to motilin whereas ouabain completely blocked it, suggesting that the action of 13-Nle-motilin is in some way associated with electrogenic Na^+ transport (RUPPIN 1977).

13-Nle-motilin (up to 240 pmol/min) was found to have no effect on the peristalsis of the isolated guinea pig ileum (HOLZER and LEMBECK 1979). In contrast to other peptides, motilin seems to affect only the gut muscle, whereas it is inactive on smooth muscle of other than gastrointestinal origin (e.g., uterine or vascular; STRUNZ et al. 1975).

II. In Vivo Studies

1. Action on the Lower Esophageal Sphincter

Whereas, as already said, isolated muscle strips taken from canine LES were unresponsive to motilin, in anesthetized and in conscious dogs, the peptide (10–1,000 ng/kg), given by intravenous injection or infusion, induced phasic contractions of the LES, which however, were considered to be related to the remarkable pressure increase in the stomach (JENNEWEIN et al. 1975, 1976). The effect of motilin was antagonized by atropine and hexamethonium (MEISSNER et al. 1976). Duodenal alkalinization, which is known to represent an effective stimulus for motilin release in the dog (DRYBURGH and BROWN 1975), caused only a slight and not significant LES pressure increase. Results obtained with a different technique in conscious dogs, showed that motilin administered during the interdigestive period (0.3–2.7 μg kg^{-1} h^{-1}) induced a peculiar motor activity which was indistinguishable from the naturally occurring interdigestive contractions in the LES and the stomach (ITOH et al. 1978 a).

The motilin-induced contractions were instantly abolished by ingestion of food and there was a close correlation between the increase in plasma motilin concentration and the LES motor activity during the interdigestive state (AIZAWA et al. 1978 a, b). The authors suggested that motilin controls the motor activity of the LES during the interdigestive phase. Motilin was also shown to stimulate LES contraction in the opossum, being approximately as effective as gastrin; the response was dose dependent (0.05–1 μg/kg, i.v.) and was inhibited by secretin (0.65 U kg^{-1} h^{-1}; GUTIÉRREZ et al. 1977).

Studies performed in humans showed that 13-Nle-motilin caused a dose-related increase in LES pressure; peak values (with maximum pressure exceeding basal levels by 160%) were achieved with 0.2 μg kg^{-1} h^{-1} i.v. infusion and were about one-half of those obtained with 0.6 μg/kg pentagastrin. The LES response to motilin was markedly lessened, though not completely abolished, by concomitant atropine infusion (LUX et al. 1976; RÖSCH et al. 1976). However, contrasting findings were reported as to the physiologic role of motilin in regulating LES motor activity. HELLEMANS et al. (1975, 1976) found quite variable relations between changes in LES pressure and plasma levels of motilin following alkalinization and subsequent acidification of the antrum or duodenum and concluded that a role of endogenous motilin in the regulation of LES activity is either nonexistent or overwhelmed by other influences. ECKARDT and GRACE (1976) were also unable to find any consistent correlation between plasma motilin changes and LES pressure. On other hand, DOMSCHKE et al. (1976) found a good correlation between the increase in plasma motilin following acidification of the duodenum and the increase in LES pressure and suggested a role for this peptide in the intrinsic regulation of the LES.

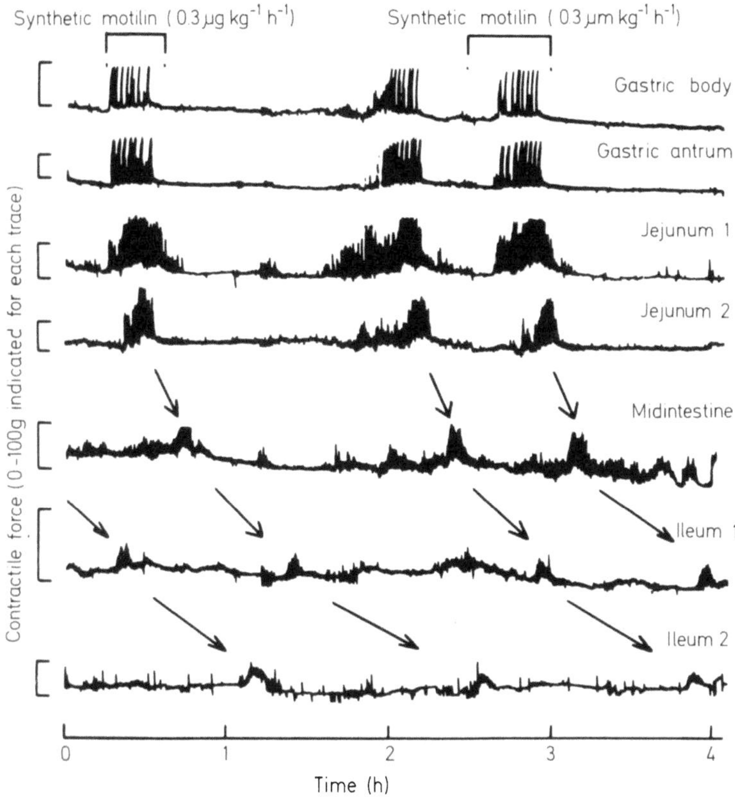

Fig. 2. Effect of i.v. infusion of motilin in a dose of 0.3 μg kg^{-1} h^{-1} during the interdigestive state. Paper speed was adjusted to 1 mm/min to show changes over a 4-h period in one diagram. (ITOH et al. 1976)

It is possible, of course, that these conflicting results reflect differences in measurements which could have been made in different states of motor activity (digestive or interdigestive) or under different conditions of gastric distension (caused by the varying amounts of liquid necessary to acidify or alkalinize), which could affect LES pressure.

2. Action on the Motility of the Stomach and the Intestine

The effect of motilin on the dog stomach was peculiar and differed according to the physiologic condition of the animals. When it was administered in the digestive state it had no effect upon the motor activity, even when doses were increased up to 6 μg kg^{-1} h^{-1}. On the other hand, when motilin was infused, even in low doses (0.3 μg kg^{-1} h^{-1}), during the interdigestive state it induced a motility pattern precisely like the naturally occurring interdigestive contractions (Fig. 2). Moreover, motilin (0.5 μg kg^{-1} h^{-1}), administered 10 min after the termination of naturally occurring contractions during the interdigestive phase, produced contractions similar to those occurring naturally. Increasing the dose of motilin (up to

2.7 μg kg^{-1} h^{-1}) shortened the time necessary for the onset of the reaction (ITOH et al. 1977). The motility pattern was identical to that of "hunger contractions", which in its turn appears to be phase III of the interdigestive migrating myoelectric complex. Motilin-induced contractions and naturally occurring contractions were both inhibited by ingestion of food or an infusion of pentagastrin. In addition, the effect of duodenal acidification, which in the interdigestive state inhibited the regular cycle of the natural contractions, was counteracted by motilin. These findings suggest that interdigestive motor activity is, at least partly, regulated by circulating motilin, which can be considered to be a true interdigestive hormone (ITOH et al. 1975, 1976). During the interdigestive state, it was found that the plasma motilin concentration increased in complete accordance with the cyclic interdigestive contractions of the stomach (ITOH et al. 1978b). These mechanical changes found counterparts in the myoelectric changes (WINGATE et al. 1976; CASTRESANA et al. 1978; LEE et al. 1977, 1978). Whereas the peptide did not change the frequency of slow waves, it produced a dose-related (0.06–0.25 μg/kg i.v.) increase in the incidence of spike potentials on slow waves. The stimulatory effect of motilin was inhibited by secretin (0.25 and 0.5 U/kg) or gastric inhibitory polypeptide (GIP; 0.25 and 0.5 μg/kg).

In the dog, somatostatin was found to delay the onset of the motilin response and to decrease its effect on motor activity in the stomach and the jejunum. Moreover, during somatostatin infusion, the motilin-induced contractions did not migrate to the jejunum (ORMSBEE et al. 1978). WINGATE et al. (1976) actually suggested that motilin interacts with a control center for interdigestive state motor activity by stimulating receptors in the duodenum, which in turn send afferent impulses to the control center. This complex neurohumoral regulation of gastrointestinal motility and, more exactly, the interaction between cholinergic nerves and motilin activity were carefully investigated by ORMSBEE and MIR (1978) in conscious dogs with chronically implanted electrodes placed from the antrum to the jejunum. They found that bolus injections of motilin (100 ng/kg) were followed by a pattern of contractile activity which closely resembled the natural interdigestive burst period.

In other studies performed in the dog, no precise correlation was found between serum motilin levels and duration of gastric contractions (NAKATAKE et al. 1980); gastric contractions were intermittent in spite of continuous infusion of motilin (0.5 μg kg^{-1} h^{-1}). However, serum motilin levels was found to be increased when interdigestive contractions were seen. Intravenous glucose (20% solution 1.2 ml/min) did not influence the interdigestive contractions and thus apparently did not suppress the release of motilin. The motilin-induced burst period appeared to migrate down the length of the small intestine and was abolished by administration of atropine or hexamethonium. Vagotomy significantly influenced neither the interdigestive contractile complexes nor the motilin-induced motor activity. Therefore a preganglionic cholinergic site of action for motilin in the conscious dog with chronically implanted electrodes was suggested. Motilin could, therefore, stimulate preganglionic cholinergic neurons in the myenteric plexus to initiate an interdigestive complex in the stomach and proximal duodenum, as shown by THOMAS et al. (1979a) who were also able to demonstrate that motilin speeded interdigestive motor cycles in transplanted fundic pouches of the dog (THOMAS et al. 1979b). After this, a series of neurohumoral mechanisms could be involved in the migration of the complex. The ileal propagation of the activity front is apparently independent of motilin blood levels (POITRAS et al. 1979).

Motilin antiserum specific for porcine motilin, infused into pigs with an in vivo concentration of 1/2,000, failed to affect the onset of interdigestive myoelectric complexes in the duodenum (BORODY et al. 1980b). From this immunoneutralization study the authors concluded that motilin is not essential for the initiation of migrating myoelectric complexes in the pig. Motilin showed only very feeble, if any, stimulatory activity on the stomach of the anesthetized rat (BERTACCINI and CORUZZI 1977).

The effect of motilin on gastric emptying is controversial and, again, some discrepancies might be explained on the basis of methodological differences or of species differences. DEBAS et al. (1977) found that motilin enhances gastric emptying of liquids in dogs through a stimulant action on the proximal stomach. This result is in accordance with the work of VALENZUELA (1976) who observed a dose-related increase in intragastric pressure after motilin (62–1,000 ng kg^{-1} h^{-1}) administration, whereas RUPPIN et al. (1975) found that 13-Nle-motilin inhibits gastric evacuation of liquids in humans.

In the isolated perfused canine stomach (COOK et al. 1973), it was shown that motilin infusion (5–20 nmol/h) caused a transient slowing of electrical control activity, followed by a return to normal frequencies, along with a substantial increase in response and mechanical activity.

Atropine (0.2 mg/h), but not tetrodotoxin (2 µg/kg) apparently blocked the response to motilin. This again indicated a certain interference between the peptide and the cholinergic system, which, however, seems to be different under the various experimental conditions. In a similar preparation which included the duodenum, the effect of intra-arterial injections of 13-Nle-motilin (40–640 ng) on both intraluminal pressure and myoelectric activity was investigated (GREEN et al. 1976a, b), in a search for an explanation for the effects on gastric emptying. It was found that, whereas pressure changes in the antrum were small and not dose related, a remarkable dose-dependent increase in pressure occurred in the pylorus and in the duodenum, which was twice as sensitive as the pylorus. 13-Nle-motilin decreased the frequency of antral slow waves and disturbed their normal propagation. Conversely, the duodenal slow wave frequency was not altered by motilin which, however, caused a dose-dependent increase in spike activity. Atropine (100 µg/h) completely inhibited the effects of motilin. According to these data, the effect of motilin on gastric emptying in the dog may be explained as being the consequence of a disturbance in the coordination between antral, pyloric, and duodenal motor activity. The difference in the response of the isolated and innervated intestine is again in favor of the hypothesis that motilin interacts with the center controlling interdigestive activity which is extraenteric (RUPPIN et al. 1976c). It is obvious that the experimental conditions play a remarkable role in determining situations which, though interesting from a theoretical point of view, are far from anything considered as physiologic.

According to LEE et al. (1980) the peak increase in plasma motilin concentration coincided with phase III of the interdigestive myoelectric activity (activity front) in the proximal duodenum. Ingestion of a meat meal resulted in a decrease in the plasma motilin level accompanied by phase II-like myoelectric activity of the duodenum (digestive pattern). Changes of plasma motilin were not related to gastrin, cholecystokinin (CCK), or secretin.

Recent studies (Bloom et al. 1978b; Christofides et al. 1979c) showed that in humans, gastric emptying of solids was increased by administration of natural porcine motilin, even in very low doses (0.34–0.6 pmol kg^{-1} min^{-1}), which gave plasma motilin concentrations of the same order of magnitude as those achieved after gastric distension (one of the few natural stimuli known to increase gastric emptying). Even a dose of 0.2 pmol kg^{-1} min^{-1} was able to abolish the initial slow phase of gastric emptying, inducing a significant acceleration in the rate of gastric emptying of glucose (Christofides et al. 1979b). The simultaneous increase of plasma motilin was similar to the normal postprandial increment (Long et al. 1980). However, intraduodenal instillation of 0.1 *M* HCl or ingestion of fat (both of which cause a significant rise in plasma motilin) inhibit gastric emptying, thus suggesting that control of gastric emptying is not primarily dependent on motilin. Rees et al. (1978) demonstrated that interdigestive motor cycles and cyclic release of motilin also occur in achlorhydria (induced by cimetidine): thus entry of gastric acid into the duodenum does not seem to be essential for generation of interdigestive cycles of motor activity.

Other human studies (Vantrappen et al. 1978; Lux et al. 1978, 1979) confirmed that 13-Nle-motilin (0.4 μg kg^{-1} h^{-1}) initiated extra activity similar to the naturally occurring interdigestive complexes within the esophageal body, LES, and stomach; on the whole the effect was similar to that reported in dogs. Motilin i.v. infusions (0.4–6.4 pmol kg^{-1} min^{-1}) induced an activity front in 12 of 16 normal volunteers (Vantrappen et al. 1979). The mean activity front was significantly reduced in comparison with control subjects to 46 min and this was found even at the lowest dose of porcine motilin, producing an increase in plasma levels of the peptide of 57 pmol/l. These results supported the suggestion that a cyclic rise in plasma motilin level is one of the factors involved in producing the activity front in the human migrating myoelectric complex. Human colonic motility was also shown (Rennie et al. 1979) to be affected by motilin; a very low dose (0.16 pmol kg^{-1} min^{-1}) achieving plasma levels similar to those recorded postprandially (Christofides et al. 1979a; Rennie et al. 1980), caused significant increases in the electrical line integral in intraluminal pressure and motility index. Maximal myoelectric and pressure changes correlated with peak motilin levels achieved (62 ± 13 pmol/l). The authors concluded that the peptide may be a factor in the control of gastrocolic reflex. As in the dog, so in humans, a close relationship between motilin plasma levels and interdigestive motor activity was observed; both changes appeared to be controlled by a cholinergic influence since they were abolished by atropine (0.6 mg as a bolus; You et al. 1980).

Though 13-Nle-motilin was shown to cause a marked acceleration of intestinal transit time in humans (a decrease of 50% was observed after 0.4 μg kg^{-1} h^{-1} of the peptide), to induce interdigestive motor complexes, and to stimulate intestinal fluid (Ruppin et al. 1976b, 1979), the same dose of the peptide did not significantly influence the manifestation and duration of postoperative ileus in six female patients (Ruppin et al. 1976a). However, according to a recent report (Bloom et al. 1978a) motilin plasma levels was found to be significantly higher, from

56 pmol/l in control subjects to over 150 pmol/l in patients suffering from diarrhea of various origins. In contrast, patients with constipation had normal levels of motilin. Thus, the peptide may well play a role in the upper gastrointestinal motor changes associated with diarrhea.

C. Conclusions

In conclusion, motilin seems to affect mainly, but not exclusively, the proximal part of the gastrointestinal tract. The peptide has no significant influence upon the gut's contractile activity during the digestive state. Conversely, in the interdigestive state it induces the cyclic recurrent episodes of caudad-moving bands of strong contractions that move from the lower esophageal sphincter to the terminal ileum. Plasma motilin concentrations were shown to fluctuate periodically in complete accordance with occurrence of gastric and jejunal contractions (PEETERS et al. 1979). The definition of "interdigestive hormone" seems to be quite appropriate. Since most of the studies were performed in the dog, further studies on human subjects are needed. So far, diseases due to hypermotilinemia or hypomotilinemia are not known and this of course respresents another limit to our knowledge on the physiologic importance of this gastrointestinal peptide.

References

Aizawa I, Hiwatashi K, Itoh Z (1978a) Physiological role of motilin in the lower esophageal sphincter (Abstr). VIth World Congr Gastroenterol, Madrid, June 5–9, p 37
Aizawa I, Hiwatashi K, Takahashi I, Itoh Z (1978b) Control of motor activity in the lower oesophageal sphincter by motilin. In: Duthie HL (ed) Gastrointestinal motility in health and disease. Lancaster, MTP Press, pp 101–109
Bertaccini G, Coruzzi G (1977) Action of some natural peptides on the stomach of the anaesthetized rat. Naunyn Schmiedebergs Arch Pharmacol 230:163–166
Bertaccini G, Coruzzi G, Scarpignato C (1980) Exogenous and endogenous compounds which affect the contractility of the lower esophageal sphincter (LES). In: Stipa S, Belsey R, Moraldi A (eds) Int Symp Med and Surg Problems of the Esophagus, Rome, May 7–9. Academic Press, New York, pp 22–29
Bloom SR, Christofides ND, Besterman HS (1978a) Raised motilin in diarrhoea. Gut 19:A959
Bloom SR, Christofides ND, Modlin I, Fitzpatrick ML (1978b) Effect of motilin on gastric emptying of solid meals in man. Gastroenterology 74:A1010
Borody T, Byrnes D, Henderson L (1980a) Mechanism of motilin release by metoclopramide. In: Bloom SR, Polak JM (eds) Regulatory peptides, Suppl 1. Elsevier/North-Holland Biomedical. Amsterdam Oxford New York, p S 13a
Borody T, Byrnes D, Slowiaczek J, Titchen D (1980b) Effect of motilin antiserum infusion on porcine idmcs. In: Bloom SR, Polak JM (eds) Regulatory peptides, Suppl 1. Elsevier/North-Holland Biomedical, Amsterdam Oxford New York, p S 13b
Brown JC, Mutt V, Dryburgh JR (1971) The further purification of motilin, a gastric motor activity stimulating polypeptide from the mucosa of the small intestine of dogs. Can J Physiol Pharmacol 49:399–405
Castresana M, Lee KY, Chey WY, Yajima H (1978) Effects of motilin and octapeptide of cholecystokinin on antral and duodenal myoelectric activity in the interdigestive state and during inhibition by secretin and gastric inhibitory polypeptide. Digestion 17:300–308

Christofides ND, Bloom SR, Besterman HS, Adrian TE, Ghatei MA (1979a) Release of motilin by oral and intravenous nutrients in man. Gut 20:102–106
Christofides ND, Long RG, Fitzpatrick ML, Bloom SR (1979b) Motilin increases the rate of gastric emptying of glucose. Gut 20:A924
Christofides ND, Modlin IM, Fitzpatrick ML, Bloom SR (1979c) Effect of motilin on the rate of gastric emptying and gut hormone release during breakfast. Gastroenterology 76:903–907
Cook MA, Kowalewski K, Daniel EE, (1973) Electrical and mechanical activity recorded from the isolated perfused canine stomach: the effects of some G.I. polypeptides. Fourth Int Symp Gastrointest Motility Rend Gastroenterol 5:A136
Debas HT, Yamagishi T, Dryburgh JR (1977) Motilin enhances gastric emptying of liquids in dogs. Gastroenterology 73:777–780
Domschke W, Lux G, Mitznegg P et al. (1976) Relationship of plasma motilin response to lower esophageal sphincter pressure in man. Scand J Gastroenterol [Suppl 39] 11:81–84
Dryburgh JR, Brown JC (1975) Radioimmunoassay for motilin. Gastroenterology 68:1169–1176
Eckardt W, Grace ND (1976) Lower esophageal sphincter pressure and serum motilin levels. Am J Dig Dis 21:1008–1011
Fox JE, Tranck N, Daniel EE (1980) Motilin: its presence and function in muscle layers of the gastrointestinal tract (Abstr 10). In: Christensen J (ed) Gastrointestinal motility. Raven, New York, pp 59–65. Seventh Int Symp Gastrointest Motility, Iowa, Sept 11–14, 1979
Green WER, Ruppin H, Wingate DL, Domschke W, Wünsch E, Demling L, Ritchie HD (1976a) Effect of 13-Nle-motilin on the electrical and mechanical activity of the isolated perfused canine stomach and duodenum. Gut 17:362–370
Green WER, Ruppin H, Wingate DL, Wünsch E (1976b) Direct effects of 13-norleucine-motilin on the electrical and mechanical activity of the isolated perfused canine stomach and duodenum. J Physiol (Lond) 256:48P–49P
Gutiérrez JG, Thanik KD, Chey WY, Yajima H (1977) The effect of motilin on the lower esophageal sphincter of the opossum. Am J Dig Dis 22:402–405
Hellemans J, Vantrappen G, Bloom SR (1975) The hormonal control of lower esophageal sphincter pressure. In: Vantrappen G (ed) Fifth International Symposium on Gastrointestinal Motility. Typoff, Herentals, pp 43–77
Hellemans J, Vantrappen G, Bloom SR (1976) Endogenous motilin and the LES pressure. Scand J Gastroenterol [Suppl 39] 11:67–73
Holzer P, Lembeck F (1979) Effect of neuropeptides on the peristaltic reflex. Naunyn Schmiedebergs Arch Pharmacol [Suppl] 307:R51
Itoh Z, Aizawa I, Takeuchi S, Couch EF (1975) Hunger contractions and motilin. In: Vantrappen G (ed) Fifth International Symposium on Gastrointestinal Motility. Typoff, Herentals, pp 48–55
Itoh Z, Honda R, Hiwatashi K, Takeuchi S, Aizawa I, Takayanagi R, Couch EF (1976) Motilin-induced mechanical activity in the canine alimentary tract. Scand J Gastroenterol [Suppl 39] 11:93–110
Itoh Z, Takeuchi S, Aizawa I, Takayanagi R (1977) Effect of synthetic motilin on gastric motor activity in conscious dogs. Am J Dig Dis 22:813–819
Itoh Z, Aizawa I, Honda R, Katsutoshi H, Hiwatashi K, Couch EF (1978a) Control of lower-esophageal-sphincter contractile activity by motilin in conscious dogs. Am J Dig Dis 23:341–345
Itoh Z, Takeuchi S, Aizawa I et al. (1978b) Changes in plasma motilin contraction and gastrointestinal contractile activity in conscious dogs. Am J Dig Dis 23:929–935
Itoh Z, Takeuchi S, Aizawa I et al. (1978c) Recent advances in motilin research: its physiological and clinical significance. In: Grossman M, Speranza V, Basso N, Lezoche E (eds) Gastrointestinal hormones and pathology of the digestive system. Plenum, New York, pp 241–257
Jennewein HM, Hummelt H, Siewert R, Waldeck F (1975) The motor-stimulating effect of natural motilin and the lower esophageal sphincter, fundus, antrum, and duodenum in dogs. Digestion 13:246–250

Jennewein HM, Bauer R, Hummelt H, Lepsin G, Siewert R, Waldeck F (1976) Motilin effects on gastrointestinal motility and esophageal sphincter (LES) pressure in dogs. Scand J Gastroenterol [Suppl 39] 11:63–65
Lee KY, Chey WY, Tai HH, Wagner D, Yajima H (1977) Cyclic changes in plasma motilin levels and interdigestive myoelectric activity of canine antrum and duodenum. Gastroenterology 72:A139/1162
Lee KY, Chey WY, Tai HH, Yajima H (1978) Radioimmunoassay of motilin: validation and studies on the relationship between plasma motilin and interdigestive myoelectric activity of the duodenum of dog. Am J Dig Dis 23:789–795
Lee KY, Kim MS, Chey WY (1980) Effects of a meal and gut hormones on plasma motilin and duodenal motility in dog. Am J Physiol 238:G280–G283
Long RG, Christofides ND, Fitzpatrick ML, Mitchenere P, Bloom SR (1980) Somatostatin and motilin increase the rate of gastric emptying of glucose. Eur J Clin Invest 10:23
Lux G, Rösch W, Domschke S, Domschke W, Wünsch E, Jaeger E, Demling L (1976) Intravenous 13-Nle-motilin increases the human lower esophageal sphincter pressure. Scand J Gastroenterol [Suppl 39] 11:75–79
Lux G, Strunz U, Domschke S, Femppel J, Rösch W, Domschke W (1978) 13-Nle-motilin and interdigestive motor and electrical activity of human small intestine. Gastroenterology 74:A1058
Lux G, Lederer P, Femppel J, Rosch W, Domschke W (1980) Spontaneous and 13-Nle-motilin-induced interdigestive motor activity of esophagus, stomach, and small intestine in man (Abstr 45). In: Christensen J (ed) Gastrointestinal motility. Raven, New York, p 219. Seventh Int Symp Gastrointest Motility, Iowa, Sept 11–14, 1979
Meissner AJ, Bowes KL, Zwick R, Daniel EE (1976) Effect of motilin on the lower esophageal sphincter. Gut 17:925–932
Morgan KG, Go VLW, Szurszewski JH (1980) Motilin increases the influence of excitatory myoenteric plexus neurons on gastric smooth muscle in vitro (Abstr 19). In: Christensen J (ed) Gastrointestinal motility. Seventh Int Symp Gastrointest Motility, Iowa, Sept 11–14, 1979. Raven, New York, p 28
Nakatake N, Noda H, Takamine Y, Mori T, Nagamine S, Tobe T, Yajima H (1980) Release of motilin and interdigestive gastric contractions in dog. Abstracts XI th Int Congr Gastroenterol Hamburg, June 8–13, pp E10–E11
Ormsbee HS, Mir SS (1978) The role of the cholinergic nervous system in the gastrointestinal response to motilin *in vivo*. In: Duthie HL (ed) Gastrointestinal motility in health and disease. MTP Press, Lancaster, pp 113–122
Ormsbee HS, Hoehler SL, Telford GL (1978) Somatostatin inhibits motilin-induced interdigestive contractile activity in the dog. Dig Dis Sci 23:781–788
Peeters TL, Vantrappen G, Janssens J (1980) Fluctuations of motilin and gastrin levels in relation to the interdigestive motility complex in man (Abstr 47). In: Christensen J (ed) Gastrointestinal motility. Raven, New York, p 287. Seventh Int Symp Gastrointest Motility, Iowa, Sept 11–14, 1979
Poitras P, Steinbach J, Van Deventer G, Walsh JH, Code CF (1979) Effect of somatostatin on interdigestive myoelectric complexes and motilin blood levels. Gastroenterology 76:1218
Rees WDW, Miller LJ, Malagelada JR, Go VLW (1978) Role of gastric acid secretion in the generation of human interdigestive motor activity. Gut 19:A997
Rennie JA, Christofides ND, Bloom SR, Johnson AG (1979) Stimulation of human colonic activity by motilin. Gut 20:A912
Rennie JA, Christofides ND, Ellis MR, Michener P, Johnson AG, Bloom SR (1980) Effect of motilin on human colonic activity. Clin Sci 58:12
Riemer J, Kolling K, Mayer CJ (1977) The effect of motilin on the electrical activity of rabbit circular duodenal muscle. Eur J Physiol 372:343–350
Rösch W, Lux G, Domschke S, Domschke W, Wünsch E, Jaeger E, Demling L (1976) Effect of 13-NLE-motilin on lower esophageal sphincter pressure in man. Gastroenterology 70:A931
Ruppin H (1977) Ouabain-sensitive contractile response to 13-norleucine motilin of rabbit duodenal muscle. Gastroenterology 72:A1123

Ruppin H, Domschke S, Domschke W, Wünsch E, Jaeger E, Demling L (1975) Effects of 13-Nle-motilin in man – inhibition of gastric evacuation and stimulation of pepsin secretion. Scand J Gastroenterol 10:199–202
Ruppin H, Kirndorfer D, Domschke S, Domschke W, Schwemmle K, Wünsch E, Demling L (1976a) Effect of 13-Nle-motilin in postoperative ileus patients: a double-blind trial. Scand J Gastroenterol [Suppl 39] 11:89–92
Ruppin H, Sturm G, Westhoff D, Domschke S, Domschke W, Wünsch E, Demling L (1976b) Effect of 13-Nle-motilin on small intestinal transit time in healthy subjects. Scand J Gastroenterol [Suppl 39] 11:85–88
Ruppin H, Thompson HH, Wingate DL, Wünsch E (1976c) 13-norleucine-motilin (NLEM) and the control of interdigestive intestinal myoelectric activity in the conscious dog. J Physiol (Lond) 263:225P–226P
Ruppin H, Soergel KH, Dodds JW, Wood CM, Domschke W (1979) Effects of the interdigestive motor complex (IMC) and 13-norleucine motilin (NLEM) on fasting intestinal flow rate and velocity in man. Gastroenterology 76:1231
Schubert H, Brown JC (1974) Correction to the amino acid sequence of porcine motilin. Can J Biochem 52:7–8
Schubert E, Mitznegg P, Strunz U et al. (1975) Influence of the hormone analogue 13-NLE-motilin and of 1-methyl-3-isobutylxanthine on tone and cyclic 3′, 5′-AMP content of antral and duodenal muscles in the rabbit. Life Sci 16:263–272
Segawa T, Nakano M, Kai Y, Kawatani H, Yajima H (1976) Effect of synthetic motilin and related polypeptides on contraction of gastrointestinal smooth muscle. J Pharm Pharmacol 28:650–651
Strunz U, Domschke W, Mitznegg P et al. (1975) Analysis of the motor effects of 13-norleucine motilin on the rabbit, guinea pig, rat, and human alimentary tract in vitro. Gastroenterology 68:1485–1491
Strunz U, Domschke W, Domschke S, Mitznegg P, Wünsch E, Jaeger E, Demling L (1976a) Potentiation between 13-Nle-motilin and acetylcholine on rabbit pyloric muscle in vitro. Scand J Gastroenterol [Suppl 39] 11:29–33
Strunz U, Domschke W, Domschke S, Mitznegg P, Wünsch E, Jaeger E, Demling L (1976b) Gastroduodenal motor response to natural motilin and synthetic position 13-substituted motilin analogues: a comparative in vitro study. Scand J Gastroenterol [Suppl 39] 11:199–203
Strunz U, Mitznegg P, Domschke S, Domschke W, Wünsch E, Demling L (1978) VIP antagonizes motilin-induced antral contractions *in vitro*. In: Duthie HL (ed) Gastrointestinal motility in health and disease. MTP Press, Lancaster, pp 125–131
Strunz U, Neeb S, Mitznegg P (1979) Somatostatin but not atropine inhibits motilin secretion in vitro. Gastroenterology 76:1256
Thomas PA, Kelly KA, Go VLW (1979) Motilin regulation of interdigestive activity in the transplanted proximal stomach. Gut 20:A912
Thomas PA, Kelly KA, Go VLW (1980) Hormonal regulation of gastrointestinal interdigestive motor cycles (Abstr 44). In: Cjristensen J (ed) Gastrointestinal motility. Raven, New York, p 267. Seventh Int Symp Gastrointest Motility, Iowa, Sept 11–14, 1979
Valenzuela JE (1976) Effects of intestinal hormones and peptides on intragastric pressure in dogs. Gastroenterology 71:766–769
Vantrappen G, Janssens J, Peeters TL, Bloom S, Van Tongeren J, Hellemans J (1978) Does motilin have a role in eliciting the interdigestive migrating motor complex (MCM) in man? Gastroenterology 74:A1149
Vantrappen G, Janssens J, Peeters TL, Bloom SR, Christofides ND, Hellemans J (1979) Motilin and the interdigestive migrating motor complex in man. Dig Dis Sci 24:497–500
Wingate DL, Ruppin H, Green WER et al. (1976) Motilin-induced electrical activity in the canine gastrointestinal tract. Scand J Gastroenterol [Suppl 39] 11:111–118
Wünsch E (1976) Synthesis of motilin analogues. Scand J Gastroenterol [Suppl 39] 11:19–24
Yajima H, Kay Y, Kawatani H (1975) Synthesis of the decosapeptide corresponding to the entire amino acid sequence of porcine motilin. JCS Chem Commun 159–160
You CH, Chey WY, Lee KY (1980) Studies on plasma motilin concentration and interdigestive motility of the duodenum in humans. Gastroenterology 79:62–66

Neurotensin

A. Introduction

Neurotensin (NT) is a tridecapeptide originally isolated from bovine hypothalamus extracts by CARRAWAY and LEEMAN (1973). Subsequently it became evident that the gastrointestinal tract represented both the major source of neurotensin (according to CARRAWAY and LEEMAN 1976, about 90% of the total immunoreactive neurotensin of the rat came from the gut; see also ORCI et al. 1976; KITABGI et al. 1976) and an important target organ for this peptide. The recently isolated human peptide (HAMMER et al. 1980) has been found to be identical to the neurotensin originally discovered in bovine hypothalamus and ileum. NT is active as a peptidergic transmitter in neural tissue, where it is localized in the synaptosomal fraction, and it may also be a circulating hormone since it has been identified in a typical endocrine cell in the ileal mucosa and in rat plasma. Neurotensin-like immunoreactivity has also been recently found in human plasma (BLACKBURN et al. 1978). The structure of neurotensin is the following:

1 2 3 4 5 6 7 8 9 10 11 12 13
pGlu-Leu-Tyr-Glu-Asn-Lys-Pro-Arg-Arg-Pro-Tyr-Ile-Leu-OH.

B. Structure–Activity Relationships

Studies of structure–activity relationships have been reported from a number of laboratories (CARRAWAY and LEEMAN 1975; FOLKERS et al. 1976; RÖKAEUS et al. 1977; SEGAWA et al. 1977; LEEMAN et al. 1977). It was shown that the biologic activity of neurotensin resides almost exclusively in the COOH terminal hexapeptide (20%–30% as active as the whole molecule) when assessed by bioassay in guinea pig preparations. The COOH terminal pentapeptide retained approximately 1% of the activity of the hexapeptide. The NH_2 terminal decapeptide (NT 1–10) was absolutely inactive and modification of the NT molecule in positions 2–7 apparently had little effect on either biologic potency of binding to mast cells.

The two arginine residues at positions 8 and 9 are apparently indispensable, perhaps because of ionic interactions between their positively charged side chains and the receptor binding site. DArg^8-NT was found to be almost as potent as NT whereas DArg^9-NT retained only 5% of the activity of the parent peptide. Both modified sequences had greater binding to mast cells than NT (LAZARUS et al. 1977). However, the pharmacologic "efficacies" of these peptides were very similar. Surprisingly, DPhe^{11}-NT and DTyr^{11}-NT were actually more potent than neurotensin (RIVIER et al., 1977). The addition to the COOH terminal hexapeptide of the 2–7 NH_2 terminal sequence doubled the peptide's activity and this may be due to increased stability of the larger peptides.

When the Glu residue at position 4 was replaced with a Gln residue no difference in the smooth muscle activities of the two peptides was observed. Moreover, the two compounds were indistinguishable by radioimmunoasay and FOLKERS et al. (1976) even suggested that Gln^4-NT, rather than the Glu^4 analog, may be the naturally occurring peptide.

Neurotensin-NH_2 and Gln^4 – neurotensin-NH_2 had less than 1% of the activity of NT. In a recent study (KITABGI et al. to be published), a highly significant correlation was found when the biologic potencies of NT and NT analogs were compared with their binding affinities in either the neural or the extraneural radioreceptorassay. The positive charges on both arginyl residues 8 and 9 and the L configuration of Arg^9 were important for both binding and biologic activity. An aromatic residue in the L configuration was required in position 11 of the NT molecule. The side chain methyl groups of Ile^{12} and COOH terminal residue Leu^{13} as well as the presence of Leu^{13} in the L configuration, were required for activity.

It is of interest that, although the NT sequence is not contained within the sequence of other known mammalian peptides, there is a close chemical resemblance between the COOH terminal active region of NT and a peptide discovered in amphibian skin, xenopsin (Pyr-Glu-Gly-Lys-Arg-Pro-Trp-Ile-Leu-OH) which has similar pharmacologic effects (ARAKI et al. 1973).

C. Effects on the Gastrointestinal Tract

I. In Vitro Studies

The early, preliminary paper about the contraction of guinea pig ileum and the relaxation of rat duodenum (CARRAWAY and LEEMAN 1973) made it possible to consider that neurotensin resembles peptides of the bradykinin family (BERTACCINI 1976). In subsequent very accurate investigations, neurotensin appeared to have specific effects on motor activity of isolated preparations which characterized this peptide as completely different from the other brain–gut peptides (KITABGI and FREYCHET 1978, 1979a, b; KITABGI et al. 1979; RÖKAEUS et al. 1977; BISSETTE et al. 1978).

On the isolated lower esophageal sphincter (LES) of the rat, NT showed a remarkable spasmogenic effect starting from a threshold dose of 6×10^{-9} M; this action differed from that of bradykinin which, in the same experimental conditions, always had a biphasic effect (Fig. 1). Conversely NT always caused a relaxation of the guinea pig LES. In both rat and guinea pig preparations, tachyphylaxis was a common feature (BERTACCINI et al. 1980; CORUZZI and BERTACCINI 1980).

In the isolated rat fundus strip, NT and Gln^4-NT caused dose-dependent contractions from a threshold dose of 0.24 nM. The neurotensins induced a slow contraction, like 5-HT, rather than a fast response, like acetylcholine. With an interval between doses of 12 min or more, no tachyphylaxis was seen, this was present only with shorter intervals. Responses to neurotensin were not changed by administration of atropine, morphine, methysergide, or hexamethonium. According to RÖKAEUS et al. (1977), the rat fundus strip is a suitable tool for studies of structure–activity relations among the neurotensins. It is very sensitive to these peptides, gives a rather steep concentration–response curve, with very modest tachyphylaxis. In subsequent studies (QUIRION et al. 1980a) the effect of neurotensin on rat stomach was shown, to be independent of the intramural release of histamine or prostaglandins. Moreover, the myotropic action of the peptide was not influenced by

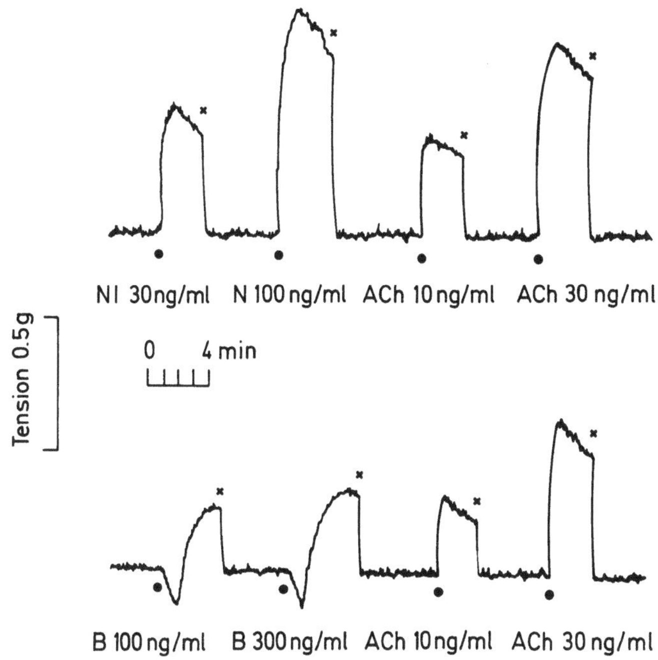

Fig. 1. Lower esophageal sphincter of the rat. *NT*, neurotensin; *ACh*, acetylcholine; *B*, bradykinin. *Crosses* indicate washout

8-Leu-angiotensin II (10^{-6} *M*), a well-characterized angiotensin antagonist, nor by somatostatin (3×10^{-7} *M*), nor glucagon (2×10^{-6} *M*), two peptides known to be present in gastric tissues. In addition, rat stomach strips desensitized with bradykinin (6×10^{-6} *M*) or substance P (7.4×10^{-6} *M*) were found to maintain their sensitivity to neurotensin. All these data seem to suggest the existance of specific NT receptors in the smooth muscle of rat stomach; of course, further studies with specific (not yet available) NT antagonists are needed to support this view. In this connection (D-Trp^{11})-NT which behaved as a relatively specific antagonist of NT in perfused rat heart, was found to have no inhibitory effect toward NT on the rat stomach (QUIRION et al. 1980b). Rat stomach strip responded dose-dependently not only to NT (1.3×10^{-9}–5.4×10^{-7} *M*) but also to NT fragments; the minimum structure required for the full stimulation was H-Arg^9-Pro^{10}-Tyr^{11}-Ile^{12}-Leu^{13}-OH. The chemical groups responsible for the full activation (intrinsic activity) of NT receptors seemed, however, to be located in the sequence -Arg^9-Pro^{10}-Tyr^{11} (QUIRION et al. 1980a). The rat duodenum was relaxed and its spontaneous activity inhibited by NT, at a concentration of 24 n*M*.

Rat ileum, at its basal low tone was not affected by NT, even at a concentration of 100 n*M*. On the contrary, when it was spontaneously hypertonic or during acetylcholine-induced contractions, it was relaxed by neurotensin in a dose-dependent fashion (1–60 n*M*). This effect appeared to be myogenic in origin, since it was unaffected by the common inhibitors, including tetrodotoxin.

The effect on the guinea pig ileum appeared to be more complex. A good dose-related contractile effect was present (1–60 n*M*), though the maximum response

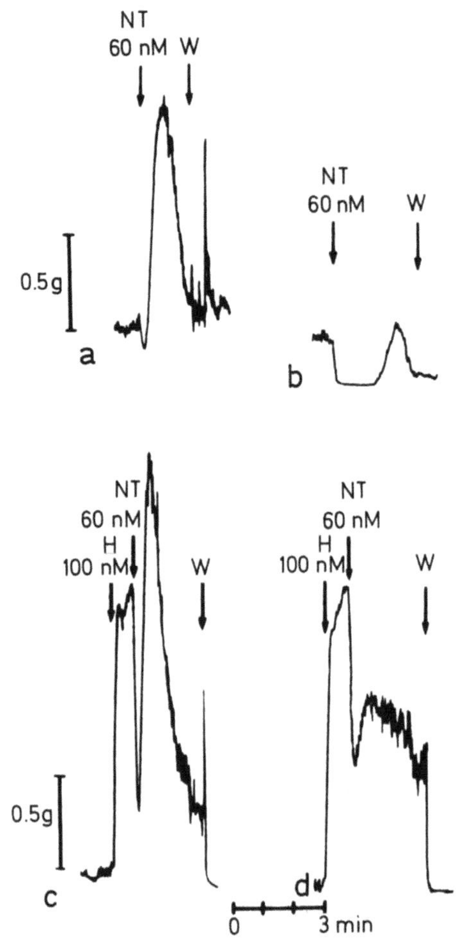

Fig. 2 a–d. Effect of neurotensin *NT* on longitudinal muscle strips of the guinea pig ileum. **a** response of the muscle to 60 n*M* NT; W, indicates washout; **b** as **a** in the presence of 0.3 μ*M* TTX; **c** effect of 60 n*M* NT on the muscle contracted by 100 n*M* histamine *H;* **d** as **c** in the presence of 0.3 μ*M* TTX. (KITABGI and FREYCHET 1979 a)

was noticeably lower than that to acetylcholine, histamine, or other peptides like bradykinin or substance P. (Gln^4)-NT and NT were equipotent in increasing both tone and motility of the ileum. Tachyphylaxis was found to be present if the time interval between two doses of the peptides was less than 12 min. Atropine inhibited and tetrodotoxin (TTX) blocked this spasmogenic effect, while chlorpheniramine was completely ineffective. However, if NT was given when the ileum was contracted by histamine, it produced a biphasic response, consisting of a quick relaxation followed by a contraction. TTX blocked this contracting effect while leaving unaffected the initial relaxation which was therefore considered to be myogenic in origin (Fig. 2). Also, morphine and opioid peptides were shown to shift and depress the concentration–response curve to neurotensin, an effect which was completely prevented by naloxone (ZETLER 1980), allowing us to conclude that in this preparation the contractile effect of NT is mediated by the release of acetylcholine from postganglionic nerve endings. Apparently NT was unable to change the levels of cyclic AMP and cyclic GMP in longitudinal muscle of the guinea pig ileum, suggesting that cyclic nucleotides are not involved in motor effects of the peptide. Binding studies of NT and some synthetic analogs, performed by KITABGI and FREYCHET (1969a), showed that these peptides bind to a crude membrane preparation of longitudinal smooth muscle. The authors suggested that the binding is to receptor sites which mediate the effect of NT on smooth muscle.

Finally, neurotensin strongly contracted the guinea pig taenia coli, being more potent in terms of threshold doses (1–2 n*M*) and less active in terms of maximum effect than histamine. This effect, which was unaffected by TTX, was never preceded by a relaxation, even when the muscle was first contracted by histamine. In contrast to the effect on guinea pig ileum, which tended to decrease spontaneously, that on the taenia coli lasted for several minutes.

The effect of NT on membrane potential and conductance on the guinea pig taenia coli was recently investigated (KITABGI et al. 1979; HAMON et al. 1979). In spontaneously active preparations, at 37 °C neurotensin (0.5–10 n*M*) caused a membrane depolarization, decreased the size of the spikes, and increased their frequency. This caused an increase in the frequency of phasic contractions, which was followed by a tonic contraction with the highest doses of the peptide. At low temperature (20 °C), when the taenia coli had little or no spontaneous activity, NT (50 n*M*) depolarized the smooth muscle membrane and increased its conductance, with consequent appearance of a tonic contraction. This effect seemed to be primarily due to an increase in Na^+ and Ca^{2+} conductances. Neurotensin also had a peculiar effect on the rat isolated ileum (KITABGI and FREYCHET 1978): the peptide had no effect when the intestine had a basal low tone, however it produced a quick dose-dependent relaxation when added to a preparation with a spontaneously increased tone or in preparations contracted by acetylcholine (Fig. 3).

II. In Vivo Studies

Very few data are available so far about the action of neurotensin or Gln^4-neurotensin in vivo. Recent studies were performed in healthy volunteers with (Gln^4)-neurotensin (6, 12, and 18 pmol kg^{-1} min^{-1}). LES pressure decreased significantly from 13.7 to 5.3 mm Hg. This decrease occurred at plasma neurotensin-like immunoreactivity of approximately 50 p*M*, i.e., at levels below those obtained in humans after a meal, thus at absolutely physiologic plasma concentrations of neurotensin or a neurotensin metabolite (THOR et al. 1980). Gln^4-NT, tested in the dog, was shown to have a remarkable inhibitory effect on the spontaneous motor activity of canine fundic and antral pouches (ANDERSSON et al. 1977). This inhibition occurred after a short latency period (2–6 min). It was dose related from 6 to 100 ng kg^{-1} min^{-1}, and was more striking in innervated antral pouches than in denervated Heidenhain pouches. Apparently, duodenal and intestinal pouches did not respond to the peptide, the threshold dose for the gastric inhibitory effect was lower than those required to cause blood pressure changes or an increase in blood glucose concentration (ROSELL et al. 1976), and the authors concluded that the gastrointestinal tract may be a target organ for neurotensin or Gln^4-NT.

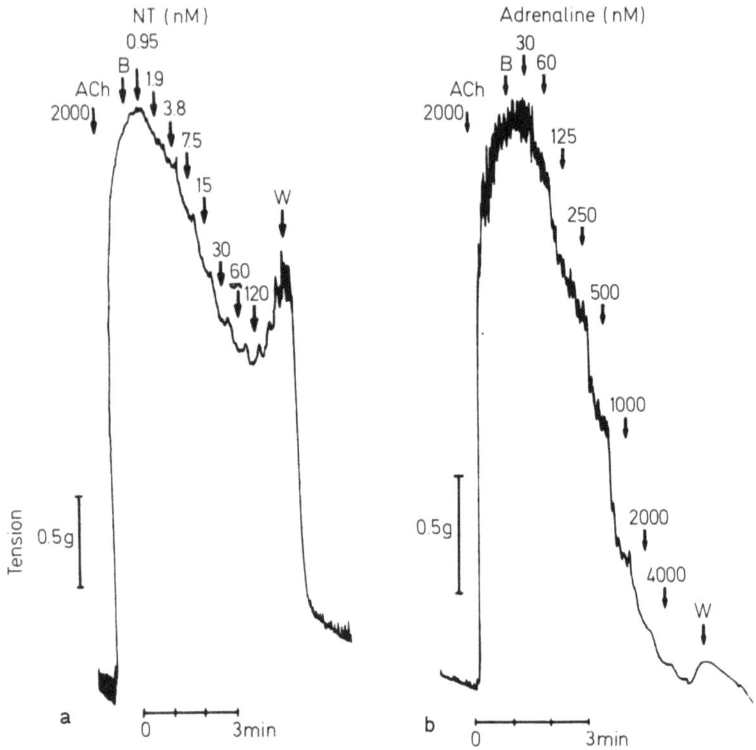

Fig. 3 a, b. Cumulative dose–response curves of the relaxing effect of neurotensin *NT* **a** and adrenaline **b** on the rat ileum contracted by acetylcholine *ACh*. Drugs were added to give the final concentrations indicated (in n*M*). *B*, indicates buffer solution; *W*, indicates washout. (KITABGI and FREYCHET 1978)

Neurotensin appeared to be endowed with a striking spasmogenic action on the rat pylorus (G. BERTACCINI and G. CORUZZI unpublished work 1980); its threshold dose was about 10 ng/kg i.v., a value which is only slightly higher than those of cerulein and bombesin which were shown to be the most potent peptides in this particular region (for review see BERTACCINI 1976). However, tachyphylaxis was a common feature for neurotensin and also the maximum duration of the spasmogenic effect (6–8 min obtained with 100–200 ng/kg) was decidedly lower than that of cerulein or bombesin (20–30 min).

In a recent investigation, infusion of neurotensin (2.4 ± 0.6 pmol kg^{-1} min^{-1}) into healthy volunteers caused a significant rise in plasma levels of the peptide, together with a significant delay ($15 \pm 6\%$) in gastric emptying of a test solution (BLACKBURN et al. 1980). Since, in the same investigation, NT was also shown to inhibit gastric acid and pepsin output, the peptide was considered, together with other intestinal peptides, as a candidate for the identity of "enterogastrone." Finally, similar low doses of the peptide (6 pmol kg^{-1} min^{-1}) administered in healthy volunteers, were found to inhibit the interdigestive migrating myoelectric complex in the duodenum and in the jejunum. In all the subjects examined, during infusion of (Gln^4)-neurotensin, the motility pattern changed from the interdigestive pattern to pressure waves resembling the activity seen after ingestion of food (THOR et al. 1980).

According to preliminary data, NT is released in excess in the dumping syndrome and may thus be responsible for some of the so far unexplained aspects of this condition (BLOOM et al. 1978). It is obvious, however, that data available at present are not sufficient for drawing any conclusion about the role of this peptide in the gastrointestinal tract.

References

Andersson S, Rosell S, Hjelmquist U, Chang D, Folkers K (1977) Inhibition of gastric and intestinal motor activity in dogs by (Gln^4)-Neurotensin. Acta Physiol Scand 100:231–235

Araki K, Takibana S, Uchiyama M, Nakajma T, Yasuhata Y (1973) Isolation and structure of a new active peptide "xenopsin" on the smooth muscle expecially on a strip of fundus from a rat stomach, from the skin of *Xenopus leavis*. Chem Pharm Bull (Tokyo) 21:2801–2804

Bertaccini G (1976) Active polypeptides of nonmammalian origin. Pharmacol Rev 28:127–177

Bertaccini G, Coruzzi G, Scarpignato C (1981) Exogenous and endogenous compounds which affect the contractility of the lower esophageal sphincter (LES). In: Stipa S, Belsey R, Moraldi A (eds) Int Symp Med and Surg Problems of the Esophagus, Rome, May 7–9, 1980, Academic Press, New York

Bissette G, Manberg P, Nemeroff CB, Prange AJ Jr (1978) Neurotensin, a biologically active peptide. Life Sci 23:2173–2182

Blackburn AM, Bloom SR, Polak JM (1978) Neurotensin: a new peptide hormone in the circulation of man. J Endocrinol 79:P26

Blackburn AM, Bloom SR, Long RG, Fletcher DR, Christofides ND, Fitzpatrick ML, Baron JH (1980) Effect of neurotensin on gastric function in man. Lancet 1:987–989

Bloom SR, Blackburn AM, Ebeid FH, Ralphs DNL (1978) Neurotensin and the dumping syndrome. Gastroenterology 74:A1011

Carraway R, Leeman SE (1973) The isolation of a new hypotensive peptide, neurotensin, from bovine hypothalamus. J Biol Chem 248:6854–6861

Carraway R, Leeman SE (1975) The aminoacid sequence of a hypothalamic peptide, neurotensin. J Biol Chem 250:1907–1911

Carraway R, Leeman SE (1976) Characterization of radioimmunoassayable neurotensin in the rat. J Biol Chem 251:7045–7052

Coruzzi G, Bertaccini G (1980) Effect of some vasoactive peptides on the lower esophageal sphincter. Pharmacol Res Commun 12:965–973

Folkers K, Chang KD, Humphries J, Carraway R, Leeman SE, Bowers CY (1976) Synthesis and activities of neurotensin and its acid and amide analogs: possible natural occurrence of (Gln^4)-neurotensin. Proc Natl Acad Sci USA 73:3833–3837

Hammer RA, Leeman SE, Carraway R, Williams RH (1980) Isolation of human intestinal neurotensin. J Biol Chem 255:2476–2480

Hamon G, Kitabgi P, Worcel M (1979) Neurotensin: electrophysiological studies of its action on the guinea-pig taenia coli. Br J Pharmacol 66:122P–123P

Kitabgi P, Freychet P (1978) Effects of neurotensin on isolated intestinal smooth muscles. Eur J Pharmacol 50:349–357

Kitabgi P, Freychet P (1979a) Neurotensin: contractile activity, specific binding, and lack of effect on cyclic nucleotides in intestinal smooth muscle. Eur J Pharmacol 55:35–42

Kitabgi P, Freychet P (1979b) Neurotensin contracts the guinea-pig longitudinal ileal smooth muscle by inducing acetylcholine release. Eur J Pharmacol 56:403–406

Kitabgi P, Carraway R, Leeman SE (1976) Isolation of a tridecapeptide from bovine intestinal tissue and its partial characterization as neurotensin. J Biol Chem 251:7053–7058

Kitabgi P, Hamon G, Worcel M (1979) Electrophysiological study of the action of neurotensin on the smooth muscle of the guinea-pig taenia coli. Eur J Pharmacol 56:87–93
Kitabgi P, Poustis C, Granier C, Van Rietschoten J, Morgat JL, Freychet P (to be published) Neurotensin binding to extraneural and neural receptors: comparison with biologic activity and structure-activity relationship. Mol Pharmacol
Lazarus LH, Perrin MH, Brown MR, Rivier JE (1977) Verification of both the sequence and conformational specificity of neurotensin in binding to mast cells. Biochem Biophys Res Commun 76:1079–1085
Leeman SE, Mroz EA, Carraway R (1977) Substance P and neurotensin. In: Gainer H (ed) Peptides in neurobiology. Plenum, New York, pp 99–144
Orci L, Baetens O, Rufener C, Brown M, Wale W, Guillemin R (1976) Evidence for immunoreactive neurotensin in dog intestinal mucosa. Life Sci 19:559–562
Quirion R, Regoli D, Rioux F, St Pierre S (1980a) The stimulatory effect of neurotensin and related peptides in rat stomach strips and guinea-pig atria. Br J Pharmacol 68:83–91
Quirion R, Rioux F, Regoli D, St Pierre S (1980b) Selective blockade of neurotensin-induced coronary vessel constriction in perfused rat hearts by a neurotensin analogue. Eur J Pharmacol 61:309–312
Rivier JE, Lazarus JH, Perrin MH, Brown MR (1977) Neurotensin analogues. Structure-activity relationship. J Med Chem 10:1409–1412
Rökaeus Å, Burcher E, Chang D, Folkers K, Rosell S (1977) Actions of neurotensin and (Gln^4)-neurotensin on isolated tissues. Acta Pharmacol Toxicol (Copenh) 41:141–147
Rosell S, Burcher E, Chang D, Folkers K (1976) Cardiovascular and metabolic actions of neurotensin and (Gln^4)-neurotensin. Acta Physiol Scand 98:484–491
Segawa T, Hosokawa M, Kitagawa K, Yajima H (1977) Contractile activity of synthetic neurotensin and related polypeptides on guinea pig ileum. J Pharm Pharmacol 29:57–58
Thor K, Rosell S, Rokaeus A, Nyquist O, Levenhaupt A, Kager L, Folkers K (1980a) Plasma concentrations of neurotensin-like immunoreactivity (NTLI) and lower esophageal sphincter (LES) pressure in man following infusion of (Gln^4)-neurotensin. Abstr XIth Int Congr Gastroenterol. Thieme, Stuttgart, p 28
Thor K, Rökaeus Å, Kager L, Folkers K, Rosell S (1980b) (Gln^4)-neurotensin inhibits the interdigestive migrating motor complex in man. In: Bloom SR Polak JM (eds) Regulatory peptides, suppl 1. Elsevier/North-Holland Biomedical, Amsterdam Oxford New York, p S114
Zetler G (1980) Antagonism of the gut-coutracting effects of bombesin and neurotensin by opioid peptides, morphine, atropine or tetrodotoxin. Pharmacology 21:348–354

Bombesin

A. Introduction

Bombesin is a prototype of a series of peptides of amphibian origin whose structure is shown in Table 1. Bombesin was first isolated from amphibian skin, then bombesin-like peptides were found to be present in avian and mammalian gut and brain (ERSPAMER and MELCHIORRI 1976; WALSH and DOCKRAY 1978; LECHAGO et al. 1978). Quite recently two molecular forms with COOH terminal bombesin immunoreactivity have been demonstrated (DOCKRAY et al. 1979). They were found both in myenteric plexuses and in mucosal endocrine cells. Probombesins, large biologically inactive precursor molecules giving the active forms after acid hydrolysis, probably occur in the rat and guinea pig stomach; a clear-cut heterogeneity

Table 1. Bombesin and bombesin-like peptides in amphibian skin[a]

Trivial name	Structure[b]
Bombesin	pGlu-Gln-Arg-Leu-Gly-Asn-Gln-Trp-Ala-Val-Gly-His-Leu-Met-NH_2
Alytensin	pGlu-Gly-Arg-Leu-Gly-Thr-Gln-Trp-Ala-Val-Gly-His-Leu-Met-NH_2
Litorin	pGlu-Gln-Trp-Ala-Val-Gly-His-Phe-Met-NH_2
$Glu(OMe)^2$-litorin	pGlu-Glu(OMe)-Trp-Ala-Val-Gly-His-Phe-Met-NH_2
$Glu(OEt)^2$-litorin	pGlu-Glu(OEt)-Trp-Ala-Val-Gly-His-Phe-Met-NH_2
Ranatensin	pGlu-Val-Pro-Gln-Trp-Ala-Val-Gly-His-Phe-Met-NH_2
Ranatensin C	X-Glx-Thr-Pro-Gln-Trp-Ala-Val-Gly-His-Phe-Met-NH_2
Ranatensin R	Ser-Asp-Ala-Thr-Leu-Arg-Arg-Tyr-Asn-Gln-Trp-Ala-Thr-Gly-His-Phe-Met-NH_2

[a] For review see ERSPAMER (1980)
[b] X = unidentified residue; Glx = either Gln or Glu

is also apparent for the bombesin-like peptide of the human gastric mucosa (ERSPAMER et al. 1979). In this connection, a heptacosapeptide with potent gastrin-releasing activity has been isolated from porcine nonantral gastric and intestinal tissue (McDONALD et al. 1979). The suggested amino acid sequence is:
Ala-Pro-Val-Ser-Val-Gly-Gly-Gly-Thr-Val-Leu-Ala-Lys-Met-Tyr-Pro-Arg-Gly-Asn-His-Trp-Ala-Val-Gly-His-Leu-Met-NH_2.
Striking homology in the COOH terminal region may be seen with bombesin; in addition another bombesin-like peptide has so far only been purified from canine intestinal muscle (REEVE et al. 1980). The amino acid sequence has not yet been established.

Studies on gastrointestinal motility were mainly carried out with bombesin, litorin, or the synthetic COOH terminal nonapeptide, which was shown to posses all the prerequisites of an excellent substitute for bombesin in experimental and clinical investigations. Studies on structure–activity relationships carried out with natural compounds or synthetic analogs have enabled us to draw the following general conclusions

1) A minimum COOH terminal sequence of seven amino acid residues is necessary for detectable bombesin-like activity. The COOH terminal hexapeptide had less than 0.1% of the activity of bombesin.
2) The COOH terminal octapeptide retained 10%–30% of the activity of the parent substance and the nona-, deca-, and undecapeptides were approximately as potent as bombesin.
3) Compounds of lesser importance were obtained by substitution of some of the amino acid residues in the bombesin molecule.

However, all the octapeptides examined had a more rapid onset of action but a less-sustained action, indicating faster metabolism or weaker binding to receptor sites.

B. Effects on the Motility of the Gastrointestinal Tract

I. In Vitro Studies

The first extensive paper describing the effects of bombesin on isolated preparations of the gastrointestinal tract from various animal species, was that by ERSPA-

Table 2. Stimulatory effect of bombesin on isolated preparations of gastrointestinal tract from different laboratory animals

Target[a]	Threshold doses (ng/ml)	Tachyphylaxis[b]
Kitten ileum	0.1 – 0.5	–
Guinea pig duodenum	5 – 20	+
Guinea pig ileum		
LM	1 – 5	+ –
CM	250 –500	+ –
Guinea pig colon	0.03– 0.5	+
Rat LES	25 – 50	+
Rat pylorus	2 – 10	+ +
Rat duodenum	5 – 50 R[c]	+ +
Rat colon	0.03– 0.1	+
Hamster ileum	2 – 10	+
Hamster colon	2 – 10	+
Rabbit duodenum	10 – 50	+
Rabbit ileum	0.1 – 5	+ +
Rabbit colon	0.1 – 2	+ +
Fowl ileum	0.1 – 1	+

[a] LM, CM = longitudinal and circular muscle, respectively
[b] + +, +, –, + – = strong, moderate, absent, or irregular
[c] R = relaxation

MER et al. (1972). In the small intestine of 10–30-day-old kittens, bombesin had a remarkable dose-dependent stimulant action, causing an increase in tone accompanied by a less remarkable reinforcement of the phasic movements. Its activity exceeded by several times that of other peptide and nonpeptide substances and was unaffected by atropine or by hexamethonium.

The guinea pig ileum responded in a quite different way inasmuch as it showed a less evident increase in tone along with an enormous increase in phasic movements which persisted for 6–12 h but were promptly abolished by washing. Tachyphylaxis was always present. According to a very recent study by ZETLER (1980), atropine caused a depression of the concentration–response curve to bombesin whilst morphine, Met-enkephalin and β-endorphin depressed but also shifted the response curve to bombesin, the effect of opioids being completely prevented by naloxone. Apparently bombesin stimulated intramural neurons via receptors that are inhibited by the activation of opioid.

In a recent study (BERTACCINI et al. 1980) bombesin was found to contract the lower esophageal sphincter in both rats (threshold dose 1.8×10^{-8} *M*) and guinea pigs (threshold dose 6×10^{-7} *M*). Tachyphylaxis was a common feature in both isolated preparations. The guinea pig colon was more sensitive to bombesin and less prone to tachyphylaxis. The only peptide whose potency paralleled that of bombesin was bradykinin.

Variable results were obtained with the rat large intestine. However in this preparation too, bombesin appeared to be by far the most active compound examined. Rat duodenum, unlike all the other preparations examined, showed an atropine-resistant relaxation which was similar to the well-known relaxation induced

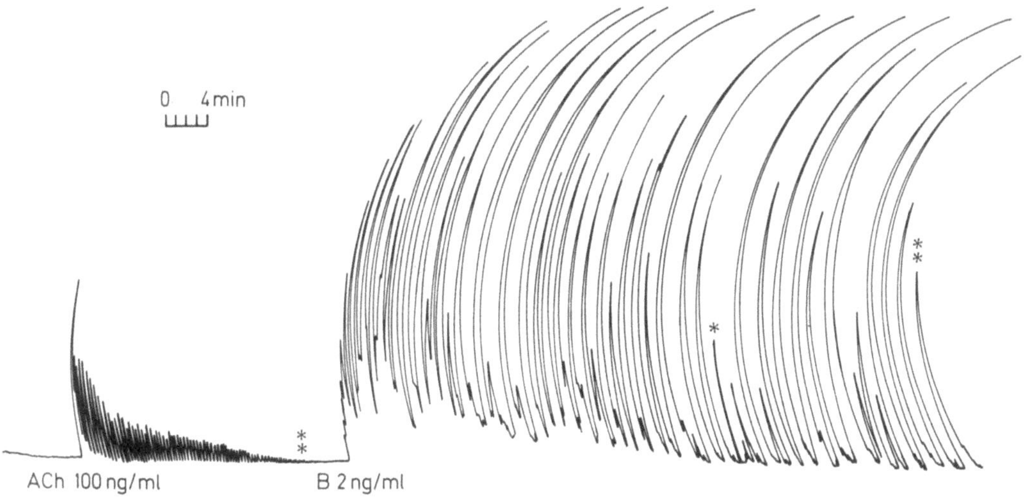

Fig. 1. Human stomach antrum: effect of acetylcholine *ACh* and of bombesin *B*. *Asterisk*, kymograph stopped for 2 h; *double asterisk*, washout. (BERTACCINI et al. 1974b)

by bradykinin but less striking. In small and large intestine from other animal species (hamster, rabbit, chicken, and tortoise) bombesin had stimulant effects which were, however, erratic in kind and intensity. Tachyphylaxis was a common feature in all the experiments, though in various degrees. A synopsis of the effects of bombesin on isolated preparations of gastrointestinal smooth muscle is shown in Table 2 which summarizes data by ERSPAMER et al. (1972), by BERTACCINI et al. (1979) and by G. BERTACCINI (unpublished work 1980).

In comparison with bombesin, alytesin showed only minor quantitative differences in the various preparations. Litorin behaved essentially in the same way as bombesin and was 1.5–8 times as active as bombesin in various preparations. The action of litorin was more prompt and the relaxation after washing was more rapid than after bombesin. Also, tachyphylaxis was less frequent and less intense with the nonapeptide (ENDEAN et al. 1975; BROCCARDO et al. 1975).

Extensive investigations were carried out by BERTACCINI et al. (1974a, c, 1979) on segments of human gastrointestinal tract removed during surgery. Bombesin was found to cause the appearance or reinforcement of rhythmic movements, together with a remarkable increase in tone in all the segments of the gastrointestinal tract, from the stomach to the rectum. After washing, the return to basal conditions usually took 5–15 min. When there was no washout, the effect was much more prolonged than that of other peptide and nonpeptide substances and sometimes the increased peristalsis lasted for several hours (Fig. 1). The threshold stimulatory dose was often extremely low (20–50 pg/ml), the most sensitive tissues being the taenia coli and the appendix. This sensitivity actually increased after the strips had been stored in the cold for 24 h. The circular and longitudinal muscle layers showed approximately the same sensitivity to the peptide. The response was dose dependent in many preparations, but sometimes tachyphylaxis appeared at the

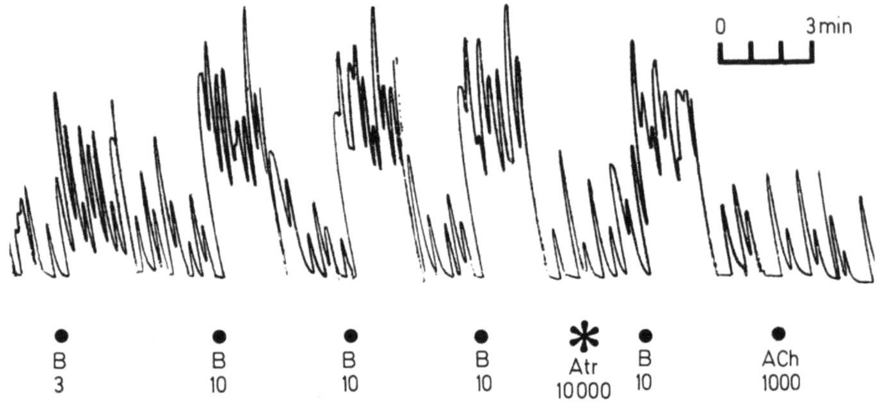

Fig. 2. Human ileum longitudinal layer; effects of bombesin *B*, atropine *Atr*, and acetylcholine *ACh*. Doses in ng/ml. (BERTACCINI et al. 1974c)

third or the fourth consecutive administration of bombesin. The appendix was less prone to tachyphylaxis than the other tissues.

The usual inhibitors (atropine, hexamethonium, tetrodotoxin, dibenamine, methysergide, and mepyramine) did not significantly modify the effect of bombesin (Fig. 2). Results obtained in isolated preparations of human gastrointestinal tract are summarized in Table 3.

II. In Vivo Studies

1. Effects on the Lower Esophageal Sphincter

Bombesin was found (MUKHOPADHYAY and KUNNEMANN 1979) to exert a potent stimulant effect on the opossum lower esophageal sphincter (LES) which was dose dependent (5–100 ng/kg in vivo or 10^{-9}–10^{-8} M in vitro), rapid in onset, and lasted 5–10 min. Repeated administrations of high doses of the peptide caused rapid tachyphylaxis which, however, did not modify the response to pentagastrin. Atropine and hexamethonium did not modify the response to bombesin, which was significantly antagonized by tetrodotoxin, phentolamine, and reserpine. A direct effect on the smooth muscle as well as an indirect effect through postganglionic adrenergic neurons was suggested. In humans, bombesin (10 μg kg^{-1} min^{-1}) was found to increase LES pressure in both normal subjects and antrectomized patients (E. CORAZZIARI et al. unpublished work). No correlation was found in any subject between plasma gastrin levels and the degree of the LES pressure increase. This is in sharp contrast with results reported by MARLETTA et al. (1979) who infused bombesin (15 ng kg^{-1} min^{-1}) into ten normal subjects and found a linear correlation between the increase in LES pressure and serum gastrin values during bombesin infusion. At present we have no explanation for this discrepancy and further data on this interesting subject are needed. Of course the usual reservation concerning the different antibodies used for the radioimmunoassay and the different molecular forms of gastrin which could be detected in these investigations must be kept in mind.

Table 3. Action of bombesin on different isolated preparations from human alimentary tract

Tissue[a]	Number of strips	Threshold dose (ng/ml)	No effect
Stomach body			
CM	35	0.05–10	2
LM	30	0.02–10	2
Stomach antrum			
CM	25	0.1 – 6	2
LM	22	0.3 –20	2
Duodenum LM	3	5 –20	—
Small intestine			
CM	5	1 –20	1
LM	7	0.5 –20	—
Large intestine CM	10	1 –12	3
Taenia coli LM	25	0.05– 5	3
Appendix (children) LM	54	0.02– 2	—

[a] CM = circular muscle; LM = longitudinal muscle

2. Effects on the Stomach

An interesting experiment was performed by KOWALEWSKI and KOLODEJ (1976) with the isolated ex vivo perfused canine stomach, with simultaneous recording of myoelectric and mechanical activity. Under these experimental conditions, bombesin induced premature control potentials and disruption of the regular electrical control activity (ECA) pattern with uncoupling of the ECA cycle and marked mechanical response. On the whole, the response to bombesin was not dissimilar from those to pentagastrin or methacholine. Atropine (0.2 mg/h), hexamethonium (100 mg/h), and tetrodotoxin (100 μg/kg) strongly decreased or abolished the response of both electrical and mechanical activity to bombesin and this suggested that a neural release of acetylcholine mediates the effects of the peptide.

In the conscious dog, the body and the fundus of the innervated stomach were relaxed by bombesin (0.3–3 μg/kg i.v.) whereas the antrum was always contracted. The denervated Heidenhain pouch was also contracted by bombesin (0.1–0.5 μg/kg i.v.), with a marked degree of tachyphylaxis (BERTACCINI and IMPICCIATORE 1975). A decrease in canine intragastric pressure caused by bombesin (1–5 ng kg^{-1} min^{-1}) has also been observed by BROCCARDO (1978). Since somatostatin, in doses (40–160 ng/kg^{-1} min^{-1}) which block the release of gastrin induced by bombesin, did not abolish the effect of bombesin, it was concluded that this was not mediated by gastrin release.

In the anesthetized rat, bombesin has been shown to contract the whole stomach and the pylorus (with a threshold stimulant intravenous dose of 1–5 ng/kg). This effect was not blocked by the common inhibitors, but showed a remarkable tachyphylaxis (BERTACCINI and IMPICCIATORE 1975). Recent experiments (M. IMPICCIATORE and F. BERTI unpublished work 1980) have shown that pretreatment of

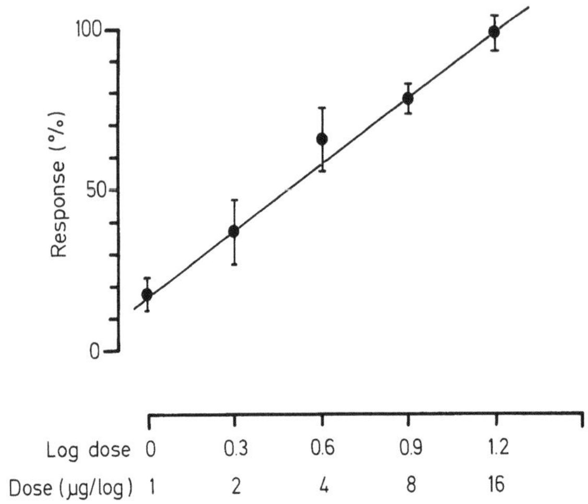

Fig. 3. Dose–response relationship of bombesin on gastric emptying in conscious rats. Each value represents the mean of the values obtained from five or six rats. Vertical bars are standard errors. The line is the least-squares regression line (y, $18.6 \pm 68.9\,x$; r, 0.5201; N, 28, $P<0.01$). Maximum response taken as 100

rats with indomethacine partially prevented the effect of bombesin which was then found, by a biologic technique, to release a prostaglandin of the F type. In preliminary experiments it was shown that bombesin delayed gastric emptying in the conscious rat dose-dependently (1–16 µg/kg intraperitoneally; SCARPIGNATO and BERTACCINI 1981; Fig. 3).

3. Effects on the Small and Large Intestine

In conscious dogs with electrodes chronically implanted on different segments of the gut, bombesin (0.3–1 µg kg^{-1} h^{-1}) produced a remarkable increase in the frequency of pacemaker potentials in the antrum, duodenum, jejunum, and ileum, with no consistent change in the colon. In the duodenum and jejunum, the increase in frequency of gastrointestinal basic electric rhythm (BER) was correlated with the decrease in pacemaker potential amplitude. The propagation velocity of the pacemaker potential was approximately halved. In the antrum and ileum, spikes were not affected, whereas they were abolished in the duodenum and jejunum. The highest doses used caused disappearance of the rhythmicity of contractions of the duodenum and proximal jejunum with appearance of an irregular sequence of slow and small potentials and of a true disorganization of electrical activity (Fig. 4). This was probably due to the failure of coupling between relaxation oscillators over critical maximal frequencies. During recovery, electrical activity gradually returned towards the preinfusion pattern (CAPRILLI et al. 1975). Like bombesin, litorin caused disappearance of spikes, accompanied by complete arrest of mechanical activity of the upper small intestine. The secondary hypermotility which followed the interruption of the peptide infusion was even more remarkable for litorin than for bombesin. In conscious fasted dogs, bombesin (2–5 ng kg^{-1} min^{-1}) provoked an immediate termination of the interdigestive migrating myoelectric com-

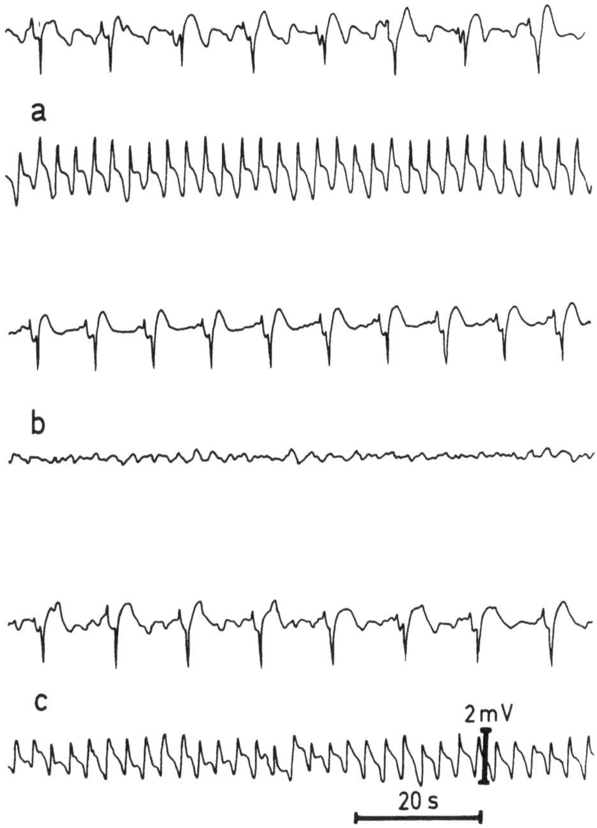

Fig. 4 a–c. Gastric and duodenal electric activity in the dog recorded before **a,** during infusion of bombesin (10 ng kg^{-1} min^{-1}) **b,** and during recovery **c.** Electric disorganization of the duodenal recording is evident in **b.** (R. CAPRILLI unpublished work 1978)

plex; after the infusion was discontinued there was an increase in the frequency and propagation velocity of the interdigestive migrating myoelectric complex (MELCHIORRI 1978).

The activity of bombesin on the human gastrointestinal tract was investigated by X-ray examination (BERTACCINI et al. 1974c) or by recording intraluminal pressure in the duodenum and jejunum (CORAZZIARI et al. 1974). The results obtained by both methods were very similar. The peptide (5–20 ng kg^{-1} min^{-1}) was shown to act differently on the various segments of the gastrointestinal tract. The body and the fundus of the stomach completely lost their basal motility. The antrum and the pylorus were immediately contracted as was the ileocecal valve. The motilities of duodenum, jejunum, and ileum were depressed or totally inhibited (Fig. 5). In four of six subjects, colonic motility was also inhibited (Fig. 6). All these changes lasted 15–20 min, then tended to disappear, even if the infusion was prolonged. As soon as the infusion was discontinued there was an immediated relaxation of the pylorus, followed by a remarkable hyperactivity of the whole gastrointestinal tract, especially the duodenum and the jejunum, lasting 10–15 min. These changes were accompanied by a significant ($P < 0.01$) acceleration of transit measured by means

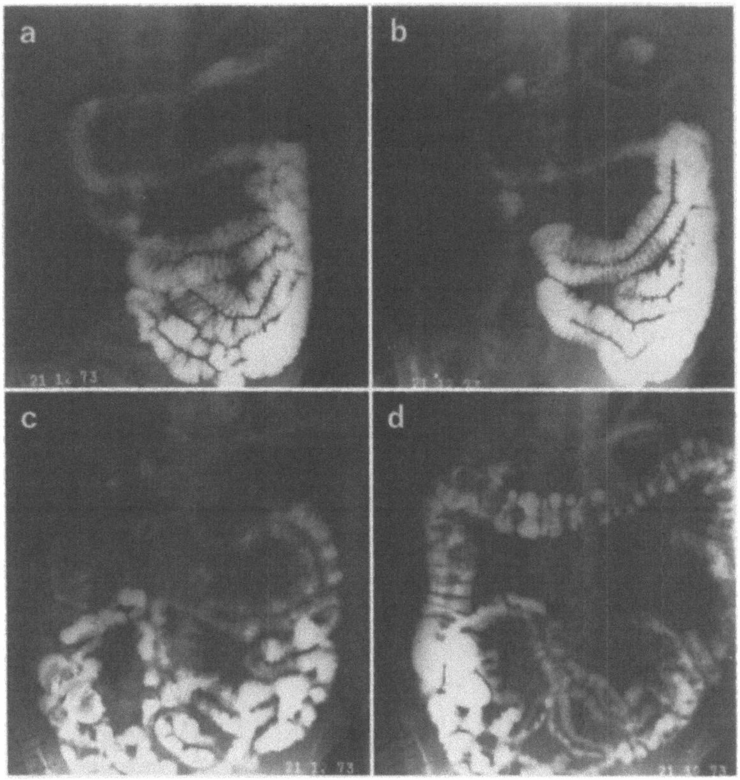

Fig. 5a–d. X-ray examination of the digestive tract. Radiograms taken 5 min **a** and 10 min **b** from the beginning of bombesin infusion (20 ng kg^{-1} min^{-1}) and 5 min **c** and 10 min **d** after the end of the infusion

of radiopaque markers. Apparently, the possibility of reducing gut motility during infusion of bombesin was appreciated by radiologists and ORLANDINI (unpublished work) actually speculated on the practical application of this phenomenon in radiologic diagnosis of particular diseases of the alimentary canal. All these effects were also obtained with the synthetic COOH terminal nonapeptide, given at the same doses and infusion rates. Side effects, represented by nausea and abdominal pain, were present only in a few subjects treated with the highest doses tested; they disappeared as soon as the infusion was discontinued.

C. Conclusions

From all the data reported here it is clear that bombesin exerts a quite peculiar activity on the gut: a predominantly stimulatory effect in the in vitro preparations (with the exception of the rat duodenum) and a predominantly inhibitory effect in the in vivo experiments (with the exception of rat stomach and of some sphincter muscles such as the LES, pylorus and ileocecal valve) which appeared to be con-

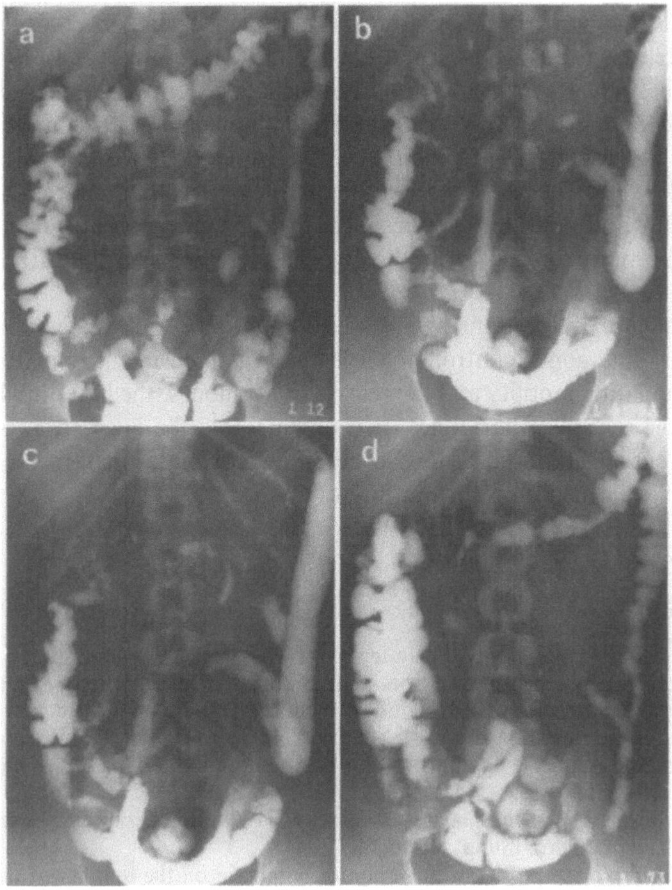

Fig. 6 a–d. X-ray examination of the large intestine. Basal radiogram **a**, 5 min **b**, and 10 min **c** after the beginning of bombesin infusion (15 ng kg^{-1} min^{-1}) and 5 min **d** after discontinuing the infusion

tracted. Though differences between in vitro and in vivo observations are fairly common, since the former reflect the activities of compounds which diffuse into the tissues from the surrounding fluid with only local effects, and the latter concern the activities of compounds reaching the muscle layer through its vascular supply, it is difficult to find an acceptable explanation for the striking discrepancies observed with bombesin. The only hypothesis which can be suggested is that the final effect of bombesin represents the algebraic sum of different effects, some directed towards the smooth muscle (these are prominent in the isolated preparations) and some mediated through the release of known and/or unknown stimulatory or inhibitory substances. Indeed, bombesin has been shown to be one of the most effective and polyvalent "releasing factors" so far known: it releases gastrin (BERTACCINI et al. 1974 b; BASSO et al. 1976), cholecystokinin (ERSPAMER et al. 1974; FENDER et al. 1976), pancreatic polypeptide (TAYLOR et al. 1978), glucagon (FALLUCCA et al. 1977), gastric inhibitory polypeptide (BECKER et al. 1978), prolactin and growth hormone (RIVIER et al. 1978), motilin and neurotensin (BLOOM et al. 1979), while it inhibits release of vasoactive intestinal peptide (MELCHIORRI et al. 1975). Moreover, bombesin was shown to release acetylcholine (KOWALEWSKI and KOLODEJ 1976) catecholamines (S. E. VIZI personal communication 1974) and as already mentioned a prostaglandin of the F type (M. IMPICCIATORE and F. BERTI unpublished work 1980). The latest observation on this topic is that reported by AKANDE et al. (1980) who found that bombesin (17 ng kg^{-1} min^{-1}) is able to release substance P-like immunoreactivity in the dog. This release is partially atropine sensitive.

As in the case of secretions, so in the case of motility, there appears to be a classical agonist–antagonist control system between bombesin and somatostatin: the former stimulating motility and the release of hormones, the latter inhibiting motility and the release of hormones. It is obvious that the interaction between all these different effects at the various levels of the gastrointestinal tract may be seen as its peculiar influence on the motility of the gut.

References

Akande B, Modlin IM, Reilly P, Jaffe BM (1980) Release of substance P-like immunoreactivity by a meal and bombesin. In: Bloom SR, Polak JM (eds) Regulatory peptides, suppl 1. Elsevier/North-Holland Biomedical, Amsterdam Oxford New York, p 51

Basso N, Giri S, Lezoche E, Materia A, Melchiorri P, Speranza V (1976) Effect of secretin, glucagon, and duodenal acidification on bombesin-induced hypergastrinemia in man. Am J Gastroenterol 66:448–451

Becker HD, Börger HW, Schafmayer A, Werner M (1978) Bombesin releases GIP in dogs. Scand J Gastroenterol [Suppl 49] 13:14

Bertaccini G, Impicciatore M (1975) Action of bombesin on the motility of the stomach. Naunyn Schmiedebergs Arch Pharmacol 289:149–156

Bertaccini G, Erspamer V, Melchiorri P, Sopranzi N (1974a) Gastrin release by bombesin in the dog. Br J Pharmacol 52:219–225

Bertaccini G, Impicciatore M, Molina E, Zappia L (1974b) Action of some natural and synthetic peptides on the motility of human gastrointestinal tract in vitro. In: Daniel EE (ed) Fourth Int Symp Gastrointest Motility. Mitchell, Vancouver, pp 287–292

Bertaccini G, Impicciatore M, Molina E, Zappia L (1974c) Action of bombesin on human gastrointestinal motility. Rend Gastroenterol 6:45–51

Bertaccini G, Zappia L, Molina E (1979) "In vitro" duodenal muscle in the pharmacological study of natural compounds. Scand J Gastroenterol [Suppl 54] 14:87–93

Bertaccini G, Coruzzi G, Scarpignato C (1981) Exogenous and endogenous compounds which affect the contractility of the lower esophageal sphincter (LES). In: Stipa S, Belsey R, Moraldi A (eds) Int Symp Med and Surg Problems of the Esophagus, Rome, May 7–9, 1980. Academic Press, New York, pp 22–29

Bloom SR, Chatei MA, Christofides ND et al. (1979) Bombesin infusion in man, pharmacokinetics, and effect on gastrointestinal and pancreatic hormonal peptides. J Endocrinol 83:P51

Broccardo M (1978) Effect of bombesin and somatostatin on intragastric pressure in dogs (Abstr 531). 7th Int Congr Pharmacol, Paris, July 1978. Pergamon, Oxford

Broccardo M, Falconieri Erspamer G, Melchiorri P, Negri L, De Castiglione R (1975) Relative potency of bombesin-like peptides. Br J Pharmacol 55:221–227

Caprilli R, Melchiorri P, Improta G, Vernia P, Frieri G (1975) Effects of bombesin and bombesin-like peptides on gastrointestinal myoelectric activity. Gastroenterology 68:1228–1235

Corazziari E, Torsoli A, Delle Fave GF, Melchiorri P, Habib I, Fortunée (1974) Effects of bombesin on the mechanical activity of the human duodenum and jejunum. Rend Gastroenterol 6:55–59

Dockray GJ, Vaillant C, Hutchison J, Dimaline R, Gregory RA (1979) Characterization of molecular forms of cholecystokinin (CCK), vasoactive intestinal peptide (VIP), and bombesin-like immunoreactivity (BLI) in nerves and endocrine cells. In: Rosselin G, Fromageot P, Bonfils S (eds) Hormone receptors in digestion and nutrition. Elsevier/North-Holland Biomedical, Amsterdam Oxford New York, pp 501–511

Endean R, Erspamer V, Falconieri Erspamer G, Improta G, Melchiorri P, Negri L, Sopranzi N (1975) Parallel bioassay of bombesin and litorin, a bombesin-like peptide from the skin of *Litoria aurea*. Br J Pharmacol 55:213–219

Erspamer V (1980) Peptides of the amphibian skin active on the gut. II. Bombesin-like peptides: isolation, structure, and basic functions. In: Jerzy Glass GB (ed) Gastrointestinal hormones. Raven, New York, pp 343–361

Erspamer V, Melchiorri P (1976) Amphibian skin peptides active on the gut. J Endocrinol 70:12P–13P

Erspamer V, Falconieri Erspamer G, Inselvini M, Negri L (1972) Occurrence of bombesin and alytesin in extracts of the skin of three european discoglossid frogs and pharmacological actions of bombesin on extravascular smooth muscle. Br J Pharmacol 45:333–348

Erspamer V, Improta G, Melchiorri P, Sopranzi N (1974) Evidence of cholecystokinin release by bombesin in the dog. Br J Pharmacol 52:227–232

Erspamer V, Falconieri Erspamer G, Melchiorri P, Negri L (1979) Occurrence and polymorphism of bombesin-like peptides in the gastrointestinal tract of birds and mammals. Gut 20:1047–1056

Fallucca F, Delle Fave G, Gambardella S, Mirabella C, De Magistris L, Carratù R (1977) Glucagon secretion induced by bombesin in man. In: Speranza V, Basso N, Lezoche E (eds) Int Symp Gastrointest Horm Dig Pathol, Rome, June 13–15. Arti Grafiche Tris, Rome, p A131

Fender HR, Curtis PJ, Rayford PHL, Thompson JC (1976) Effect of bombesin on serum gastrin and cholecystokinin in dogs. Surg Forum 37:414–416

Kowalewski K, Kolodej A (1976) Effect of bombesin, a natural tetradecapeptide, on myoelectrical and mechanical activity of isolated, *ex vivo* perfused, canine stomach. Pharmacology 14:8–19

Lechago J, Holmquist AL, Walsh JH (1978) Localization of a bombesin-like peptide in frog gastric mucosa by immunofluorescence and RIA. Gastroenterology 74:A1054

Marletta F, Monello S, Catalano F, Mandala ML, Daniele S, Blasi A (1979) Relationship between lower oesophageal sphincter pressure and serum gastrin levels during bombesin infusion. Ital J Gastroenterol 11:9–11

McDonald RJ, Jörnvall H, Nilsson G, Vagne M, Ghatei M, Bloom SR, Mutt V (1979) Characterization of a gastrin releasing peptide from porcine non-antral gastric tissue. Biochem Biophys Res Commun 90:227–233

Melchiorri P (1978) Bombesin and bombesin-like peptides of amphibian skin. In: Bloom SR (ed) Gut hormones. Churchill Livingstone, Edinburgh London, pp 534–540

Melchiorri P, Improta G, Sopranzi N (1975) Inibizione della secrezione di VIP da parte della bombesina nel cane, nel gatto e nell'uomo. Rend Gastroenterol [Suppl 1] 7:57

Mukhopadhyay AK, Kunnemann M (1979) Mechanism of lower esophageal sphincter stimulation by bombesin in the opossum. Gastroenterology 76:1409–1414

Reeve JR, Chew P, Walsh J (1980) Amino acid composition of a canine bombesin-like peptide. In: Bloom SR, Polak JM (eds) Regulatory peptides, suppl 1. Elsevier/North-Holland Biomedical, Amsterdam Oxford New York, p 590

Rivier C, Rivier J, Vale W (1978) The effect of bombesin and related peptides on prolactin and growth hormone secretion in the rat. Endocrinology 102:519–522

Scarpignato C, Bertaccini G (1981) Bombesin delays gastric emptying in the rat. Digestion 21:104–106

Taylor IL, Walsh JH, Carter DC, Wood J, Grossman MI (1978) Effect of atropine and bethanechol on release of pancreatic polypeptide (PP) and gastrin by bombesin in dog. Scand J Gastroenterol [Suppl 49] 13:183

Walsh JH, Dockray GJ (1978) Localization of bombesin-like immunoreactivity (BLI) in gut brain of rat. Gastroenterology 74:A1108

Zetler G (1980) Antagonism of the gut-contracting effects of bombesin and neurotensin by opioid peptides, morphine, atropine or tetrodotoxin. Pharmacology 21:348–354

CHAPTER 2c

Peptides: Pancreatic Hormones

G. BERTACCINI

Glucagon

A. Introduction

The pancreatic hormone glucagon, well known essentially for its metabolic effects, has also been used as a pharmacologic tool in different conditions: as a provocative test for pheochromocytoma, as a stimulus for growth hormone release, in the treatment of uncomplicated insulin-induced and sulfonylurea-induced hypoglycemia, and in some cases of acute heart failure in which myocardial tissue is essentially healthy. From a chemical point of view glucagon is a member of the so-called secretin family and it shares 14 positionally identical amino acids with secretin (see Table 1 in Chap. 2a, Secretin), suggesting that these two peptides may have a common ancestral gene and that their structure may contain a still undeciphered message of phylogenetic and physiologic significance (for reviews see LEFEBVRE and UNGER 1972; FOÀ et al. 1977). No wonder that their effects have so many points in common: both stimulate the secretion of insulin, inhibit gastric secretion, and exert a predominant inhibitory effect on gastrointestinal motility. This latter effect will be described in detail.

B. Effects on the Lower Esophageal Sphincter

Glucagon was shown to reduce lower esophageal sphincter (LES) pressure in dogs and in humans when given as a bolus (1–100 μg/kg) or by continuous infusion (0.5–0.75 $\mu g\ kg^{-1}\ h^{-1}$). The maximum effect lasted about 30 min and was obtained with 60 μg/kg in humans and with 100 μg/kg in dogs. The effect was dose dependent and was observed both under basal conditions and during pentagastrin-increased LES pressure (JENNEWEIN et al. 1973; HOGAN et al. 1975). In contrast to that of secretin, glucagon-induced inhibition was apparently noncompetitive (WALDECK et al. 1973; JAFFER et al. 1974). Similar results were obtained with isolated canine LES preparations with concentrations of glucagon as low as 10^{-8}–10^{-6} g/ml. In the conscious baboon, glucagon was found to have a very weak relaxant effect on the LES. Its activity was only 1/32 that of VIP for reduction of basal LES pressure and 1/64 that of VIP for reduction of pentagastrin-stimulated LES pressure (SIEGEL et al. 1979).

Quite different results were obtained in the cat (BEHAR 1978). In this species, intravenous glucagon (1–80 μg/kg) caused LES contraction, the maximal response being obtained with 20 and 40 μg, threshold dose being as low as 1 μg/kg. The magnitude of the LES-induced contraction after administration of glucagon was two-thirds of the rise in pressure observed after a maximal dose of pentagastrin (1 μg/kg). Hexamethonium, phentolamine, and tetrodotoxin as well as pretreatment with reserpine or surgical bilateral adrenalectomy blocked the effect of glucagon, indicating that the hormone may stimulate the preganglionic neuron of the sympathetic neural pathway to the LES, requiring intact ganglionic cholinergic transmission and the release of noradrenaline (BEHAR et al. 1979).

In recent studies in humans (CHRISTIANSEN et al. 1977), it was shown that endogenously released glucagon (after i.v. infusion of L-arginine, which resulted in plasma concentrations of pancreatic glucagon comparable to those seen after a meal) caused a significant reduction of pentagastrin-stimulated (0.5 μg kg^{-1} h^{-1}) LES pressure. Exogenous glucagon (1.6 μg kg^{-1} h^{-1}) lowered LES pressure to a lesser degree, in spite of higher plasma glucagon levels (CHRISTIANSEN et al. 1977). This probably indicates either that arginine releases other inhibitory substances or that endogenously released glucagon has activity quantitatively different from that of exogenously administered porcine glucagon. There was no interaction between glucagon and secretin on the pentagastrin-stimulated LES (CHRISTIANSEN and BORGESKOV 1974).

Glucagon was also shown to decrease elevated resting LES pressure in patients with achalasia (JENNEWEIN et al. 1973) and the same effect was obtained in one patient with Zollinger–Ellison syndrome and LES pressure enhanced by the consequent hypergastrinemia (HOGAN et al. 1975). Doses of 60–100 μg/kg were necessary to obtain these effects. In one patient with hyperglucagonemia due to a pancreatic carcinoma, the LES resting pressure and the LES responses to a variety of stimuli were normal before and after the operation (with consequent return to normal levels of glucagon; TOLIN et al. 1979). All these observations suggest that the hormone plays no physiologic role in the regulation of LES tone, and that therefore the LES relaxation after relatively large doses of glucagon should be considered a truly pharmacologic effect of the hormone. The usefulness of glucagon (1 mg i.v.) in a case of severe esophageal obstruction secondary to food impaction in the lower third of the esophagus was recently reported, with the demonstration of the rapid passage of the meat bolus into the stomach consequent to the visible relaxation of the LES (PILLARI et al. 1979).

C. Effect on the Stomach

I. In Vivo Studies

The inhibitory effect of glucagon on gastric hunger contractions in normal subjects was first described by STUNKARD et al. (1955). NECHELES et al. (1966) demonstrated a decrease in intraluminal pressure in the stomach after glucagon administration and stated that the inhibition was related to the arteriovenous blood sugar difference. In the dog, decrease in intragastric pressure by a low (6.3 μg kg^{-1} h^{-1}) but not by a high (25 μg kg^{-1} h^{-1}) dose of glucagon has also been reported (VALENZUELA 1976). The doses necessary to induce these effects appeared to be "pharmacologic" rather than "physiologic" since they produced plasma glucagon levels (more than 3,000 pg/ml) far in excess of those encountered in physiologic circumstances.

In the isolated perfused canine stomach, glucagon (5 mg/h) inhibited mechanical activity and electrical response activity. The hormone was also able to decrease but not to suppress changes induced by perfusion with pentagastrin and methacholine (KOWALEWSKI and KOLODEJ 1975). The action of glucagon lasted for 20–30 min after interruption of infusion suggesting a rather slow catabolism of the peptide. Similar results were obtained in the same kind of preparation from the pig (KOWALEWSKI et al. 1976). These experiments did not suffice to establish whether the effect of glucagon was a direct one on the stomach muscle or was mediated through release of catecholamines in the supporting animal, with a consequent hypercatecholaminemia in the perfusion blood. On the other hand, since the vasodilatory effect of glucagon lasted only during the infusion of the hormone, the hemodynamic effect did not seem to be directly correlated with the effect on electrical and mechanical activity.

In the conscious dog with chronically implanted electrodes, glucagon (5 μg/kg i.v.) caused a inhibition of gastric contractions, with a reduction or cessation of spike activity. This effect was abolished only by bivagotomy or by pretreatment with dihydroergotamine, suggesting that glucagon has two modes of action: an activation of vagal inhibitory fibers and a release of catecholamines from the adrenal medulla (MIOLAN and ROMAN 1975). Similar findings were reported by WATANABE et al. (1979). Glucagon (1 and 10 μg/kg i.v.) administered both in the fasted and in the fed state did not affect the amplitude of the initial potential but completely suppressed the second potential. The intervals between the initial potentials were prolonged. The duration of the glucagon inhibitory effect lasted for 10–28 min.

Studies in humans indicated that both motility and gastric emptying were decreased by glucagon (HRADSKY et al. 1973; MILLER et al. 1974a, 1978a; CHERNISH et al. 1978a). Changes in the number of contractions of the antrum and in the size of the pylorus after intravenous glucagon (1 mg) were quite similar to those elicited by Buscopan (20 mg; KILL et al. 1976). According to BORTOLOTTI et al. (1975), glucagon (0.05–1 $\mu g^{-1}\ kg^{-1}\ h^{-1}$), induced dose-related inhibition of basic electrical rhythm (BER) frequency, together with an inhibition of antral motor activity, followed at the end of infusion, by an increase in motor activity remarkable more than that of the preinfusion period. On the whole, the effects of glucagon were qualitatively similar to those of secretin though quantitatively smaller. The inhibition of gastric motility caused, as a logical consequence, a remarkable delay in gastric emptying which was highly significant after i.v. administration of 0.5–2 mg glucagon (MEVES et al. 1975; CHERNISH et al. 1978a). This effect was probably also connected to the increase in pyloric pressure which was demonstrated in humans after glucagon infusion, as well as after secretin infusion (PHAOSAWASDI et al. to be published).

II. In Vitro Studies

Glucagon in concentrations as high as 1 μg/ml had no effect on contraction amplitude or isotonic tone of strips from human stomach (in either antrum or corpus;

CAMERON et al. 1970). Higher concentrations (10 μg/ml) were tried on the isolated guinea pig stomach (GERNER and HAFFNER 1975) and found to have a direct inhibitory effect. Both motility index and basal pressure were decreased in the fundus, whereas in the antrum the pressure effect was seen only in distended preparations. In the same preparation, glucagon (12×10^{-6} *M*) was shown to inhibit the antral contractions induced by cholecystokinin (CCK). The inhibition seemed to be specific, since acetylcholine response was not modified by glucagon. Moreover the flattening and the shifting of the dose–response curve to CCK suggested an antagonism of noncompetitive type (GERNER and HAFFNER 1978).

D. Effects on the Small Intestine

I. Studies in Experimental Animals

Conflicting results have been reported for the intestinal effects of glucagon, which was sometimes found to inhibit and sometimes to increase intestinal motility. In a few experiments, both effects were observed, depending on the dose employed. In the anesthetized cat, glucagon (10–100 μg kg^{-1} min^{-1}) was found to cause marked inhibition of motility in both the jejunum and the colon, an effect which was abolished by the exclusion of the adrenals, suggesting the mediation of endogenous catecholamines (FASTH and HULTEN 1971).

One of the early experiments (GRANATA et al. 1974), in the conscious dog, showed that glucagon (20–40 μg/kg i.v.) caused an increase in the amplitude of spontaneous jejunal contractions which sometimes preceded, sometimes followed, and at times completely masked the well-known inhibitory effect of the hormone. These motor effects were accompanied by an increase in heart rate and mesenteric vasodilatation. The effects of glucagon in the absence (Fig. 1) or in the presence (Fig. 2) of spontaneous jejunal motility are shown. Slight intestinal hypermotility in the conscious dog has been confirmed in recent experiments (LIN 1980). Moreover, stimulation, lasting 3–5 min, of both mechanical and electrical activity in the duodenum and the distal small intestine was observed after a bolus i.v. injection of glucagon (0.05 mg/kg). When an i.v. infusion (0.5–1 mg/h) was given, the mechanical contraction of the circular muscle and spike potential activity continued throughout the period of infusion (EVANS et al. 1978; FOSTER et al. 1979). In the anesthesized dog, the opposing effects of glucagon were apparently related to the doses administered, low doses (10–20 μg/kg) causing increased motor activity in the small intestine and increased electrical activity in the stomach and small intestine, and large doses (200 μg/kg) causing inhibition of motor and electrical activity (NICOLOV and DELEVA 1977).

Fig. 1 a–f. Effects of glucagon in the anesthesized dog. Recordings of **a** pneumogram; **b** arterial pressure; **c** mean flow in the superior mesenteric artery; **d, e** intraluminal pressures recorded from two points of the jejunum (10 cm apart). The *cross* on the baseline **f** indicates the end of the injection of glucagon. Time from the beginning of the injection is indicated at the top of the tracings. Vertical lines indicate 1 s; *HR*, heart rate; *RM*, vascular resistance in the mesenteric artery (average arterial pressure in mm Hg divided by flow in the mesenteric artery in ml/min). (GRANATA et al. 1974) ▶

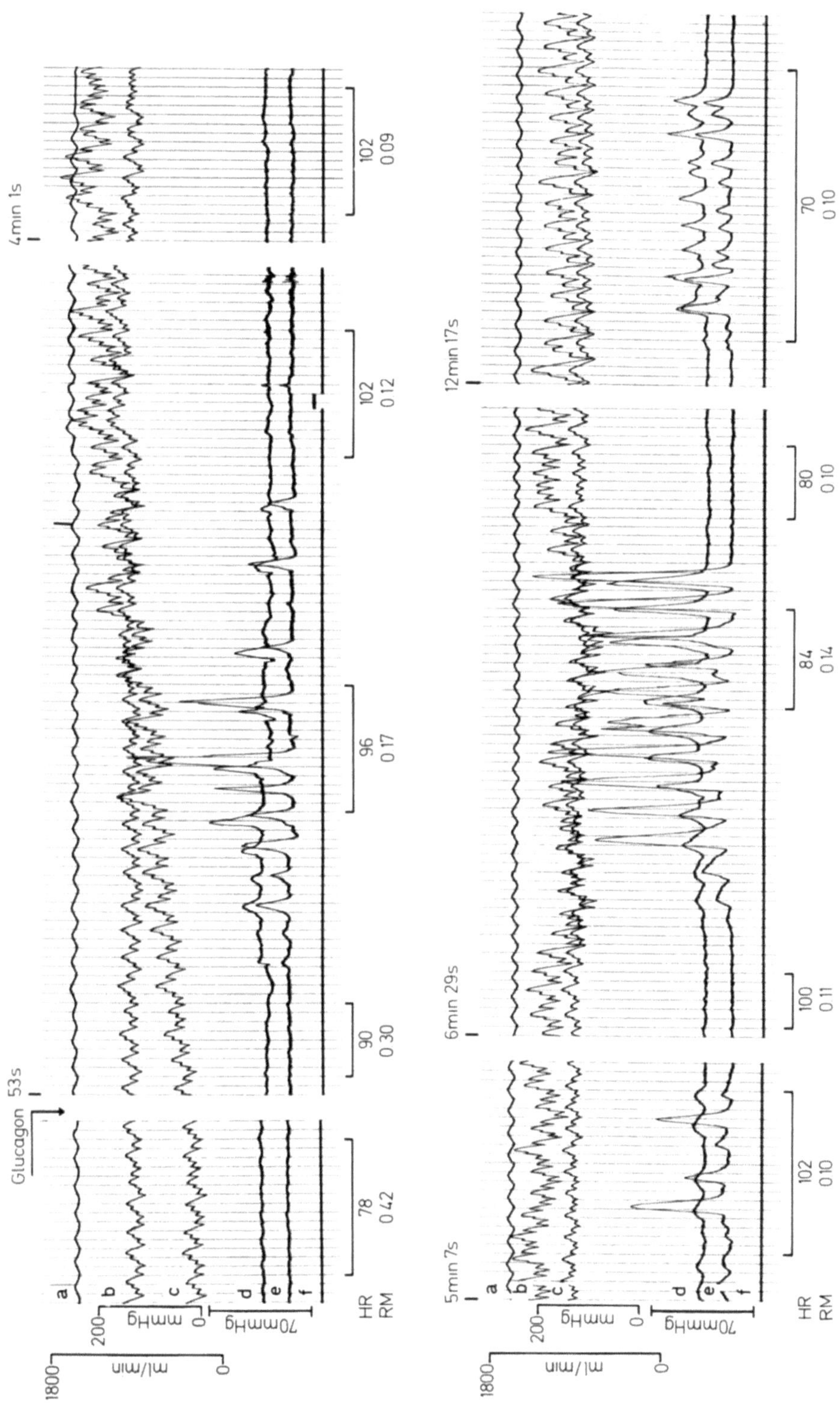
1800
ml/min
0
200
mmHg
0
70mmHg
a
b
c
d
e
f
HR
RM
Glucagon
53s
4min 1s
78
0.42
90
0.30
96
0.17
102
0.12
102
0.09
5min 7s
6min 29s
12min 17s
102
0.10
100
0.11
84
0.14
80
0.10
70
0.10

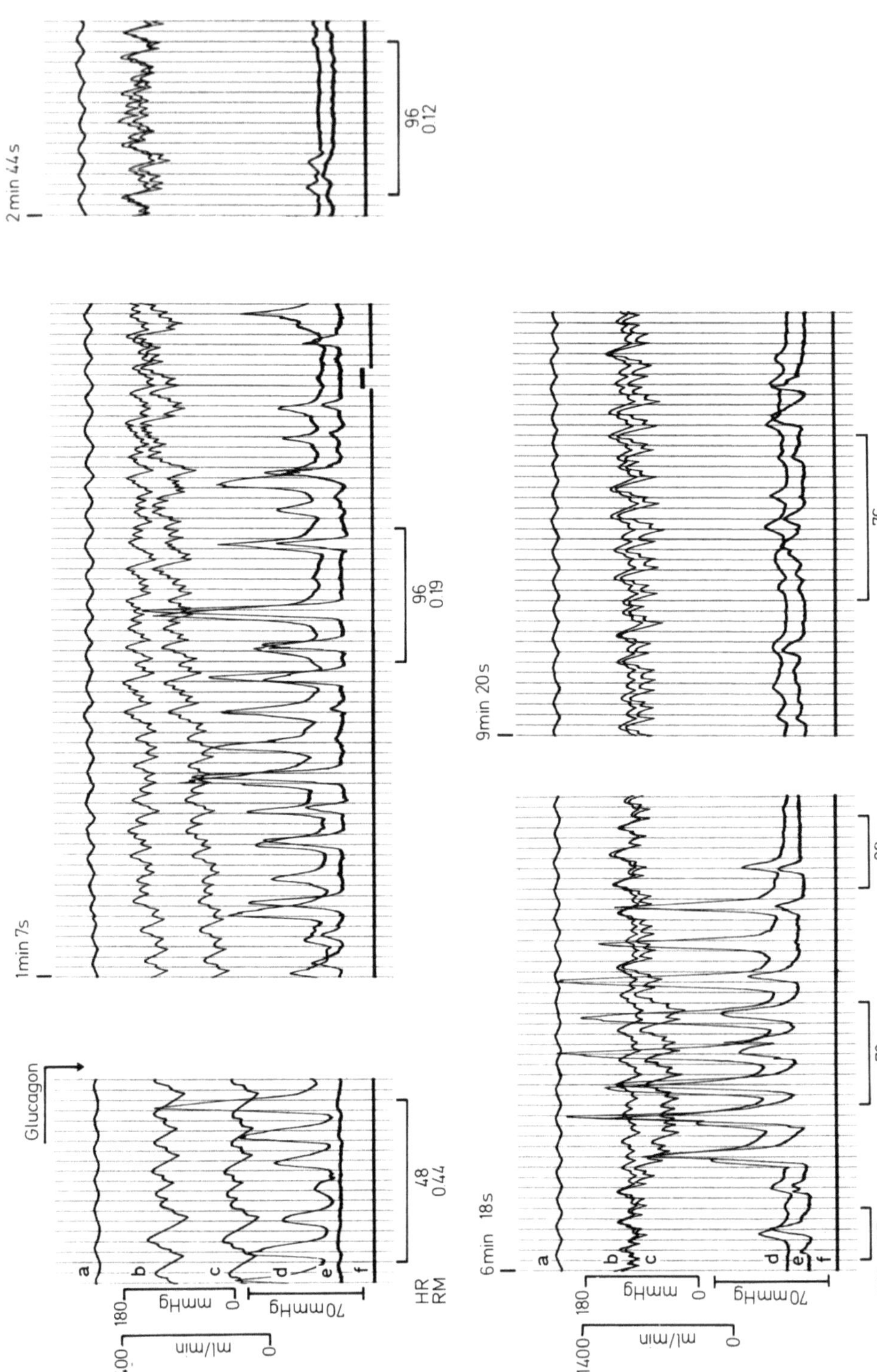

Fig. 2. Effects of glucagon in the anesthetized dog during spontaneous jejunal motility. Traces and symbols as in Fig. 1

In the isolated vascular-perfused small intestine of the dog, rapid intra-arterial injection of glucagon (15–100 μg) produced phase-locked spike bursts with visible contractions, with the maximal response in the midjejunum as reported by WINGATE et al. (1978). The same authors showed that in the conscious dog with chronically implanted electrodes, 1 mg/kg glucagon inhibited duodenal and jejunal spike activity when given by a bolus whereas 1 mg/h i.v. infusion, abolished migrating complexes and increased total spike activity at all levels of the small intestine. Glucagon infusion induced hyperglycemia and hyperinsulinemia, but infusions of insulin or glucose were without effect. In the light of all these observations that indicate possible stimulatory effects of glucagon in the dog, it is possible that the watery diarrhea, which followed administration of high doses of glucagon in combination with gastrin, was not only due to increased secretion of electrolytes in the jejunum and decreased absorbtion of electrolytes in the ileum, but could also have involved the stimulatory effect of glucagon on gut muscle.

In the conscious rat, high doses of i.v. glucagon (10 and 100 $\mu g\ kg^{-1}\ min^{-1}$) inhibited basal contractions in the jejunum up to complete suppression and significantly delayed transit without causing significant changes in absorption or secretion of fluids within the intestine (SCOTT and SUMMERS 1976). Also, the contractility of the intestinal villi was shown to be depressed in the dog by glucagon (0.12–5 μg intra-arterially) and this effect was thought to be connected to a competitive antagonism with secretin, which increases villous motility, and/or to circulation changes in villous blood capillaries (IHASZ et al. 1976).

Finally, in one in vitro study, glucagon was shown to lower tension in the circular and longitudinal muscle layers of the opossum duodenum and to decrease acetylcholine-induced contractions; however, rather high concentrations (10^{-5} *M*) had to be used in both cases (ANURAS and COOKE 1978). Rabbit jejunum was more sensitive to glucagon which dose-dependently (10^{-7}–10^{-5} *M*) inhibited spontaneous contractions, even after blockade of neuronal conduction by tetrodotoxin. However, glucagon appeared to be about 100 times less potent than somatostatin (COHEN et al. 1979).

II. Studies in Humans

Early studies with glucagon showed a constant inhibitory effect of the hormone on motor activity as recorded by balloon or observed by X-ray examination (DOTEVAL and KOCH 1963; CHERNISH et al. 1972; HICKS and TURNBERG 1974; WHALEN 1974). The effects were usually dose-related and could be observed even after intraportal administration (0.025–0.1 mg; KOCH et al. 1967). More recent studies showed that glucagon (0.5 and 1 $\mu g\ kg^{-1}\ min^{-1}$) inhibited myoelectric and mechanical activity in the duodenum, inducing dilatation and stasis (CORAZZIARI 1976; LABÒ and BORTOLOTTI 1976). This effect was more remarkable than those of other peptides, such as secretin, cholecystokinin, or cerulein. Glucagon shortened the intervals between successive migrating motor complexes even when administered as a bolus i.v. injection (1 mg; FOSTER et al. 1979). A similar inhibitory effect was observed in the jejunum after administration of 1.2 $\mu g\ kg^{-1}\ h^{-1}$, which significantly increased mean transit time. However, changes in fluid absorption and secretion were also noted, with a consequent increase in jejunal volume (HICKS and TURNBERG 1974).

According to PATEL et al. (1979) the effects of glucagon on human small intestine are mainly connected with changes in plasma insulin and glucose concentrations rather than with direct activity on the smooth muscle. In humans, a paradoxical stimulatory effect of glucagon, though very short lasting, was also observed after intravenous injection (MILLER et al. 1978 b). The slight increase in gut motility appeared just before the onset of hypotonicity or atonicity. The duodenum was the first to manifest the effect and the last to recover.

The relaxing properties of glucagon, overcoming functional spasm and permitting more detailed evaluation of organic narrowing, were applied clinically for hypotonic duodenography or endoscopic and radiologic examination of the gastrointestinal tract, usually with encouraging results, also considering the few side effects of the hormone compared with the anticholinergics used for the same purposes, which can precipitate cardiac arrhythmias, urinary retention, and glaucoma. Intravenous or intramuscular glucagon (0.5–2 mg), because of its rapid onset (1–5 min) and short duration of action (10–30 min), depending on the dose and the route of administration, was found to be useful tool in the diagnosis of occult small neoplasms, early Crohn's disease, Meckel's diverticulum, occult upper gastrointestinal bleeding, etc. (MLECKO 1974; GOHEL et al. 1975; CARSEN and FINBY 1976; FERRUCCI et al. 1977; BERTRAND et al. 1977; VECCHIOLI et al. 1977; MILLER et al. 1974 a, 1978 a, b; CHERNISH et al. 1978 b; HECHT et al. 1979).

An accurate study performed in infants and children allowed RATCLIFFE (1980) to establish the best dosage of glucagon to be used in double contrast barium examinations. A dose of 0.5–1 μg/kg i.v., producing an atonic period of 3–5 min, was suggested for double contrast meals. A larger dose of 0.8–1.25 μg/kg was recommended for barium enemas for which an atonic period of about 10 min was found to be satisfactory. No undesirable side effect was found in the twenty subjects examined.

E. Effects on the Large Intestine

Motor activities, whether recorded with pressure transducers, balloons, or intraluminal catheters, were all decreased in the dog by glucagon (LIN 1980). Apparently, doses of 5–10 μg kg^{-1} h^{-1} were always followed by an inhibitory effect, whereas i.v. bolus administration (0.1–0.5 μg/kg) was followed in 40% of the experiments by a stimulatory effect similar to that observed in the small intestine (GARCIA-VILAR 1979). As in the case of the small intestine, data from human studies are much more numerous.

In humans, both mechanical activity, recorded with balloons or intraluminal catheters, and myoelectrical activity, recorded with intraluminal, serosal, and surface electrodes, were remarkably decreased. Glucagon inhibited not only motility under basal conditions but also that stimulated by food, morphine, prostigmine, or cholecystokinin.

According to TAYLOR et al. (1975 a, b), glucagon inhibition of both slow wave electrical activity and motility throughout the colon and rectum (Fig. 3) was not related to the hyperglycemic effect of the hormone nor to a possible release of catecholamines, and a "direct" effect of the hormone on the smooth muscle was suggested. However, a certain degree of tachyphylaxis seen after successive adminis-

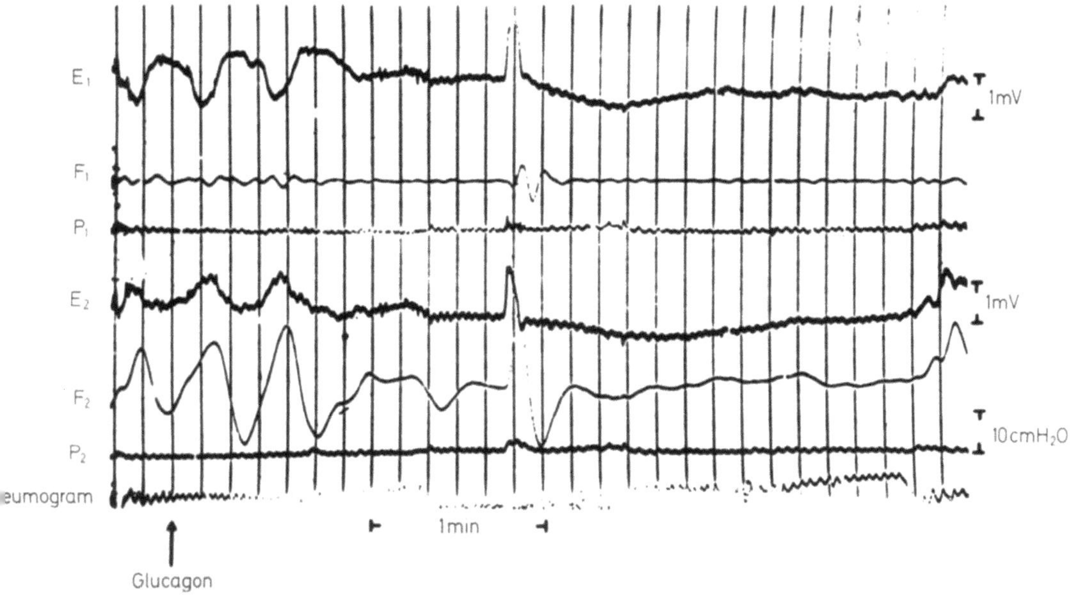

Fig. 3. Recording obtained by intraluminal electrodes 13 and 8 cm from the anus, showing a predominant 3 cycles/min slow wave electrical rhythm (E_1 and E_2). Approximately 60 s after the administration of glucagon (10 μg/kg) a complete inhibition of both electrical and pressure activity (P_1 and P_2) occurs, lasting for 3 min 40 s (10 s markers). The figure also shows traces from two filters, 6–9 cycles/min (F_1) and 3 cycles/min and (at the bottom) the pneumogram. (TAYLOR et al. 1975a)

trations of glucagon would be consistent with the idea that there is a possible release of known and/or unknown inhibitory mediators. Glucagon (0.5 mg/kg followed by 30 μg kg^{-1} h^{-1}) caused a strong inhibition of cholecystokinin-induced and prostigmine-induced motor activity in the colon and the rectum (CHOWDURY and LORBER 1975), and it also inhibited food-increased or morphine-increased motor activity in the colon, but not in the anal sphincter (CHOWDURY and LORBER 1977). Conversely, the unstimulated internal anal sphincter was inhibited by a pulse dose of the hormone (GARDNER et al. 1973). Surprisingly, glucagon (1–10 μg/ml) was found to contract the human taenia coli, an effect which was not modified by atropine (0.1 μg/ml; EGBERTS and JOHNSON 1977).

The relaxant properties of glucagon in the large intestine (Fig. 4) suggested that it could be used in radiologic examination of the colon and many authors have claimed that glucagon should be preferred to other drugs, such as propantheline or atropine, which have numerous side effects and contraindications in comparison with glucagon (MILLER et al. 1974b; GOHEL et al. 1975; MEEROFF et al. 1975; HARNED et al. 1976).

F. Conclusions

In conclusion, the action of glucagon appears to be predominantly an inhibitory one, at least in humans, whereas in experimental animals stimulatory effects can

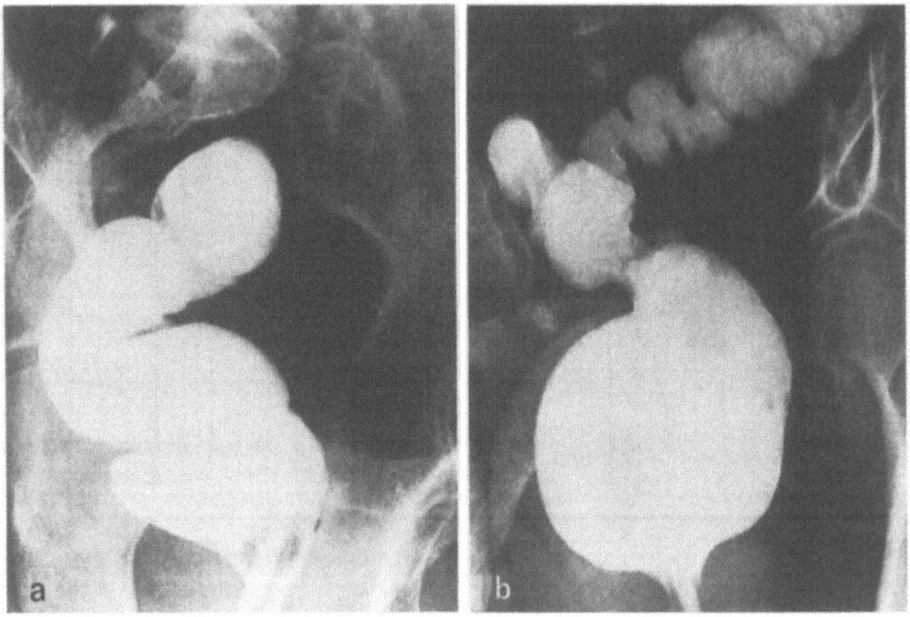

Fig. 4 a, b. Effects of glucagon on human intestine. The flow of barium appears to be obstructed **a** at the rectosigmoid; 7 min after i.m. injection of 2 mg of glucagon, **b** spasm is relieved. No organic disease is seen. (GOHEL et al. 1975)

occur in some segments of the gastrointestinal tract, indicating marked species differences in the effects of the hormone. The mechanism of action of the hormone is poorly understood so far, since some in vitro data are apparently in favor of direct activity on the smooth muscle while in vivo experiments seem to suggest a release of catecholamines from the adrenal glands as being responsible for the relaxant effects. Of course, the release of other known and/or unknown humoral mediators cannot be totally excluded.

In all of the studies, the doses required for the effects on gastrointestinal motility far exceeded those required for the hyperglycemic activity of glucagon, which can be considered the primary action of the hormone. Moreover, the serum level of glucagon during inhibition of gut motility was far in excess of that encountered under physiologic circumstances (VALENZUELA 1976). In any case, with other endogenous substances affecting gut motility, we can hypothesize that glucagon, perhaps not by itself, may contribute in the physiologic regulation of motility of the gastrointestinal tract by interacting with the very many stimulatory or inhibitory endogenous substances which may be released under physiologic conditions.

Recently, glucagon-like immunoreactive substances have been found to be present in tissues other than the pancreas (UNGER et al. 1961). Later on, gastric glucagon-like and enteric glucagon-like substances were described (LEFEBVRE and LUYCKX 1978; HOLST 1978), mainly in the stomach and the ileum but also in the jejunum and the colon (BLOOM and POLAK 1978). They must be structurally related to pancreatic glucagon, to explain their cross-immunoreactivity with it, but of course more precise studies are needed to assess the relation between the plasma levels of pancreatic and enteroglucagon released by physiologic stimuli and their biologic effects on gut motility. It is, however, interesting that preliminary data have shown that "purified enteroglucagon" is able to inhibit antral and duodenal motility in the conscious dog at very low doses (LIN 1980).

References

Anuras S, Cooke RA (1978) Effects of some gastrointestinal hormones on two muscle layers of duodenum. Am J Physiol 234:E60–E63
Behar J (1978) Effect of glucagon on the feline lower esophageal sphincter (LES) in vivo. Gastroenterology 74:A1116
Behar J, Field S, Marin C (1979) Effect of glucagon, secretin, and vasoactive intestinal polypeptide on the feline lower esophageal sphincter: mechanism of action. Gastroenterology 77:1001–1007
Bertrand G, Linscheer WG, Raheja KL, Woods RE (1977) Double-blind evaluation of glucagon and propantheline bromide (probanthine) for hypotonic duodenography. Am J Roentgenol 128:197–200
Bloom SR, Polak JM (1978) Gut hormone overview. In: Bloom SR (ed) Gut hormones. Churchill Livingstone, Edinburgh London, pp 3–18
Bortolotti M, Sanavio C, Sansone G, Labò G (1975) Modifications in human gastric motility induced by secretin and by glucagon. Rend Gastroenterol 7:240
Cameron AJ, Phillips SF, Summerskill WHJ (1970) Comparison of effects of gastrin, cholecystokinin-pancreozymin, secretin, and glucagon on human stomach muscle in vitro. Gastroenterology 59:539–545
Carsen GM, Finby N (1976) Hypotonic duodenography with glucagon. A clinical comparison study. Radiology 118:529–533
Chernish SM, Miller RE, Rosenak BD, Schulz NE (1972) Hypotonic duodenography with the use of glucagon. Gastroenterology 63:392–398
Chernish SM, Brunelle RR, Rosenak BD, Ahmadzai S (1978a) Comparison of the effects of glucagon and atropine sulfate on gastric emptying. Am J Gastroenterol 70:581–586
Chernish SM, Miller RE, Brunell RL, Rosenak BD (1978b) Dose-response to intravenous glucagon as measured by roentgenography. Radiology 127:55–59
Chowdhury AR, Lorber SH (1975) Effect of glucagon on cholecystokinin and prostigmin-induced motor activity of the distal colon and rectum in humans. Gastroenterology 68:875
Chowdhury AR, Lorber SH (1977) Effects of glucagon and secretin on food- or morphine-induced motor activity of the distal colon, rectum, and anal sphincter. Dig Dis Sci 22:775–780
Christiansen J, Borgeskov S (1974) The effect of glucagon and the combined effect of glucagon and secretin on lower esophageal sphincter pressure in man. Scand J Gastroenterol 9:615–618
Christiansen J, Lauritzen K, Moesgaard J, Holst JJ (1977) Effect of endogenous and exogenous glucagon on pentagastrinstimulated lower esophageal sphincter pressure in man. Scand J Gastroenterol 12:33–36
Cohen ML, Wiley KS, Yaden E, Slater IH (1979) *In vitro* actions of somatostatin, D-Val^1-Trp^8-somatostatin and glucagon in rabbit jejunum and guinea pig ileum. J Pharmacol Exp Ther 211:423–429
Corazziari E (1976) Mechanical activity of the second portion of human duodenum. Rend Gastroenterol 8:64
Doteval G, Koch NG (1963) The effect of glucagon on intestinal motility in man. Gastroenterology 45:364–367
Egberts EH, Johnson AG (1977) The effect of cholecystokinin on human *taenia coli*. Digestion 15:217–222
Evans DF, Foster GE, Hardcastle JD, Johnson F, Wright J (1978) The effect of glucagon on the canine duodenum and small intestine. Br J Pharmacol 64:475P

Fasth S, Hulten L (1971) The effect of glucagon on intestinal motility and blood flow. Acta Physiol Scand 83:169–173
Ferrucci JT, Long JA (1977) Radiologic treatment of esophageal food impacting using intravenous glucagon. Radiology 125:25–28
Foà PP, Bajaj JS, Foà NL (eds) (1977) Glucagon: its role in physiology and clinical medicine. Springer, Berlin Heidelberg New York
Foster GE, Hardcastle JD, Evans DF, Wright J, Johnson F (1979) Action of glucagon on the human and canine duodenum. Gut 20:A439–A440
García-Vilar R Recherches sur la motricité colique chez le chien. Master's thesis, Institut National Polytechnique de Toulouse, pp 1–136
Gardner JD, Malloy RG, Hogan WJ (1973) Pentagastrin and glucagon effects on the internal anal sphincter pressure in man. Clin Res 21:826
Gerner T, Haffner JFW (1975) The significance of distention for the effect of glucagon on the fundic and antral motility in isolated guinea-pig stomach. Scand J Gastroenterol 10:51–53
Gerner T, Haffner JFW (1978) The inhibitory effect of secretin and glucagon on pressure responses to cholecystokinin-pancreozymin in isolated guinea-pig stomach. Scand J Gastroenterol 13:537–544
Gohel VK, Dalinka MK, Coren GS (1975) Hypotonic examination of the colon with glucagon. Radiology 115:1–4
Granata L, Leone D, Paccione F, Ruccia D (1974) Effetti del glucagone sulla motilità del digiuno nel cane non narcotizzato. Boll Soc Ital Biol Sper 50:780–785
Harned RK, Stelling CB, Williams S, Wolf GL (1976) Glucagon and barium enema examinations: a controlled clinical trial. Am J Roentgenol 126:981–984
Hecht HL, Hollenberg GM, Pradham AR (1979) Glucagon-induced small intestinal hypotonia demonstrating bleeding lymphoma. Gastrointest Radiol 4:61–63
Hicks T, Turnberg LA (1974) Influence of glucagon on the human jejunum. Gastroenterology 67:1114–1118
Hogan WJ, Dodds WJ, Hoke SE, Reid DP, Kalkhoff RK, Arndorfer RC (1975) Effect of glucagon on esophageal motor function. Gastroenterology 69:60–65
Holst JJ (1978) Physiology of enteric glucagon-like substances. In: Bloom SR (ed) Gut hormones. Churchill Livingstone, London Edinburgh, pp 383–386
Hradsky M, Stockbrügger R, Oestberg H (1973) The effect of glucagon on gastric motility, the pylorus and reflux of bile into the stomach during gastroscopic examination. Scand J Gastroenterol [Suppl 20] 8:26
Ihasz M, Koiss I, Németh EP, Folly G, Papp M (1976) Action of caerulein, glucagon or prostaglandin E_1 on the motility of intestinal villi. Pfluegers Arch 364:301–304
Jaffer SS, Makhlouf GM, Schorr BA, Zfass AM (1974) Nature and kinetics of inhibition of lower esophageal sphincter pressure by glucagon. Gastroenterology 67:42–46
Jennewein HM, Waldeck F, Siewert R, Weiser F, Thimm R (1973) The interaction of glucagon and pentagastrin on the lower oesophageal sphincter in man and dog. Gut 14:861–864
Kill J, Andersen D, Weinreich J (1976) A double-blind comparison of gastric relaxation after buscopan and glucagon Novo. Scand J Gastroenterol [Suppl 38] 11:58
Koch NG, Darle N, Doteval G (1967) Inhibition of intestinal motility in man by glucagon given intraportally. Gastroenterology 53:88–92
Kowalewski K, Kolodej A (1975) Effect of glucagon on myoelectrical activity recorded from the isolated homologous perfused canine stomach. Arch Int Pharmacodyn Ther 218:186–195
Kowalewski K, O'Sullivan G, Kolodej A (1976) Effect of glucagon on myoelectrical and mechanical activity of the isolated homologous perfused porcine stomach. Pharmacology 14:115–124
Labò G, Bortolotti M (1976) Effect of gut hormones on myoelectric and manometric activity of the duodenum in man. Rend Gastroenterol 8:64
Lefebvre PJ, Luyckx AS (1978) Gastric-glucagon: physiology and pathology. In: Grossman M, Speranza V, Basso N, Lezoche E (eds) Gastrointestinal hormones and pathology of the digestive system. Plenum, New York, pp 173–181

Lefebvre PJ, Unger RH (1972) Glucagon. Pergamon, Oxford
Lin TS (1980) Effects of insulin and glucagon on secretory and motor function of the gastrointestinal tract. In: Jerzy Glass GB (ed) Gastrointestinal Hormones. Raven, New York, pp 639–691
Meeroff JC, Jorgens J, Isenberg JI (1975) The effect of glucagon on barium-enema examination. Radiology 115:5–7
Meves M, Beger HG, Hüthwohl B (1975) The effect of some gastrointestinal hormones on gastric evacuation in man. In: Vantrappen G (ed) Fifth International Symposium on Gastrointestinal Motility. Typoff, Herentals, pp 76–81
Miller RE, Chernish SM, Skucas J, Rosenak BD, Rodda BE (1974a) Hypotonic roentgenography with glucagon. Am J Roentgenol Radium Ther Nuc Med 121:264–274
Miller RE, Chernish SM, Skucas J, Rosenak BD, Rodda BE (1974b) Hypotonic colon examination with glucagon. Radiology 113:555–562
Miller RE, Chernish SM, Brunelle RL, Rosenak BD (1978a) Dose response to intramuscular glucagon during hypotonic radiography. Radiology 127:49–53
Miller RE, Chernish SM, Brunelle RL, Rosenak BD (1978b) Double-blind radiographic study of dose-response to intravenous glucagon for hypotonic duodenography. Radiology 127:55–59
Miolan JP, Roman C (1975) Mechanisms of the inhibitory effect of glucagon on gastric motility. In: Vantrappen G (ed) Fifth International Symposium on Gastrointestinal Motility. Typoff, Herentals, pp 70–75
Mlecko LM (1974) Hypotonic duodenoscopy using glucagon. Gastroenterology 66:A164/818
Necheles H, Sporn J, Walker L (1966) Effect of glucagon on gastrointestinal motility. Am J Gastroenterol 45:34–39
Nicolov NA, Deleva JI (1977) Effects of glucagon on the motor and mio-electrical activity of the gastrointestinal tract in dogs. Riv Farmacol Ter 8:275–280
Patel GK, Whalen GE, Soergel KH, Wu WC, Meade RC (1979) Glucagon effects on the human small intestine. Dig Dis Sci 24:501–508
Phaosawasdi K, Boden G, Kolts B, Fisher RS (to be published) Hormonal effects on pyloric sphincter pressure: are they of physiological importance? Clin Res
Pillari G, Bank S, Katzka I, Fulco JD (1979) Meat bolus impaction of the lower esophagus associated with a paraesophageal hernia. Successful noninvasive treatment with intravenous glucagon. Am J Gastroenterol 71:287–289
Ratcliffe JF (1980) Glucagon in barium examination in infants and children: special reference to dosage. Br J Radiol 53:860–862
Scott LD, Summers RW (1976) Correlation of contractions and transit in rat small intestine. Am J Physiol 230:132–137
Siegel SR, Brown FC, Castell DO, Johnson LF, Said SI (1979) Effects of vasoactive intestinal polypeptide (VIP) on lower esophageal sphincter in awake baboons-comparison with glucagon and secretin. Dig Dis Sci 24:345–349
Stunkard SJ, Van Itallie TB, Reis BB (1955) The mechanism of satiety. Effect of glucagon on gastric hunger contraction in man. Proc Soc Exp Biol Med 89:258–261
Taylor I, Duthie HL, Cumberland DC, Smallwood R (1975a) Glucagon and the colon. Gut 16:973–978
Taylor I, Duthie HL, Smallwood R (1975b) The effect of glucagon on colonic myoelectric activity. In: Vantrappen F (ed) Fifth International Symposium on Gastrointestinal Motility. Typoff, Herentals, pp 76–81
Tolin RD, Boden G, Fisher RS (1979) Effects of endogenous hyperglucagonemia on lower esophageal sphincter pressure and gastric acid secretion. Dig Dis Sci 24:296–304
Unger RH, Eisentraut A, Sims K, McCall MS, Madison LL (1961) Sites of origin of glucagon in dogs and humans. Clin Res 9:53
Valenzuela JE (1976) Effect of intestinal hormones and peptides on intragastric pressure in dogs. Gastroenterology 71:766–769
Vecchioli A, Aluffi A, Parrella RE, Colagrande C (1977) Glucagon in gastric and duodenal roentgenology. In: Speranza V, Basso N, Lezoche E (eds) Int Symp Gastrointestinal Horm and Pathol Dig Syst, Rome, June 13–15, 1977. Arti Grafiche Tris, Rome, p 104

Waldeck F, Siewert R, Jennewein HM, Weiser F (1973) Das Druckprofil im unteren Ösophagussphinkter beim Menschen und seine Beeinflussung durch Gastrin, Calcitonin und Glucagon. Dtsch Med Wochenschr 98:1059–1063
Watanabe O, Atobe Y, Atsutaka Mori K, Akagi M, Nishi K (1979) Effects of feeding and glucagon on electrical activity of the stomach in the conscious dog: Proc 8 th Symposium on Pharmacological Activity and Mechanism, Kumamoto, Oct. 25–26. p S-4
Whalen GA (1974) Glucagon and the small gut. Gastroenterology 67:1284–1286
Wingate DL, Pearce EA, Thomas PA, Boucher BJ (1978) Glucagon stimulates intestinal myoelectric activity. Gastroenterology 74:A1152

Insulin

A. Introduction

As was mentioned in Chap. 1, it has been known for a long time that some gastrointestinal hormones can influence endocrine pancreatic secretions and vice versa. This complex relationship was named the "enteroinsular axis" (UNGER and EISENTRAUT 1969) and in its turn this represents the endocrine component of an even more complex system which could be called the "enteropancreatic axis" (FELBER and DICK 1975), that includes all the interactions of the gastrointestinal tract, endocrine, and exocrine pancreas. There are comprehensive and analytic reviews concerning the effects of insulin on motor and secretory functions of the digestive tract by BACHRACH (1953) and by LIN (1980). In this chapter, only the effects of insulin on the motility of the gastrointestinal tract will be considered.

B. Effects on the Lower Esophageal Sphincter

Apparently insulin has no direct effect on the lower esophageal sphincter (LES; GOYAL and RATTAN 1978), but insulin-induced hypoglycemia was reported to decrease LES pressure in humans, probably because of the consequent suppression of gastrin release by acid secreted in response to insulin. Indeed, in subjects whose gastric contents were continuously neutralized with $NaHCO_3$, insulin increased the LES pressure. These data suggest that there may be effects of insulin on the LES, mediated by changes in gastrin levels, but these effects were only hypothesized, not demonstrated (CASTELL 1971; GROSSMAN 1971).

C. Effects on the Stomach

The action of insulin on gastric motility is quite complex and both stimulatory and inhibitory effects have been described since the very early work on the topic (BULATAO and CARLSON 1924; QUIGLEY 1928, 1929; QUIGLEY et al. 1929; QUIGLEY and BARNES 1930). A great majority of the investigators reported that the effect of insulin-induced hypoglycemia was predominantly excitatory in the dog (QUIGLEY and BARNES 1930; TEMPLETON and QUIGLEY 1929, 1930; LA BARRE 1931; WILDER and SCHULTZ 1932; LALICH et al. 1937; LORBER and SHAY 1962), in humans

(QUIGLEY et al. 1929; MANVILLE and CHUINARD 1934), in rats (BOGACH et al. 1974), in mice (MONIUSZKO-JAKONIUK 1974), and in sheep (HILL 1954). In sheep, not only intravenous insulin, but also insulin released subsequent to i.v. infusion of volatile fatty acids, provokes continuous irregular spiking activity, resembling the postprandial pattern seen in dogs (RUCKEBUSCH and FIORAMONTI 1975). In both sheep and dogs, insulin (3 and 1 IU/kg), respectively) induced a high level of spiking activity on both the antrum and the duodenum, masking the migrating myoelectric complexes (MMC) on the latter and related episodes of antral inhibition (RUCKEBUSCH 1979).

Increased tone, type A contractions, and prolonged hunger periods were reported, together with accelerated gastric emptying of barium (SIMICI et al. 1927) and of a test meal (FELDMAN and MORRISON 1948). Also in the buffalo calf *(Bubalus arnee bubalis)*, insulin (1–5 IU/kg i.v.) was shown to stimulate the frequency and amplitude of rumen movements dose-dependently. All dosages lowered plasma glucose and increased plasma lactic acid concentrations (SINGH et al. 1972). However, other authors described a primary gastric inhibitory effect of insulin-induced hypoglycemia in dogs and humans (HEINZ and PALMER 1930; MULINOS 1933; NECHELES et al. 1941; SCHAPIRO and WOODWARD 1959; JANHBERG et al. 1977). Finally, a few investigators have even reported a biphasic effect, with an initial depression followed by hypermotility in dogs, rabbits, fish, and sheep (REGAN 1933; POSTLETHWAITE et al. 1948; HILL 1954; BOWEN 1962; GZGZYAN and KUZINA 1973; GZGZYAN et al. 1973; ALI et al. 1976). Doses employed in the different experiments were in the ranges 0.5–5 IU/kg in dogs, 0.1–0.25 IU/kg in humans, 1.5–5 IU/kg in rabbits, and 1–3 IU/kg in sheep. The question of the relation of blood sugar level to gastric motility was carefully reviewed by LIN (1980), to whom the reader is referred. In these studies, the sugar concentration in the blood was not always determined. However, most studies support the view that insulin-induced hypermotility was inhibited by glucose administration and that the blood sugar level during insulin-induced hypoglycemia must be a critical factor in the initiation of hunger contractions. Also, the inhibitory effect on motility of insulin-induced hypoglycemia could apparently be reversed by intravenous administration of glucose, as was observed in the forestomach of the sheep (ALI et al. 1976), in the Heidenhain pouch of the dog (LORBER and SHAY 1962), and in humans (NECHELES et al. 1941). According to BACHRACH (1953), the motor effect in humans was neither as striking nor as consistent as that in dogs and in a few cases (QUIGLEY et al. 1929) hypoglycemic symptoms were not accompanied by the typical gastric response.

D. Effect on the Small Intestine

A predominantly stimulatory effect of insulin on the motility of the small intestine was reported. QUIGLEY and SOLOMON (1929–1930) showed an increase in motility in the human duodenum, even in the absence of gastric contraction. In the rat, insulin was also found to increase intestinal motility (BOGACH et al. 1974); apparently these effects were abolished by atropine or by double vagotomy. In the dog, contractions in a Thiry–Vella ileal loop were reported by MEYTHALER and GRAESER (1935) and later by BUENO and RUCKEBUSCH (1975); insulin (1 IU/kg) was shown to induce a pattern of uniform spiking activity, resembling that of the fed state, which lasted 4–5 h. In the sheep, the latter authors observed that MMC were disrupted by exogenous insulin or by its release by an infusion of volatile fatty acids and continuous irregular spiking activity was recorded for 1–2 h. In both species, alloxan treatment altered the MMC pattern, but insulin was able to restore it to normal (Bueno and Ruckebusch 1975, 1976). The authors suggested that insulin levels are of importance in the control of the jejunal motor profile and may mediate, at least partially, the postprandial disappearance of MMC in dogs.

As in the case of gastric motility, intestinal motility has also been shown in some investigations to be depressed instead of increased by insulin. A primary inhibition of human duodenal motility was described by Schapiro and Woodward (1959). Insulin was also shown to decrease ileal motility in the dog (Bogach et al. 1973) and ileal and colonic motility in the guinea pig (Meythaler and Graeser 1935), after intravenous or intracardiac administration. An inhibitory effect of insulin was also observed in isolated intestinal transplants of the dog, in which decreases of both rate and strength of peristaltic contractions were noted (Kleitsch and Puestow 1939).

E. Effects on the Large Intestine

The motility of the colon has also been shown to be influenced by insulin in several ways. Together with inhibitory effects in the guinea pig (Meythaler and Graeser 1935) and in humans (Shapiro and Woodward 1959; Killenberger and Cornwell 1964), there is stimulatory activity in the dog (Quigley and Solomon 1929–1930; Nga et al. 1973) which is antagonized by atropine or oral administration of glucose. In very recent and precise experiments, however, the remarkable stimulatory effect of insulin (0.05–0.1 IU/kg), causing a noticeable increase in migrating spike bursts and in short spike burst frequency, was *not* affected by the simultaneous perfusion of isotonic glucose (García-Vilar 1979), suggesting that the mechanism is at least in part independent of the metabolic changes induced by the hormone.

I. In Vitro Studies

In the few in vitro esperiments reported in the literature, both stimulatory and inhibitory effects of insulin were observed. Winter and Smith (1924), Barlow (1931), and Prasad (1934), saw inhibitory effects of insulin on gut motility, while increases in amplitude, tonus, and frequency of contraction of rabbit intestine, which were antagonized by atropine, were observed by other investigators (Pavel and Milcou 1932). It is difficult to establish whether these in vitro effects are connected with a direct effect of insulin on the smooth muscle or represent the consequence of the metabolic action of the hormone. In this connection it must be mentioned that insulin (0.1 IU/ml) was shown to have a noticeable effect on the metabolism of isolated rabbit colon and human jejunum, causing an increase in glucose uptake, glycogen content, incorporation of leucine into protein, and also increasing the membrane transport of α-aminoisobutyric acid and 3-*0*-methylglucose (Arnqvist 1974; Arnqvist and Lundstrom 1976). However, these effects appeared after incubation times of 120–180 min.

F. Mechanism of Action

An important observation was made by LA BARRE (1931) and by LA BARRE and DESTREE (1930), who found that the gastric motor effect of insulin in the dog was not influenced by extirpation of the cerebral hemispheres, but was abolished by extirpation of the lower autonomic centers, confirming that the action of insulin-induced hypoglycemia was mediated through the vagal centers, as had been suggested by QUIGLEY and TEMPLETON (1929–1930). The importance of vagal integrity for the effects of insulin on gastrointestinal motility was subsequently confirmed in the dog (LALICH et al. 1937), the cat (MULINOS 1933), the rabbit (POSTLETHWAITE et al. 1948), and in vagotomized patients (FELDMAN and MORRISON 1948). The importance of the mediation of vagal mechanisms was also supported by the action of atropine, which was shown by several investigators to inhibit the effects of insulin in humans, dogs, and sheep (QUIGLEY et al. 1929; WILDER and SCHULTZ 1932; HILL 1954). Of course, if we insert into the picture vagal stimulation by insulin, we cannot ignore a series of effects deriving from this situation: vagal stimulation releases not only gastrin, but also VIP, somatostatin (SCHWARTZ 1978), glucagon (KANETO et al. 1974), pancreatic polypeptide (ADRIAN et al. 1978; MARCO et al. 1978; SIVE et al. 1978), perhaps secretin (LEE et al. 1978), and other kinds of paracrine secretions which can affect gastrointestinal motility (DE FRONZO et al. 1977).

There are only a few studies dealing with the effects of insulin on the sympathetic system, but it is well known that insulin-induced hypoglycemia stimulates both the parasympathetic and the sympathetic autonomic systems in experimental animals and in humans (CHRISTENSEN 1974). Of course, catecholamines released by insulin exert an inhibitory effect on intestinal motility, both through stimulation of β-receptors on the smooth muscle and by acting on the cholinergic nerve terminals of intestine through α-receptors, to prevent acetylcholine release (PATON and VIZI 1969). In addition, insulin-induced hypoglycemia may release histamine from the gastric mucosa (CODE 1956; KAHLSON et al. 1964) and whether or not insulin-released histamine has an effect on gastric motility is still unknown.

From these considerations, it is clear that the final action of insulin represents the net effect of a complicated chain of responses, involving the autonomic nervous systems (both parasympathetic and sympathetic), the endocrine and, possibly, the paracrine functions, each of which exerts an effect of its own. This could be the explanation for the conflicting results obtained in different studies performed under different experimental conditions. It is often hard to find acceptable explanations for the contrasting data in the abundant literature about insulin and gastrointestinal motility. The possibility that commercially available insulins used in different experiments may not be absolutely identical must be kept in mind. Monocomponent insulin and synthetic insulin were not available in the early experiments and different contaminants, endowed with some degrees of biologic activity, were quite possibly present. Moreover, it has been recognized that pancreatic islets produce not only insulin and glucagon, but also other very active substances, such as somatostatin, pancreatic polypeptide, and thyrotropin-releasing hormone, all of which can affect gut motility to different degrees. Thus, it is also possible that, in some experiments, an effect which was attributed to insulin was really the algebraic sum of effects of different interacting substances. Some apparently paradoxical effects of insulin may find an explanation in the light of these observations, especially if high doses were administered by intravenous bolus in experiments in vivo, or high concentrations were added to isolated in vitro preparations, as was brilliantly pinpointed quite recently by LIN (1980).

Finally, the recent data of GARCÍA-VILAR (1979), together with the few available in vitro data, seem to suggest that insulin may have some effects on motor activity of the digestive tract which are not entirely mediated through changes in blood sugar levels. Furthermore, it has been known for a long time that spontaneous motility of the bowel could not be significantly modified by intravenous injection of glucose or correlated with spontaneous changes in blood sugar levels (QUIGLEY and HALLARAN 1932; MULINOS 1933). Experiments with 2-deoxy-D-glucose, which are numerous in the field of gastric secretion, scarcely exist in the field of motility, and they could be of considerable help in the interpretation of the results so far available. Probably, when we refer to the motor effects of insulin on the alimentary tract, we need additional accurate studies in order to assess for each experimental situation whether we are speaking of an "insulin-induced hypoglycemia effect" or simply of an "insulin effect."

References

Adrian TE, Besterman HS, Christofides ND, Bloom SR (1978) Interaction of gastrointestinal hormones and cholinergic innervation on the release of pancreatic polypeptide. Scand J Gastroenterol [Suppl 49] 13:1

Ali TM, Nicholson T, Singleton AG (1976) Stomach motility in insulin-treated sheep. Q J Exp Physiol 61:321–329

Arnqvist HJ (1974) Action of insulin on vascular and intestinal smooth muscle. Effects on aminoacid transport, protein synthesis, and accumulation of glucose carbon. Acta Physiol Scand 90:132–142

Arnqvist HJ, Lundstrom B (1976) Effects of insulin on human intestinal smooth muscle. Acta Endocrinol [Suppl 203] 82:10

Bachrach WH (1953) Action of insulin hypoglycemia on motor and secretory functions of the digestive tract. Physiol Rev 33:566–592

Barlow OW (1931) Effect of insulin on perfused heart and on isolated rabbit intestine. J Pharmacol Exp Ther 41:217–228

Bogach PG, Nga CS, Groisman SD (1973) Effect of insulin hypoglycemia on the motility of the dog jejunum and ileum. Fiziol Zh 19:471–476

Bogach PG, Groisman SD, Chan SN (1974) Effect of varying degree of parasympathetic denervation of the stomach, the duodenum and the jejunum on the motor reactions induced by insulin hypoglycemia. Fiziol Zh SSSR 60:1446–1453

Bowen JM (1962) Effect of insulin hypoglycemia on gastrointestinal motility in the sheep. Am J Vet Res 23:948–954

Bueno L, Ruckebusch Y (1975) Evidence for a role of endogenous insulin on intestinal motility. In: Vantrappen G (ed) Fifth International Symposium on Gastrointestinal Motility. Typoff, Leuven, pp 64–69

Bueno L, Ruckebusch M (1976) Insulin and jejunal electrical activity in dogs and sheep. Am Physiol 230:1538–1544

Bulatao E, Carlson AJ (1924) Influence of experimental changes in blood sugar levels on gastric hunger contraction. Am J Physiol 69:108–115

Castell DO (1971) Changes in lower esophageal sphincter pressure during insulin-induced hypoglycemia. Gastroenterology 61:10–15

Christensen NJ (1974) Plasma norepinephrine and epinephrine in untreated diabetics during fasting and after insulin administration. Diabetes 23:1–8

Code CF (1956) Histamine and gastric secretion. Ciba Foundation Symposium. In: Wolstenholme GEW, O'Connor CM (eds) Histamine. Churchill Livingstone, Edinburgh London, pp 189–219
De Fronzo RA, Andres R, Bledsoe TA, Boden G, Faloona GA, Tobin JD (1977) A test of the hypothesis that the rate of fall in glucose concentration triggers counterregulatory hormonal responses in man. Diabetes 26:445–452
Felber JP, Dick J (1975) L'axe entéro-pancréatique. Med Hyg 33:82–83
Feldman M, Morrison S (1948) The effect of insulin on motility of the stomach following bilateral vagotomy. Am J Dig Dis 15:175A
García-Vilar R (1979) Recherches sur la motricité colique chez le chien. Master's Thesis, Institut National Polytechnique de Toulouse, pp 1–136
Goyal RK, Rattan S (1978) Neurohumoral, hormonal, and drug receptors for the lower esophageal sphincter. Gastroenterology 74:598–619
Grossman MI (1971) How does insulin stimulate the lower esophageal sphincter? Gastroenterology 61:119–120
Gzgzyan DM, Kuzina MM (1973) Stomach motor activity in the black sea ray *Daeyatis paetinaca*. Zh Evol Biokhim Fiziol 9:536–539
Gzgzyan DM, Kuzina M, Tanaschuk OF (1973) The effect of hypophysical hormons and insulin on motor activity of the stomach in the scorpion fish *Scorpaena porpus*. Zh Evol Biokhim Fiziol 9:301–303
Heinz TE, Palmer WL (1930) A study of the effect of insulin on gastric motility. Proc Soc Exp Biol Med 27:1047–1049
Hill KJ (1954) Insulin hypoglycemia and gastric motility in the sheep. Q J Exp Physiol 39:253–260
Jahnberg T, Abrahamson H, Jansson G, Martinson J (1977) Gastric relaxation response to insulin before and after vagotomy. Scand J Gastroenterol 12:229–233
Kahlson G, Rosengren E, Svahn D, Thunberg R (1964) Mobilization and formation of histamine in the gastric mucosa as related to gastric secretion. J Physiol (Lond) 174:400–416
Kaneto A, Miki E, Kosaka K (1974) Effects of vagal stimulation on glucagon and insulin secretion. Endocrinology 95:1005–1010
Killenberg PG, Cornwell GG (1964) Effect of insulin hypoglycemia on the human sigmoid colon. Am J Dig Dis 9:221–228
Kleitsch WP, Puestow CB (1939) Studies of intestinal motility: the effect of intravenous solutions and of insulin upon peristalsis. Surgery 6:687–696
La Barre J (1931) Influence of insulin hypoglycemia of the central nervous system on gastric motility. C R Soc Biol (Paris) 107:258–260
La Barre J, Destree P (1930) Role des centres nerveux supérieurs dans l'hypermotilité gastrique consécutive aux états d'hypoglycémie. C R Soc Biol (Paris) 104:112–113
Lalich J, Youmans WB, Meek WJ (1937) Insulin and gastric motility. Am J Physiol 120:554–558
Lee KY, Chey WY, Tai HH (1978) Roles of the vagus in endogenous release of secretin and exocrine pancreatic secretion in dog. In: Grossman M, Speranza V, Basso N, Lezoche E (eds) Gastrointestinal hormones and pathology of the digestive system. Plenum, New York, pp 211–216
Lin TM (1980) Effects of insulin and glucagon on secretory and motor function of the gastrointestinal tract. In: Jerzy Glass GB (ed) Gastrointestinal hormones. Raven, New York, pp 639–691
Lorber SH, Shay H (1962) Effect of insulin and glucose on gastric motor activity of dogs. Gastroenterology 43:564–574
Manville IA, Chuinard EG (1934) Studies on gastric hunger mechanisms. Am J Dig Dis 1:688–693
Marco J, Hedo JA, Villanueva ML (1978) Control of pancreatic polypeptide secretion by glucose in man. J Clin Endocrinol Metab 46:140–145
Meythaler F, Graeser F (1935) Die Wirkung des Insulins auf den Darm. Arch Exp Pathol Pharmakol 178:27–35

Moniuszko-Jokaniuk J (1974) Influence of insulin on the effect of neostigmine in healthy mice and mice with alloxan-induced diabetes mellitus. Acta Physiol Pol 25:497–508
Mulinos MG (1933) The gastric hunger mechanism. IV. The influence of experimental alterations in blood sugar concentration on the gastric hunger contractions. Am J Physiol 104:371–378
Necheles H, Olson WH, Morris R (1941) Depression of gastric motility by insulin. Am J Dig Dis 8:270–273
Nga CS, Bogach PG, Groisman SD (1973) Mechanisms of the effect of insulin hypoglycemia on colon motility. Byull Eksp Biol Med 76:12–15
Paton WDM, Vizi ES (1969) The inhibitory action of noradrenalin and adrenalin on acetylcholine output by guinea-pig ileum longitudinal muscle strip. Br J Pharmacol 35:10–29
Pavel I, Milcou SM (1932) Action de l'insuline sur l'intestin. C R Soc Biol (Paris) 109:776–779
Postlethwaite RW, Hill HV, Chittum JR, Grimson KS (1948) Effect of vagotomy and of drugs on gastric motility. Ann Surg 128:184–194
Prasad S (1934) Effect of insulin on the contraction of the intestinal muscle. Indian J Med Res 21:563–567
Quigley JP (1928/1929) Action of insulin on the gastric motility of man. Proc Soc Exp Biol Med 26:769–770
Quigley JP, Barnes BO (1930) Action of insulin on the motility of the gastrointestinal tract. VI. Antagonistic action of posterior pituitary lobe preparations. Am J Physiol 95:7–12
Quigley JP, Hallaran WR (1932) The independence of spontaneous gastrointestinal motility and blood sugar levels. Am J Physiol 100:102–110
Quigley JP, Solomon EI (1929/1930) Action of insulin on the motility of the gastrointestinal tract. V. a. Action on the human duodenum. b. Action on the colon of dogs. Am J Physiol 91:488–495
Quigley JP, Templeton RD (1929/1930) Action of insulin on the motility of the gastrointestinal tract. IV. Action on the stomach following double vagotomy. Am J Physiol 91:482–487
Quigley JP, Johnson V, Solomon EI (1929) Action of insulin on the motility of the gastrointestinal tract. Am J Physiol 90:89–98
Regan JF (1933) The action of insulin on the motility of the empty stomach. Am J Physiol 104:91–95
Ruckebusch Y (1979) Interaction of duodenal and antral activity in sheep and dogs. J Physiol (Lond) 254:79P–80P
Ruckebusch M, Fioramonti J (1975) Insuline-secretion et motricité intestinale. C R Soc Biol (Paris) 169:435–439
Schapiro H, Woodward ER (1959) The action of insulin hypoglycemia on the motility of the human gastrointestinal tract. Am J Dig Dis 4:787–791
Schwartz TW (1978) Pancreatic polypeptide (PP). In: Grossman M, Speranza V, Basso N, Lezoche E (eds) Gastrointestinal hormones and pathology of the digestive system. Plenum, New York, pp 165–168
Simici D, Giurea G, Dimitriu C (1927) L'action de l'insuline sur la motilité et l'évacuation de l'estomac à l'état normal et pathologique. Arch Mal Appar Dig Mal Nutr 17:17–18
Singh RV, Sud SC, Bahga HS, Soni BK (1972) Effect of insulin on rumen motility, blood glucose and blood lactic acid in male buffalo-calves *(Bubalus bubalis)*. Indian J Anim Sci 42:784–788
Sive AA, Vinik AI, Hickman-Van Hoorn R, Van Tonder S (1978) Secretory response of pancreatic polipeptide in man and pigs. Scand J Gastroenterol [Suppl 49] 13:A169
Templeton RD, Quigley JP (1929/1930) The action of insulin on the motility of the gastrointestinal tract. II. Action on the Heidenhain pouch. Am J Physiol 91:467–474
Unger RH, Eisentraut AM (1969) Entero-insular axis. Arch Intern Med 123:261–266
Wilder RL, Schultz FW (1932) The action of atropine and adrenalin on gastric tonus and hypermotility induced by insulin hypoglycemia. Am J Physiol 96:54–58
Winter LB, Smith W (1924) On the effect of insulin on the isolated intestine of the rabbit. J Physiol (Lond) 58:12

Pancreatic Polypeptide

A. Introduction

The discovery of pancreatic polypeptide (PP) is a classical example of serendipity, since it was isolated and sequenced before anything was known of its action or function. In 1968, KIMMEL et al., while purifying chicken insulin, found in the final stage of preparation a contaminating peptide which they called avian pancreatic peptide (APP). Later, similar peptides were found in the bovine, (BPP), porcine, ovine, and human pancreas (LIN and CHANCE 1974a; CHANCE et al. 1976). Avian and bovine pancreatic peptides are homologous peptides, each containing 36 amino acid residues in a straight chain and being identical in 15 of the 36 positions (Table 1).

According to LIN (1980), the PP isolated from the pancreas of pig, sheep, or human are very similar to BPP and the structures of these peptides differ from that of BPP in only one or two residues, at positions 2, 6, 11, or 23. Whereas there is a certain similarity between the structure of APP and that of chicken glucagon, (when the sequences of APP and chicken glucagon are aligned 8 identities can be found in positions 3, 4, 6, 10, 16, 19, 22, and 25), the structures of the mammalian PP isolated are unrelated to any of the gastrointestinal hormones known so far.

B. Structure–Activity Relationships

The data on structure–activity relationships available so far concern mainly the effects of PP on gastric and pancreatic secretion. It has been found that the COOH terminal tyrosyl amide residue is of crucial importance for the maintenance of PP activity. Des-C-Tyr-NH_2 BPP (BPP 1–35), the fragment of BPP devoid of the Tyr-amide in position 36, was absolutely inactive on the stomach and the pancreas. The COOH terminal hexapeptide (fragment 31–36) was found to be active in inhibiting gastric secretion and stimulating gut motility, though its effect was less than that of the whole molecule. The minimal effective fragment to mimic the effects of BBP is not yet known (LIN 1980).

Table 1. Amino acid sequence of BPP and APP[a]

	1 5 10
BPP	Ala-*Pro*-Leu-Glu-*Pro*-Gln-*Tyr*-*Pro*-*Gly*-*Asp*-Asn-*Ala*-
APP	Gly-*Pro*-Ser-Gln-*Pro*-Thr-*Tyr*-*Pro*-*Gly*-*Asp*-Asp-*Ala*-
	15 20
	-Thr-Pro-*Glu*-Gln-Met-Ala-Gln-Tyr-Ala-Ala-Glu-*Leu*-
	-Pro-Val-*Glu*-Asp-Leu-Ile-Arg-Phe-Tyr-Asp-Asn-*Leu*-
	25 30 35
	-Arg-Arg-*Tyr*-Ile-*Asn*-Met-Leu-*Thr*-*Arg*-Pro-Arg-*Thr*-NH_2
	-Gln-Gln-*Tyr*-Leu-*Asn*-Val-Val-*Thr*-*Arg*-His-Arg-*Tyr*-NH_2

[a] Identical amino acid residues at identical positions of BPP and APP are *italicized*

C. Effect on Gastrointestinal Motility

The action of PP on gastrointestinal motility was rather erratic, varying greatly in different animal species and according to the different doses employed. In the anesthetized opossum, intra-arterial but not intravenous administration of BPP caused a dose-related (0.15–5 μg/kg) increase in lower esophageal sphincter pressure. The antagonistic effect of TTX and of atropine suggested an effect at least partly mediated through activation of cholinergic neurons (RATTAN and GOYAL 1979).

BPP given intravenously to conscious dogs in large amounts (50–100 μg/kg) caused violent contractions of the gut which resulted in vomiting and evacuation of formed stools. It is not known whether vomiting and defecation were caused by a central or a peripheral mechanism.

When motility was measured by means of chronically implanted electrodes or intraluminal catheters, BPP was shown to decrease intraluminal pressure in the antrum, duodenum, ileocecal sphincter, and descending colon, whether administered by slow intravenous infusion or intramuscularly (5–10 μg/kg; LIN and CHANCE 1974b). With higher doses, BPP initially increased the motility from the antrum to the colon, at the same time increasing the frequency of the action potentials. These phenomena had a rapid onset, lasted between 1–5 min and 30–45 min, and were followed by a prolonged period of quiescence. BPP also enhanced gastric emptying in the rat when doses of 1–100 μg/kg were injected intraperitoneally. The maximal effect was seen up to 45 min (according to the dose) after administration of the peptide. Apparently PP infusion in a dose mimicking the normal response to a meal did not significantly change the gastric half-emptying time from that in control subjects (ADRIAN et al. 1979).

Conflicting results have been reported about the effects of BPP on bowel movement and intestinal transit in rodents. In one study in the rat (GUSTAVSON et al. 1977), BPP (10 or 50 $\mu g\ kg^{-1}\ h^{-1}$) was found to have no effect on the transit time of a test substance containing $^{51}CrO_4$. In another study (LIN and CHANCE 1978), movement of a charcoal meal in mice was enhanced by intraperitoneal injection of 10 μg/kg of BPP given 15–60 min before the meal. Species differences and administration of bovine PP to rodents might explain the different results obtained.

Finally, APP has been found to inhibit the amplitude and frequency of contraction of the turkey gizzard (DUKE and KIMMEL 1978), at 8–30 μg/kg intravenously. Only the largest doses employed were also able to inhibit the lower gut. No attempt to explain the mechanism of action of PP in the gut has yet been made. The fact that PP may be released not only by administration of food (FLOYD et al. 1978) but also by gastrointestinal hormones, candidate hormones, or nerve mediators would suggest that PP might be involved in the effects of other physiologic stimulatory or inhibitory substances. An increase in serum PP levels was found (together with an increase in vasoactive intestinal peptide, VIP) in patients suffering from watery diarrhea syndrome and for this reason it has been proposed that it and VIP may be pathogenic factors in this disease. It is obvious that further studies are needed to establish the possible effects of PP in humans and to assess whether or not PP, interacting with other intestinal mediators, may play a physiologic role in regulating the motor function of the gastrointestinal tract.

References

Adrian TE, Greenberg GR, McCloy RF, Fitzpatrick ML, Bloom SR (1979) How to assess the physiological role of a new peptide hormone: pancreatic polypeptide infusion in man. J Endocrinol 81:154P–155P

Chance RE, Root MA, Galloway JA (1976) The immunogenicity of insulin preparations. Acta Endocrinol 83(S-205):185–196

Duke GE, Kimmel JR (1978) Inhibition of gastric motility in turkey by avian pancreatic peptide (Abstr 849). Fed Proc 37:373

Floyd JC, Fajans SS, Pek S (1978) Physiologic regulation of plasma levels of PP in man. In: Bloom SR (ed) Gut hormones. Churchill Livingstone, Edinburgh London, pp 247–253

Gustavson S, Johansson H, Lundquist G, Nilsson F (1977) Effects of vasoactive intestinal peptide and pancreatic polypeptide on small bowel propulsion in the rat. Scand J Gastroenterol 12:993–997

Kimmel JR, Pollock HG, Hazelwood RL (1968) Isolation and characterization of chicken insulin. Endocrinology 83:1323–1330

Lin TM (1980) Pancreatic polypeptide: isolation, chemistry, and biological function. In: Jerzy Glass GB (ed) Gastrointestinal hormones. Raven, New York, pp 275–303

Lin TM, Chance RE (1974a) Bovine pancreatic polypeptide (BPP) and avian pancreatic peptide (APP); candidate hormones of the gut. Gastroenterology 67:737–738

Lin TM, Chance RE (1974b) Gastrointestinal actions of a new bovine pancreatic peptide (BPP). In: Chey WY, Brooks FP (eds) Endocrinology of the gut. Thorofare, NJ, pp 143–145

Lin TM, Chance RE (1978) Spectrum of gastrointestinal actions of bovine PP. In: Bloom SR (ed) Gut hormones. Churchill Livingstone, Edinburgh London, pp 242–246

Rattan S, Goyal RK (1979) Effect of bovine pancreatic polypeptide on the opossum lower esophageal sphincter. Gastroenterology 77:672–676

CHAPTER 2d

Peptides: Other Hormones

G. BERTACCINI

Vasopressin

A. Introduction

The hypothalamus of most vertebrate species secretes two main peptides whose activities, though overlapping, fall into two different categories: pressor and uterine-contracting substances. In addition some gastrointestinal motor effects have been described and they will be reported here.

The structures of these peptides with the small chemical differences which are peculiar to the different species are listed in Table 1. All are nonapeptides with a disulfide bond between the cysteines at position 1 and 6. All have a COOH terminal glycine which is amidated; differences in amino acid residues occur only at positions 3, 4, and 8. From a chemical point of view they have a definite historical interest inasmuch as they were the first small peptide hormones to be synthesized (DU VIGNEAUD et al. 1953, 1954).

Table 1. Structure of vasopressin and oxytocin in different species[a]

	1	2	3	4	5	6	7	8	9
Arg-vasopressin (Mammals)	Cys-	Tyr-	Phe-	Gln-	Asn-	Cys-	Pro-	Arg-	Gly-NH_2
Lys-vasopressin (Mammals)								-Lys-	
Vasotocin (Vertebrates)			-Ile-						
Oxytocin (Mammals, ratfish)			-Ile-					-Leu-	
Phenypressin[b] (Marsupials)		-Phe-							
Mesotocin (Birds, reptiles, amphibians)			-Ile-					-Ile-	
Isotocin (Bony fishes)				-Ser-				-Ile-	
Glumitocin (Rays)				-Ser-				-Gln-	
	1	2	3	4	5	6	7	8	9

[a] Blank spaces indicate that the amino acid residues are the same as in Arg-vasopressin
[b] See CHAUVET et al. (1980)

B. Effects on the Motility of the Gastrointestinal Tract

Very few data are available on the in vivo effects of vasopressin on gastrointestinal motility. The peptide was described (BRAZEAU 1975) as a substance capable of inducing a remarkable increase of bowel motility when given in doses of 5–20 IU. Peristaltic activity, rather than the tone, was increased and apparently the effect was greater on the large than on the small intestine. However nothing was reported about animal species or experimental conditions. These data would agree with results which are very interesting from a radiologic point of view (elimination of intestinal gas and good visualization of the bowel) and which were reported in an extensive study of more than 500 patients (GÖTHLIN 1972a, b). In spite of some moderate side effects, results were satisfactory in more than 70% of the subjects. These observations confirmed early data in the literature dealing with the effects of pitressin in the radiologic examination of the abdomen (COLLINS and ROOT 1936; JUTRAS and CANTERO 1936; SCHEIBEL 1936; PAUL and BEATTY 1937). In more recent studies abdominal discomforts and intense bowel movements were reported to occur in patients treated with 5 IU i.m. of vasopressin (FORSSMAN et al. 1973). Moreover lysin-8-vasopressin (50 μIU kg^{-1} min^{-1}) caused a significant increase in human lower esophageal sphincter (LES) pressure, apparently by a direct effect on the smooth muscle (BOESBY and PEDERSEN 1974).

Surprisingly, data obtained in experimental animals were quite different. According to previous studies (LEVY 1963), both vasopressin and oxytocin (0.1–0.3 IU/kg i.v.) produced a transient but marked inhibition of intestinal motility in the anesthesized dog, which was only occasionally followed by a transient phase of increased motility. In other studies (HIATT et al. 1966; KOWALEWSKI and KOLODEJ 1976; SCHUURKES and CHARBON 1978), vasopressin ($\leq$0.12 IU/kg) was found to be completely ineffective on canine gastric and intestinal motility, though it caused a conspicuous reduction in regional blood flow. The degree of purity of the peptides used, the presence of preservatives (like chlorbutanol) in some commercial preparations, and the possible difference in experimental conditions do not seem to represent an acceptable explanation for these discrepancies which remain largely obscure. Of course the early experiments performed with purified hypophyseal extracts (for review see VAUGHAN WILLIAMS and STREETEN 1952) can be easily criticized for the possible occurrence of active contaminants in the old preparations.

In other species, different results were obtained. In the rabbit, intravenous injections or infusions of Lys-vasopressin (0.1–2 IU/kg = 0.37–7.4 μg/kg) or Phe^2-Lys-vasopressin (0.1–2 IU/kg = 1.82–36.4 μg/kg) increased the motility of the small intestine for a short period. In the cat, neither peptide had a clear-cut effect at the same dose (BAUER et al. 1966). In the sheep, i.m. injection of 75 IU oxytocin was followed by a slight increase in the frequency of contractions of the ruminoreticulum; surprisingly, injection of 150 IU had no recognizable effect (PESSOA and SOUZA 1978).

In vitro studies of the action of vasopressin on the gut are substantially less equivocal than in vivo studies. In the proximal colon of the guinea pig, which was described as a good tool for the bioassay of vasopressin and its analogs (BOTTING 1965), vasopressin showed a potent, dose-related (1 μIU to 1 mIU/ml) contractile effect and was found to be twice as potent as vasotocin and about 20 times as potent as oxytocin. The contractile effect was inhibited by ganglion-blocking agents but surprisingly only slightly affected by atropine; cooling the tissue, anoxia, pretreatment with tetrodotoxin, and reduction of the calcium content of the bath fluid, all inhibited vasopressin-induced contractions, suggesting an indirect action of the peptide, probably through stimulation of intrinsic ganglion cells (BOTTING and TURNER 1966, 1969).

In the rat colon, Lys-vasopressin had different effects according to the doses employed: small doses (50 μIU/ml increased the tone and amplitude of spontaneous movements; on the contrary, very high doses (0.3 IU/ml) caused a complete block of spontaneous motility with a marked reduction in basal tone. These changes were reversible after washing the preparation (LE GOFF and THOUVENOT 1970). Vasopressin (10 mIU/ml) was shown to have a diphasic effect on isolated rings of rabbit colon, consisting of inhibition of spontaneous activity and relaxation of the preparation followed by a slight contraction (WOO and SOMLYO 1967). Atropine and a mixture of α-adrenergic and β-adrenergic blocking agents were ineffective, but pronethalol alone potentiated the inhibitory effect of vasopressin. Both inhibitory and excitatory effects of vasopressin were potentiated by magnesium. Longitudinal strips of rabbit colon showed only a contraction in response to vasopressin.

Unlike rabbit intestinal smooth muscle, both types of guinea pig preparations (rings and taenia coli), when responsive to vasopressin, were contracted by the peptide without a preliminary phase of inhibition. However the effect was erratic and high doses (50–250 mIU/ml) had to be used (WOO and SOMLYO 1967). These data are in sharp contrast with those reported on the proximal colon of the guinea pig (BOTTING 1965). Probably the different experimental conditions are responsible for the discrepancy; the particular region of the colon used by BOTTING, which corresponds to the sacculus rotundus in other animals, is indeed the only portion of the guinea pig colon extremely sensitive to vasopressin.

In a subsequent study (GILMORE and VANE 1970) the effect of vasopressin was investigated on a number of gastrointestinal preparations from rats, gerbils, guinea pigs, chickens, rabbits, and dogs. Of those smooth muscle preparations tested, the longitudinal muscle of the isolated rectum of the rabbit was the most satisfactory for the biologic assay of vasopressin. The peptide was active in concentrations of 4–100 μIU/ml (0.01–0.25 ng/ml) and was 20–30 times more active than oxytocin. Unlike other peptides (angiotensin II and bradykinin) which caused contraction of rabbit rectum, vasopressin caused a dose-dependent relaxation of this preparation which never showed tachyphylaxis. The failure of α- and β-adrenoceptor blocking agents to prevent the relaxation induced by vasopressin suggested that the peptide acted on receptors different from those for cathecholamines. A possible nonadrenergic nervous pathway was hypothesized by the partial inhibition induced by administration of lignocaine, but not bretylium.

Vasopressin was recently found to be very effective in causing contraction of the lower esophageal sphincter in vitro. Threshold doses were 0.1 ng/ml in the guinea pig and 1 μg/ml in the rat. A good dose–response curve was obtained and tachyphylaxis occurred only in some preparations and when high doses were used (CORUZZI and BERTACCINI 1980). The "potency" of vasopressin was remarkably greater than that of acetylcholine whereas the "efficacy" was about 50% of that

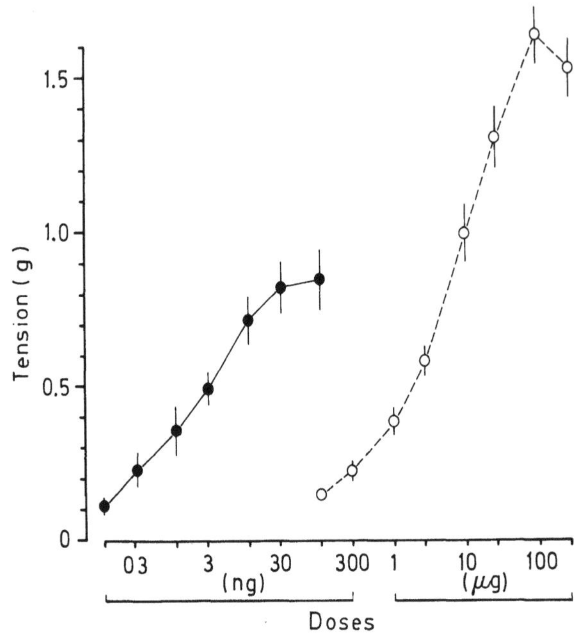

Fig. 1. Isolated preparation of the lower esophageal sphincter from the rat. *Closed circles*, vasopressin; *open circles*, acetylcholine. Mean values obtained from 5–10 experiments; vertical bars are standard errors. Doses are in ng/ml or in μg/ml

of acetylcholine (Fig. 1). Lys^8-vasopressin also had a stimulant effect on the kitten intestine, threshold doses ranging between 10 and 50 μg/ml (ERSPAMER et al. 1972).

From these results it can be seen that vasopressin does not have a particularly outstanding effect on the motility of the digestive tract, but nevertheless it can be added to the long list of peptides which affect contractility of smooth muscle, even though the gastrointestinal tract does not represent the most important target.

References

Bauer G, Gmeiner R, Winkler H (1966) Über die Wirkung synthetischer Polypeptide auf den Darm in situ. Arch Int Pharmacodyn Ther 159:373–385

Boesby S, Pedersen SA (1974) The effect of vasopressin on resting gastroesophageal sphincter pressure in man. Scand J Gastroenterol 9:587–590

Botting JH (1965) An isolated preparation with a selective sensitivity to vasopressin. Br J Pharmacol 24:156–162

Botting JH, Turmer AD (1966) Mode of action of vasopressin on isolated proximal colon of the guinea pig. Br J Pharmacol 28:197–206

Botting JH, Turmer AD (1969) Studies on the mode of action of vasopressin on the isolated proximal colon of the guinea pig. Br J Pharmacol 37:306–313

Brazeau P (1975) Agents affecting the renal conservation of water. In: Goodman LS, Gilman A (eds) The pharmacological basis of therapeutics. Macmillan, New York, pp 848–859

Chauvet MT, Hurpet D, Chauvet J, Acher A (1980) Phenypressin (Phe^2-Arg^8-vasopressin), a new neurohypophysial peptide found in marsupials. Nature 287:640–642

Collins E, Root J (1936) Elimination of confusing gas shadow during cholecystography by the use of pitressin. JAMA 107:32–35

Coruzzi G, Bertaccini G (1980) Effect of some vasoactive peptides on the lower esophageal sphincter. Pharm Res Commun 12:965–973

Du Vigneaud V, Ressler C, Swan JM, Roberts CW, Katsoyannis PG, Gordon S (1953) The synthesis of an octapeptide amide with the hormonal activity of oxytocin. J Am Chem Soc. 75:4879–4880
Du Vigneaud V, Gish DT, Katsoyannis PG (1954) A synthetic preparation possessing biological properties associated with arginine-vasopressin. J Am Chem Soc 76:4751–4752
Erspamer V, Falconieri Erspamer G, Inselvini M, Negri L (1972) Occurrence of bombesin and alytesin in extracts of the skin of three European discoglossid frog and pharmacological actions of bombesin on extravascular smooth muscle. Br J Pharmacol 45:333–348
Forssman O, Leczinski CG, Mulder J (1973) Synthetic lysine-vasopressin in herpetic neuralgia. Acta Derm Venereol (Stockh) 53:359–362
Gilmore NJ, Vane JR (1970) A sensitive and specific assay for vasopressin in the circulating blood. Br J Pharmacol 38:633–652
Göthlin J (1972a) Use of vasopressin to eliminate intestinal gas during abdominal roentgenography. Forsk Praktik 4:30–35
Göthlin J (1972b) Vasopressin in the elimination of intestinal gas. Acta Radiol Diagn 12:100–112
Hiatt RB, Goodman I, Bircher R (1966) Control of motility in Thiry-Vella ileal segments in dogs. Am J Physiol 210:373–378
Jutras A, Cantero A (1936) Le pitressin, hormone antipneumatosique, son emploi dans le radiodiagnostic abdominal. J Radiol 20:443–445
Kowalewski K, Kolodej A (1976) The effect of pitressin on secretion, motor activity and blood circulation of the totally isolated canine stomach perfused extracorporeally. Rend Gastroenterol 8:76–82
Le Goff P, Thouvenot J (1970) Action de la lysine-vasopressine sur l'activité motrice du colon proximal. Etude in vitro chez le rat. C R Soc Biol (Paris) 164:2091–2093
Levy B (1963) The intestinal inhibitory response to oxytocin, vasopressin, and bradykinin. J Pharmacol Exp Ther 140:356–366
Paul L, Beatty S (1937) The use of pitressin for the elimination of intestinal gas in roentgenography of the genito-urinary tract and gallbladder. Am J Roentgenol 38:776–779
Pessoa JM, Souza R (1978) Effect of drugs on motility of the ruminoreticulum of sheep. III. Oxytocin. Arq Esc Vet Univ Fed Minas Gerais 30:257–259
Scheibel O (1936) Concerning pitressin in roentgen examination of the abdomen as an agent for reducing shadow caused by intestinal gas. Acta Radiol 17:511–515
Schuurkes JA, Charbon GA (1978) Motility and hemodynamics of the canine gastrointestinal tract. Stimulation by pentagastrin, cholecystokinin, and vasopressin. Arch Int Pharmacodyn Ther 236:214–227
Vaughan Williams EM, Streeten DHP (1952) The action of posterior pituitary extracts upon propulsion in the small intestine of conscious dogs. Br J Pharmacol 7:47–57
Woo CY, Somlyo AP (1967) Interaction of magnesium with vasopressin in intestinal smooth muscle. J Pharmacol Exp Ther 155:357–366

Calcitonin

A. Introduction

Calcitonin is a hypocalcemic hormone with an effect opposite to that of parathyroid hormone. It was discovered and named by Copp (1964), who at first thought that it was secreted by the parathyroid glands. Foster et al. (1964) presented evidence that calcitonin originated in the thyroid gland. Calcitonin was then isolated from thyroids of different species including humans; it was characterized chemically and synthesized. Calcitonin is a polypeptide with molecular weight 3,600 daltons and contains 32 amino acid residues. A cystine disulfide bridge exists in the 1–7 position at the NH_2 terminus and is essential for biologic activity. Calcitonin isolated from human "C"-cell tumors differs from the porcine hormone in as many as 18 amino acid residues. Thus, to be reliable, immunoassay of human tissues and fluids must be done with antibodies to human thyroid material.

B. Effects on Gastrointestinal Motility

Data concerning calcitonin and gastrointestinal motility are scarce and incomplete, but they are of some interest because, apparently, the hormone can affect gut motility independently of its action on calcium metabolism.

I. In Vivo Studies

Calcitonin (1 IU kg^{-1} h^{-1} synthetic salmon calcitonin) was shown to have no effect on human lower esophageal sphincter (LES) under resting conditions when administered to healthy subjects (WALDECK et al. 1973) or to achalasia patients (DEBAT et al. 1976). However, the peptide was able to suppress the sphincteric reactivity to gastrin in normal subjects, though it was ineffective in achalasia patients. This was interpreted as being due to an action of calcitonin mediated through an inhibitory nerve pathway, which would be lost or deficient in achalasia. Endogenous calcitonin released by infusion of calcium (6 mg kg^{-1} h^{-1}) was also ineffective in modifying human LES resting pressure (DANIELIDES and MELLOW 1978). Calcitonin was found to slow down gastric emptying in rats in a dose-dependent manner (BOBALIK et al. 1974): salmon and porcine calcitonin were equiactive, whereas human calcitonin at equivalent hypocalcemic doses was remarkably less effective in slowing gastric emptying, suggesting that the gastric effect of the hormone was not mediated by changes in serum calcium.

Motility studies in the rat (SEGERSTROM 1973b), with intragastric deposition of the test meal containing a nonabsorbable isotope, showed that gastrointestinal propagation was not significantly affected by intravenous administration of porcine thyrocalcitonin. The same investigator (SEGERSTROM 1973a) found that parathyroid hormone increased gastrointestinal motility (especially gastric emptying) in intact rats but not in parathyroidectomized animals. Rats treated with vitamin D had a significantly slower gastric evacuation rate than rats treated with parathyroid hormone. All these data suggest that changes in calcium level are not essential for changes in gastrointestinal motility.

Apparently, calcitonin (2–10 IU/kg i.v. bovine calcitonin) was devoid of any effect on canine intestinal peristalsis, even when the levels of the serum calcium fell by as much as 20% (LEBEDEV and BRISKIN 1975). On the other hand, calcitonin was shown to cause diarrhea as a consequence of changes in electrolyte and fluid transport across the ileum (WALLING et al. 1977). Since similar effects were induced by administration of 5-hydroxytryptamine (5-HT) and since administration of pig calcitonin (10 IU/kg) to rats was shown to decrease the 5-HT content of the antrum, duodenum, and ileum, causing a simultaneous increase in concentration of 5-HT in the blood, it was hypothesized that the action of calcitonin is mediated through a release of 5-HT (NAKHLA and LATIF 1978).

II. In Vitro Studies

Some interesting effects were observed in isolated preparations from rabbit and guinea pig intestine (DREYFUS et al. 1976). Calcitonin (0.25 μ*M*) was found to antagonize contractile responses to electrical field stimulation. This hormonal effect was relatively specific for the muscarinic receptor sites since it was not observed at nicotinic receptors or adrenoceptors; neither did calcitonin act as a local anesthetic nor directly on the contractile machinery of smooth muscle. However, calcitonin showed a weak antihistaminic effect (on H_1-receptors) at much higher concentrations (2.5 μ*M*).

It seems unlikely that calcitonin exerts these antimuscarinic effects (which could account for the well-known action of the hormone on glandular secretion) at the concentrations at which it normally circulates in blood (about 50–250 p*M*). It is more probable that gastrointestinal effects might be found when calcitonin is given in large pharmacologic doses for therapeutic purposes or when it is autonomously hypersecreted by medullary carcinoma of the thyroid.

References

Bobalik GR, Kleszynski RR, Aldred JP, Bastian JW (1974) Differential effects of salmon, porcine, and human calcitonin on gastric secretion and gastric emptying in rats. Proc Soc Exp Biol Med 147:284–288

Copp HD (1964) Parathyroids, calcitonin, and control of plasma calcium. Recent Prog Horm Res 20:59–88

Danielides IC, Mellow MH (1978) Effect of acute hypercalcemia on human esophageal motility. Gastroenterology 75:1115–1119

Debat J, Couturier D, Roze C, Debray C (1976) Effects of thyrocalcitonin on pentagastrin induced contraction of the lower esophageal sphincter in normal and in patients with achalasia. Gastroenterology 70:876

Dreyfus CF, Gershon MD, Haymovits A, Nunez E (1976) Calcitonin: antagonism at intestinal muscarinic receptors. Br J Pharmacol 57:155–157

Foster GB, Baghdiantz A, Kumar MA, Slack E, Soliman HA, MacIntyre I (1964) Thyroid origin of calcitonin. Nature 202:1303–1305

Lebedev NN, Briskin AI (1975) The effect of thyrocalcitonin on the periodic motor activity of the gastrointestinal tract. Byul Eksp Biol Med 80:10–12

Nakhla AM, Latif A (1978) A possible role for 5-hydroxytryptamine as mediator for calcitonin actions on the gastrointestinal tract and pancreas in rats. Biochem J Cell Aspects 176:339–342

Segerstrom A (1973 a) Effect of parathyroid hormone on the propulsive gastrointestinal motility of the rat. Acta Chir Scand 139:55–59

Segerstrom A (1973 b) Thyrocalcitonin and gastrointestinal propulsive motility: an experimental study in the rat. Acta Chir Scand 139:180–183

Waldeck F, Siewert R, Jennewein HM, Weiser F (1973) Das Druckprofil im unteren Ösophagussphinkter beim Menschen und seine Beeinflussung durch Gastrin, Calcitonin und Glucagon. Dtsch Med Wochenschr 98:1059–1063

Walling MW, Brasitus TA, Kimberg DU (1977) Effects of calcitonin and substance P on the transport of Ca, Na and Cl across rat ileum in vitro. Gastroenterology 73:89–94

Coherin

A. Introduction

Coherin is a peptide, isolated from bovine posterior pituitary gland, for which the aminoacid analysis has been reported (Ala_1 Asp_4 Cys_5 Glu_4 Gly_5 Ile_3 Leu_3 Lys_1 Phe_1 Pro_5 Tyr_3) but the sequence has not (GOODMAN and HIATT 1972). Subsequent studies have revealed that a coherin complex dissociates during continuous electrophoresis to yield three subfractions: coherins A and B, two very active peptides, and a third having little, if any, activity, named coherin C. Undissociated coherin, used in most of the studies described below, designated coherin G-25, consists of approximately 5% fraction A, 10% fraction B, and 85% fraction C, probably a carrier peptide. The name "coherin" derives from the observation that it causes "coherence," i.e., peristaltic waves which propagate over the entire length of the intestinal segment under study. Basic electrical rhythm (BER) organization was indeed described by the term "electrical coherence," which was characterized by a constant phase relationship, or phase lock, between BER minima recorded from pairs of adjacent electrodes (HIATT et al. 1977).

B. Effects of Coherin

In the fasting dog, a high degree of phase locking and mainly caudad propagation of the BER in the upper small intestine have been demonstrated. By contrast, the ileum was shown to exhibit a more random and variable pattern of phase locking with only a few propagative patterns, caudad in direction. For this reason the action of coherin was studied in both isolated perfused canine jejunum (intra-arterial administration of 250–500 ng peptide) and in conscious dogs with chronically implanted electrodes (intravenous administration of coherin A and B, 1 µg/kg, and coherin G-25, 5, and 10 µg/kg). Under both experimental conditions, coherin (co-

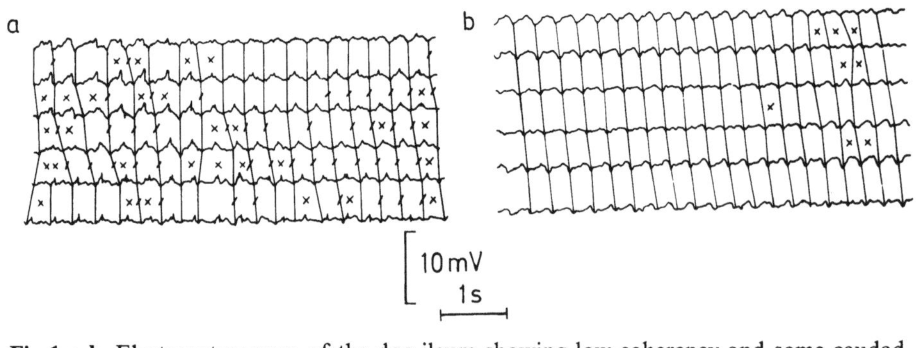

Fig. 1 a, b. Electroenterogram of the dog ileum showing low coherency and some caudad propagation before **a** and after **b** injection of coherin A. *Crosses* indicate nonparallel pairs of lines connecting BER minima; *oblique strokes* indicate caudad propagation. (HIATT et al. 1977)

herin A was the most effective fraction) caused a significant increase in coherency, or phase locking (Fig. 1) and significantly changed propagation from mainly cephalad or no propagation (simultaneous BER) to mostly caudad in direction. The obvious consequence was a net increase in caudad propulsive contractions (HIATT et al. 1974, 1977; MENDEL et al. 1975). The effect of coherin began about 15 min after injection, reaching a peak after 60 min. The action of coherin might be exerted through myogenic or neurogenic factors or a combination of these, but the real mechanism of action has not yet been determined.

The effect of coherin on the myoelectric activity of the jejunum in humans was also investigated during the postoperative period. The peptide (1 μg/kg intravenously) caused an increase in the regulatory index of the BER, associated with a marked increase in the amplitude of the slow waves, with a slight and nonsignificant increase in spiking activity (DAUCHEL et al. 1975). The occurrence of regular and ample slow waves after administration of coherin was associated with improved synchronization of the contraction of the intestinal muscular coats, with a consequently effective propulsive peristaltic activity, thus bringing about a significant shortening of the duration of the physiologic postoperative ileus.

Coherin was also administered to patients suffering from acute or chronic postgastrectomy obstructions and from regional ileitis and was found to relieve symptoms in a high percentage of cases. In some patients, the treatment was prolonged for years without evidence of any serious side effects. The therapeutic effect of the peptide in treatment of physiologic obstructions was interpreted as a consequence of its activity in organizing the propagative characteristics of intestinal BER, which in turn control mechanical propulsive efficiency, while in ileitis, coherin appeared to be useful in the control of episodes of cramps and diarrhea (HIATT and GOODMAN 1976, 1979). However, evaluation of the data was based only on the observations that during treatment patients felt better, and that symptoms reappeared soon after discontinuing coherin administration. It is obvious that the lack of controlled trials by double-blind techniques limits the validity of these interesting observations. Moreover, coherin given by single i.m. administration (100 μg) or by repeated consecutive injections (twice daily for 3 days) failed to normalize the abnormal slow wave patterns in patients with irritable colon syndrome, although the hormone did increase basal colonic spike activity and basal intraluminal pressure (SNAPE et al. 1978).

C. Conclusions

Coherin is apparently a very interesting substance endowed with real and unique biologic effects. It is clear that such terms as "increased motility" or "decreased motility" fail to describe its action on the gut, which consists essentially in changing the patterns of activity. In this sense, coherin cannot be classified together with any other endogenous compound affecting gut motility. However, sufficient amounts of pure coherin or of a synthetic analog endowed with the same biologic activity must become available as an obvious prerequisite for establishing all the possible actions of the peptide in different species, under different experimental conditions, and its possible interaction with other endogenous mediators acting directly and/or indirectly on the gut muscle. Of course, only when it is possible to correlate the plasma levels of coherin with its effects on the gastrointestinal tract will we be able to establish whether or not a physiologic role in the regulation of mechanical and electrical activity of the gut can be hypothesized for this peptide.

References

Dauchel J, Schang JC, Pousse A, Hiatt RB, Grenier JF (1975) Electromyographic study of the effects of coherin, a posterior pituitary extract, on the intestinal motility in man. In: Vantrappen G (ed) Fifth International Symposium on Gastrointestinal Motility. Typoff, Herentals, pp 88–94

Goodman I, Hiatt RB (1972) Coherin: a new peptide of the bovine neurohypophysis with activity on gastrointestinal motility. Science 178:419–421

Hiatt RB, Goodman I (1976) Peptide treatment of postgastrectomy obstruction. Arch Surg 111:997–999

Hiatt RB, Goodman I (1979) The physiologic properties and therapeutic potential of coherin. Am J Surg 137:82–86

Hiatt RB, Grenier J, Mendel C, Goodman I (1974) Action of coherin on the basic electrical rhythm and propagation in the isolated perfused canine jejunum. In: Daniel EE (ed) Fourth International Symposium on Gastrointestinal Motility. Mitchell, Vancouver, pp 61–62

Hiatt RB, Goodman I, Sandler B, Cheskin H (1977) The effect of coherin on the basic electrical rhythm of the dog ileum "in vivo." Am J Dig Dis 22:108–112

Mendel C, Jaeck D, Grenier JF, Hiatt RB, Goodman I, Sandler B (1975) Action of coherin on the basic electrical rhythm and propagation in the isolated perfused canine jejunum. J Surg Res 19:403–409

Snape WJ Jr, Sullivan MA, Cohen S (1978) The effect of coherin on colonic myoelectrical activity in the irritable bowel syndrome. Gastroenterology 74:1097

Thyrotropin-Releasing Hormone

A. Introduction

Thyrotropin-releasing hormone (TRH), the first of the hypothalamic-releasing factors to be identified and synthesized (BOWERS et al. 1970), is a tripeptide (pyroglutamyl-histidyl-prolineamide). The existance of TRH immunoreactivity in the brain, the gastrointestinal tract, and the pancreas of mammals was reported (JACKSON and REICHLIN 1974; MORLEY et al. 1977). As already observed for many other peptides of the so-called gut–brain–skin triangle (ERSPAMER 1978) TRH was found also to occur in amphibian skin (YAJIMA et al. 1975; JACKSON and REICHLIN 1977).

Besides its typical endocrine effect, which was the first to be demonstrated, it was recently shown that TRH exerts some interesting actions outside the central nervous system. In addition to an inhibitory effect on pentagastrin-induced acid secretion in humans (DOLVA et al. 1979a, b), some interesting, but so far insufficiently investigated effects on gastrointestinal motility have been described.

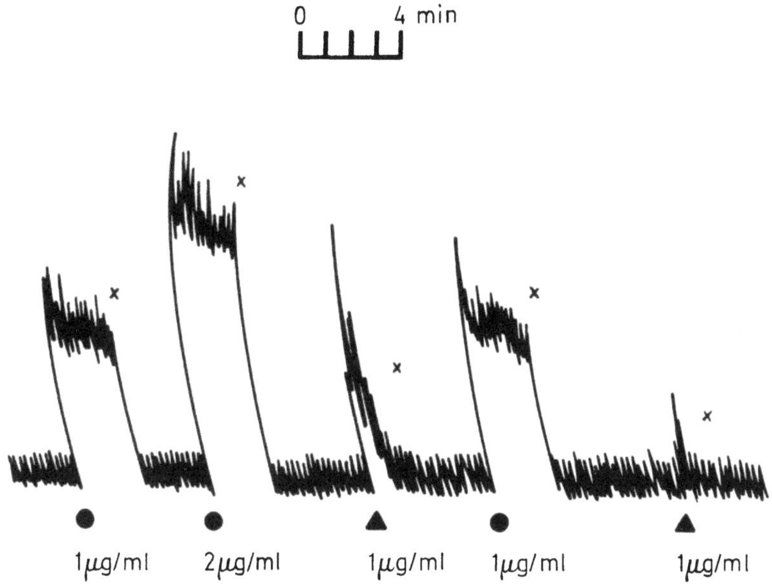

Fig. 1. Isolated pyloric sphincter from the guinea pig. *Circles*, histamine; *triangles*, TRH, *Crosses*, washout

B. In Vitro Studies

In vitro studies in the rat (BRUCE et al. 1977, 1979) showed that TRH (5.5 μ*M*) when tested for its effects on the mechanical activity of antral, pyloric sphincter, and colonic tissue did not affect the frequency of contractions, but had dramatic effects on the force of contraction in all the tissues examined, the antrum being the most sensitive. The contractile effect, which exceeded that of bethanechol (6.4 μ*M*), lasted more than 30 min. In the antrum and in the pylorus, TRH was able to potentiate the stimulatory effect of bethanechol significantly. Atropine (10 μ*M*) was ineffective in blocking TRH-induced contractions. Conversely, antral response to TRH was markedly inhibited by cimetidine (150 μ*M*), suggesting that histamine H_2-receptors may be involved in the antral contraction induced by TRH. Pyrilamine may also reduce the effect of the tripeptide, but to a lesser extent than cimetidine. In our personal experience (BERTACCINI et al. 1979), TRH had an erratic spasmogenic effect on isolated pyloric muscle from rats and guinea pigs (Figs. 1,2). Threshold stimulatory doses in both preparations ranged between 0.1 and 1 μg/ml. Complete dose–response curves could not be obtained because of the rapid appearance of tachyphylaxis. Guinea pig ileum was stimulated by TRH, but its effectiveness was less than 1/1,000 of that of histamine; tachyphylaxis was a common feature in this preparation also. TRH was ineffective on the lower esophageal sphincter from rats and guinea pigs (up to 1 μg/ml was used; G. BERTACCINI and G. CORUZZI unpublished work 1980).

Recent studies (TONOUE et al. 1979), showed that TRH (5×10^{-8} *M*) induces a distinct, dose-dependent, relaxant response in the isolated duodenum of the rat. This effect, which was absent in the jejunum and the ileum, was not blocked by tetrodotoxin, phenoxybenzamine or propranolol, suggesting a direct influence of the

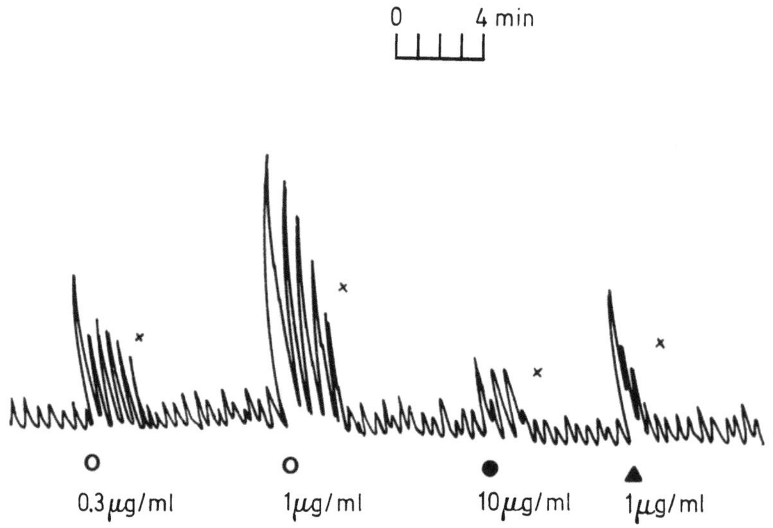

Fig. 2. Isolated pyloric sphincter from the rat. *Open circles*, acetylcholine; *full circle*, histamine; *full triangle*, TRH; *Crosses*, washout

tripeptide on the smooth muscle. Also, preincubation with indomethacin did not affect the duodenal response to TRH, indicating that prostaglandins are not involved in this response. Summing up, the effect of TRH on rat duodenum resembles that elicited by bradykinin and by bombesin, even though a common mechanism of action for the three peptides may be only hypothesized. The same group of investigators (FURUKAWA et al. 1980) observed similar stimulatory effects of TRH on the duodenum ($pD_2 = 8.0$) and the taenia coli ($pD_2 = 8.9$) of the guinea pig. These responses were inhibited by tetrodotoxin and by hyoscine, which was able to reverse the response of the duodenum to a relaxation. Hexamethonium was always ineffective. Apparently these neurogenic actions of the tripeptide on the guinea pig bowel are in sharp contrast with the myogenic nature of the response to TRH in the rat duodenum.

C. In Vivo Studies

In experiments performed in anesthetized rabbits, TRH was completely ineffective when administered intravenously (up to 1 mg/kg), but it increased both the frequency and the force of contractile activity in the proximal colon after intraventricular administration (0.5–100 µg). Administration of atropine or of ganglion-blocking agents or bilateral vagotomy antagonized the increase in the colon's motor activity. Apparently this is a unique example of a neuropeptide affecting central mechanisms responsible for the regulation of gastrointestinal motor activity (LA HANN and HORITA 1977; SMITH et al. 1977). The central injection of another tripeptide, melanocyte-releasing hormone inhibitory factor (MIF), failed to elicit any gastrointestinal motor stimulation (LA HANN 1978). TRH (2 nmol/100 g) administered intraventricularly into anesthetized rats caused, after a short latency, an increase in the amplitude and a decrease in the frequency of basic electric rhythm

(BER) and the association of bursts of spike potentials with nearly every cycle of BER in the duodenum. This effect was maximal in the proximal duodenum, tended to decrease in the distal part, and was absent in the ileum. Hypophysectomy, cord-transection, or injection of 6-hydroxydopamine did not block the duodenal response to TRH, which was, however, abolished by vagotomy or atropine administration (TONOUE and NOMOTO 1979). Thus, TRH seems to stimulate the neuronal system that controls the vagus efferents involved in regulation of the duodenal enteric nervous system, which in turn modulates the myogenic excitability of the duodenum.

In conscious dogs, TRH (2–16 μg/kg i.v.) caused a dose-related increase in the number of slow biphasic antral potentials. This stimulatory effect was blocked by somatostatin, naloxone, or dopamine and appears to be compatible with either a local or a central effect (MORLEY et al. 1979). On the whole, these data do not enable us to speculate on the mechanism of the effects of TRH on gastrointestinal motility and detailed in vitro and in vivo investigations are needed before any definite conclusions can be drawn. In experiments carried out in healthy volunteers, TRH (40 and 1,000 μg/h) was shown to inhibit gastric motility stimulated by distension of the stomach wall significantly (DOLVA et al. 1978) and to stimulate motility under basal conditions (1 mg/h was required; DOLVA and STADAAS 1979). The effect of TRH was similar to that observed after proximal vagotomy, suggesting that the tripeptide might act by a mechanism involving the vagal nerve and/or intramural cholinergic ganglion cells. Moreover, it is known that the majority of human subjects injected with synthetic TRH complain of mild nausea and abdominal discomfort (CARLSON and HERSHMAN 1975). Data available so far leave completely open the question of any possible physiologic action of the tripeptide outside the brain. The distribution and functions of the extrahypothalamic thyrotropin-releasing hormone were recently reviewed by MORLEY (1979).

References

Bertaccini G, Coruzzi G, Zappia L (1979) Azione del TRH sulla motilità gastrointestinale „in vitro." Ateneo Parmense [Acta Biomed] 50:149–152

Bowers CY, Schally AV, Enzmann F, Boler J, Folkers K (1970) Porcine thyrotropin-releasing hormone is (pyro)glu-his-pro(NH_2). Endocrinology 86:1143–1153

Bruce LA, Behsudi FM, Fawcett CP (1977) The effect of TRH on gastrointestinal smooth muscle in vitro. IRCS Med Sci 5:469

Bruce LA, Behsudi FM, Fawcett CP (1979) Histaminergic involvement in thyrotropin-releasing hormone stimulation of antral tissue in the rat. Gastroenterology 76:908–912

Carlson HE, Hershman JM (1975) The hypothalamic-pituitary-thyroid axis. Med Clin North Am 59:1045–1053

Dolva LØ, Stadaas JO (1979) Action of thyrotropin-releasing hormone on gastrointestinal functions in man. III. Inhibition of gastric motility in response to distension. Scand J Gastroenterol 14:419–423

Dolva LØ, Hanssen KF, Stadaas J, Berstad A (1978) Thyrotropin releasing hormone inhibits the pentagastrin stimulated gastric secretion and gastric motility in man. Scand J Gastroenterol [Suppl 49] 13:49

Dolva LØ, Hanssen KF, Berstad A (1979a) Actions of thyrotropin-releasing hormone on the gastrointestinal function in man. Scand J Gastroenterol 14:33–34

Dolva LØ, Hanssen KF, Berstad A, Frey HMM (1979b) Thyrotropin-releasing hormone inhibits the pentagastrin stimulated gastric secretion in man. A dose-response study. Clin Endocrinol 10:281–286

Erspamer V (1978) Correlation between active peptides of the amphibian skin and peptides of the avian and mammalian gut and brain. The gut-brain-skin triangle. In: Abstr 19th Congr Ital Pharmacol Soc. Grafiche Bellomo, Ancona, pp 109–156
Furukawa K, Nomoto T, Tonoue T (1980) Effects of thyrotropin-releasing hormone (TRH) on the isolated small intestine and taenia coli of the guinea pig. Eur J Pharmacol 64:279–287
Jackson I, Reichlin S (1974) Thyrotropin-releasing hormone (TRH): distribution in the brain, blood, and urine of the rat. Life Sci 14:2259–2266
Jackson I, Reichlin S (1977) Thyrotropin-releasing hormone: abundance in the skin of the frog, Rana pipiens, Science 198:414–415
La Hann TR (1978) Studies on the gastrointestinal motor activity evoked by central administration of thyrotropin-releasing hormone. PhD dissertation, University of Washington. Abstr Int B38, 4182
La Hann TR, Horita A (1977) Thyrotropin-releasing hormone and the gastrointestinal tract: the effect of central administration on colonic smooth muscle activity. Proc West Pharmacol Soc 20:305–306
Morley JE (1979) Extrahypothalamic thyrotropin-releasing hormone (TRH); its distribution and its functions. Life Sci 25:1539–1550
Morley JE, Garvin TJ, Pekary AE, Hersham JM (1977) Thyrotropin-releasing hormone in the gastrointestinal tract. Biochem Biophys Res Commun 79:314–318
Morley JE, Steinback JH, Feldman EJ, Solomon TE (1979) The effects of thyrotropin-releasing hormone (TRH) on the gastrointestinal tract. Life Sci 24:1059–1066
Smith JR, La Hann TR, Chesnut RM, Carino MA, Horita A (1977) Thyrotropin-releasing hormone: stimulation of colonic activity following intracerebroventricular administration. Sciences 196:660–662
Tonoue T, Nomoto T (1979) Effect of intracerebroventricular administration of thyrotropin-releasing hormone upon the electroenteromyogram of rat duodenum. Eur J Pharmacol 58:369–377
Tonoue T, Furukawa K, Nomoto T 1979) The direct influence of thyrotropin-releasing hormone (TRH) on the smooth muscle of rat duodenum. Life Sci 25:2011–2016
Yajima H, Kitagawa K, Segawa T, Nakano M, Kataoka K (1975) Occurrence of Pyr-His-Pro-NH_2 in the frog skin. Chem Pharm Bull (Tokyo) 23:3301–3303

CHAPTER 2e

Peptides: Locally Active Peptides ("Vasoactive Peptides")

G. BERTACCINI

Angiotensin

A. Introduction

Angiotensin may be considered the prototype of the so-called vasoactive peptides inasmuch as its predominant effect is on vascular smooth muscle, which is constricted by both direct and indirect effects of the peptide. However, angiotensin may affect contractility of much extravascular smooth muscle with a predominantly, if not exclusively, stimulatory effect. Here, only the effects on gastrointestinal smooth muscle will be considered.

Between 1954 and 1957, two major peptides, which corresponded to the "pressor substance" observed by BRAUN-MENÉNDEZ et al. (1940) in blood from animals with renal artery stenosis, were isolated, sequenced, and synthesized (SKEGGS et al. 1954, 1955, 1956; SCHWARZ et al. 1957; SCHWYZER et al. 1958). The larger peptide (angiotensin I) was shown to be a decapeptide which could be transformed by a plasma peptidase (converting enzyme), which cleaved off the COOH terminal dipeptide histidyl-leucine, into the active octapeptide (angiotensin II). The amino acid sequence was determined as:

1 2 3 4 5 6 7 8 9 10
Asp-Arg-Val-Tyr-Ile-His-Pro-Phe-His-Leu
Angiotensin I (residues 1–10)
Angiotensin II (residues 1–8)

This structure is common to horse, pig, rat, and human angiotensins, while ox angiotensin I has a valine residue in position 5.

B. Structure–Activity Relationships

After the synthesis of angiotensin, a number of analogs were synthesized and tested in attempts: (a) to define each of the specific parts of the angiotensin molecule that are necessary for biologic activity; (b) to identify the minimum number of amino acid residues required for the activity; and (c) to find specific inhibitors of angiotensin. Most of the results of these studies are reported in several excellent reviews (RE-

GOLI et al. 1974b; KHOSLA et al. 1974; BUMPUS and KHOSLA 1977; PEACH 1979). Conclusive results may be summarized as follows:

1) The aromatic ring of phenylalanine (COOH terminus) is essential for high intrinsic activity. Removal of the eighth residue results in an inactive heptapeptide.
2) The proline at position 7 is important for high receptor affinity and also protects angiotensin II from hydrolysis by converting enzyme.
3) A β-aliphatic or alicyclic side chain at position 5 is required to maintain activity. Apparently, Ile (human, horse, and pig) or Val (ox) residues exert rigid constraint on the peptide backbone which is important for activity.
4) The minimum peptide chain required for full biologic activity is the 3–8 COOH terminal hexapeptide. However, its potency in some preparations is strikingly diminished compared with the parent molecule (pD_2 of the hexapeptide in the rat stomach strip $=5.2$; pD_2 of angiotensin II $=7.75$).
5) The structural importance of the NH_2 terminus is connected with susceptibility to aminopeptidase and to receptor kinetics, and substitution with different residues strongly influences the duration of action of angiotensin analogs. On the basis of these data, several angiotensin inhibitors were synthesized, the most important being saralasin (CASTELLION and FULTON 1978; GAVRAS et al. 1978), which has the following structure:

1 2 3 4 5 6 7 8
Sar-Arg-Val-Tyr-Val-His-Pro-Ala

The crucial amino acid residues in this molecule are represented by sarcosine (position 1), which imparts resistance to "angiotensinases" (aminopeptidases) and alanine (position 8), which markedly reduces intrinsic activity with minimal effect on receptor affinity.

Quite recently it was found that frog *(Crinia georgiana)* skin contains an undecapeptide (150–550 μg/g) similar to mammalian angiotensins but with a tripeptide (Ala-Pro-Gly) attached to the NH_2 terminal Asp residue of the conventional angiotensin. The structure of this peptide, named "crinia-angiotensin II" (ERSPAMER et al. 1979; FALCONIERI-ERSPAMER et al. 1979), is the following:

Ala-Pro-Gly-Asp-Arg-Ile-Tyr-Val-His-Pro-Phe

This new angiotensin is approximately as potent as Val^5-angiotensin II-Asp^1-amide (Hypertensin, Ciba) in the guinea pig ileum, the rat colon, and the rat stomach. This peptide is another interesting example of the well-known similarities of mammalian and amphibian peptides.

C. Effects on the Gastrointestinal Tract

I. In Vitro Studies

In the guinea pig intestine, for both the usual whole ileum and the longitudinal muscle preparations, angiotensin II was shown to exert a dose-dependent stimulatory effect (starting from very low threshold doses: 10^{-10}–10^{-9} *M*), which was re-

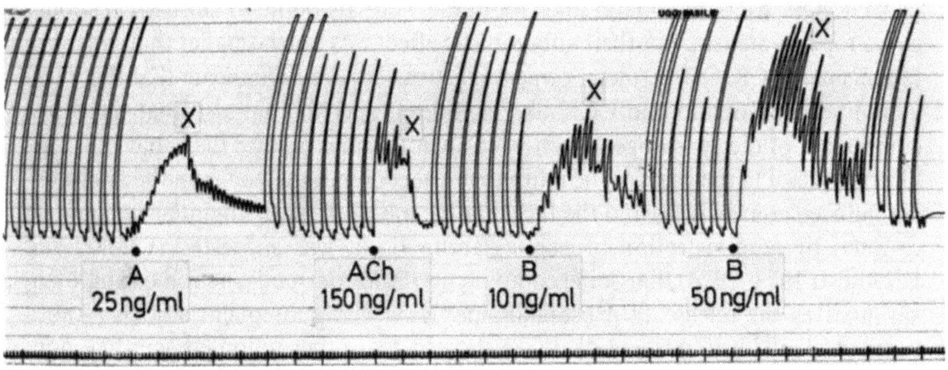

Fig. 1. Longitudinal muscle strip from guinea pig ileum electrically stimulated (0.1 Hz, 1 ms, 6 V/cm). Isometric recording. *A*, angiotensin; *ACh*, acetylcholine; *B*, bombesin. *Crosses* indicate washout

duced by atropine and morphine, but not by hexamethonium. Moreover, it was potentiated by acetylcholinesterase inhibitors (KHAIRALLAH and PAGE 1961, 1963; ROBERTSON and RUBIN 1962). Therefore, angiotensin may stimulate parasympathetic nerve tissues and elicit a contractile response at least partly mediated by acetylcholine. The peptide apparently falls into the class of non-nicotinic ganglion stimulants since the response was blocked by ganglion-blocking agents (LEWIS and REIT 1965; TRENDELENBURG 1966). According to GODFRAIND et al. (1966a, b) angiotensin has a fast indirect acetylcholine-mediated action (release of mediator from cholinergic nerve terminals blocked by atropine) and a slow direct myotropic effect, inhibited only by lidoflazine, a noncompetitive antagonist. Apparently the indirect action of angiotensin is peculiar to the guinea pig ileum. Tachyphylaxis was present only when high doses were used without a sufficient time interval between two subsequent administrations. In the longitudinal preparations, angiotensin evoked a slow contraction followed by slow relaxation after washing, resembling the effect of peptides of the bradykinin or bombesin family (G. BERTACCINI unpublished work 1980; Fig. 1). Angiotensin I also has a high relative potency in the guinea pig ileum, being one-third as active as angiotensin II (VANE 1974). This shows that converting enzyme is also present in isolated preparations. Indeed, the activity of angiotensin I was virtually abolished by the pentapeptide inhibitor of converting enzyme.

Contractile responses of guinea pig ileum varied directly with sodium concentrations of the nutrient solution: a decrease in sodium content decreased the sensitivity and, conversely, an increase in sodium content increased the sensitivity, even in the presence of atropine (KHAIRALLAH et al. 1965; BLAIR-WEST and MCKENZIE 1966; BERGMAN et al. 1971). Contractile responses to angiotensin were lessened by decreases in calcium concentration (KHAIRALLAH et al. 1965) and increased by alkalinization of the bath fluid (HUIDOBRO and PALADINI 1963). In recent experiments (ZETLER 1979), tetrodotoxin (6×10^{-8} *M*) was found to shift and depress the concentration–response curve to angiotensin. However, the pA_2 values indicated that angiotensin was only 1/30 as sensitive to tetrodotoxin (TTX) as cerulein or CCK OP. Met-enkephalin and morphine were also able to shift the response curve for angiotensin, but their antagonistic effect was much smaller than their antagonism of CCK OP, cerulein, or pentagastrin. This could indicate that the interaction between opioid and CCK-like peptides is specific, but also that the direct component of the spasmogenic action of angiotensin is greater than that of CCK-like peptides. On the basis of the inhibitory effect of indomethacin on the angiotensin-induced contractions and the fact that the initial effect of angiotensin could be restored by administration of prostaglandin E_2, it was suggested (CHONG and DOWNING 1973, 1974) that some component of the contractile action of angiotensin involves the release of prostaglandins. However, subsequent studies (ABOU-LAFIA et al. 1976; FAMAEY et al. 1978) showed that other indomethacin-like nonsteroidal and steroidal anti-inflammatory drugs inhibit angiotensin, but do so nonspecifically (other compounds like bradykinin, acetylcholine and histamine were found to be similarly inhibited). The same nonspecific potentiation was found to occur after prostaglandin administration. Thus, it appears more probable that indomethacin and prostaglandins act on the smooth muscle themselves, affecting one of the steps of the excitation–concentration coupling.

In a study of the metabolic requirements for the contractile action of angiotensin (CROCKER and WILSON 1974), it was found that the angiotensin-induced response was far more dependent upon the presence of glucose than was the response to acetylcholine; anoxia and oxidative inhibition preferentially reduced the angiotensin-induced response. The authors concluded that the response to angiotensin was dependent upon an ATP source different from that required by the contractile process. This energy-dependent stage cannot be identified with the indirect, cholinergic component of the angiotensin response in the guinea pig ileum. The guinea pig taenia coli was found to be fairly sensitive to angiotensin, with threshold doses ranging between 10 and 100 ng/ml in the different investigations. CESSI et al. (1977) observed that in this preparation angiotensin is able to stimulate electrical and mechanical activity, even when they are depressed by a lack of or an excess of Ca^{2+} ions. In addition, they showed (1978) that angiotensin decreased the frequency of action potentials induced by acetylcholine. The authors suggested that the peptide has a depolarizing effect and acts synergistically with K^+ and increasing Ca^{2+} influx.

The rat stomach strip is considered one of the most suitable tissues for accurate studies of angiotensin: it is quite sensitive to the peptide, which elicits a good fast contraction that is complete in less than 3 min. It does not usually show any spontaneous activity which could interfere in detecting the action of angiotensin and it can be used equally well in the classical bath or in a cascade superfusion system. Tachyphylaxis does not occur if sufficient time is allowed to elapse between doses.

Contrasting findings were reported for the action of angiotensin which was completely direct on the smooth muscle, according to REGOLI et al. (1974a), but was at least partially mediated by release of prostaglandins, according to CHONG and DOWNING (1973), who found a decrease in the angiotensin effect after administration of indomethacin, and according to ERCAN and TÜRKER (1977), who observed a similar decrease after giving acetylsalicylic acid or a synthetic competitive blocker of prostaglandin (SC 19220). The latter authors observed that (despartic acid)^1-angiotensin II (so-called angiotensin III) had a greater prostaglandin-releasing activity than the parent peptide in the rat stomach fundal strip, exactly as it had in the rabbit mesenteric arterial muscle (BLUMBERG et al. 1976). The action of angiotensin on the isolated rat stomach was found to be decreased by depolarization provoked by K^+, whereas the peptide potentiated the contracting effect of Ca^{2+}. It was suggested that the angiotensin effect depends on the membrane potential and consists of an increased permeability to calcium ions (CESSI and BETTINI 1974).

Rat pylorus was contracted by angiotensin, but only at very high (2–5 μg/ml) concentrations of the peptide (G. BERTACCINI unpublished work 1980). Rat duodenum responded to angiotensin (10^{-8} *M*) with a remarkable increase in tone and even more in the amplitude of spontaneous contractions (CLINESCHMIDT et al. 1971).

In test preparations of rat colon, angiotensin exerted a direct spasmogenic effect, starting from very low threshold doses (0.3–1 ng/ml). However, in disagreement with some previous statements (REGOLI and VANE 1964; POGGLITSCH and HOLZER 1971; GAGNON and SIROIS 1972), subsequent studies demonstrated that rat colon should not be considered the most suitable test material for bioassay of angiotensin, since high doses of the peptide produced variable effects and stable contraction plateaux were not maintained (REGOLI et al. 1974a). All of the investigators agreed that the action of angiotensin is a direct one on the colonic muscle. The well-known inhibitor of oxidative metabolism, 2,4-dinitrophenol reduced the response of the rat colon to angiotensin more than the response to acetylcholine; this indicates that the action of the peptide is more dependent upon energy than is that of acetylcholine, therefore suggesting that there is an energy-dependent step in the angiotensin response, which is distinct from the actual contraction process (CROCKER and WILSON 1975). The angiotensin effect was found to be dependent on the calcium concentration in the nutrient fluid; an increase in calcium concentration potentiated the responses to angiotensin and calcium-free Tyrode solution reduced the response to angiotensin, as did an increase in the intracellular concention of cyclic AMP (CROCKER et al. 1979). Differences in response to angiotensin and KCl suggested that part of the response to the peptide involves an influx of calcium, independent of depolarization, confirming the previous observations by CESSI and BETTINI (1974) for rat stomach. The dose-related contractions induced by angiotensin in the rat colon were competitively inhibited by synthetic analogs (aminophenylisobutyric acid)^8-angiotensin II, and Ala^8-angiotensin II (TÜRKER et al. 1971, 1973). The contractions of rat colon and rat ileum preparations induced by angiotensin I indicated 4% conversion (VANE 1974), in contrast to the high degree of conversion demonstrated in the guinea pig ileum.

Angiotensin was found to have a remarkable effect on the isolated lower esophageal sphincter (LES) from rats and guinea pigs (CORUZZI and BERTACCINI 1980). In the rat, threshold stimulatory doses varied between 5 and 50 ng/ml with a maximum response at 30 μg/ml. In the guinea pig, surprisingly enough, angiotensin exerted a constant relaxation (0.5–10 μg/ml). This is, so far, the only example of an inhibitory effect of angiotensin in isolated smooth muscle preparations (Fig. 2). In both species, tachyphylaxis was a common feature.

In the isolated perfused terminal ileum of the cat (TÜRKER 1973), angiotensin II was found to potentiate the inhibitory response to periarterial nerve plexus stim-

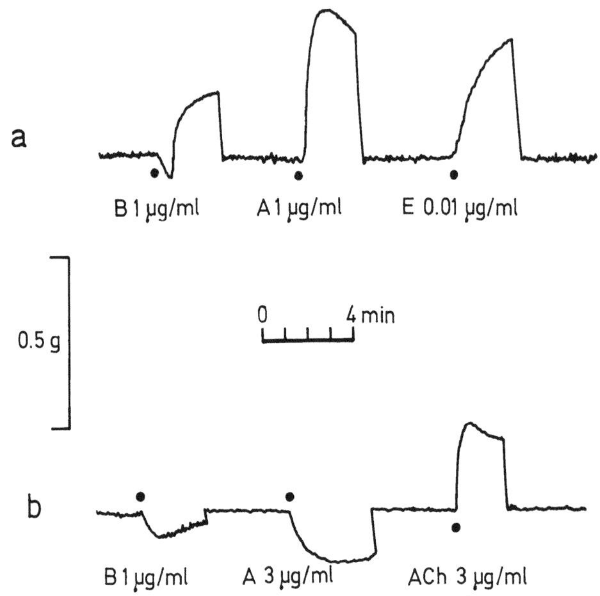

Fig. 2a, b. Effect of angiotensin and other compounds on the isolated LES from the rat **a** and the guinea pig **b** measured by a transducer and a microdynamometer. *B*, bradykinin; *A*, angiotensin; *E*, eledoisin; *ACh*, acetylcholine

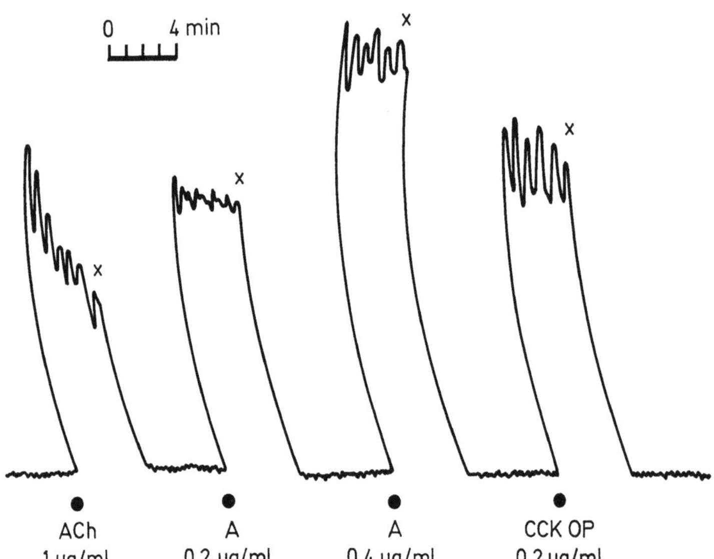

Fig. 3. Human stomach antrum in vitro, isotonic recording. *ACh*, acetylcholine; *A*, angiotensin; *CCK OP*, cholecystokinin COOH terminal octapeptide. *Crosses* indicate washout

ulation without changing the effect of noradrenaline. Thus, a cocaine-like effect was excluded and a facilitation of the release of noradrenaline from adrenergic nerve endings in response to sympathetic stimulation was suggested.

Isolated preparations from human gastrointestinal tract responded fairly well to angiotensin (Fig. 3): threshold doses were of the order of 1–5 ng/ml for all the

Table 1. Contractile activity of angiotensin II on a series of isolated preparations from the gastrointestinal tract of different species

Target	Threshold dose (ng/ml)[a]	Mechanism of action[b]	Reference
Rat LES	100 – 300	NT	CORUZZI and BERTACCINI (1980)
Rat stomach	1 – 10	D	REGOLI and VANE (1964)
	1 – 2	D	CESSI and BETTINI (1973, 1974)
	5	D, I	ERKAN and TÜRKER (1977)
Rat pylorus	1,000	NT	CORUZZI and BERTACCINI (1980)
Rat duodenum	1,000	NT	REGOLI and VANE (1964)
	50 – 100	NT	CLINESCHMIDT et al. (1971)
Rat ileum	100 –1,000	NT	REGOLI and VANE (1964)
Rat colon	1 – 10	D	REGOLI and VANE (1964)
	0.3– 1	D	GAGNON and SIROIS (1972)
	5	D	ERCAN and TÜRKER (1977)
Guinea pig LES	1,000 –3,000 R	NT	CORUZZI and BERTACCINI (1980)
Guinea pig ileum	0.4– 0.8	NT	BISSET and LEWIS (1962)
	10 – 100	NT	REGOLI and VANE (1964)
	1 – 10	D, I	GODFRAIND et al. (1966a)
	0.2– 0.5	D, I	ZETLER (1979)
Guinea pig taenia coli	10 – 100		REGOLI and VANE (1964)
	50		CESSI et al. (1977)
Pigeon rectum	10 – 100	NT	REGOLI and VANE (1964)
Hen rectal cecum	1,000	NT	BISSET and LEWIS (1962)
Human stomach	2 – 20	D	BERTACCINI et al. (1974) BERTACCINI unpublished work
Human small intestine	5 – 50	D	BERTACCINI et al. (1974)
Human large intestine	5 – 25	D	BERTACCINI et al. (1974)
	10	D	FISHLOCK and GUNN (1970)

[a] R = relaxation
[b] NT = not tested; D or I = direct or indirect effect on the smooth muscle

tissues examined and tachyphylaxis was present rarely, if at all. The stimulatory effect of the peptide appeared to be a direct one on the smooth muscle (FISHLOCK and GUNN 1970; BERTACCINI et al. 1974; G. BERTACCINI unpublished work 1979). A synopsis of the effects of angiotensin on different segments of the gastrointestinal tract in vitro is given in Table 1, where experiments with both animal and human tissues are considered.

II. In Vivo Studies

Very few studies concerning the in vivo action of angiotensin on gastrointestinal motility are available in the literature. In the opossum *(Didelphis marsupialis virginiana)*, angiotensin II produced a dose-related (0.03–1 μg/kg i.v.) increase (maximum 270%) in LES pressure. This effect, unaffected by atropine or hexamethonium, was blocked by saralasin and significantly inhibited by tetrodotoxin injected into the wall of the esophagus. Phentolamine and verapamil were also able to antagonize the spasmogenic effect of angiotensin. Therefore, it was suggested that the peptide acts both directly on the receptors in the LES and indirectly via the adrenergic nervous system. It is likely that the effect of angiotensin involves a calcium-dependent pathway (MUKHOPADHYAY and LEAVITT 1978).

Angiotensin II was recently shown to cause graded increases in human LES pressure when administered in doses of 1–5 ng kg^{-1} min^{-1}. This effect was not modified by administration of atropine, but was competitively antagonized by saralasine. An action connected with stimulation of specific receptors was hypothesized (HAULICA et al. 1980). In the ileum of the anesthetized dog (SHEHADEH et al. 1969; BERTACCINI et al. 1970; G. BERTACCINI unpublished work 1979), angiotensin was found to induce the appearance of or to reinforce rhythmic movements; the effect was dose related, from threshold doses of 25–50 ng/kg i.v. up to 1 µg/kg, and the amplitude of the contractions was increased more than the tone. Of course, the stimulant effects on the intestine were accompanied by dose-related increases in blood pressure, the opposite of what happened with the CCK-like peptides (Fig. 4). These findings were confirmed by subsequent studies (DELEVA and NICOLOV 1977) which showed that angiotensin stimulates mechanical and electrical activity in the canine stomach, duodenum, and jejunum. Only very high doses of the peptide (more than 1 µg/kg by bolus or 2 µg kg^{-1} min^{-1}) produced inhibitory effects on both mechanical and electrical activity. The same authors (DELEVA and NICOLOV 1979) showed that, in vagotomized dogs, angiotensin II constantly increased gastric slow rhythmic potential (SRP) frequency but decreased the SRP conduction velocity. The amplitude of jejunal contractions was simultaneously increased in both intact and denervated animals with the latter showing higher and longer-lasting values.

Interesting findings were reported about the effects of angiotensin in the anesthetized, adrenalectomized cat. In previous experiments, angiotensin was shown to increase ileal intraluminal pressure when given by close arterial injection, causing a short-lived increase in tone and, to a lesser extent, in the amplitude of spontaneous contractions. However, when given intravenously, angiotensin induced an inhibition of motility which was abolished by dihydroergotamine (TÜRKER and KAYAALP 1967; TÜRKER 1969; TÜRKER and KAYMAKCALAN 1971). In subsequent studies, the same group (TÜRKER and ERCAN 1978) reported only that angiotensin II (50–2,000 ng/kg) caused dose-related decreases in the intraluminal pressure of the terminal ileum. A similar effect was elicited by angiotensin III, although doses 200 times as high had to be given. The inhibitory effect was attributed to activation of sympathetic ganglia. The effects of both peptides were competitively antagonized by an i.v. infusion of Sar^1-Ile^8-angiotensin II (10^{-8} mol kg^{-1} min^{-1}). Finally, angiotensin was found to modify the fluid transport in the rat jejunum remarkably: small doses (0.59 ng kg^{-1} min^{-1}) stimulated the rate of fluid absorption (consistent with the view that angiotensin has an important role as a sodium-retaining peptide); very high doses (590 ng kg^{-1} min^{-1}) reduced fluid transport, giving rise simultaneously to an enormous increase in the plasma angiotensin level,

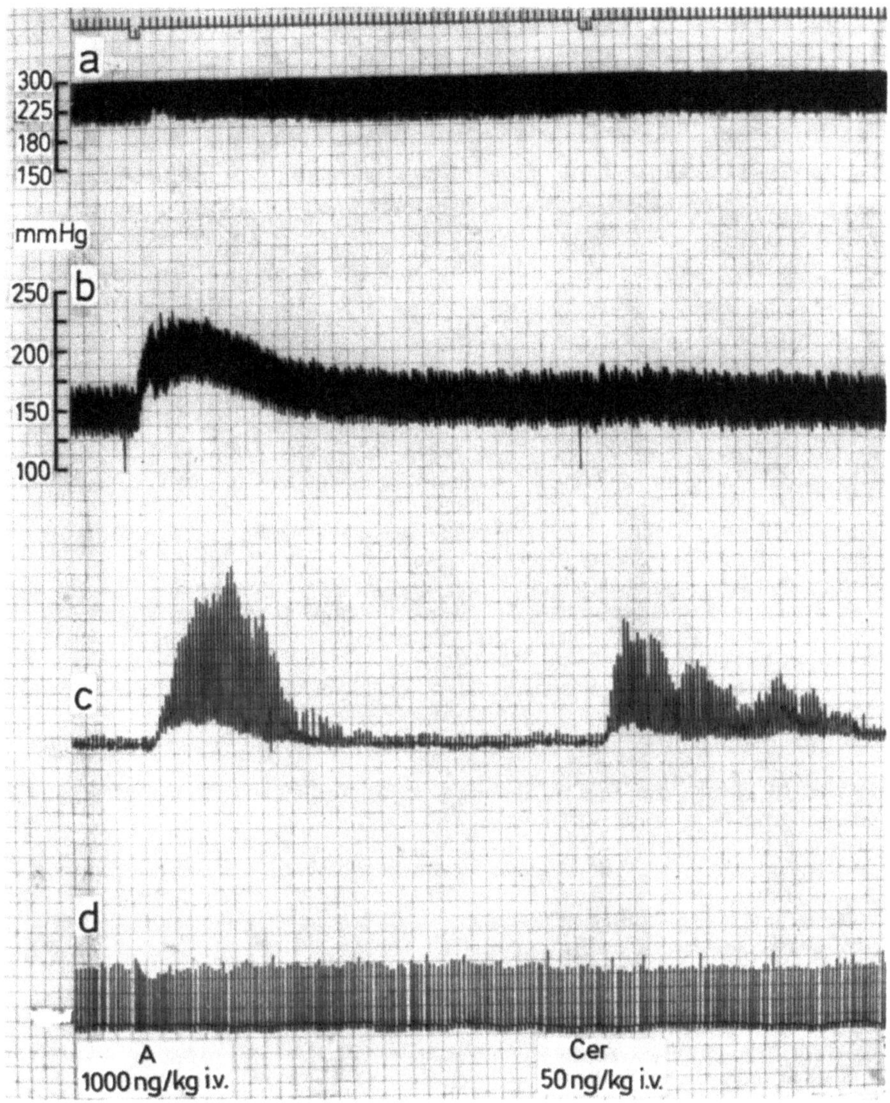

Fig. 4 a–d. Effects of angiotensin in the anesthesized dog. Time marks 20 s. Traces shown are: tachogram **a**; arterial pressure **b**; ileal motility **c**; and pneumogram **d**. *A*, angiotensin; *Cer*, cerulein. (BERTACCINI et al. 1970)

to one which is unlikely to be achieved under physiologic conditions (LEVENS et al. 1975; BOLTON et al. 1976). Of course these doses may alter the motility of the alimentary canal by different mechanisms.

D. Conclusions

The importance of angiotensin as a stimulatory peptide for a number of isolated preparations from the gastrointestinal tract seems to be established. The direct activity on in vitro strips of digestive tract from the rat and the mixed effects on the guinea pig ileum, together with the high sensitivity of these preparations to angiotensin, allow us to consider the peptide as a useful tool for many kinds of pharmacologic study. The availability of selective antagonists must also be considered as providing an interesting tool for pharmacologic studies. It seems unlikely that angiotensin can play a role under physiologic conditions in the regulation of intestinal motility. However, the previously mentioned possibility of its interaction with other endogenous humoral and/or nerve mediators cannot be excluded. Of course, it is also possible that the high blood levels of angiotensin which may be reached in pathologic conditions might per se affect the motor activity of the alimentary canal.

References

Aboulafia J, Mendes GB, Miyamoto ME, Paiva ACM, Paiva TB (1976) Effect of indomethacin and prostaglandin on the smooth muscle contracting activity of angiotensin and other agonists. Br J Pharmacol 58:223–228

Bergman J, Oehme P, Jelinek J (1971) Potentiation of angiotensin and eledoisin activities by sodium chloride. Life Sci 17:969–975

Bertaccini G, Mantovani P, Piccinin GL (1970) Activity ratio between intestinal and cardiovascular actions of caerulein and related substances in the anaesthetized dog. In: Sicuteri F, Rocha e Silva M, Back N (eds) Bradykinin and related kinins. Plenum Press, New York London, pp 213–220

Bertaccini G, Impicciatore M, Molina E, Zappia L (1974) Action of bombesin on human gastrointestinal motility. Rendic, Gastroenterol 6:45–51

Bisset GW, Lewis GP (1962) A spectrum of pharmacological activity in some biologically active peptides. Brit J Pharmacol 19:168–182

Blair-West JR, MacKenzie JS (1966) Sodium concentration and the effect of angiotensin II on ileal smooth muscle. Experientia 22:291

Blumberg A, Denny S, Nishigawa K, Pure E, Marshall GR, Needleman P (1976) Angiotensin III-induced prostaglandin release. Prostaglandins 11:195–197

Bolton JE, Munday KA, Murley C, Parsons BJ, Poat JA (1976) The relationship between plasma angiotensin II concentrations and fluid transport by rat jejunum in vivo. J Physiol (Lond) 254:81P–82P

Braun-Menéndez E, Fasciolo JC, Leloir LR, Munoz JM (1940) The substance causing renal hypertension. J Physiol (Lond) 98:283–298

Bumpus FM, Khosla MC (1977) Angiotensin analogs as determinants of the physiologic role of angiotensin and its metabolites. In: Genest J, Koiw O (eds) Hypertension: physiopathology and treatment. McGraw-Hill, New York, pp 183–201

Castellion AW, Fulton RW (1978) Preclinical pharmacology of saralasin. Kidney Int 15:5–11

Cessi C, Bettini V (1973) Sulla presenza di recettori per l'angiotensina nello stomaco di ratto. Boll Soc Ital Biol Sper 24:433–437

Cessi C, Bettini V (1974) Sull'interazione K^+ angiotensina nello stomaco isolato e denervato di ratto. Boll Soc Ital Biol Sper 50:1231–1234

Cessi C, Bettini V, Rausse A, Legrenzi E (1977) Interazione angiotensina II-Ca^{++} sulla „taenia coli" di cavia. Boll Soc Ital Biol Sper 53:850–855

Cessi C, Bettini V, Perera E, Legrenzi E (1978) Interazioni acetilcolina-angiotensina sull'attività elettrica della „Taenia-coli". Boll Soc Ital Biol Sper 54:2444–2449

Chong EKS, Downing OA (1973) Selective inhibition of angiotensin induced contractions of smooth muscle by indomethacin. J Pharm Pharmacol 25:170–171

Chong EKS, Downing OA (1974) Reversal by prostaglandin E of the inhibitory effect of indomethacin on contractions of guinea-pig ileum induced by angiotensin. J Pharm Pharmacol 26:729–730

Clineschmidt BV, Geller RG, Govier WC, Pisano JJ, Tanimura T (1971) Effects of ranatensin, a polypeptide from frog skin, on isolated smooth muscle. Br J Pharmacol 41:622–628
Coruzzi G, Bertaccini G (1980) Action of some vasoactive peptides on the isolated lower esophageal sphincter. Pharmacol Res Commun 12:965–973
Crocker AD, Wilson KA (1974) A study of the metabolic requirements for the contractile action of angiotensin upon guinea pig ileum. Br J Pharmacol 51:73–79
Crocker AD, Wilson KA (1975) A further investigation into the energy dependence of angiotensin II-induced contractions of isolated smooth muscle preparations. Br J Pharmacol 53:59–66
Crocker AD, Mayeka IM, Wilson KA (1979) The role of calcium and cyclic AMP in the contractile action of angiotensin II upon rat descending colon. Eur J Pharmacol 60:121–129
Deleva JI, Nicolov NA (1977) Effect of angiotensin II on motility and mioelectrical activity of the gastrointestinal tract in dogs. Riv Farmacol Ter 8:211–218
Deleva JI, Nicolov NA (1979) Effect of angiotensin II on the electric and motor activity of stomach and jejunum after complete vagotomy. Agressologie 20:161–166
Ercan ZS, Türker RK (1977) A comparison between the prostaglandin releasing effects of angiotensin II and angiotensin III. Agents Actions 7:569–572
Erspamer V, Melchiorri P, Nakajima T, Yasuhara T, Endean R (1979) Aminoacid composition and sequence of crinia-angiotensin, an angiotensin II-like endecapeptide from the skin of the Australian frog *Crinia georgiana*. Experientia 35:1132–1133
Falconieri Erspamer G, Nakajima T, Yasuhara T (1979) Pharmacological data on crinia-angiotensin II. J Pharm Pharmacol 31:720
Famaey JP, Fontaine J, Seaman I, Reuse J (1978) Inhibition of angiotensin-induced contractions of guinea pig isolated ileum by high concentrations of non-steroidal antiinflammatory drugs and various steroids and its reversal by prostaglandin E1. Prostaglandins 16:725–732
Fishlock DJ, Gunn A (1970) The action of angiotensin on the human colon "in vitro." Br J Pharmacol 39:34–39
Gagnon DJ, Sirois P (1972) The rat isolated colon as a specific assay organ for angiotensin. Br J Pharmacol 46:89–93
Gavras H, Gavras I, Brunner HR, Liang CS (1978) Physiologic studies with saralasin in animals. Kidney Int 15:5–20
Godfraind T, Kaba A, Polster P (1966a) Specific antagonism to the direct and indirect action of angiotensin on isolated guinea-pig ileum. Br J Pharmacol 28:93–104
Godfraind T, Kaba A, Polster P (1966b) Dissociation in two contractile components on the isolated guinea-pig ileum response to angiotensin. Arch Int Pharmacodyn Ther 163:227–229
Haulica I, Stanciu CW, Frasin M, Cijevschi C, Balan G, Pancu D (1980) Effects of angiotensin on the human lower esophageal sphincter. Abstr XI Int Congr Gastroenterol. Thieme, Stuttgart, p 28
Huidobro HV, Paladini AC (1963) Potentiation of angiotensin action on smooth muscle by alkaline pH. Experientia 19:572
Khairallah PA, Page IH (1961) Mechanism of action of angiotensin and bradykinin on smooth muscle in situ. Am J Physiol 200:51–54
Khairallah PA, Page IH (1963) Effect of bradykinin and angiotensin on smooth muscle. Ann NY Acad Sci 104:212–220
Khairallah PA, Vandaparampil GJ, Page IH (1965) Effect of ions on angiotensin interaction with smooth muscle. Arch Int Pharmacodyn Ther 158:155
Khosla MC, Smeby RR, Bumpus FM (1974) Structure-activity relationship in angiotensin II analogs. In: Page IH, Bumpus FM (eds) Angiotensin. Springer, Berlin Heidelberg New York (Handbook of experimental pharmacology, vol 37, pp 126–161)
Levens NR, Munday KA, York B (1975) Effect of angiotensin II on fluid transport, transmural potential difference, and resistance in the rat distal colon in vivo. J Endocrinol 67:64P–65P

Lewis GP, Reit E (1965) The action of angiotensin and bradykinin on the superior cervical ganglion of the cat. J Physiol (Lond) 179:538
Mukhopadhyay AK, Leavitt L (1978) Evidence for an angiotensin receptor in esophageal smooth muscle of the opossum. Am J Physiol 235:E738–E742
Peach MJ (1979) Structural features of angiotensin II which are important for biological activity. Kidney Int 15:53–56
Pogglitsch H, Holzer H (1971) Die Bestimmung von Angiotensin am isolierten Rattencolon. Wien Klin Wochenschr 83:894–898
Regoli D, Vane JR (1964) A sensitive method for the assay of angiotensin. Br J Pharmacol 23:351–359
Regoli D, Park WK, Rioux F (1974a) Pharmacology of angiotensin. Pharmacol Rev 25:69–123
Regoli D, Rioux F, Park WK, Choi C (1974b) Role of the N-terminal amino acid for the biological activities of angiotensin and inhibitory analogues. Can J Physiol Pharmacol 52:39–60
Robertson PA, Rubin D (1962) Stimulation of intestinal nervous elements by angiotensin. Br J Pharmacol 19:5–12
Schwarz H, Bumpus FM, Page IH (1957) Synthesis of a biologically active octapeptide similar to natural isoleucine angiotonin octapeptide. J Am Chem Soc 79:5697–5703
Schwyzer R, Riniker B, Iselin B, Rittel W, Kapperler H, Zuber H (1958) Val-Hypertensin I and II. Chimia 12:91
Shehadeh Z, Price WE, Jacobson ED (1969) Effect of vasoactive agents on intestinal blood flow and motility in the dog. Am J Physiol 216:386–392
Skeggs LT, Marsh WJ, Kahn JR, Shumway NP (1954) The existence of two forms of hypertensin. J Exp Med 99:275–283
Skeggs LT, Marsh WH, Kahn JR, Shumway NP (1955) Amino acid composition and electrophoretic properties of hypertensin I. J Exp Med 102:435–440
Skeggs LT, Lentz KE, Shumway NP, Woods KR (1956) The amino acid sequence of hypertensin II. J Exp Med 104:193–197
Trendelenburg U (1966) Observations on the ganglion-stimulating action of angiotensin and bradykinin. J Pharmacol Exp Ther 154:418–425
Türker RK (1969) Possible postganglionic adrenergic effect of angiotensin in the isolated perfused cat intestinal segment. Arch Int Physiol Biochim 77:587–596
Türker RK (1973) Effect of angiotensin on the response to norepinephrine and periarterial stimulation of the isolated perfused cat terminal ileum. Eur J Pharmacol 21:171–177
Türker RK, Ercan ZS (1978) A comparative study with angiotensin II and (Des-aspartic acid)[1]-angiotensin II in the anaesthetized cats. Res Commun Chem Pathol Pharmacol 21:15–24
Türker RK, Kayaalp SO (1967) Inhibitory effect of angiotensin on intestinal motility of the cat and its relation to sympathetic nervous system. Arch Int Physiol Biochim 75:735–744
Türker RK, Kaymakcalan S (1971) Effect of morphine and nalorphine on the intestinal motility of the cat. Arch Int Pharmacodyn Ther 193:397–404
Türker RK, Yamamoto M, Khairallah PA, Bumpus FM (1971) Competitive antagonism of 8-Ala-angiotensin II to angiotensin I and II on isolated rabbit aorta and rat ascending colon. Eur J Pharmacol 15:285–291
Türker RK, Yamamoto M, Bumpus FM (1973) A new short-acting antagonist of angiotensin II. Arch Int Pharmacodyn Ther 201:162–169
Vane JR (1974) The fate of angiotensin I. In: Page IH, Bumpus FM (eds) Angiotensin. Springer, Berlin Heidelberg New York (Handbook of experimental pharmacology, vol 37, pp 17–40)
Zetler G (1979) Antagonism of cholecystokinin-like peptides by opioid peptides, morphine or tetrodotoxin. Eur J Pharmacol 60:67–77

Bradykinin

A. Introduction

Bradykinin and its analogs are probably the most widely diffused polypeptides in the animal kingdom. They have been found in mammals, reptiles, amphibia, and insects, very often in exceedingly large amounts. Since the discovery of bradykinin by ROCHA E SILVA et al. (1949), the structures of 14 additional naturally occurring kinins have been reported (Table 1) and it is probable that many more exist. The latest discovered bradykinin is Hyp^3-bradykinin found by NAKAJIMA et al. (1979) in the skin of the South African frog *Heleophryne purcelli* (20–500 µg/g fresh tissue).

The history of bradykinins, the problems of structure–activity relationships in natural and synthetic bradykinins, the biosynthesis and inactivation of these peptides (kininogen–kallikrein–kininase system), the kinin-potentiating factors, and the wide spectrum of activities of the bradykinins are exaustively reviewed in two volumes edited by ERDÖS (1970, 1979) and in several review articles(ANASTASI et al. 1966b; ERSPAMER and ANASTASI 1966; PISANO 1968; ROCHA E SILVA and ROTHSCHILD 1974; BERTACCINI 1976). Here as far as the structure–activity relationship is concerned, I want only to mention that the basic structure is nearly always the same in all the natural bradykinins (Table 1).

Apart from some substitutions in the bradykinin molecule, other peptides have one or more amino acid residue attached to the NH_2 or the COOH terminus. Some of these latter compounds may be considered precursors or kininogens because they release bradykinin after digestion with trypsin. The spectra of activities of all these peptides are qualitatively similar, if not identical.

As to synthetic analogs, more than 300 compounds were tabulated by SCHRÖDER (1970) and by STEWART (1979). The aims of this enormous effort were several

a) To identify the groups in the molecule responsible for receptor binding (affinity) and for activation of the receptor (intrinsic activity)
b) To identify the amino acid residues responsible for determining the shape of the peptide molecule in solution and in combination with a possible receptor
c) To synthesize analogs with enhanced or prolonged or more selective activity
d) To synthesize analogs with the same affinity for bradykinin receptors, but devoid of stimulant activity and therefore useful as specific antagonists

Most of these goals have so far remained unachieved.

As far as gut motility is concerned, some important phenomena were observed in the guinea pig ileum, one of the classic preparations for bradykinins: some bradykinin analogs of higher molecular weight ("pachykinins," ROCHA E SILVA 1972), obtained by attaching increasing numbers of amino acid residues to the NH_2 terminus, which were more potent than the parent molecule in increasing permeability, were much less potent on the guinea pig ileum. By contrast, another similar kinin (polysteskinin) was found to be twice as potent in the ileum on a molar basis. Another peculiar behavior was that of phyllokinin, which was found in the guinea pig ileum to be less potent but more "brady" (Greek *bradus* slow) than true bra-

Table 1. Naturally occurring kinins

Trivial name	Structure	Source
Bradykinin	Arg-Pro-Pro-Gly-Phe-Ser-Pro-Phe-Arg	Mammals[a]
Lys-bradykinin (kallidin)	Lys-Arg-Pro-Pro-Gly-Phe-Ser-Pro-Phe-Arg	Mammals
Met-Lys-bradykinin	Met-Lys-Arg-Pro-Pro-Gly-Phe-Ser-Pro-Phe-Arg	Mammals
Polisteskinin	Glu-Thr-Asn-Lys-Lys-Lys-Leu-Arg-Gly-Arg-Pro-Pro-Gly-Phe-Ser-Pro-Phe-Arg	Insects
Vespulakinin 1[b]	Carb Carb Thr-Ala-Thr-Thr-Arg-Arg-Arg-Gly-Arg-Pro-Pro-Gly-Phe-Ser-Pro-Phe-Arg	Insects
Vespulakinin 2[b]	Carb Carb Thr-Thr-Arg-Arg-Arg-Gly-Arg-Pro-Pro-Gly-Phe-Ser-Pro-Phe-Arg	Insects
Polisteskinin R	Ala-Arg-Arg-Pro-Pro-Gly-Phe-Thr-Pro-Phe-Arg	Insects
Vespakinin X	Ala-Arg-Pro-Pro-Gly-Phe-Ser-Pro-Phe-Arg-Ile-Val	Insects
Vespakinin M	Gly-Arg-Pro-Hyp-Gly-Phe-Ser-Pro-Phe-Arg-Ile-Asp	Insects
Thr^6-bradykinin	Arg-Pro-Pro-Gly-Phe-Thr-Pro-Phe-Arg	Reptiles
Phyllokinin	Arg-Pro-Pro-Gly-Phe-Ser-Pro-Phe-Arg-Ile-Tyr(SO_3H)	Amphibians
Val^1, Thr^6-bradykinin	Val-Pro-Pro-Gly-Phe-Thr-Pro-Phe-Arg	Amphibians
Bombinakinin O	Arg-Pro-Pro-Gly-Phe-Ser-Pro-Phe-Arg-Gly-Lys-Phe-His	Amphibians
Ranakinin N	Arg-Pro-Pro-Gly-Phe-Ser-Pro-Phe-Arg-Val-Ala-Pro-Ala-Ser	Amphibians
Ranakinin R	Arg-Pro-Pro-Gly-Phe-Thr-Pro-Phe-Arg-Ile-Ala-Pro-Glu-Ile-Val	Amphibians

[a] Also present in amphibians
[b] Carb indicates carbohydrate residues

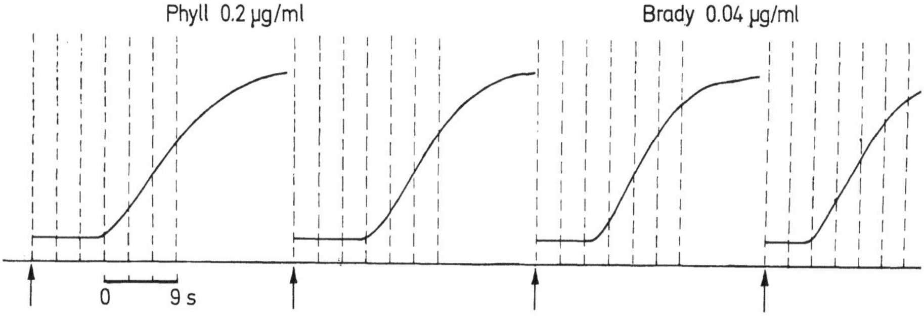

Fig. 1. Guinea pig ileum preparation suspended in 10 ml Krebs solution at 32 °C. Spasmogenic response to approximately equiactive doses of phyllokinin *Phyll* and bradykinin *Brady*. Drum speed was relatively high, and the distance between two consecutive broken vertical lines was run in 3 s. It may be seen that the latency period, i.e., the time elapsing between the introduction of the peptide into the bath *(arrows)* and the start of contraction, was longer for phyllokinin than for bradykinin. Moreover, the ascent of the contraction curve was somewhat more rapid for bradykinin than for phyllokinin. (ANASTASI et al. 1966b)

dykinin itself (Fig. 1; ANASTASI et al. 1966a). Though the available evidence suggests that phyllokinin acts as an intact molecule, the possibility that it may affect smooth muscle contractility through the release of bradykinin cannot be totally excluded. The activity of phyllokinin and the subsequent observations with bombinakinin O and ranakinins N and R are especially interesting since organic chemists have never been able to prepare highly active homologs with substituents at the carboxyl end of the bradykinin molecule (SCHRÖDER 1970). As to relaxation of the rat duodenum, results in this assay roughly paralleled those with the rat uterus (see STEWART 1979).

Another interesting problem which might throw light on the relationship between the kallikrein–kinin system and the renin–angiotensin system (kininase II of plasma and tissues is identical with the converting enzyme of angiotensin I) is that of the bradykinin-potentiating factors (BPF). These peptides, which were found in the venoms of crotalid snakes (for review see STEWART 1979), were shown to potentiate the action of bradykinin, both by inhibition of kininases (particularly evident in vivo) and by a direct effect on tissue in vitro, probable a mixed action. According to TOMINAGA et al. (1975) and SABIA et al. (1977) another mechanism is possible, since they observed that some BPF may increase the response of the ileum to bradykinin for several hours, even though the tissue was washed out; they spoke about "sensitization," but this mechanism was not elucidated. Two synthetic peptides (Val-Glu-Ser-Ser-Lys and Pyr-Lys-Trp-Ala-Pro) were also shown to potentiate the effects of bradykinin strongly, probably through a sensitization of bradykinin receptors owing to an increased affinity of the receptor for the peptide (UFKES et al. 1976, 1977). Other natural peptides (byproducts of the action of thrombin on fibrinogen; GLADNER 1966) were found to potentiate the action of bradykinins, and so do some synthetic peptides (for review see STEWART 1979).

Sulphydryl compounds have also been shown to potentiate the bradykinin-induced contractions of isolated guinea pig ileum. This was interpreted as either an inhibition of the tissue kininases that degrade bradykinin (PICARELLI 1962; SHER-

MAN and GAUTIERI 1969; Iso et al. 1979) or a sensitization of bradykinin receptors (CAMARGO and FERREIRA 1971; UFKES et al. 1977). The possibility that thiol compounds such as cysteine might potentiate the effect of bradykinin by facilitating the release of acetylcholine from nerve endings was also reported (POTTER and WALASZEK 1972).

The bulk of the experiments on bradykinin potentiation refer to the contractile more than to the relaxant effects, however, potentiation of the relaxation has also been studied (CAMARGO and FERREIRA 1971; BONTA and HALL 1973). On the whole, potentiation of bradykinin stimulatory activity, which occurred in various degrees with the different BPF and in the different preparations, was more frequently observed than was relaxation, this being consistent with the idea that at least two different receptor sites are involved in the action of bradykinin.

B. Effects on the Gastrointestinal Tract

I. In Vitro Studies

In vitro studies are much more numerous than in vivo studies because of the extraintestinal side effects induced by bradykinin, whose primary role is probably the one it plays in inflammatory processes. Most of the experiments were performed with bradykinin. However, when kallidin was used very similar effects were observed. The results shown in Tables 2 and 3, which are largely derived from our personal experience, clearly demonstrate that bradykinin exerts a predominantly stimulatory effect on the gastrointestinal tracts of different experimental animals. However, inhibitory responses are also possible and in a few cases a biphasic response may occur, i.e., an initial relaxation followed by a contraction. Not all of

Table 2. Contracting activity of bradykinin on a series of isolated preparations of the gastrointestinal tract from different experimental animals

Preparation	Threshold dose (ng/ml)
Guinea pig ileum	0.5– 2
Guinea pig large intestine	20 – 100[a]
Rat LES	50 – 200[a]
Rat stomach	5 – 50
Cat jejunum	0.5– 2
Rabbit duodenum	10 – 50
Rabbit ileum	10 – 50[a]
Rabbit large intestine	> 100
Dog duodenum	0.5– 40
Dog large intestine	0.5– 50
Frog stomach	1,000 –4,000
Pigeon duodenum	2,000 –5,000
Ox reticuloomasal sphincter	50 – 100

[a] Biphasic response – short-lasting relaxation followed by longer-lasting increase in tone

Table 3. Relaxant activity of bradykinin on a series of isolated preparations of the gastrointestinal tract from different experimental animals

Preparation	Threshold dose (ng/ml)
Rat duodenum	0.1– 1[a]
Rat colon	10 – 50[a]
Hen rectal cecum	500 –1,000[b]
Guinea pig LES	100 – 300
Monkey ileum	>100

[a] Biphasic response (relaxation followed by contraction) also possible
[b] A stimulatory response was also reported

these isolated preparations can be used for the biologic assay of bradykinin and its analogs: some of them are not sufficiently sensitive, some others are not reliable because of the rapid appearance of tachyphylaxis or because the response is not constant, etc.

The contractile effect of bradykinin in the guinea pig ileum is quite special, since it is considerably slower than those of other stimulatory substances, such as histamine or acetylcholine, and begins after a short latency period. This particular behavior led to the name given to the peptide. The slow contraction of the guinea pig ileum, the dose-related relaxant effect on the rat duodenum, and the contractile action on rat stomach strip, have usually been utilized to characterize peptides of the bradykinin family (GADDUM and HORTON 1959; BISSET and LEWIS 1962; STÜRMER and BERDE 1953; VANE 1964; BERTACCINI et al. 1979). A predominant relaxation was also demonstrated in the chicken rectal cecum and in the rat colon (HORTON 1959; STÜRMER and BERDE 1963). A relaxant effect of bradykinin on the guinea pig ileum or a biphasic response (relaxation followed by contraction) after inducing a contraction with acetylcholine or histamine was also demonstrated (HALL and BONTA 1972, 1973a, b). Apparently, this effect was absolutely independent of the sympathetic nervous system and is likely to be due to a direct action on muscle cell membrane. Since it was demonstrated only in the whole ileum preparation and not in the longitudinal muscle strip, a stimulatory effect on the circular muscle layers, which would simulate a longitudinal relaxation, could not be excluded. A similar situation for the relaxant effect of cerulein on the contraction induced by histamine in the guinea pig ileum was reported (MANTOVANI and VIZI (1974).

Bradykinin (1–10 μg/ml), applied to the serosal surface or introduced into the lumen of the isolated guinea pig ileum, depressed or abolished the peristaltic reflex. This effect was antagonized by physostigmine, but not by 5-hydroxytryptamine or substance P (BELESLIN et al. 1964). The authors suggested that the probable site of action of bradykinin is the cholinoceptive synapses in the peristaltic reflex arc.

An interesting relationship between steroid hormones and the sensitivity of the guinea pig ileum to bradykinin was recently pointed out (WEINBERG et al. 1976): female or castrated male guinea pigs were found to be more sensitive to bradykinin than intact males. Testosterone reversed this effect of castration, whereas treatment with β-estradiol resulted in bradykinin sensitivity closely approaching that in females. There are two possible explanations for these findings: (a) modified receptors were synthesized as a result of steroid action; or (b) the conformation of bradykinin receptors can be changed by the presence of some steroid hormones.

On the guinea pig taenia coli the effect of bradykinin was mostly biphasic: an acute initial phase characterized by spike inhibition and decreased isometric tension, followed by a second phase with an increased frequency and amplitude of the spikes and membrane depolarization, accompanied by an increase in the isometric tension. Exclusion of sodium, in the presence of normal calcium concentrations strengthened the first phase and abolished the second. Lowering the calcium concentration had the opposite effect. When the concentrations of both electrolytes were reduced, the spontaneous spike activity disappeared (AARSEN and VAN CASPEL-DE BRUYN 1970). Probably, bradykinin acts on different sites of the cell membrane which are involved in the spike generation and in the depolarization. In contrast to bradykinin, which can have both inhibitory and stimulatory effects, the

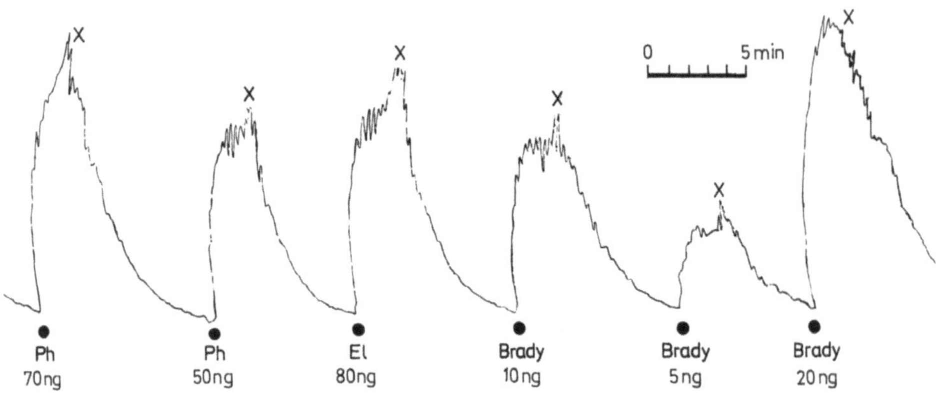

Fig. 2. Dog large intestine preparation suspended in 10 ml Tyrode solution at 37 °C. Responses to physalaemin *Ph*, eledoisin *El*, and bradykinin *Brady*. *Crosses* indicate washout. Note the similarity of contractions produced by the three polypeptides. In this preparation, bradykinin was the most active polypeptide, and eledoisin was the least active. (BERTACCINI et al. 1965)

bradykinin potentiating factor BPP 5a has only a stimulatory effect which is probably different in origin from that of bradykinin (AARSEN 1977).

Recent studies, in which theoretical dose–response curves were constructed from experimental pD_2 values by the Clark equation, were found to be identical with experimental curves obtained with cat jejunum and terminal ileum, indicating that these preparations are highly specific for bradykinin and are the most reliable test system for studies of the structure–activity relationships for this type of peptide (BARABÉ et al. 1975).

The rat ileum also responded fairly well to bradykinin with a good concentration–response curve between 10^{-10} and 10^{-8} *M*. In a particular preparation in which bradykinin could be perfused by the serosal or mucosal surface, the former application was found to be more effective than the latter (WALKER and WILSON 1979). The lower esophageal sphincter responded predominantly with contraction in the rat and with relaxation in the guinea pig, however, the sensitivity of both preparation was rather low (10^{-7} *M*; CORUZZI and BERTACCINI 1980). Dog duodenum and dog large intestine were, in some cases, extremely sensitive but did not represent good tools for bradykinin assay, because of the variability in the response. However, dog large intestine was the only segment of the gastrointestinal tract in which bradykinin was much more potent than the tachykinins (Fig. 2).

On the reticuloomasal sphincter of the ox, bradykinin exerted a spasmogenic effect (threshold doses 10–100 ng/ml) being 3–7 times less effective than eledoisin but 10–20 times more potent than acetylcholine (FAUSTINI et al. unpublished work). A marked dose-related contraction of goat ruminal strips was observed by VEENENDAAL et al. (1980). The threshold dose of bradykinin was 0.2 ng/ml; maximal contraction was obtained with 26 μg/ml. The effect of the peptide was antagonized by sodium meclofenamate (10 μg/ml).

Data obtained in vitro for the human gastrointestinal tract are summarized in Table 4, which is a synopsis of the results obtained in different investigations (FISHLOCK 1966; ZAPPIA et al. 1972; BERTACCINI et al. 1974; G. BERTACCINI unpublished work 1980). It is evident from Table 4 that different segments of human gastrointestinal tract were sensitive to bradykinin. Generally, the longitudinal muscle

Table 4. Action of bradykinin on isolated preparations of human gastrointestinal tract

Tissue[a]		Number of strips	Threshold dose (ng/ml)	Kind of response[b]
Stomach	LM	6	0.2 - 20	+
Jejunum	LM	26	0.02- 5	+
	CM	15	500 - 100	−+
Ileum	LM	14	0.02- 0.5	+
	CM	12	0.5 - 5	−
Appendix (children)	LM	20	0.5 - 50	+
Colon	LM	20	{ 5 - 100	−
			{ 500 -1,000	+
	CM	14	10 -1,000	−

[a] LM = longitudinal muscle; CM = circular muscle
[b] Contraction indicated by +; relaxation indicated by −

layer was the more sensitive to the peptide and responded with contraction, with the exception of that of the colon, which could be relaxed with low doses and contracted with high doses. The circular muscle layer was usually relaxed by bradykinin. Tachyphylaxis was a common feature in all the different segments of the gut. Contractions appeared to be connected by a direct effect of bradykinin, since they were not affected by the common inhibitors (Fig. 3), but relaxations were greatly reduced by pronethalol or propanolol, suggesting interference with the sympathetic system.

II. In Vivo Studies

Compared with the amount of data for the in vitro effects of bradykinin, there are relatively few data on gastrointestinal motility in vivo. This is probably connected, as is the case for other kinins, with the strong hypotensive effect and with the bronchoconstriction induced by bradykinin, which in most cases overwhelm the gastrointestinal effects. In addition, most of the data in the literature were obtained with anesthetized animals and therefore possible interactions with general anesthetics cannot be excluded. In the anesthetized dog, bradykinin (0.1–5 μg/kg i.v.) was found to inhibit intestinal motility, an effect which was lessened by very high doses of diphenhydramine (10 mg/kg) or atropine (1 mg/kg). In contrast both α- and β-sympatholytic agents were ineffective (LEVY 1963). In other experiments, bradykinin was either inactive or even moderately increased intestinal motility when high doses were given (6 μg/kg intra-arterially, HIATT et al. 1966; 0.5 μg kg^{-1} min^{-1}, SHEHADEH et al. 1969; 2–5 μg/kg i.v., BERTACCINI et al. 1970; MANTOVANI and BERTACCINI 1971). Intestinal spasm in intact dogs or in Thiry–Vella loops and in canine colon nerve preparation in vivo was reported (GRAY and YANO 1975).

In a canine jejunal loop in situ, low doses of bradykinin (1–10 nmol/l) did not alter spontaneous motility, though it increased regional blood flow. Higher levels of the peptide (20–100 nmol/l) significantly augmented rhythmic contractions. Whereas atropine did not modify the effects of bradykinin, pretreatment with indomethacin (2–10 mg/kg i.v. 1 h prior to the experiment) reduced the increased

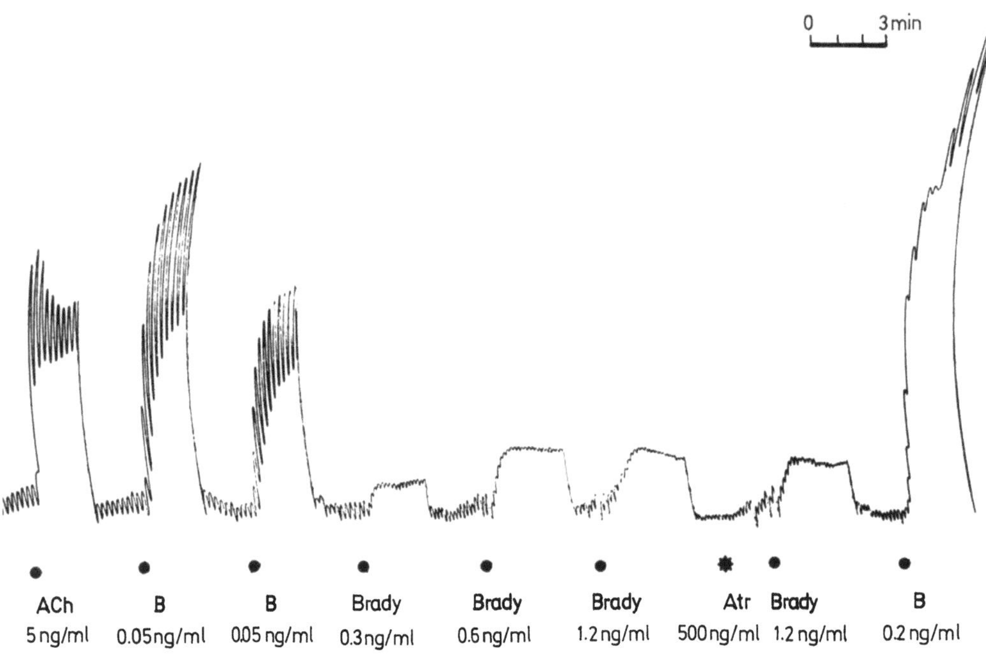

Fig. 3. Effect of bradykinin *Brady* on the circular layer of the human stomach body in vitro compared with that of acetylcholine *ACh* and bombesin *B*. *Atr*, atropine. (G. BERTACCINI unpublished work)

blood flow and intestinal motility, thus suggesting an at least partial mediation of prostaglandin-like substances (PYTKOWSKI 1979).

In cats and rabbits, 0.25–8 µg/kg bradykinin or kallidin injected into the aorta caused inhibition followed by an increase of intestinal motility (VON KLUPP et al. 1964; WINKLER et al. 1965). The initial relaxation could be blocked by local anesthetic ganglion-blocking agents and atropine, suggesting a nerve-mediated effect (WINKLER et al. 1965). In the anesthetized cat, the same inhibition and transient dose-related relaxation of the intestine were observed after intravenous administration (TÜRKER et al. 1964). The inhibitory response disappeared when the cats were pretreated with reserpine. Other investigators observed different effects with different kinds of administration. An intravenous bolus injection of bradykinin or kallidin (2–16 µg/kg) elicited a biphasic response in rabbits and cats (primary inhibition and secondary stimulation of intestinal motility). Continuous infusion of the same peptides (1–3 $\mu g\ kg^{-1}\ min^{-1}$) caused only inhibition of motility without the subsequent stimulation (BAUER et al. 1966a).

When administered intra-arterially to the cat, bradykinin (1–8 µg/kg) had a biphasic effect on the ileum with a short inhibition of the tonus and the amplitude of spontaneous contractions, followed by a more prolonged phase of stimulation (VON KLUPP et al. 1964). In subsequent studies, the peptide at the intra-arterial dose of 10 µg was shown to cause a profound and prolonged gastric relaxation, together with a marked and equally prolonged colonic contraction. Changes in gastric tone were quite similar to those elicited by vagal stimulation in the presence of atropine and were not blocked by antiadrenergic drugs. On the other hand, the colonic motor response mimicked the atropine-resistant expulsive contraction elicited by activation of the pelvic nerves. Intravenous bradykinin caused very moderate and short-lasting gastric relaxation and profound small intestine relaxation which were abolished by antiadrenergic drugs or by adrenalectomy. Colonic motility appeared to be increased, considering the tonus and not the amplitude of spontaneous contractions (FASTH and HULTÉN 1973; FASTH et al. 1975). It must be noted that the effect on gut motility was not the "primary" effect of the peptide, since threshold doses for inducing intestinal changes were more than ten times those which evoked vasodilatation.

Bradykinin was also shown to affect canine villous motility, not when applied locally (1–10 μg/ml) but when injected into the mesenteric artery (1 μg/min). The effect was biphasic: initially the peptide decreased or abolished the villous motility, then it noticeably increased the motility. The first phase was interpreted to be a nerve reflex long-distance effect, which was prevented by atropine or novocain administration; the second, stimulatory phase was apparently a direct effect (LUDÁNY et al. 1967).

In humans, bradykinin (10–20 μg/min for 3–5 min) generally reduced the motility of the distal colon in both normal subjects and patients with organic or functional disorders. The motor activity induced by prostigmine was abolished by bradykinin, but no attempt was made to investigate the mechanism of action of the peptide (MURRELL and DELLER 1967).

If the bowel wall is as sensitive in vivo as it has been demonstrated to be under particular experimental conditions in vitro, there is the possibility that increased intestinal movement and spasm of the longitudinal muscle layers may be caused by very small amounts of bradykinin. The general question of possible reciprocal interactions among the different endogenous active substances leaves completely open the question of the hypothetical role of bradykinins in regulation of gut motility. The carcinoid syndrome, one symptom of which is diarrhea, is associated with elevated blood kinins (OATES et al. 1964). It can be hypothesized that the latter may contribute to the diarrhea by inducing a net secretory state in the intestine. Of course, a complex interaction of bradykinin with 5-hydroxytryptamine (5-HT) may be also responsible for the different symptoms of carcinoid syndrome.

In the veterinary field, fluctuations of bradykinin and 5-HT blood levels and inhibition of the ruminal contractions occurring in the goat infected with *Trypanosom vivax* or inoculated with a pyrogenic dose of lipopolysaccharide did not appear to be significantly correlated (VEENENDAL et al. 1976). However, intravenous injection of bradykinin (0.5–4 μg/kg) in the goat, caused a constant dose-dependent inhibition of ruminal contractions. This effect was prevented by administration of phenylbutazone (30 mg/kg) and sodium meclofenamate (2 mg/kg) (VEENENDAL et al. 1980).

C. Mechanism of Action

Considerable efforts have been made by several investigators to explain the mechanism of action of bradykinin, which we have already said may stimulate or inhibit or produce biphasic responses in the smooth muscles of different preparations. Stimulatory effects of bradykinin on the gut are generally said to be direct effects on the smooth muscle, since they are unaffected by the common inhibitors (hexamethonium, atropine, antihistamines, morphine, tetrodotoxin), at least in most of the commonly used isolated preparations. In some preparations in which an initial decrease in tone was observed before the contraction (rabbit small intestine, rat ileum, rat LES) (KONZETT and STÜRMER 1960; BAUER et al. 1966b; CORUZZI and BERTACCINI 1980), the primary inhibitory phase was diminished or abolished by pretreatment with morphine (probably by a neurotropic action in rabbit but not in rat intestine, suggesting different mechanisms for the two species (BAUER et al. 1966b).

The interpretation of the peculiar relaxant effect of bradykinin on the rat duodenum is controversial. Some investigators claim that this phenomenon is independent of the release of catecholamines and of stimulation of β-adrenoceptors (ANTONIO 1968; UFKES et al. 1975) whereas others favor a sympathomimetic mechanism (TÜRKER et al. 1964; MONTGOMERY 1968; TÜRKER and OZER 1970; BOGDANIK et al. 1971). According to a more recent study (PAEGELOW et al. 1977), there may be a link between the cyclic AMP system and the relaxant activity of bradykinin on the rat duodenum, since the peptide was found to stimulate adenyl cyclase in the rat duodenum at the same low dosage that relax the isolated organ.

Finally, it must be mentioned that the alteration in smooth muscle tone induced by bradykinin may be due to complex molecular interactions; bradykinin is, in fact, able to enhance the formation of prostaglandins in the rat duodenum, PGE_2 being the largely predominant type. There is an increasing body of evidence suggesting relationships between prostaglandins and bradykinin in several systems. Leaving aside problems concerning tissues outside the gastrointestinal tract (for review see ERDÖS 1979), there are important pieces of information that suggest that prostaglandin may participate in the contractile effect of bradykinin on some districts of the gut, at least in some animal species. In rat terminal ileum, aspirin and indomethacin (which are known to inhibit prostaglandin synthesis) reduced the response to bradykinin by 50%–70%, and so did the prostaglandin antagonist, polyphloretin phosphate; all these agents left the contractions induced by acetylcholine unaffected, suggesting the action to be specific against bradykinin (mediated through the negative effects on prostaglandins; CROCKER and WILLAVOYS 1976). In addition, it was demonstrated that contractions of rat fundus strip by bradykinin were potentiated by a prostaglandin-like substance released during perfusion of both the mucosal and the serosal surface of rat terminal ileum with bradykinin (CROCKER et al. 1978). Subsequent studies (WALKER and WILSON 1979) demonstrated that contractions of the rat ileum to bradykinin involve prostaglandin synthesis only with mucosal and not serosal perfusion with the peptide. A confirmation of the interaction of bradykinin with prostaglandins was also reported by HARDCASTLE et al. (1978). They found that bradykinin strongly increased the potential difference across both the jejunum and the colon of the rat and this effect was significantly lowered by indomethacin. However indomethacin failed to affect the contractions of rat stomach and cat small intestine induced by bradykinin (BARABÉ et al. 1975) and this suggested that the involvement of prostaglandins is not a general phenomenon for bradykinin in all smooth muscles.

Moreover, both stimulatory and inhibitory responses to bradykinin are associated with sodium-dependent depolarization and a decrease in membrane resistance. In addition, bradykinin was shown to increase the intracellular calcium concentration in isolated guinea pig ileum (JOHNSON 1979), indicating the possible importance of intracellular ion exchange.

D. Conclusions

The obvious question which arises when considering the direct effect of bradykinin on smooth muscle is whether or not there are specific receptor sites for the peptide. Serious difficulties, however, were encountered by the investigators who confronted this problem:

1) Studies on structure–activity relationships with fragments and analogs of bradykinin did not serve for precise distinction of the groups responsible, for affinity, or for activation of receptors and, in fact, in the cat ileum they showed that 1-Arg, 4-Gly, 5-Phe, 8-Phe, and 9-Arg are all essential for the interaction (BARABÉ et al. 1977). In the cat ileum, bradykinin and kallidin were shown (by the criterion of desensitization) to act on the same receptor (DROUIN et al. 1979a), which was called receptor B_2 and found to be different from receptor B_1 occurring on rabbit aorta strips and in numerous other tissues of various species (DROUIN et al. 1979b). Some compounds containing a chain extension at the amino end are potent stimulants of the B_2-receptors, the extension with the Met-Lys appearing particularly favorable.

2) As we have already said, potentiating factors were able to potentiate the effect of bradykinin, but to different degrees in different preparations.

3) The most important criterion for classification (namely, the apparent affinity constants of competitive antagonists) could not be used, since no such inhibitors, are available for bradykinin. In fact, the claim by GARCÍA-LEME and ROCHA E SILVA (1965) that methixene competes with bradykinin in the guinea pig ileum was not confirmed (VAN RIEZEN 1966).

4) Direct binding studies were performed with uterine, but not gut muscle and, in addition, the study of receptor binding can give erroneous results because of the presence in the tissues of kininase, which presumably have lower affinities for kinins, but higher binding capacities (ODYA and GOODFRIEND 1979).

In conclusion, though bradykinin is one of those peptides which have been more throughly investigated for their obvious physiopathologic importance, not only the physiologic role, but also the mechanism of its pharmacologic effects on the digestive system are not completely understood as yet.

References

Aarsen PN (1977) The effects of bradykinin and the bradykinin potentiating peptide BPP_{5a} on the electrical and mechanical responses of the guinea pig taenia coli. Br J Pharmacol 61:523–532

Aarsen PN, Van Caspel-De Bruyn M (1970) Effect of changes in ionic environment on the action of bradykinin on the guinea-pig taenia coli. Eur J Pharmacol 12:348–358

Anastasi A, Bertaccini G, Erspamer V (1966a) Pharmacological data on phyllokinin (bradykinyl-isoleucyl-tyrosine O-sulphate) and bradykinyl-isoleucyl-tyrosine. Br J Pharmacol 27:479–485

Anastasi A, Ersparmer V, Bertaccini G, Cei GM (1966b) Isolation, amino acid sequence, and biological activity of phyllokinin (bradykinyl-isoleucyl-tyrosine O-sulphate), a bradykinin-like endecapeptide of the skin of *Phyllomedusa rohdei*. In: Erdös EG, Back N, Sicuteri F (eds) Hypotensive peptides. Springer, Berlin Heidelberg New York, pp 76–84

Antonio A (1968) The relaxing effect of bradykinin on intestinal smooth muscle. Br J Pharmacol 32:78–86
Barabé J, Park WK, Regoli D (1975) Application of drug receptor theories to the analysis of the myotropic effects of bradykinin. Can J Physiol Pharmacol 53:345–353
Barabé J, Drouin JN, Regoli D, Park WK (1977) Receptors for bradykinin in intestinal and uterine smooth muscle. Can J Physiol Pharmacol 55:1270–1285
Bauer G, Gmeiner R, Winkler H (1966a) Über die Wirkung synthetischer Polypeptide auf den Darm in situ. Arch Int Pharmacodyn Ther 159:373–385
Bauer G, Ziegler E, Konzett H (1966b) Zur Hemmwirkung von Kininen an isolierten Darmpräparaten. Naunyn Schmiedebergs Arch Pharmacol 254:235–244
Beleslin DB, Bogdanović SB, Radmanović BZ (1964) The possible site of action of bradykinin on the peristaltic reflex of the isolated guinea pig ileum. Arch Int Pharmacodyn Ther 147:43–52
Bertaccini G (1976) Active polypeptides of nonmammalian origin. Pharmacol Rev 28:127–177
Bertaccini G, Cei GM, Erspamer V (1965) Occurrence of physalaemin in extract of the skin in *Physalaemus fuscumaculatus* and its pharmacological actions on extravascular smooth muscle. Br J Pharmacol 25:363–379
Bertaccini G, Mantovani P, Piccinin GL (1970) Activity ratio between intestinal and cardiovascular actions of caerulein and related substances in the anaesthetized dog. In: Sicuteri F, Rocha e Silva M, Back N (eds) Bradykinin and related kinins. Plenum, New York London, pp 213–220
Bertaccini G, Impicciatore M, Molina E, Zappia L (1974) Action of bombesin on human gastrointestinal motility. Rend Gastroenterol 6:45–51
Bertaccini G, Zappia L, Molina E (1979) "In vitro" duodenal muscle in the pharmacological study of natural compounds. Scand J Gastroenterol [Suppl 54] 14:87–93
Bisset GW, Lewis GP (1962) A spectrum of pharmacological activity in some biologically active peptides. Br J Pharmacol 19:168–182
Bogdanik T, Straczkowski W, Stasiewicz J, Szalaj W (1971) The influence of alfa and beta-adrenergic blockade on the duodenal motility; effects of calcium and magnesium ions and bradykinin. In: Union Intern. Thérapeutique (ed) Xe Congrès international de thérapeutique. Paris 2–4 Octobre 1969. Doin, Paris, pp 407–415
Bonta IL, Hall DWR (1973) Potentiation of the biphasic bradykinin response of the guinea-pig ileum. Br J Pharmacol 49:161P–162P
Camargo A, Ferreira SH (1971) Action of bradykinin potentiating factor (BPF) and dimercaprol (BAL) on the response to bradykinin of isolated preparations of rat intestines. Br J Pharmacol 42:305–307
Coruzzi G, Bertaccini G (1980) Action of some vasoactive peptides on the isolated lower esophageal sphincter. Pharmacol Res Commun 12:965–973
Crocker AD, WalkerR, Wilson KA (1978) Prostaglandins and the contractile action of bradykinin on the longitudinal muscle of the rat isolated ileum. Br J Pharmacol 64:441P
Crocker AD, Willavoys SP (1976) Possible involvement of prostaglandins in the contractile action of bradykinin on rat terminal ileum. J Pharm Pharmacol 28:78
Drouin JN, St-Pierre SA, Regoli D (1979a) Receptors for bradykinin and kallidin. Can J Physiol Pharmacol 57:375–379
Drouin JN, Gaudreau P, St-Pierre S, Regoli D (1979b) Biological activities of kinins modified at the N- or at the C-terminal end. Can J Physiol Pharmacol 57:1018–1023
Erdös EG (ed) (1970) Handbook of experimental pharmacology, vol XXV: Bradykinin, kallidin, and kallikrein. Springer, Berlin Heidelberg New York
Erdös EG (ed) (1979) Handbook of experimental pharmacology, vol XXV Suppl: Bradykinin, kallidin, and kallikrein. Springer, Berlin Heidelberg New York
Erspamer V, Anastasi A (1966) Polypeptides active on plain muscle in the amphibian skin. In: Erdös EG, Back N, Sicuteri F (eds) Hypotensive peptides. Springer, Berlin Heidelberg New York, pp 63–75
Fasth S, Hultén L (1973) The effect of bradykinin on intestinal motility and blood flow. Acta Chir Scand 139:699–705
Fasth S, Hultén L, Jahnberg T, Martinson J (1975) Comparative studies on the effects of bradykinin and vagal stimulation on motility in the stomach and colon. Acta Physiol Scand 93:77–84

Fishlock J (1966) Effect of bradykinin on the human isolated small and large intestine. Nature 212:1533–1535
Gaddum JH, Horton EW (1959) The extraction of human urinary kinin (substance Z) and its relation to the plasma kinins. Br J Pharmacol 14:117–124
García Leme J, Rocha e Silva M (1965) Competitive and non-competitive inhibition of bradykinin on the guinea pig ileum. Br J Pharmacol 25:50–58
Gladner JA (1966) Potentiation of the effect of bradykinin. In: Erdös EG, Back N, Sicuteri F (eds) Hypotensive peptides. Springer, Berlin Heidelberg New York, p 344
Gray GW, Yano BL (1975) A study of the actions of methampyrone and of a commercial intestinal extract preparation on intestinal motility. Am J Vet Res 36:201–208
Hall DWR, Bonta IL (1972) Neurogenic factors involved in the relaxing effect of bradykinin on the isolated guinea-pig ileum. Arch Int Pharmacodyn Ther 197:380–381
Hall DWR, Bonta IL (1973 a) Effects of adrenergic blockers on the relaxation of the guinea pig ileum by bradykinin and adrenaline. Eur J Pharmacol 21:139–146
Hall DWR, Bonta IL (1973 b) The biphasic response of the isolated guinea pig ileum by bradykinin. Eur J Pharmacol 21:147–154
Hardcastle J, Hardcastle PT, Flower RJ, Sanford PA (1978) The effect of bradykinin on the electrical activity of rat jejunum. Experientia 34:617–618
Hiatt RB, Goodman I, Bircher R (1966) Control of motility in thiry-vella ileal segments in dogs. Am J Physiol 210:373–378
Horton EW (1959) Human urinary kinin excretion. Br J Pharmacol 14:125–132
Iso T, Nishimura K, Oya M, Iwao JI (1979) Potentiating mechanism of bradykinin action on smooth muscle by sulphydryl compounds. Eur J Pharmacol 54:303–305
Johnson AR (1979) Effects of kinins on organ systems. In: Erdös EG (ed) Bradykinin, kallidin, and kallikrein. Springer, Berlin Heidelberg New York (Handbook of experimental pharmacology, vol XXV Suppl., pp 357–399)
Konzett H, Stürmer E (1960) Biological activity of synthetic polypeptides with bradykinin-like properties. Br J Pharmacol 15:544–551
Levy B (1963) The intestinal inhibitory response to oxytocin, vasopressin, and bradykinin. J Pharmacol Exp Ther 140:356–366
Ludány G, Ihász M, Karika J (1967) Bradykinin and motility of the intestinal villi. Med Pharmacol Exp 17:311–314
Mantovani P, Bertaccini G (1971) Action of caerulein and related substances on gastrointestinal motility of the anesthetized dog. Arch Int Pharmacodyn Ther 193:362–371
Mantovani P, Vizi ES (1974) Further observations on the relaxant effect of caerulein on the guinea-pig ileum. J Pharm Pharmacol 26:461–462
Montgomery EH (1968) The response of the rat duodenum to bradykinin. Proc West Pharmacol Soc 11:51–52
Murrell TGC, Deller DJ (1967) Intestinal motility in man: the effect of bradykinin on the motility of the distal colon. Dig Dis Sci 12:568–576
Nakajima T, Yasuhara T, Falconieri Erspamer G, Visser J (1979) Occurrence of Hyp^3-bradykinin in methanol extracts of the skin of the South African leptodactylid frog *Heleophrine purcelli.* Experientia 35:1133
Oates JA, Melmon K, Sjoerdsma A, Gillespie L, Mason DT (1964) Release of a kinin peptide in the carcinoid syndrome. Lancet 1:514–517
Odya CE, Goodfriend TL (1979) Bradykinin receptors. In: Erdös EG (ed) Bradykinin, kallidin, and kallikrein. Springer, Berlin Heidelberg New York (Handbook of experimental pharmacology, vol XXV Suppl, pp 287–300)
Paegelow I, Reissmann S, Vietinghoff G, Römer W, Arold H (1977) Bradykinin action in the rat duodenum through the cyclic AMP system. Agents Actions 7/4:447–451
Picarelli ZP (1962) Kininases. Ciencia Cult (Sao Paulo), 14:232–236
Pisano JJ (1968) Vasoactive peptides in venoms. Fed Proc 27:58–62
Potter DE, Walaszek EJ (1972) Potentiation of the bradykinin response by cysteine: mechanism of action. Arch Int Pharmacodyn Ther 197:338–349
Pytkowski B (1979) On the contribution of prostaglandin-like substances to the action of bradykinin on intestinal motility and blood flow in canine jejunal loop in situ. Eur J Clin Invest 9:391–396
Rocha e Silva M (1972) The kinin trail. Possible significance of bradykinin and related kinins to auto-pharmacology. In: Abstr Fifth Int Congr Pharmacol, San Francisco, p 21

Rocha e Silva M, Rothschild HA (1974) A bradykinin anthology. Sociedade Brasileira de Farmacologia e Terape'utica Experimental, Sao Paulo, pp 1–335
Rocha e Silva M, Beraldo WT, Rosenfeld G (1949) Bradykinin, a hypotensive and smooth muscle stimulating factor released from plasma globulin by snake venoms and by trypsin. Am J Physiol 156:261–273
Sabia EB, Tominaga M, Paiva ACM, Paiva TB (1977) Bradykinin potentiating and sensitizing activities of new synthetic analogues of snake venom peptides. J Med Chem 20:1679–1681
Schröder E (1970) Structure-activity relationships of kinins. In: Erdös EG (ed) Bradykinin, kallidin, and kallikrein. Springer, Berlin Heidelberg New York (Handbook of experimental pharmacology, vol XXV, pp 324–350)
Shehadeh Z, Price WE, Jacobson ED (1969) Effects of vasoactive agents on intestinal blood flow and motility in the dog. Am J Physiol 216:386–392
Sherman WT, Gautieri RF (1969) Cardiovascular and gastrointestinal effect of bradykinin and its potentiation by thiols in rats. J Pharm Sci 58:971–975
Stewart JM (1979) Chemistry and biologic activity of peptides related to bradykinin. In: Erdös EG (ed) Bradykinin, kallidin, and kallikrein. Springer, Berlin Heidelberg New York (Handbook of experimental pharmacology vol XXV, Suppl, pp 227–272)
Stürmer E, Berde B (1963) A comparative pharmacological study of synthetic eledoisin and synthetic bradykinin. J Pharmacol Exp Ter 140:349–355
Tominaga M, Stewart JM, Paiva TB, Paiva ACM (1975) Synthesis and properties of new bradykinin potentiating peptides. J Med Chem 18:130–133
Türker RK, Ozer A (1970) The effect of prostaglandin E_1 and bradykinin on normal and depolarized isolated duodenum of the rat. Agents Actions 1:124–127
Türker K, Kiran BK, Kaymakcalan S (1964) The effects of synthetic bradykinin on intestinal motility in different laboratory animals and its relation to catecholamines. Arch Int Pharmacodyn Ther 151:260–268
Ufkes JGR, Van Der Meer C (1975) The effect of catecholamine depletion on the bradykinin-induced relaxation of isolated smooth muscle. Eur J Pharmacol 33:141–144
Ufkes JGR, Aarsen PN, Van Der Meer C (1976) The bradykinin potentiating activity of two pentapeptides on various isolated smooth muscle preparations. Eur J Pharmacol 40:137–144
Ufkes JGR, Aarsen PN, Van Der Meer C (1977) The mechanism of action of two bradykinin-potentiating peptides on isolated smooth muscle. Eur J Pharmacol 44:89–97
Vane JR (1964) The use of isolated organs for detecting active substances in the circulating blood. Br J Pharmacol 23:360–373
Van Riezen H (1966) Methixene: a non-competitive antagonist of bradykinin. J Pharm Pharmacol 18:688
Veenendal GH, Van Miert AS, Van Den Ingh TS, Scotman AJ, Zwart D (1976) A comparison of the role of kinins and serotonin in endotoxin induced fever and *Trypanosoma vivax* infections in the goat. Res Vet Sci 21:271–279
Veenendaal GH, Woutersen Van Nijnanten FMA, Van Miert ASJPAM (1980) Responses of goat ruminal musculature to bradykinin and serotonin in vitro and in vivo. Am J Vet Res 41:479–483
Von Klupp H, Konzett H, Winkler H (1964) Zur Wirkung von Bradykinin auf die Darmmotilität in situ. Arch Exp Pathol Pharmakol 247:325–326
Walker R, Wilson KA (1979) Prostaglandins and the contractile action of bradykinin on the longitudinal muscle of rat isolated ileum. Br J Pharmacol 67:527–533
Weinberg J, Diniz CR, Mares-Guia M (1976) Influence of sex and sexual hormones in the bradykinin-receptor interaction in the guinea pig ileum. Biochem Pharmacol 25:433–437
Winkler H, Bauer G, Gmeiner R (1965) Zur Wirkung von Bradykinin, Kallidin und Eledoisin auf den Katzen- und Kaninchen-Darm in situ. Naunyn Schmiedebergs Arch Exp Pathol Pharmakol 250:459–468
Zappia L, Molina E, Violini A, Bassani F (1972) Ricerche preliminari sull'azione del nuovo polipeptide bombesina sull'appendice umana „in vitro". Ateneo Parmense [Acta Biomed] 43:3–8

CHAPTER 3

Amines: Histamine

G. BERTACCINI

A. Introduction

Physiologic roles of histamine have not yet been clarified. Its distribution in the gastrointestinal tract is consistent with the idea that it has a function in secretion rather than in motility, but there are many important factors which cannot be disregarded: the turnover rate of histamine, the number and susceptibility of receptors at the specific targets, the interaction with other humoral and nervous mediators, etc. Of course, detailed consideration of histamine distribution, synthesis, and metabolism is beyond the scope of this review.

In 1966, ASH and SCHILD showed for the first time the existence of different types of histamine receptors. They defined as H_1-receptors those which could be blocked by the classical antihistaminics and they pointed out the existence of at least one other class of receptors for which no specific antagonist was available. Most of the spasmogenic effects of histamine on smooth muscle involved H_1-receptors. The discovery of H_2-receptors (BLACK et al. 1972) and of their selective agonists and antagonists provided fresh impetus to the investigation of the histamine effects, but problems multiplied in logarithmic progression and it soon became apparent that the more histamine was investigated the more problems remained to be resolved.

Much of what was known about histamine before the discovery of H_2-receptors is contained in two exhaustive volumes edited by ROCHA E SILVA (1966, 1978), and the specific effects of the amine on gut motility were carefully reviewed by DANIEL in 1968. The recent history of histamine, especially that related to the H_2-receptors, is summarized in five symposium reports (WOOD and ALISON SIMKINS 1973; BURLAND and ALISON SIMKINS 1977; CREUTZFELDT 1978; WASTELL and LANCE 1978; LUCCHELLI 1978) and in a recent review (HIRSCHOWITZ 1979), which deal mainly with the function of histamine in gastric secretion. Paradoxically, the H_2-receptor antagonists, which were so useful in the understanding of the physiology of gastric secretion, have so far probably contributed in a negative sense to the understanding of the physiologic role of histamine in gastrointestinal motility. In fact, several effects of the H_2-blockers were immediately attributed to the antagonism at the H_2-receptor level without any consideration of the possible intrinsic nonspecific actions which were found to be present, though in different degrees, with the H_2-blockers available so far: burimamide, metiamide, cimetidine, and ranitidine (BERTACCINI and DOBRILLA 1980). Some effects of burimamide on the guinea pig ileum or of cimetidine on the lower esophageal sphincter (LES) or on gastric emptying were immediately taken as evidence for a certain physiologic role of H_2-receptors in those particular areas (ileum, LES, or stomach, respectively) whereas no definite proofs for these statements were given and actually, they were disproved by subsequent studies, as will be discussed in the rest of this chapter.

B. Activity on the Lower Esophageal Sphincter

Conflicting results have been reported about the action of histamine on the LES, probably due to differences in the technique used or to species differences. In addition, most of the available papers are not about the action of histamine, but rather that of cimetidine, because of the obvious clinical interest of this new drug.

In the pig-tailed macaque, *Macaca nemestrina*, and in the bush-tailed phalanger *Trichosurus vulpecula*, histamine (5–50 μg/kg) relaxes the LES by way of both H_1- and H_2-receptors and this effect is blocked by a combination of H_1- and H_2-antagonists (DE CARLE and GLOVER 1975). In the North American opossum, *Didelphis marsupialis virginiana*, which belongs to a different genus from the Australian opossum, the results were different; in vitro studies showed that histamine, 2-(2-pyridyl)-ethylamine (a selective stimulant of the H_1-receptors) and compound 48/80 (a well-known histamine releaser) caused dose-related increases in LES basal tension as well as in the amplitude of the "off response" of the esophageal body. Mepyramine abolished or even reversed the action of the three compounds. Metiamide given alone had no effect, whereas in combination with mepyramine it completely abolished the responses to all agonist drugs (DE CARLE et al. 1976). Exhaustive studies performed with H_1- and H_2-receptor agonists and antagonists and also with the neural inhibitors tetrodotoxin, (RATTAN and GOYAL 1978; GOYAL and RATTAN 1978) suggested that stimulation of H_1-receptors on the sphincter muscle causes contraction, whereas activation of H_1-receptors on intramural inhibitory neurons causes inhibition of the sphincter. Activation of H_2-receptors on the sphincter muscle causes inhibition of the sphincter. These data suggest that in these species the LES contains predominantly excitatory H_1- and also inhibitory H_2-receptors for histamine, which is a situation identical to that found by WALDMAN et al. (1977) and by SCHOETZ et al. (1978) in the guinea pig and baboon gallbladder, respectively. The above results confirmed the observations made in the opossum by COHEN and SNAPE (1975), who showed that metiamide is able to augment the maximal LES muscle response to histamine in vitro and also to increase the LES pressure in vivo in a dose-dependent fashion up to 2 mg kg^{-1} h^{-1} i.v. Similar and even clearer results were obtained with the isolated guinea pig LES (TAKAYANAGI and KASUYA 1977); contractions induced by histamine (10^{-6} g/ml) were reversed by pretreatment with chlorpheniramine (3×10^{-7} g/ml) and potentiated by cimetidine (10^{-4} g/ml). Under the same experimental conditions, histamine (3×10^{-5} g/ml) failed to contract the rat LES.

However other studies (BERTACCINI et al. 1981 a) reported that histamine is able to contract the LES from rats (threshold dose = 1.6×10^{-5} *M*) as well as guinea pigs (threshold dose = 3×10^{-6} *M*). The effect was blocked in both species by chlorpheniramine.

In the conscious baboon, increasing i.v. boluses of histamine caused an increase in LES pressure with a maximum response at a dose of 12 μg/kg. Chlorpheniramine did not alter basal LES pressure, but did abolish the contractile effect of histamine. Conversely, cimetidine was absolutely ineffective, both on the LES basal pressure and on increased LES pressure after histamine, suggesting that only H_1-receptors are involved in the stimulant action of exogenous histamine (BROWN et al. 1978). Contrasting findings were reported on the effects of histamine on human LES in vitro; MISIEWICZ et al. (1969) found the amine to cause either contractions or a biphasic response, BURLEIGH (1979), on the contrary, reported only a relaxant effect of histamine under similar experimental conditions. Probably the different pathology of the specimens of human esophagogastric junction was responsible for these discrepancies. However in neither study was the problem of histamine receptors clarified.

In our department (CORUZZI and BERTACCINI 1982) isolated preparations of human LES responded with a contraction to histamine or to the selective H_1-agonist, 2-aminoethylthiazole (threshold doses were 1 and 10 μg/ml respectively). This effect was probably connected with a stimulation of H_1-receptors since it was inhibited by H_1-antagonists; moreover both H_2-agonists and H_2-antagonists had erratic effects causing (only at very high doses) contraction, relaxation and/or biphasic effects thus suggesting an action related to the specific molecules and not to the excitation or the blockade of the H_2-receptors.

Histamine at doses of 2–40 μg kg^{-1} h^{-1} i.v., was also shown (KRAVITZ et al. 1978) to cause graded increases in pressure of the human LES in vivo. This contractile effect was unaffected by diphenhydramine (50 mg i.v.), whereas it was completely blocked by cimetidine, given by i.v. infusion (4 mg kg^{-1} h^{-1}) or orally (300 mg). It is of interest that cimetidine alone did not change LES basal pressure. These data apparently confirmed previous reports (CASTELL and HARRIS 1970) that betazole (a substance known to stimulate the H_2-receptors selectively) caused contraction of the LES in humans. As for the effects of cimetidine, they will be considered in a subsequent chapter. Here, I want only to emphasize that most of the investigators have found this H_2-blocker to be ineffective on human LES pressure (for review see BERTACCINI et al. 1980). Only BAILEY et al. (1976) found that i.v. infusion of 150 mg cimetidine in 1 h into normal volunteers caused a slight stimulant effect during the first 15 min (low blood levels of the drug), followed by a slight inhibition in the following 45 min (higher blood levels). Also, ROESCH et al. (1976) found cimetidine to cause a significant rise in the LES basal pressure and to increase the effect of pentagastrin. The authors claim that the effect of cimetidine is related to the blockade of inhibitory H_2-receptors.

According to recent data obtained in our department (BERTACCINI et al. 1981 b), the new H_2-antagonist ranitidine, having a nitrofuran ring instead of the imidazole nucleous of cimetidine, exerts a remarkable increase in human LES pressure at doses of 0.25–1 mg/kg i.v. Surprisingly, this action seems to be connected with a stimulation of the cholinergic system since it is completely prevented by small doses of subcutaneous atropine (0.5 mg).

In conclusion, endogenous histamine seems to have no important effects on human LES, whereas exogenous histamine seems to stimulate the H_2-receptors of human LES in the direction opposite to its effect on experimental animals. In any case, it is probable that the effect of histamine on the LES represents the net effect of stimulation of different receptors. The effects of histamine on the LES, together with the different receptors involved, are summarized in Table 1.

Table 1. Histamine receptors in the lower esophageal sphincter

Species	Receptors [a] H₁	Receptors [a] H₂	Compounds used	Reference [b]
Monkey	–	–	Histamine	DE CARLE and GLOVER (1975)
	–	–	Histamine; H_1-agonists	
Australian opossum (in vivo)	–	–	Histamine; H_1- and H_2-agonists and antagonists	RATTAN and GOYAL (1978)
American opossum (in vitro and in vivo)	+	–	Histamine; H_1- and H_2-agonists; metiamide	COHEN and SNAPE (1975); DE CARLE et al. (1976)
Baboon (in vivo)	+	0	Histamine; H_1-antagonists; cimetidine	BROWN et al. (1978)
Guinea pig (in vitro)	+	–	Histamine; H_1- and H_2-antagonists	TAKAYANAGI and KASUYA (1977)
Guinea pig (in vitro)	+	0	Histamine; H_1- and H_2-antagonists	BERTACCINI et al. (1981 a)
Rat (in vitro)	0	0	Histamine	TAKAYANAGI and KASUYA (1977)
Rat (in vitro)	+	0	Histamine; H_1- and H_2-antagonists	BERTACCINI et al. (1981 a)
Human (in vivo)	0	+	Histamine; H_1-antagonists; cimetidine	KRAVITZ et al. (1978)
Human (in vivo)	+?		Betazole	CASTELL and HARRIS (1970)
Human (in vitro)	+–?		Histamine	MISIEWICZ et al. (1969)
Human (in vitro)	–?		Histamine	BURLEIGH (1979)
Human (in vitro)	+	0	Histamine; H_1- and H_2-agonists and antagonists	CORUZZI and BERTACCINI (1982)

[a] + = Contraction; – = relaxation; 0 = no effect; ? = type of receptor not established
[b] Only representative papers are cited

C. Action on the Stomach

Histamine has been shown to contract the stomach in several species. In the kitten and the guinea pig stomach in vitro and in the antrum of the dog in vivo, the action is mainly on nervous structures. In rat stomach strips, early experiments demonstrated a stimulant effect of histamine, but at concentrations of the order of 1 μg/ml. Recent data (ERCAN and TÜRKER 1977) have shown that stimulation of H_2-receptors causes relaxation of isolated rat stomach. On the other hand, the rat stomach in vivo seemed to contract through stimulation of H_1-receptors (BLACK et al. 1972). Recent studies in the guinea pig fundus and antrum showed that histamine (5×10^{-4} *M*) caused a rise in the baseline without an alteration in amplitudes. The use of mepyramine (which blocked the effect of histamine) and cimetidine (which was ineffective) suggested that the motor response to histamine is mediated via H_1-receptors (GERNER et al. 1979).

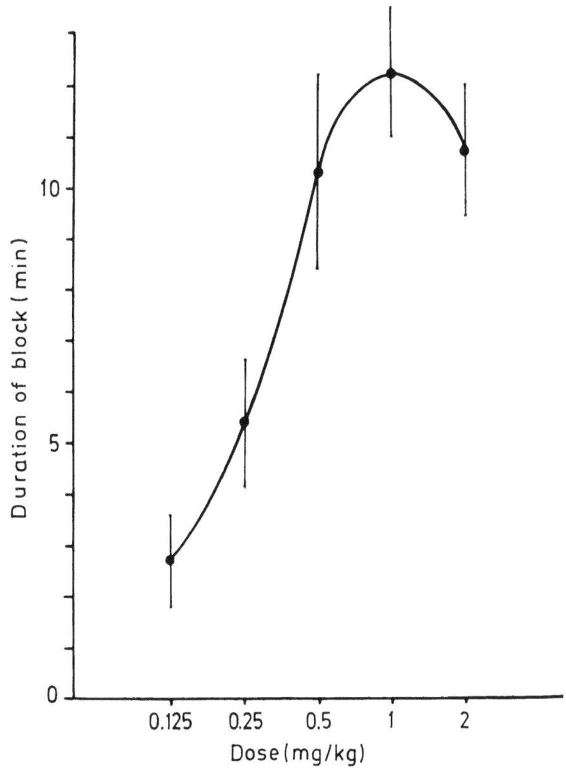

Fig. 1. Spasmogenic effect of histamine on the pylorus of the anesthetized rat, plotted as the duration of the block of the duodenal effluent versus dose. Each value represents the mean values from 5–8 experiments. *Vertical bars* show standard errors

In other studies, FARA and BERKOWITZ (1978) found that both H_1- and H_2-receptor selective agonists contracted strips from circular muscle of dog antrum; however, rather large doses were necessary for maximum responses (1×10^{-4} g/ml and 5×10^{-4} g/ml, respectively). Histamine, under the same experimental conditions, was able to potentiate the maximal stimulatory response to either gastrin or cholecystokinin octapeptide. Interesting and rather peculiar results were obtained by BERTACCINI et al. (1977) in the in situ rat pylorus, with doses of histamine equivalent to (or actually lower than) those that stimulate gastric secretion in this species (0.1–0.2 mg/kg i.v.). In this preparation, histamine caused a striking dose-related contraction of the gastroduodenal junction (Fig. 1). This effect was mimicked to a certain extent by H_1- and H_2-agonists but, surprisingly, was not abolished by H_1- or H_2-antagonists or by a combination of both types of drugs. Different kinds of blockers (atropine, hexamethonium, methysergide, etc.) failed to modify this spasmogenic effect of histamine, which appears to be a nonspecific muscular effect similar to that elicited in the same preparation by many polypeptides and can be blocked only by substances such as adrenaline, prostaglandin E_1, or papaverine which directly affect the pyloric smooth muscle. The rat pylorus seems to provide, so far, the first example in the gastrointestinal tract of an action of histamine not inhibited by the known antagonists; other examples have been

Table 2. Histamine receptors in the stomach

Species and tissue	Receptors [a]		Compounds used	Reference [b]
	H_1	H_2		
Rat stomach in vivo	+	0	Histamine; H_1-agonists	[1]
Rat stomach in vitro	NT	−	H_2-agonists	[2]
Rat pylorus in vivo	+*		Histamine; H_1- and H_2-agonists and antagonists	[3]
Guinea pig stomach in vitro	+	0	Histamine; mepyramine; cimetidine	[4]
Guinea pig pylorus in vitro	+?		Histamine	[5]
Dog antrum in vitro	+	+	H_1- and H_2-agonists	[6]
Cat stomach in vivo	−?		Histamine	[7]
Kitten fundus and ferret fundus in vitro	+?		Histamine	[8]
Cow forestomach in vitro	+	−	Histamine; mepyramine; metiamide	[9]

[a] + = Contraction; − = relaxation; NT = not tested; * = possible subtype of classical receptor; 0 = no effect; ? = type of receptor not established
[b] Only representative papers are cited

[1] BLACK et al. (1972); [2] ERCAN and TÜRKER (1977); [3] BERTACCINI et al. (1977); [4] GERNER et al. (1979); [5] BERTACCINI et al. (1979a); [6] FARA and BERKOWITZ (1978); [7] FASTH et al. (1975); [8] YATES et al. (1978); [9] OHGA and TANEIKE (1978)

found in tracheobronchial smooth muscle (FLEISCH and CALKINS 1976; CHAND and EYRE 1977), in the rat heart (DAI 1976), and in the brain (HAAS and BUCHER 1975).

Though conclusive evidence is still lacking, it was hypothesized that there is an unknown histamine receptor or, more probably, that there are different subclasses of the classical histamine receptors (BERTACCINI et al. 1977; BERTACCINI 1978a; BERTACCINI and CORUZZI 1981). Quite recent experiments (YATES et al. 1978) were performed on the gastric fundus from kittens and young ferrets, with simultaneous recording of the gastric secretion and the motility of a strip of circular muscle fibers. In this experimental situation, concentrations of histamine sufficient to produce secretory effects (10^{-6}–10^{-5} *M*) also produced modulation of motor activity, with an initial increase in the magnitude of spontaneous contractions, followed by a cessation of contractile activity and a sustained increase in tone. Apparently, the kitten was much more sensitive to histamine than the ferret. The authors suggested that modulation of gastric motility may be a physiologic action of histamine. However, no indication is given about the histamine receptors that might be involved in this phenomenon. The same may be said for the slight relaxant effect of histamine observed following intra-aortic injection (10 μg) in the atropinized cat (FASTH et al. 1975).

A recent study (MCCALLUM et al. 1979) showed that histamine caused a dose-related (1–10 μg/kg) contraction of the feline pylorus. This effect was mimicked by the H_1-receptor selective agonist, 2-(2-pyridyl)ethylamine, but not by the H_2-receptor selective agonist, dimaprit. The contractile response was strongly reduced by diphenhydramine and slightly potentiated by cimetidine, suggesting an involvement of H_1-receptors. Since tetrodotoxin was also able to cause a partial inhibition of the effects of histamine, a neural pathway together with the direct activity on the smooth muscle was hypothesized.

Quite recently histamine has also been shown (OHGA and TANEIKE 1978) to have direct excitatory and inhibitory effects on the bovine ruminal and reticular smooth muscle. Independent of the dose used (0.54–540 μM), histamine caused three different responses in the longitudinal muscle layer: contraction alone, relaxation followed by contraction, or pure relaxation. In the circular muscle layer, only contractions were seen. The responses induced by histamine were not affected by tetrodotoxin (1.6 μM), atropine (0.72 μM), or α- and β-blocking agents. However, mepyramine (0.25–2.5 μM) completely and reversibly blocked the contractile responses and metiamide (41–82 μM) competitively antagonized the relaxation induced by histamine. The parallel shifting of the dose–response curve to histamine and the pA_2 values for the antagonists suggested that H_1-receptors mediated the stimulatory and H_2-receptors the inhibitory responses to histamine in the bovine forestomach. Histamine was also shown to contract the reticuloomasal sphincter of cattle in vitro at threshold doses of 1–1.5 µg/ml. However no attempt was made to establish the receptors involved in this stimulatory effect (R. FAUSTINI et al. unpublished work). The effects of histamine on the stomach of different experimental animals together with the receptors involved is shown in Table 2.

D. Gastric Emptying

We have only a few data on the effects of histamine on gastric emptying and of course they cannot be deduced from data obtained with cimetidine, whose effects may be connected not only to muscle H_2-receptor blockade but also to acid secretion blockade, with all the consequences that this implies. However, according to a recent study (DUBOIS et al. 1977, 1978), histamine H_2-receptors may be involved in the regulation of gastric emptying, as suggested by the fact that administration of dimaprit, a selective H_2-receptor agonist (0.12–0.24 μM kg^{-1} h^{-1} i.v.) significantly increased gastric emptying in monkeys whereas cimetidine decreased it. In our department (SCARPIGNATO et al. 1981) we showed that histamine (1–30 mg/kg i.p.) delayed gastric emptying of a phenol red test meal in a dose-dependent fashion in the rat. This effect, which was not mimicked by dimaprit, and not inhibited by the H_2-blockers was mimicked by 2-aminoethylthiazole (an H_1-receptor selective stimulant) and inhibited dose-dependently, by chlorpheniramine, suggesting that H_1-receptors are responsible for the delay in gastric emptying observed in the rat (Fig. 2).

E. Action on the Intestine

Histamine caused contraction of the bowel in most species, though with consistent quantitative differences. The smooth muscle of the gut was not so sensitive to histamine as is that of other areas, such as the bronchi. However, the guinea pig ileum, because of the constancy and the reliability of its response to histamine and the

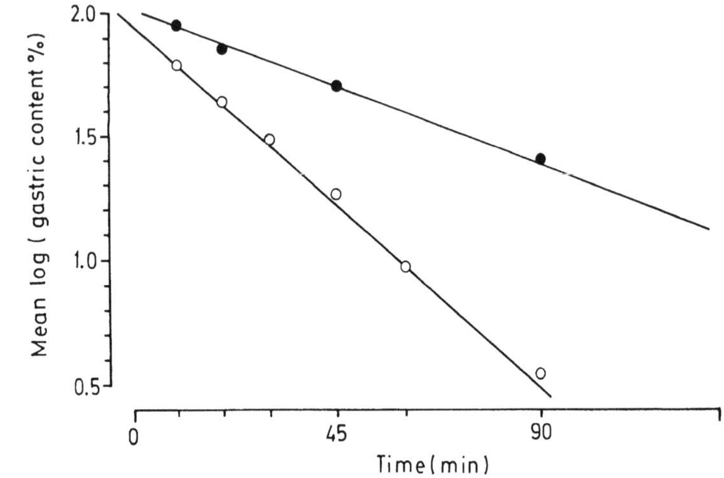

Fig. 2. Semilogarithmic plot of gastric content versus time. The lines are the calculated least-squares regression lines (*open circles*, controls; *r*, 0.8600; *n*, 27 $P < 0.001$ *full circles*, histamine-treated rats; *r*, 0.9246; *n*, 34 $P < 0.001$)

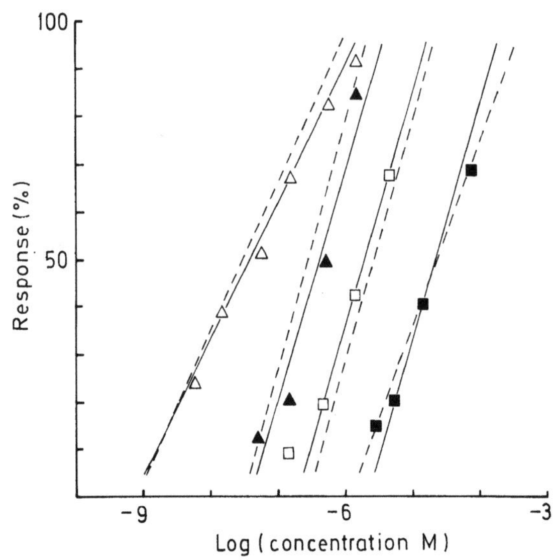

Fig. 3. Dose–response curves for histamine *(open triangles)*, 2-aminoethylthiazole *(full triangles)*; 5-ethylhistamine *(open squares)*, and 5-methylhistamine *(full squares)*. Values refer to the mean of the values obtained from 4–5 experiments on the longitudinal muscle preparation *(full lines)*. The *broken lines* refer to the whole ileum preparation for which single values were not reported

complete lack of tachyphylaxis, has been used for decades for the biologic assay of the amine. Both the commonly used whole ileum and the more sophisticated longitudinal muscle preparation (PATON and VIZI 1969) can be used satisfactorily with overlapping results. Figure 3 shows that not only histamine and 2-aminoethylthiazole but also some H_2-receptor agonists (though noticeably less potent than histamine) show a good dose–response curve for contraction on both kinds of preparations. Both an indirect and a more important direct action of histamine on the guinea pig ileum longitudinal muscle layer have been described (PARROT and THOUVENOT 1966): the first is represented by fast unsustained contractions, observed after small doses of histamine, connected with stimulation of preganglionic sites in the intrinsic nervous system since they are depressed by hexamethonium, cooling, and atropine; the second is represented by a sustained, more constant, atropine-resistant response and it is generally considered to be due to stimulation of histamine H_1-receptors.

This concept, which was based on the competitive antagonism by mepyramine (ASH and SCHILD 1966), received further confirmation in recent experiments which showed that histamine receptors in the guinea pig ileum are labeled by the specific binding of mepyramine ^3H (HILL et al. 1977). Comparing the mepyramine ^3H binding in different parts of the ileum, the highest binding was found to occur in the longitudinal muscle with values ten times those of the mucosa and more than seven times those of the circular muscle. The potency of histamine in competing for specific mepyramine ^3H binding was substantially less than biologic potency of histamine: the equilibrium constant of binding K_b of histamine for specific mepyramine ^3H binding sites in guinea pig ileum is 12 μM, about 100 times the concentration required to elicit a 50% maximal contraction. This discrepancy might be explained by the existance of spare receptors for histamine (CHANG et al. 1979). The affinity of histamine for mepyramine ^3H binding sites in the rat ileum was less than that on the guinea pig ileum in accordance with the low activity of histamine in the rat. The direct activity of histamine (threshold stimulant dose $= 10^{-9}$ M) showed a good dose–response relationship, very similar to that evoked by acetylcholine, which however, was approximately ten times as potent as histamine (G. BERTACCINI unpublished work 1980). Mepyramine and chlorpheniramine caused parallel shifts to the right of the dose–response curve to histamine and their pA_2 values were 8.71 and 7.90, respectively (ARUNLAKSHANA and SCHILD 1959).

In the circular muscle layer, the action of histamine was much weaker than in the longitudinal one and it appeared to be mediated through stimulation of the intramural plexuses; in fact, it was potentiated by cholinesterase inhibitors and antagonized by hyoscine and morphine (BROWNLEE and HARRY 1963). Of course it must be remembered that the techniques used to register the response of the circular muscle are much less reliable than those used for recording the longitudinal contractions. Both an increase in ileal intraluminal pressure during isotonic contractions of the longitudinal muscle (G. BERTACCINI unpublished work 1980) and an erratic increase (10%–15%) in peristaltic activity (which involves circular muscle contraction) in response to histamine (10^{-8}–10^{-7} M) has been observed (A. CREMA et al. personal communication 1980). Large doses of histamine (10–25 μg/ml), on the other hand, have actually been reported to produce a significant inhibition of the peristaltic reflex (BELESLIN and SAMARDZIC 1978). The circular muscle layer of the opossum duodenum was contracted by histamine only in enormous concentrations (2×10^{-2} M) in contrast to the longitudinal muscle which was contracted at concentrations of 5×10^{-6} M (FAULK et al. 1977).

The guinea pig taenia caeci was also extremely sensitive to histamine (threshold stimulant dose = 5 ng/ml), whose action was competitively inhibited by mepyramine. Only neonatal rabbit ileum (6–20 days) was contracted by histamine

(3×10^{-7} *M*) with a dose–response curve similar to that caused by acetylcholine. Histamine-induced contractions were competitively inhibited by mepyramine ($pA_2 = 8.9$) and unaffected by hyoscine (4×10^{-7} *M*) or tetrodotoxin (3×10^{-6} *M*). In the adult rabbit, even enormous amounts of histamine (3×10^{-3} *M*) caused a maximum contraction which was never greater than 25% of the maximum contraction induced by acetylcholine. The author (BOTTING 1975) suggested that neonatal rabbit intestine may possess large numbers of H_1-receptors, which are either lost or rendered ineffective in adult animals. In other studies (TUCKER and SNAPE 1979) circular muscle from both proximal and distal rabbit colon was shown to contract in response to histamine (10^{-8}–10^{-3} *M*). The spasmogenic effect was unaffected by cimetidine (10^{-4} *M*) but completely blocked by diphenhydramine (10^{-4} *M*), suggesting an action mediated through H_1-receptors.

However, the proximal colon of the rabbit was shown to respond dose-dependently to histamine (5×10^{-7}–10^{-5} *M*) with contractions which were completely blocked by mepyramine (GLOVER 1979). In this preparation, as well as in the guinea pig ileum, dithiothreitol, an agent which reduces disulfide linkages to sulphydryl groups and has no effect on basal tone or on acetylcholine-induced contractions, potentiated the effect of histamine by a factor of ten (GLOVER 1979). Since it is known that dithiothreitol has little effect on histamine metabolizing enzymes (FLEISCH et al. 1973) it was suggested that the drug caused potentiation by reducing a disulfide bridge at one of the steps in the sequence of events that connects the H_1-receptor with the contractile mechanism. In an extensive study performed with the chicken gastrointestinal tract, CHAND and EYRE (1976) found that the stimulatory effect of histamine associated with excitation of H_1-receptors varies quantitatively in the different regions of the gut. Threshold concentrations were: 10^{-7}–10^{-6} *M* in the esophagus and the crop; 10^{-7}–10^{-4} *M* in the small intestine; and 10^{-7}–10^{-6} *M* in the cecum.

In the dog duodenum, in vivo, intra-arterial histamine caused contractions which were prevented by atropine and hexamethonium. The motor activity was very moderately increased as to both amplitude and tone with a rather short-lasting effect (G. BERTACCINI unpublished work 1980). However, according to more recent experiments (KONTUREK and SIEBERS 1979, 1980), histamine alters small bowel motility of the dog via stimulation of H_1-receptors. In doses of 10–320 $\mu g\, kg^{-1}\, h^{-1}$ it caused a dose-dependent increase in the appearance rate and the propagation velocity of the interdigestive migrating myoelectric complexes. This effect was mimicked by 2-methylhistamine and abolished by tripelennamine; on the other hand 4-methylhistamine and metiamide were absolutely inactive. Recent experiments performed in anesthetized rats (SAKAI 1979) showed that histamine caused a monophasic fast contraction of the ileum which was relatively dose dependent (1–100 μg intra-arterially). This contractile effect was abolished by tetrodotoxin, hexamethonium, morphine, and high doses of mepyramine (50–100 μg), but not by atropine or methysergide. SAKAI suggested that histamine acts by a primary action on the myenteric nerve plexus involving cholinergic interneurons which, however, lead to stimulation of noncholinergic, nontryptaminergic terminal fibers. According to early papers on human bowel strips in vitro, histamine may relax human ileum (both longitudinal and circular layers); it has a biphasic effect (relaxation followed by contraction) on the circular colonic muscle, while in the taenia coli the effect is most erratic: contraction, biphasic response, or pure relaxation are possible (Fishlock and Parks 1963; Bucknell and Whitney 1964). These effects, elicited by various doses of histamine (0.1–10 μg/ml depending on the different preparations), were apparently blocked by mepyramine. No accurate dose–response studies were performed at that time. Histamine was also found to cause a dose-dependent contraction (0.1–30 μ*M*) of the ileum from the common tree shrew, *Tupaia glis*, a primitive primate. This effect was competitively inhibited by diphenhydramine (Sakai et al. 1979).

Only one paper, so far, deals with the possibility of the existence of two slightly different types of H_1-receptors (Labrid et al. 1977). This hypothesis which was based on the different behavior of three H_1-receptor antagonists (mepyramine, diphenhydramine, and eprozinol) in the dose–response curve to histamine of guinea pig ileal and tracheal smooth muscle, needs confirmation by means of the accurate use of H_1- *and* H_2-receptor selective agonists *and* antagonists.

In one of the few experiments performed in humans (Misiewicz et al. 1967), both histamine (0.04 mg $kg^{-1} h^{-1}$ i.v.) and betazole (1.5–2 mg/kg i.v.) were found to be completely ineffective in modifying motor activity in the whole alimentary tract. Histamine was also found to have a very modest, if any, activity on other segments of the human gut in vitro being 10–100 times less effective than some gastrointestinal peptides like bombesin or cholecystokinin (Bertaccini et al. 1974).

F. H_2-Receptors

There is evidence for and against the occurrence of H_2-receptors (whose stimulation causes relaxation) in the intestinal muscle. Bareicha and Rocha e Silva (1975, 1976) were the first who claimed that the duodenum and ileum of the guinea pig contain a certain amount (12.4% and 15.7%, respectively) of true H_2-receptors with relaxant activity. They based their assumption only on the potentiation caused by burimamide on the response of small doses of histamine ($< 10^{-7}$ *M*) whereas the maximum responses were absolutely unchanged, probably because of the greater effect of H_1-receptors.

One of the early papers on this topic was that of Ambache et al. (1973); they found that in the longitudinal muscle ileal preparation, histamine, in the presence of mepyramine, produced a dose-dependent inhibition of the neurogenic tetanic spasm elicited by field stimulation. This inhibitory effect was blocked by burimamide, but was not mimicked by 4-(5)-methylhistamine, suggesting that the receptors mediating histamine inhibition *resemble* H_2-receptors in their susceptibility to burimamide blockade but *differ* in being insensitive to a selective H_2-receptor selective agonist. This may represent the first indication of the existance of a heterogeneity in the population of H_2-receptors.

Further evidence for the existance of a subtype of H_2-receptors in the guinea pig ileum was suggested by Fjalland (1979); however it was based on the fact that clonidine (considered an H_2-agonist) induced suppression of electrically induced twitches, and on different antagonistic activity ratio of cimetidine and burimamide on the guinea pig ileum versus the isolated atria. A similar study was performed by Chand and De Roth (1978) using the chicken ileum. Also in this case, evidence

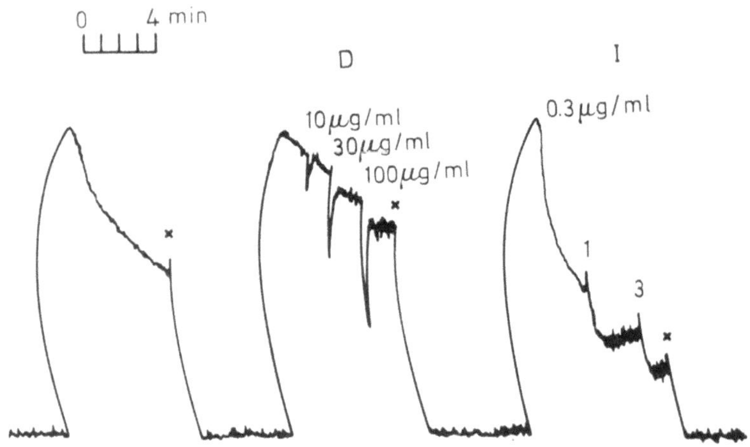

Fig. 4. Relaxations of guinea pig duodenum caused by dimaprit *D* and impromidine *I* on the histamine-induced contractions. *Crosses* indicate washout

for the occurrence of H_2-receptors consisted only in the potentiation, by high doses of metiamide (5×10^{-5} *M*), of the dose–response curve to histamine and the parallel lack of potentiation in the response to carbachol. More recently, REINHARDT et al. (1979) confirmed the occurrence of H_2-receptors in the guinea pig ileum after contracting the ileum with high concentrations of potassium (100 m*M*) and causing relaxation with histamine in the presence of mepyramine. This relaxation was prevented by high concentrations of metiamide (10^{-5} *M*). No dose–response curves were constructed and only one concentration of histamine was employed.

Evidence against the presence of H_2-receptors whose stimulation causes relaxation is strongly supported by several important data:

1) Metiamide at concentrations 2×10^{-4} *M* has been shown to have no effect on the responses of histamine (BLACK et al. 1972; KENAKIN et al. 1974; PARSONS 1977). The same behavior between metiamide and cimetidine was also reported (BERTACCINI et al. 1979 b).

2) Dimaprit and 5-methylhistamine (two selective H_2-receptor agonists) even in concentrations as high as 1.3×10^{-5} *M* have failed to inhibit the response to histamine in the guinea pig ileum (BERTACCINI et al. 1979 b), but higher doses (10^{-4} *M*) caused a relaxation which, however, was not prevented by cimetidine. On the other hand impromidine, the newest, extremely powerful H_2-receptor agonist, was shown to antagonize the effect of histamine on the ileum, but the antagonism was competitive in nature ($pA_2 = 5.47$), thus suggesting an inhibitory action on H_1-receptors rather than a stimulatory action on H_2-receptors (DURANT et al. 1978). Recent experiments (BERTACCINI and ZAPPIA 1981) showed that dimaprit and impromidine (this last compound was about 100 times more potent than dimaprit) caused a dose-dependent inhibitory effect on the contraction induced by histamine on guinea pig duodenum (Fig. 4). However, this effect was not antagonized by cimetidine or ranitidine (the most recent H_2-receptor blocker), even in the enormous amount of 30 µg/ml, suggesting the possibility of a subtype of histamine receptor which mediates relaxation, and is sensitive to the H_2-agonists but insensitive

to the H_2-antagonists. A relaxant effect quite similar to that elicited by dimaprit and impromidine was also induced by clonidine and tolazoline, both of which are known to stimulate the H_2-receptors. All the H_2-receptor agonists tested were shown to relax the guinea pig duodenum contracted not only by histamine but also by acetylcholine or excess of K^+ (BERTACCINI and ZAPPIA 1981).

3) A peculiar phenomenon was observed by KENAKIN et al. (1974), i.e., the transformation of H_1- to H_2-receptors by lowering the temperature of the nutrient fluid, whereas at 37 °C the dose–response curve to histamine was unaffected by metiamide and showed the expected shift to the right after pretreatment with a selective anti-H_1-receptor compound (tripelennamine 5×10^{-8} *M*), at 12 °C the response to histamine showed a parallel shift to the right with metiamide (7.5×10^{-5} *M*), and was virtually unaffected by tripelennamine. This obviously suggested a clear temperature-dependent interconversion of histamine H_1- and H_2-receptors, but in this case stimulation of H_2-receptors gave rise to contraction and not relaxation. Again, confirmation of these data by the use of selective H_1-agonists (which would be inactive at low temperature) and selective H_2-agonists (which would be at least as active as histamine at low temperature) is needed.

Our personal experience (G. BERTACCINI and L. ZAPPIA unpublished work 1981) provided evidence against temperature-dependent interconversion of histamine receptors, since selective agonists like dimaprit and impromidine failed to elicit any stimulatory action at 12 °C; moreover at this low temperature selective antagonists like cimetidine or tiotidine, were unable to cause any significant shifting of the dose-response curve to histamine which, on the other hand, was shifted to the right by d-chlorpheniramine (1×10^{-8}) a selective H_1-antagonist.

4) Finally, the investigations concerning the possible relaxant activity on guinea pig ileum do not report any effect of selective H_1-receptor agonists (which would *not* have to be potentiated by an H_2-antagonist); furthermore, all the experiments refer to the usual whole ileum preparation and not to the pure longitudinal muscle strip; therefore, possible interference by the circular muscle (whose stimulation could simulate a relaxation of the longitudinal contraction) could not be totally excluded.

For the mechanism of action of histamine beyond the amine–receptor interaction on motility little is known, unlike the mechanism for secretion, in which the activation of the adenyl cyclase–cyclic AMP system clearly appears to be involved. Recent papers indicate that the histamine effect on the guinea pig ileum, consisting of phasic contractions and subsequent tonic contractions, is initiated by the release and the passive influx of Ca^{2+} from storage sites containing loosely bound Ca^{2+} (OHMURA 1976).

An interaction of histamine with Ca^{2+} was also observed in the rabbit taenia coli (TAKAYANAGI et al. 1977). The contractions induced by histamine (5×10^{-5} *M*) in a calcium-free Locke–Ringer solution were less than 50% of those observed in normal Locke–Ringer solution. The response to histamine appeared to be more dependent than the response to acetylcholine on the presence of external Ca^{2+}, whereas Ca release and transport of Ca^{2+} from the binding stores in cellular membranes did not change significantly, as they did in the guinea pig ileum. The effects of histamine on the intestine, together with the receptors involved are summarized in Table 3.

Table 3. Histamine receptors in the intestine

Species and tissue	Receptors[a] H_1	Receptors[a] H_2	Compounds used	Reference[b]
Guinea pig duodenum	+	−	Histamine; burimamide	[1]
		−*	H_1- and H_2-agonists and antagonists	[2]
Guinea pig ileum		−*	Histamine; mepyramine; burimamide; 4-methylhistamine	[3]
Guinea pig ileum	+	−	Histamine; burimamide	[4]
Guinea pig ileum	+	−	Histamine; metiamide	[5]
Guinea pig ileum	+	0	Histamine	[6]
Guinea pig ileum	+	0	Histamine; tripelennamine	[7]
Guinea pig ileum	+	−* 0	Histamine; H_1- and H_2-agonists and antagonists	[8]
Guinea pig ileum	NT	−*	Clonidine; cimetidine	[9]
Chicken ileum	+	−	Histamine; metiamide	[10]
Rat ileum	+	NT	Histamine	[11]
Guinea pig taenia coli	+	NT	Histamine; mepyramine	[12]
Rabbit ileum	+	NT	Histamine; mepyramine	[13]
Rabbit colon	+	NT	Histamine; mepyramine	[14]
Tree shrew ileum	+	NT	Histamine; diphenydramine	[15]
Human colon	− +	NT	Histamine; mepyramine	[16, 17]
Dog small intestine in vivo	+	0	Histamine; H_1- and H_2-agonists and antagonists	[18]

[a] + = Contraction; − = relaxation; NT = not tested; * = possible subtype of classical receptor
[b] Only representative papers are cited

[1] BAREICHA and ROCHA E SILVA (1975); [2] BERTACCINI et al. (1979c); [3] AMBACHE et al. (1973); [4] BAREICHA and ROCHA E SILVA (1975); [5] REINHARDT et al. (1979); [6] BLACK et al. (1972); [7] KENAKIN et al. (1974); [8] BERTACCINI et al. (1979b); [9] FJALLAND (1979); [10] CHAND and DE ROTH (1978); [11] PARROT and THOUVENOT (1966); [12] PARROT and THOUVENOT (1966); [13] BOTTING (1975); [14] GLOVER (1979); [15] SAKAI et al. (1979); [16] FISHLOCK and PARKS (1963); [17] BUCKNELL and WHITNEY (1964); [18] KONTUREK and SIEBERS (1979)

G. Conclusions

In the opinion of the writer, data available so far are probably in favor of the occurrence of a subgroup of H_2-receptors in the guinea pig ileum with different "characteristics" from the classical H_2-receptors which seem to be absent in the longitudinal layer. As already pointed out (BERTACCINI 1978b) several criteria should be fulfilled in order to establish that an observed pharmacologic effect is surely connected with the specific interaction histamine-H_2 receptors:

a) The effect must be mimicked by at least two selective H_2-receptor agonists
b) The effect must be *competitively* inhibited by at least two of the known H_2-receptor antagonists
c) The effect must *not* be mimicked by selective H_1-receptor agonists and *not* be competitively inhibited by at least two of the known H_1-receptor antagonists of different structure.

So far, all these criteria have not been satisfied in the experiments on the occurrence of H_2-receptor with relaxant activity, on the guinea pig ileum. In view, not only of the occurrence and the distribution along the digestive tract of the well-established two classes of histamine receptor (H_1 predominant and mediating contraction; H_2 usually mediating relaxation, but in some cases also contraction), but also of the possibility of the existence of subtypes of these different receptors (BERTACCINI and CORUZZI 1981) and finally of the availability of rather selective agonists and antagonists of H_1- and H_2-receptors, it is obvious that most of the early results concerning the actions of histamine on gastrointestinal smooth muscle will have to be reconsidered.

The problem of a possible physiologic role of histamine in the regulation of gastrointestinal motility, is still open (BERTACCINI et al. 1980); we do not know how many endogenous substances are involved in gut motility and what could be the role of hormonal, neural, vascular, or metabolic influences on the effect of histamine. The in vitro experiments demonstrate that histamine may affect intestinal muscle even in very small amounts, whereas the in vivo studies are not sufficiently reliable because of a number of indirect, systemic actions which can mask the effect of histamine on gut motility. Summing up, it is most probable that histamine does not have a primary role in peristalsis, as it has in gastric secretion. However, the possibility that the amine may contribute to the regulation of gastrointestinal motility cannot be excluded, even if direct evidence for such a role is still lacking.

References

Ambache N, Killick SW, Zar AM (1973) Antagonism by burimamide of inhibitions induced by histamine in plexus-containing longitudinal muscle preparations from guinea pig ileum. Br J Pharmacol 48:362P–363P

Arunlakshana O, Schild HO (1959) Some quantitative uses of drug antagonists. Br J Pharmacol 14:48–58

Ash ASF, Schild HO (1966) Receptors mediating some actions of histamine. Br J Pharmacol 27:427–439

Bailey RJ, Sullivan SN, MacDougall BRD, Williams R (1976) Effect of cimetidine on lower oesophageal sphincter. Br Med J 2:678

Bareicha I, Rocha e Silva M (1975) Occurrence of H_2-receptors for histamine in the guinea-pig intestine. Biochem Pharmacol 24:1215–1219

Bareicha I, Rocha e Silva M (1976) H_1- and H_2-receptors for histamine in the ileum of the guinea pig. Gen Pharmacol 7:103–106

Beleslin DB, Samardzic R (1978) The effect of muscarine on cholinoceptive neurones subserving the peristaltic reflex of guinea pig isolated ileum. Neuropharmacology 17:793–798

Bertaccini G (1978a) Fisiologia e farmacologia dei recettori istaminergici. In: Lucchelli PE (ed) Cimetidina – farmacologia e clinica. Smith Kline & French, Milan, pp 39–46

Bertaccini G (1978b) Histamine H_2-receptors and gastric secretion. In: Grossman M, Speranza V, Basso N, Lezoche E (eds) Gastrointestinal hormones and pathology of the digestive system. Plenum, New York, pp 69–74

Bertaccini G, Coruzzi G (1981) Evidence for and against heterogeneity in the histamine H_2-receptor population. Pharmacology 23:1–13

Bertaccini G, Dobrilla G (1980) Histamine H_2-receptor antagonists: old and new generation. Ital J Gastroenterol 12:297–302

Bertaccini G, Impicciatore M, Molina E, Zappia L (1974) Action of bombesin on human gastrointestinal motility. Rend Gastroenterol 6:45–51

Bertaccini G, Coruzzi G, Molina E, Chiavarini M (1977) Action of histamine and related compounds on the pyloric sphincter of the rat. Rend Gastroenterol 9:163–168
Bertaccini G, Coruzzi G, Zappia L (1979a) Azione del TRH sulla motilità gastrointestinale *in vitro*. Ateneo Parmense [Acta Biomed] 50:149–152
Bertaccini G, Molina E, Bobbio P, Foggi E (1981b) Ranitidine increases lower oesophageal sphincter pressure in man. Ital J Gastroenterol 13:149–150
Bertaccini G, Molina E, Zappia L, Zseli J (1979b) Histamine receptors in the guinea pig ileum. Naunyn Schmiedebergs Arch Pharmacol 309:65–68
Bertaccini G, Zappia L, Molina E (1979c) "In vitro" duodenal muscle in the pharmacological study of natural compounds. Scand J Gastroenterol [Suppl 54] 14:87–93
Bertaccini G, Scarpignato C, Coruzzi G (1980) Histamine receptors and gastrointestinal motility. In: Torsoli A, Lucchelli PE, Brimblecombe RW (eds) European symposium of further experience with H_2-receptor antagonists in peptic ulcer disease and progress in histamine research. Excerpta Medica, Amsterdam London New York, pp 251–261
Bertaccini G, Coruzzi G, Scarpignato C (1981a) Exogenous and endogenous compounds which affect the contractility of the lower esophageal sphincter (LES). In: Stipa S, Belsey RHR, Moraldi A (eds) Medical and surgical problems of the esophagus. Academic, London, pp 22–29
Bertaccini G, Zappia L (1981) Histamine receptors in the guinea pig duodenum. J Pharm Pharmacol 33:590–593
Black JW, Duncan WAM, Durant CJ, Ganellin CR, Parsons EM (1972) Definition and antagonism of histamine H_2-receptors. Nature 236:385–390
Botting JH (1975) Sensitivity of neonatal rabbit ileum to histamine. Br J Pharmacol 53:428–429
Brown FC, Dubois A, Castell DO (1978)Histaminergic pharmacology of primate lower esophageal sphincter. Am J Physiol 235:E42–E46
Brownlee G, Harry J (1963) Some pharmacological properties of the circular and longitudinal muscle strips from the guinea-pig isolated ileum. Br J Pharmacol 21:544–554
Bucknell A, Whitney B (1964) A preliminary investigation on the pharmacology of the human isolated taenia coli preparation. Br J Pharmacol 23:164–175
Burland W, Alison Simkins M (eds) (1977) Cimetidine. Excerpta Medica, Amsterdam London New York, pp 1–392
Burleigh DE (1979) The effects of drugs and electrical field stimulation on the human lower esophageal sphincter. Arch Int Pharmacodyn Ther 240:169–176
Castell DO, Harris LD (1970) Hormonal control of gastroesophageal sphincter strength. N Engl J Med 282:886–889
Chand N, De Roth L (1978) Ocurrence of H_2-inhibitory histamine receptors in chicken ileum. Eur J Pharmacol 52:143–145
Chand N, Eyre P (1976) The pharmacology of anaphylaxis in the chicken intestine. Br J Pharmacol 57:399–408
Chand N, Eyre P (1977) Atypical (relaxant) response to histamine in cat bronchus. Agents Actions 7:183–190
Chang RSL, Tran VT, Snyder SH (1979) Characteristic of histamine H_1 receptors in peripheral tissues labeled with [^{3}H]mepyramine. J Pharmacol Exp Ther 209:437–442
Cohen S, Snape WJ (1975) Action of metiamide on the lower esophageal sphincter. Gastroenterology 69:911–919
Coruzzi G, Bertaccini G (1982) Histamine receptors in the lower esophageal sphincter (LES). Agents and Actions 12:1–5
Creutzfeldt W (ed) (1978) Cimetidine. Excerpta Medica, Amsterdam London New York, pp 1–319
Dai S (1976) A study of the actions of histamine on the isolated rat heart. Clin Exp Pharmacol Physiol 3:359–367
Daniel E (1968) Pharmacology of the gastrointestinal tract. In: Code CF (ed) Handbook of physiology, vol IV. American Physiological Society, Washington DC; pp 2267–2324
De Carle DJ, Glover WE (1975) Independence of gastrin and histamine receptors in the lower oesophageal sphincter of the monkey and possum. J Physiol (Lond) 245:78P–79P
De Carle DJ, Brody MJ, Christensen J (1976) Histamine receptors in esophageal smooth muscle of the opossum. Gastroenterology 70:1071–1075

Dubois A, Hamilton B, Castell DO (1977) Histamine H_2 receptor involved in the regulation of gastric emptying. Gastroenterology 72:A1051
Dubois A, Nompleggi D, Myers L, Castell DO (1978) Histamine H_2 receptor stimulation increases gastric emptying. Gastroenterology 74:A1028
Durant GJ, Duncan WAM, Ganellin CR, Parsons ME, Blakemore RC, Rasmussen AC (1978) Impromidine is a very potent and specific agonist for histamine H_2 receptors. Nature 276:403–404
Ercan ZS, Türker RK (1977) Histamine receptors in the isolated rat stomach fundus and rabbit aortic strips. Pharmacology 15:118–126
Fara JW, Berkowitz JM (1978) Effects of histamine and gastrointestinal hormones on dog antral smooth muscle in vitro. Scand J Gastroenterol [Suppl 49] 13:60
Fasth S, Hulten L, Jahnberg T, Martinson J (1975) Comparative studies on the effects of bradykinin and vagal stimulation on motility in the stomach and colon. Acta Physiol Scand 93:77–84
Faulk D, Anuras S, Christensen J (1977) The two muscle layers in duodenum differ in response to parasympathomimetic drugs, histamine, and substance P. Gastroenterology 72:A1057
Fishlock DJ, Parks AG (1963) A study of human colonic muscle in vitro. Br Med J 2:666–667
Fjalland B (1979) Evidence for the existence of another type of histamine H_2-receptor in guinea-pig ileum. J Pharm Pharmacol 31:50–51
Fleisch JH, Calkins OJ (1976) Comparison of drug-induced responses of rabbit trachea and bronchus. J Appl Physiol 41:62–66
Fleisch JH, Krzan MC, Titus E (1973) Pharmacologic receptor activity of rabbit aorta effect of dithiothreitol and N-ethylmaleimide. Circ Res 33:284–290
Gerner T, Haffner JFW, Norstein J (1979) The effect of mepyramine and cimetidine on the motor responses to histamine, cholecystokinin and gastrin in the fundus and antrum of isolated guinea pig stomachs. Scand J Gastroenterol 14:65–72
Glover WE (1979) Effect of dithiothreitol on histamine receptors in rabbit colon and guinea-pig ileum. Clin Exp Pharmacol Physiol 6:151–157
Goyal RK, Rattan S (1978) Neurohumoral, hormonal, and drug receptors for the lower esophageal sphincter. Gastroenterology 74:598–619
Haas HL, Bucher UM (1975) Histamine H_2-receptors on single central neurones. Nature 255:634–635
Hill SJ, Young JM, Marrian DH (1977) Specific binding of ^{3}H-mepyramine to histamine H_1 receptors in intestinal smooth muscle. Nature 270:361–362
Hirschowitz BI (1979) H_2 histamine receptors. Annu Rev Pharmacol Toxicol 19:203–244
Kenakin TP, Krueger CA, Cook DA (1974) Temperature-dependent interconversion of histamine H_1 and H_2 receptors in guinea pig ileum. Nature 252:54–55
Konturek SJ, Siebers R (1979) Role of histamine H_1 and H_2 receptors in the myoelectric activity of the small bowel. Gastroenterology 76:A1174
Konturek SJ, Siebers R (1980) Role of histamine H_1- and H_2-receptors in myoelectric activity of small bowel in the dog. Am J Physiol 238:G50–G56
Kravitz JJ, Snape WJ Jr, Cohen S (1978) Effect of histamine and histamine antagonists on human lower esophageal sphincter function. Gastroenterology 74:435–440
Labrid C, Dureng G, Duchenne-Marullaz P, Moleyre J (1977) Dualist or pseudo-dualist interactions of mepyramine, diphenhydramine, and eprozinol with histamine at H_2-receptors. Jpn J Pharmacol 27:491–500
Lucchelli PE (ed) (1978) Cimetidina. Smith Kline & French, Milan, pp 5–312
McCallum RW, Li Calzi LK, Biancani P (1979) Histamine receptors in the feline pylorus. Clin Res 27:455A
Misiewicz JJ, Holdstock DJ, Waller L (1967) Motor responses of the human alimentary tract to near-maximal infusions of pentagastrin. Gut 8:463–469
Misiewicz JJ, Waller SL, Anthony PP, Gummer JWP (1969) Achalasia of the cardia: pharmacology and histopathology of isolated cardiac sphincter muscle from patients with and without achalasia. Q J Med 38:17–30
Ohga A, Taneike T (1978) H_1- and H_2-receptors in the smooth muscle of the ruminant stomach. Br J Pharmacol 62:333–337

Ohmura I (1976) Action mechanisms of the contracting drugs, K, acetylcholine, histamine, and Ba and of the antispasmodics, isoproterenol, and papaverine in the isolated guinea pig ileum, particularly in relation to Ca. Folia Pharmacol Jpn 72:201–210
Parrot JL, Thouvenot J (1966) Action de l'histamine sur les muscles lisses. In: Rocha e Silva (ed) Histamine. Its chemistry, metabolism, and physiological and pharmacological actions. Springer, Berlin Heidelberg New York (Handbook of experimental pharmacology, vol XVIII/1, pp 202–224)
Parsons ME (1977) The antagonism of histamine H_2-receptors in vitro and in vivo with particular reference to the actions of cimetidine. In: Burland WL, Alison Simkins M (eds) Cimetidine. Excerpta Medica, Amsterdam London New York, pp 13–20
Paton WDM, Vizi ES (1969) The inhibitory action of noradrenaline and adrenaline on acetylcholine output by guinea-pig ileum longitudinal muscle strip. Br J Pharmacol 35:10–29
Rattan S, Goyal RK (1978) Effects of histamine on the lower esophageal sphincter *in vivo:* evidence for action at three different sites. J Pharmacol Exp Ther 204:334–342
Reinhardt D, Ritter E, Butzheinen R, Schümann HJ (1979) Relationship between histamine-induced changes of cyclic AMP and mechanical activity on smooth muscle preparations of the guinea pig ileum and the rabbit mesenteric artery. Agents Actions 9:155–162
Rocha e Silva M (ed) (1966) Histamine. Its chemistry, metabolism, and physiological and pharmacological agents. Handbook of experimental pharmacology, vol XVIII/1. Springer, Berlin Heidelberg New York, pp 1–991
Rocha e Silva M (ed) (1978) Histamine II and anti-histaminics. Handbook of experimental pharmacology, vol XVIII/2. Springer, Berlin Heidelberg New York, pp 1–700
Roesch W, Lux G, Schittenhelm W, Demling L (1976) Stimulation of lower esophageal sphincter pressure (LES) by cimetidine. A double blind study. Acta hepatogastroenterology (Stuttg) 23:423–425
Sakai K (1979) A pharmacological analysis of the contractile action of histamine upon the ileal region of the isolated blood-perfused small intestine of the rat. Br J Pharmacol 67:587–590
Sakai K, Shiraki Y, Tatsumi T, Tsuji K (1979) The actions of 5-hydroxytryptamine and histamine on the isolated ileum of the tree shrew (*Tupaia glis*). Br J Pharmacol 66:405–408
Scarpignato C, Coruzzi G, Bertaccini G (1981) Effect of histamine and related compounds on gastric emptying of the rat. Pharmacology 23:185–191
Schoetz DJ, Wise WE, LaMorte WW, Bickett DH, Williams LF (1978) Histamine receptors in the primate gallbladder. Gastroenterology 74:A1090
Takayanagi I, Hongo T, Kasuya Y (1977) Difference in the mechanisms by which acetylcholine and histamine interact with Ca^{2+} to contract the rabbit taenia coli. J Pharm Pharmacol 29:775–776
Takayanagi I, Kasuya Y (1977) Effects of some drugs on the circular muscle of the isolated lower oesophagus. J Pharm Pharmacol 29:559–560
Tucker HJ, Snape WJ (1979) Comparison of proximal and distal colonic muscle of the rabbit. Am J Physiol 237:E383–E388
Waldman DB, Zfass AM, Makhlouf GM (1977) Stimulatory (H_1) and inhibitory (H_2) histamine receptors in gallbladder muscle. Gastroenterology 72:932–936
Wastell C, Lance P (eds) (1978) Cimetidine. Churchill Livingstone, Edinburgh London, pp 1–302
Wood CJ, Alison Simkins M (eds) (1973) International symposium on histamine H_2-receptor antagonists. Smith Kline & French, Welwyn Garden City, pp 1–412
Yates JC, Schofield B, Roth SH (1978) Acid secretion and motility of isolated mammalian gastric mucosa and attached muscularis externa. Am J Physiol 234:E319–E326

CHAPTER 4

Acidic Lipids: Prostaglandins

A. Bennett and G. J. Sanger

A. Introduction

Many studies on gastrointestinal motility have dealt mainly with prostaglandins (PGs) of the E and F series (PGE and PGF) which until recently were thought to be the major PGs formed by tissues. Reviews of this work include Bennett and Fleshler (1970), Bennett (1972, 1973, 1976a, b, 1977), Wilson (1972), Main (1973), Waller (1973), Karim and Ganesan (1974), and Robert (1974). Other specialist reviews concerning PGs and the gut are referred to subsequently. PGs are formed from fatty acids which are released mainly from phospholipids of cell membranes. Metabolism by cyclooxygenase of the released precursors, of which arachidonic acid is the most abundant, can result in various PGs and related cyclic substances collectively known as prostanoids (Fig. 1). In addition, metabolism of arachidonic acid by lipoxygenase produces various straight-chain derivatives including a new group of compounds called leukotrienes of which slow-reacting substance of anaphylaxis (SRS-A) is a constituent (Samuelsson et al. 1979; Morris et al. 1980; Fig. 1). Most of the work described in this chapter concerns the prostanoids. Little is known about the formation of lipoxygenase products in the gut, but SRS-A potently contracts the longitudinal muscle of guinea-pig isolated ileum (Piper and Seale 1978).

PG endoperoxides, prostacyclin (PGI_2) and, in particular, thromboxane A_2 (TxA_2) are chemically unstable, and this hampers investigations and probably

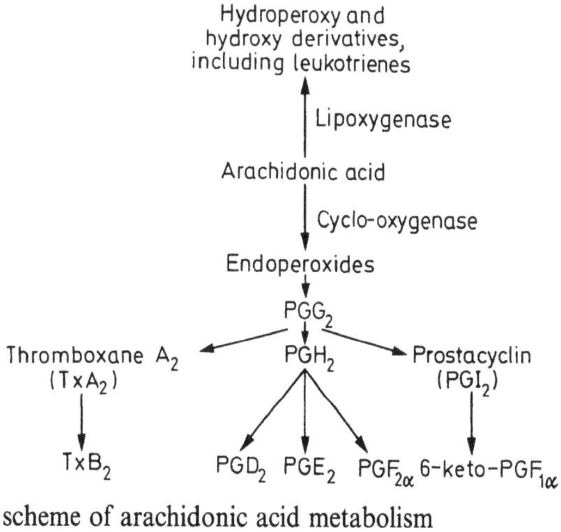

Fig. 1. Simplified scheme of arachidonic acid metabolism

underestimates their potency. To help overcome the problem, more stable analogues can be used, such as the epoxymethano analogues of PGH_2 (BUNDY 1975). However, it cannot be presumed that these substances act on the same receptors as the parent compound. There is some confusion on the extent to which epoxymethano PGH_2 analogues stimulate PGH_2 receptors or TxA_2 receptors (COLEMAN et al. 1980a) or act by increasing prostanoid synthesis (MALMSTEN 1977; SANGER et al. 1981). Such factors probably vary with the species and tissues studied.

Measurement of prostanoid synthesis may involve bioassay, chromatography, and radioimmunoassay. However, unless there is formal identification with gas chromatography–mass spectrometry, it is better to use the term PG-like material (PG-lm) as in the following text, or to use other appropriate terms.

B. Occurrence, Formation, Release, and Degradation of Prostanoids

I. Occurrence

PGE and PGF_{α} compounds occur in a wide variety of gastrointestinal tissues (see BENNETT 1976a), but some aspects of their distribution have been determined only in the rat (COLLIER 1974) and in humans (BENNETT et al. 1968c, 1977b). The latter authors extracted PG-lm (assayed on rat gastric fundus which is most sensitive to PGE compounds) from different regions of human gut muscle and mucosa, and from sections cut through the gut wall. More PG-lm occurred in mucosal extracts of stomach or terminal ileum than in the muscle, whereas the reverse was found in the colon.

More recently, PGD_2, 6-keto-$PGF_{1\alpha}$ and TxB_2 have been found in extracts of gut tissue from various animals (PACE-ASCIAK and WOLFE 1971; PACE-ASCIAK 1976; ALI et al. 1977; BENNETT et al. 1977b; SUN et al. 1977; DUPONT et al. 1978; KNAPP et al. 1978; MONCADA et al. 1978b; LE DUC and NEEDLEMAN 1980), and 6-keto-$PGF_{1\alpha}$ occurs in extracts of human rectal mucosa (SINZINGER et al. 1978). Incubation of microsomal pellets of dog gastrointestinal muscle with ^{14}C-arachidonic acid formed mainly 6-keto-$PGF_{1\alpha}$ and PGE_2, whereas when ^{14}C-PGH_2 was the substrate only 6-keto-$PGF_{1\alpha}$ was formed (LE DUC and NEEDLEMAN 1980). In contrast the mucosa formed low amounts of 6-keto-$PGF_{1\alpha}$, PGE_2, $PGF_{2\alpha}$, and TxB_2 with ^{14}C-arachidonic acid incubation, and 6-keto-$PGF_{1\alpha}$, TxB_2, and 12-hydroxyheptadecatrienoic acid on incubation with ^{14}C-PGH_2. No regional differences were found in the type of prostanoid formed.

We have now analysed the prostanoids extracted from homogenates of human gut muscle or mucosa, using gas chromatography–mass spectrometry (GC–MS) (BENNETT et al. 1980, 1981). Following homogenisation in Krebs solution to allow new prostanoid formation from released endogenous precursors, the only prostanoids detected were those formed from arachidonic acid. If derivatives of 8,11,14-eicosatrienoic acid or 5,8,11,14,17-eicosapentaenoic acid were present, their amounts were probably at most 80 ng recovered/g tissue wet weight.

All the extracts of muscle and mucosa contained arachidonic acid, 6-keto-$PGF_{1\alpha}$ and TxB_2. With gastric tissue, PGE_2 or 12-HETE were also detected in two of three specimens of muscle, whereas in the mucosa PGE_2, $PGF_{2\alpha}$ or 12-hydroxyeicosatetraenoic acid (12-HETE) were found in two of the three specimens and PGD_2 occurred in one. The muscle from terminal ileum was unusual because 6-keto-$PGF_{1\alpha}$ and TxB_2 were the only detected eicosanoids (a term which includes lipoxygenase products) except that 12-HETE was found in one of three specimens. With ileal mucosa, in contrast, 12-HETE was detected in all three specimens whereas PGE_2 and $PGF_{2\alpha}$ occurred in extracts of two specimens and PGD_2 in one of these. In the four specimens of sigmoid colon examined, PGE_2 and 12-HETE occurred in all extracts of the muscle, and $PGF_{2\alpha}$ occurred in one. 12-HETE was found in all specimens of colonic mucosa, whereas PGD_2, PGE_2 or $PGF_{2\alpha}$ occurred in two specimens each.

Although human gut muscle and mucosa seem to produce PGI_2 and TxA_2, as indicated by identification of their degradation compounds 6-keto-$PGF_{1\alpha}$, and TxB_2, the extent to which these arise from blood vessels and platelets respectively is not known. The consistent presence of the lipoxygenase product 12-HETE in the colon, compared with its occasional presence in extracts of stomach or terminal ileum, suggests synthesis by gut tissues rather than only by platelets. Thus there may be regional differences in the contributions of lipoxygenase products to gastrointestinal functions or disorders. A similar relationship may also apply to PGD_2, PGE_2, and $PGF_{2\alpha}$ which were often detected in gut mucosa but rarely in the muscle, particularly of the terminal ileum.

Using radioimmunoassay, PESKAR et al. (1980) found that incubates of the microsomal fraction or whole-cell preparations of human gastric mucosa formed more PGE_2 than 6-keto-$PGF_{1\alpha}$. Similarly, after subcutaneous injection of pentagastrin, gastric juice contained more PGE_2 than 6-keto-$PGF_{1\alpha}$.This contrasts with the mass spectrometric results of BENNETT et al. (1977b), possibly because of different methodology. Our present GC–MS results are only semiquantitative and, in most tissues where PGE_2 was found, we do not know whether its amount differed from that of 6-keto-$PGF_{1\alpha}$. Apart from the contribution of blood vessels and platelets to the 6-keto-$PGF_{1\alpha}$, TxB_2, and 12-HETE extracted, other factors may alter the amounts of various eicosanoids by affecting arachidonic acid metabolism. These include the disease for which the specimens were resected, medication, diet, anaesthesia, muscle activity, and endogenous substances which affect prostanoid synthesis or inactivation. The relative importance of the different pathways for arachidonic acid metabolism in the gut is therefore still far from clear. Nevertheless, the wide distribution of eicosanoids makes them candidates for numerous physiological and pathophysiological processes.

II. Formation and Release

It seems that PGs are not stored in tissues, but are synthesised and released when required in response to stimuli such as nerve excitation (COCEANI et al. 1967; BENNETT et al. 1967), gentle mechanical trauma such as stretch or compression (BENNETT et al. 1967, 1977b; COLLIER 1974), and chemical irritants (COLLIER et al. 1975). Damage during isolation of tissues may therefore cause excessive and inappropriate PG synthesis, and studies with such tissues might reflect diseases involving locally increased PG synthesis (BENNETT 1977). Release of PG-lm by stretching or distension does not seem to involve nerves, as shown by release from guinea-pig ileum in the presence of tetrodotoxin (TAKAI et al. 1974; YAGASAKI et al. 1974). Futhermore, release of PG-lm from distended rat stomach was not affected by the 5-hydroxytryptamine antagonist methysergide (BENNETT et al. 1967).

TONNESEN et al. (1974) found that the amount of PG-lm in human gastric juice may follow a circadian rhythm in phase with that of gastric acid secretion, PGE-lm being high at midnight, low during the early morning and high at mid-day. Release of PG-lm associated with cholinergic nerve activity occurs in rat stomach and small intestine (BENNETT et al. 1967; COCEANI et al. 1967; WOLFE et al. 1967; RADMANOVIĆ 1968). PG-lm is also released from guinea-pig ileum by high frequency electrical transmural nerve stimulation of intrinsic nerves (BOTTING and SALZMANN 1974). Release of PG-lm in response to sympathetic nerve stimulation may vary with the tissue or species. Thus, COCEANI et al. (1967) and FERREIRA et al. (1976) found no increase in PG-lm with sympathetic stimulation in rat stomach or rabbit jejunum, but PG-lm was released from guinea-pig ileum in response to noradrenaline (BOTTING 1977). PGs released in response to specific autonomic nerve stimuli may serve as feedback modulators which increase or reduce the evoked response (see Sect. D).

Hypertonic solutions stimulate PG release from rat gastric mucosa (ASSOULINE et al. 1977; KNAPP et al. 1977, 1978). The authors suggest that: (i) hypertonic solutions may be useful as an alternative approach to administration of PG analogues for gastric "cytoprotection;" (ii) PG release may partly explain the marked effects of highly osmolar gastric contents on secretion, motility and blood flow in various regions of the gut; and (iii) PGs may play a role in the hyperosmolar dumping syndrome.

Finally, prostanoid synthesis may be controlled by endogenous inhibitors of cyclooxygenase (COOK and LANDS 1976; SAEED et al. 1977). In canine gastrointestinal mucosa, synthesis of prostanoids from microsomal fractions of muscle was inhibited by mixing with microsomal fractions of mucosa, which form only low amounts of prostanoids on incubation with ^{14}C-arachidonic acid (LE DUC and NEEDLEMAN 1980). The mucosal cyclooxygenase inhibitor was found to be a fatty acid which was inactive with intact tissue.

III. Degradation

PG degradation by the gut has been studied less extensively than PG synthesis. Little information is available concerning PG metabolism in gut muscle, but polyphloretin phosphate may contract rat stomach muscle by inhibiting PG-15-hydroxydehydrogenase, the enzyme mainly responsible for PG inactivation (GANESAN and KARIM 1973). In rabbit stomach fundus and antrum muscle, SPENNEY (1979) found two PG-metabolising enzymes, PG-15-hydroxydehydrogenase and Δ^{13}-reductase.

PESKAR and PESKAR (1976) found three PG-metabolising enzymes (PG-15-hydroxydehydrogenase, Δ^{13}-reductase and 9-keto-reductase, in decreasing order of their specific activities) in the 100,000 *g* supernatant of human homogenised gastric fundus mucosa. However, the autors point out that this does not necessarily reflect their activity in vivo, since high enzyme activity may occour within a small compartment of the tissue. 9-keto-reductase could also be of great importance in vivo since it can convert PGE compounds to PGF_α compounds, and so change the type of biological activity in some tissues (see Sect. C).

In a later study, PESKAR (1978) found the same three types of enzyme in the mucosa of human oesophagus, gastric fundus, corpus and antrum, and duodenum, with similar specific activities in the various tissues. Similar unpublished results were reported for colonic and rectal mucosa. Thus mucosa throughout the human gut seems able to metabolise PGs. In contrast, rat stomach pyloric but not fundic homogenates contained PG-15-hydroxydehydrogenase and Δ^{13}-reductase (PACE-ASCIAK 1972). SPENNEY (1979) found both PG-15-hydroxydehydrogenase and Δ^{13}-reductase in rabbit stomach fundus and antrum mucosa, and less in the muscle; the activity of Δ^{13}-reductase was greater in all tissues. HOULT and MOORE (1980) recently suggested that PG-synthesising and PG-metabolising enzymes are coupled in gastrointestinal and other tissues, and that the regulation of PG activity may be under sensitive metabolic control. They produced evidence for a reduced PG-metabolising activity in certain diseases associated with increased synthesis of PG-lm.

C. Actions of Prostanoids on the Tone and Reactivity of Isolated Gastrointestinal Muscle

Most studies have concerned PGE and PGF compounds. In general, both types of compound cause contraction of gastrointestinal longitudinal muscle, whereas in circular muscle, PGF compounds usually cause contraction and PGE compounds usually cause relaxation (BENNETT and FLESHLER 1970). In addition, human isolated internal anal sphincter contracted to $PGF_{2\alpha}$ and relaxed to PGE_2 (BURLEIGH et al. 1979), whereas the longitudinal muscle from foetal small and large intestine usually contracted to PGE_2 or $PGF_{2\alpha}$ (HART 1974).

PGD_2 contracts the longitudinal muscle of rat or human stomach, rabbit jejunum and guinea-pig intestine (HORTON and JONES 1974; HAMBERG et al. 1975; BENNETT et al. 1981; BENNETT and SANGER 1980), and the circular muscle of guinea-pig colon (BENNETT and SANGER 1978; BENNETT et al. 1980c). PGG_2, PGH_2 and its epoxymethano analogues, PGI_2, 6-keto-$PGF_{1\alpha}$, 6,15-diketo-$PGF_{1\alpha}$, TxA_2-like material or TxB_2 contract the longitudinal muscle of rat stomach, rat or gerbil colon, guinea-pig ileum and chick rectum (HAMBERG et al. 1975; BUNTING et al. 1976; BOOT et al. 1977; CHIJIMATSU et al. 1977; GORMAN et al. 1977; BENNETT et al. 1978, 1980b). However in almost all of these tissues from laboratory animals (in contrast with human tissue, see later) PGE_2 seems to be the most potent prostanoid, although $PGF_{2\alpha}$, the PG endoperoxides or TxA_2 may have considerable potency in some tissues. For example, compared with PGE_2 in rat stomach, PGG_2 or PGH_2 were approximately 2–3 times, and TxA_2 was approximately 10 times, less potent (BUNTING et al. 1976). In guinea-pig ileum, epoxymethano analogues of PGH_2 were about 100–400 times less active than PGE_2 (CHIJIMATSU et al. 1977; BENNETT et al. 1978). PGI_2 seems less potent than many other prostanoids, but perhaps this is partly due to its instability at physiological pH. The stable analogue 6β-PGI_1 is less potent than PGI_2 on rat gastrointestinal and cardiovascular systems, but its efficacy may be increased in conditions where stability is important (WHITTLE et al. 1978). Finally, it has been suggested that in at least some tissues, the epoxymethano analogues act not on PGH_2 receptors but behave like TxA_2 (COLEMAN et al. 1980a). In other tissues, responses to the epoxymethano analogues of PGH_2 may be selectively reduced with indomethacin (MALMSTEN 1977; SANGER et al. 1981), but there is no similar evidence in experiments on gastrointestinal tissues (BENNETT et al. 1980, BENNETT et al. 1981).

We have recently examined the actions of several prostanoids on guinea-pig and human gastrointestinal muscle. The studies on guinea-pig intestinal circular muscle (SANGER and BENNETT 1980) confirm our earlier findings (BENNETT et al. 1968a; FLESHLER and BENNETT 1969; BENNETT and SANGER 1978), that in the colon PGE_2 causes muscle relaxation whereas $PGF_{2\alpha}$ or PGD_2 are excitatory. Contraction also occurred with an epoxymethano analogue of PGH_2 (U-46619), PGI_2 or 6-keto-$PGF_{1\alpha}$, but $PGF_{2\alpha}$ was the most potent. TxB_2 had no effect (0.001–10 µg/ml). The PG antagonist SC-19220 (SANNER 1969) reduced the muscle tone, but unmasked inhibitory effects of PGD_2, U-46619 or PGI_2 which were shown as a reduction of acetylcholine-induced contraction. These prostanoids therefore seem to exert a predominant excitatory effect which overshadows an inhibitory action in the same tissue.

The circular muscle of guinea-pig isolated ileum is unusual because it has no tone and is almost unaffected by acetylcholine. It does not contract to most of the prostanoids tested, although U-46619 sometimes caused a very small contraction. However, PGD_2, PGE_2 or PGI_2 reduced submaximal contractions to KCl, with PGE_2 being the most potent. U-46619 had a variable effect on KCl-induced contraction whereas $PGF_{2\alpha}$, 6-keto-$PGF_{1\alpha}$ or TxB_2 produced no significant change. Our results therefore show differences of circular muscle responses to prostanoids in guinea-pig ileum and colon: inhibition predominates in the ileum whereas both inhibitory and excitatory effects occur in the colon.

In the longitudinal muscle of human isolated stomach, terminal ileum or sigmoid colon (taenia), PGD_2, PGE_2, $PGF_{2\alpha}$ or U-46619 caused dose-dependent contraction (BENNETT and SANGER 1980; BENNETT et al. 1980a, 1981). These prostanoids were usually most potent in the stomach and least potent in the colon, possibly reflecting regional differences in gastrointestinal motility. U-46619 was the most potent excitatory prostanoid in all tissues, causing contraction of the stomach longitudinal muscle in concentrations as low as 0.0001–1 ng/ml; PGE_2 caused contraction in concentrations as low as 0.5–10 ng/ml. In contrast, PGI_2 caused relaxation in stomach and colon, but often weakly contracted strips of terminal ileum. 6-keto-$PGF_{1\alpha}$, 6,15-diketo-$PGF_{1\alpha}$ or TxB_2 usually had a weak and variable action on these tissues. The actions of prostanoids on the longitudinal muscle of human isolated gut therefore differ in some ways from those previously described with laboratory animals. PGI_2 can potently relax human muscle from some regions, and the most potent excitatory prostanoid was U-46619 instead of PGE_2.

In circular muscle strips of human isolated stomach or sigmoid colon, U-46619 was again the most potent agonist. Gastric contractions occurred with concentrations as low as 0.1–1 ng/ml, but colonic contractions which occurred with concentrations as low as 10 ng/ml were usually weak and not dose-dependent. PGD_2, $PGF_{2\alpha}$ or TxB_2 usually contracted the circular muscle from either region, but PGI_2 consistently, and with approximately equal potency, relaxed stomach and colon.

PGE_2 relaxed or contracted gastric circular muscle, possibly depending on the region of stomach studied, although BENNETT et al. (1968c) found that PGE_2 relaxed strips from the body or antrum. In the colon PGE_2 usually caused relaxation, but 6-keto-$PGF_{1\alpha}$ or 6,15-diketo-$PGF_{1\alpha}$ had no effect in either tissue (BENNETT et al. 1981).

Since PGI_2 consistently relaxed the human gastric and colonic muscles, we looked for possible interactions between excitatory prostanoids and PGI_2. With strips of stomach *longitudinal* muscle, sodium PGI_2 1 μg/ml lowered the tone, and this may explain why contractions to U-46619 or acetylcholine tended to increase slightly. In contrast, PGI_2 reduced submaximal contractions to PGE_2 or $PGF_{2\alpha}$ (BENNETT and SANGER 1980). However, in three specimens of stomach *circular* muscle, submaximal contractions to U-46619, but not acetylcholine, were reduced with PGI_2 1 μg/ml, so that the type of excitatory prostanoid affected by PGI_2 may vary with the muscle layer. PGI_2 was not tested against $PGF_{2\alpha}$ which was less potent and consistent than U-46619.

Isolated gastrointestinal *longitudinal* muscle from several species possesses tone which can be reduced by drugs which inhibit PG action (BENNETT and POSNER 1971) or synthesis (DAVISON et al. 1972; FERREIRA et al. 1972; BOTTING and SALZMANN 1974; BENNETT et al. 1975a; FRANKHUIJZEN and BONTA 1975; STOCKLEY and BENNETT 1976; BENNETT and STOCKLEY 1977; BURLEIGH 1977; BENNETT et al. 1980c). Isolated *circular* muscle tone and spontaneous activity is usually increased by inhibitors of PG synthesis (BENNETT et al. 1975a; STOCKLEY and BENNETT 1976; BENNETT and STOCKLEY 1977; BENNETT et al. 1980c). Similarly, indomethacin increased the electrical activity of human isolated colonic circular muscle, but slightly reduced the activity of the taenia (KIRK and DUTHIE 1977). Inhibitors of PG synthesis can correspondingly affect tissue contractions to various agonists (BENNETT 1977).

These findings are part of the considerable evidence that PGs contribute to the control of tone and responses in isolated gut muscle. The extent to which PGs released from damaged tissue contribute to the effects on tone is not known (BENNETT 1977), but PGs may have a physiological role since, in conscious human subjects, rectally administered indomethacin increased the tone of the lower oesophageal sphincter (DILAWARI et al. 1975). This response may be due to blockade of synthesis of inhibitory prostanoids. Similarly, in anaesthetised guinea-pigs, the PG synthesis inhibitor 5,8,11,14-eicosatetraynoic acid (TYA) applied serosally to the ileum, reduced spontaneous intraluminal pressure changes, although there was no effect when TYA was injected into the bloodstream, perhaps owing to poor absorption or other factors limiting its availability (WILLIS et al. 1974).

D. Prostanoids and Gastrointestinal Nerves

I. Parasympathetic and Noncholinergic Excitatory Nerves

Contractions to PGE_1, PGE_2, $PGF_{1\alpha}$ or $PGF_{2\alpha}$ in longitudinal muscle from guinea-pig ileum or colon, dog stomach or colon, and occasionally human ileum or colon, are reduced with tetrodotoxin or botulinus toxin (BENNETT et al. 1968a; HARRY 1968; BENNETT and FLESHLER 1969; AKANUMA 1970; VANASIN et al. 1970;

BENNETT et al. 1975a; KOWALEWSKI and KOTEDEJ 1975; SCHULZ and CARTWRIGHT 1976). Thus PGs may stimulate interaction with excitatory (e.g. cholinergic) nerves. In guinea-pig colon, PGE compounds activate noncholinergic excitatory nerves (BENNETT and FLESHLER 1969; BENNETT et al. 1975a). Rabbit duodenum, rat ileum and some human tissues do not respond to PGE compounds by tetrodotoxin-sensitive mechanisms (MIYAZAKI et al. 1967; BENNETT et al. 1968a), and PGE compounds do not seem to act through a neural pathway in circular gut muscle (FLESHLER and BENNETT 1969; BENNETT and FLESHLER 1970; AKANUMA 1970).

There are many experiments to determine whether PGE compounds, in concentrations too low to cause muscle contraction on their own, can affect the longitudinal muscle response to acetylcholine (ACh). In some species there is no effect on ACh-induced contractions (AKANUMA 1970; GRUBB and BURKS 1974; FRANKUIJZEN and BONTA 1975), whereas in guinea-pig ileum or stomach and in rabbit ileum, contractions to ACh are increased (HARRY 1968; KADLEC et al. 1974; SUZUKI et al. 1975; ABOULAFIA et al. 1976; SCHULZ and CARTWRIGHT 1976; SANGER 1977). In the human gut, contractions to ACh may be either increased or reduced by PGE_2, depending on the concentration of PGE_2, the gut region and on the disease (BENNETT et al. 1968c; CROFTS et al. 1979). Where PGE compounds potentiate ACh-induced contractions this could be nonselective since low concentrations of PGE compounds also increase submaximal contractions to histamine, which acts directly on the muscle (ABOULAFIA et al. 1976; SCHULZ and CARTWRIGHT 1976; LAEKEMAN and HERMAN 1978). However, GRBOVIC and RADMANOVIĆ (1978) found that PGE_2 or $PGF_{2\alpha}$ potentiated contractions of guinea-pig ileum to ACh, but not to histamine or nicotine.

The evidence relating to an involvement of PGs with ACh release from nerve terminals is confusing, probably owing to experimental difficulties. With guinea-pig ileum in the presence of eserine, PGE_1 or PGE_2 had no effect on ACh overflow (measured by bioassay or gas chromatography–mass spectrometry) from the ileum (HADHÁZY et al. 1973; ILLÉS et al. 1974; BENZ and SALZMANN 1974; HEDQVIST et al. 1980), or caused an increase (TAKAI and YAGASAKI 1976; KADLEC et al. 1978). However, PGE compounds consistently reverse drug-induced inhibition of evoked ACh overflow (HALL et al. 1975; SCHULZ and CARTWRIGHT 1976; KADLEC et al. 1978; HEDQVIST et al. 1980).

Experiments with inhibitors of PG synthesis are also confusing. High concentrations of indomethacin which antagonise contractions of guinea-pig ileum to ganglion stimulants or even to ACh (BENNETT et al. 1975b; SANGER 1977), did not affect the release of ACh in the presence of eserine (BENZ and SALZMANN 1974; BOTTING and SALZMANN 1974; HAZRA 1975). Perhaps this is because eserine or the resultant excessively high concentration of ACh at the nerve junction protect against inhibition of nerve activity by indomethacin (SANGER 1977).

In other experiments on guinea-pig ileum, HALL et al. (1975) reported that 0.25 mM acetylsalicylic acid reduced ACh overflow, but this high concentration is not selective for inhibition of PG synthesis (SMITH and DAWKINS 1971). Similarly, using gas chromatography–mass spectrometry, HEDQVIST et al. (1980) found that a high (30 µM) concentration of indomethacin reduced ACh overflow. KADLEC et al. (1978) obtained a similar effect with substantially less (1 µM) indomethacin, but one difference from previous workers is their use of a modified Krebs solution (see BENNETT et al. 1975b).

Thus most experiments are consistent with the view that in guinea-pig ileum, PGE compounds can increase ACh overflow. Important factors in the lack of agreement are probably the failure to use submaximal stimuli for ACh release, and a possible protective effect of eserine against the effects of indomethacin. In other tissues the effect may be different. PGE_1 or PGE_2 (and to a lesser extent $PGF_{2\alpha}$) strongly inhibited cholinergic contractions to field stimulation in the circular muscle of dog small intestine, whereas PGE_1 was much less active in inhibiting contractions to ACh (NAKAHATA et al. 1980). PGs may therefore exert a negative feedback on ACh release in this tissue.

II. Adrenergic and Nonadrenergic Inhibitory Nerves

In rabbit isolated jejunum or ileum PGE_1 or PGE_2, but not $PGF_{2\alpha}$, usually antagonises the inhibitory response to perivascular nerve stimulation, probably by reducing noradrenaline release from nerve terminals (PERSSON and HEDQVIST 1973; HORTON 1973; ILLÉS et al. 1973; ABDEL-AZIZ 1974; ILLÉS et al. 1974; HEDQVIST and PERSSON 1975).

Similarly, in guinea-pig taenia caecum PGE_1 or PGE_2 (but not $PGF_{2\alpha}$) antagonised the response to perivascular nerve stimulation, but the effect was due to a reduction of both noradrenaline release and action (SAKATO 1975; SAKATO and SHIMO 1976; ISHII et al. 1977). With guinea-pig ileum PGE_1 or PGE_2 acted mainly by antagonising the response to noradrenaline (GINZTLER and MUSACCHIO 1974; SANGER and WATT 1978) and partly by reducing noradrenaline release (KADLEC et al. 1978; SANGER and WATT 1980).

In rat anococcygeus muscle, low concentrations of PGE_2 inhibited sympathetic motor responses, probably by reducing noradrenaline release, whereas similar concentrations of the epoxymethano PGH_2 analogue U-46619 nonselectively potentiated sympathetic responses (AL TIMIMI et al. 1978).

Nonadrenergic inhibitory nerve responses in guinea-pig isolated taenia caecum or opossum lower oesophageal sphincter were not affected by PGE_1, PGE_2, $PGF_{2\alpha}$ or indomethacin (KADLEC et al. 1974; BURNSTOCK et al. 1975; SAKATO and SHIMO 1976; DANIEL et al. 1979). However, the contractions which followed cessation of nerve stimulation could be somewhat reduced by inhibitors of PG synthesis (KADLEC et al. 1974; BURNSTOCK et al. 1975; SAKATO 1975; BENNETT and STOCKLEY 1977).

III. Other Possible Nerves and Neurotransmitters

5-Hydroxytryptamine (5-HT) is present in the myenteric plexus of guinea-pig and mouse intestine where it may act as a neurotransmitter (TAFURI and RAICK 1964; GERSHON and ROSS 1966). PGE compounds increased the electrically evoked release of 5-HT from guinea-pig ileum (KADLEC et al. 1975), but PGE_1 or PGE_2 did not release 5-HT from the rat stomach and jejunum (THOMPSON and ANGULO 1968). "Enkephalinergic" neurones have been reported to occur in the intestine of various species (ELDE et al. 1976; HUGHES et al. 1977). Met-enkephalin or leu-enkephalin nonselectively antagonised contraction of guinea-pig ileum to PGE or PGF_α compounds (JAQUES 1977; SPRUEGEL et al. 1977). The relationship between other "peptidergic" neurones (HÖKFELT et al. 1980) and prostanoids in the gut is not known.

E. Prostanoid Antagonists and Different Types of Prostanoid Receptors

The subject of PG antagonists has been reviewed by EAKINS and SANNER (1972), BENNETT (1974), SANNER (1974), SANNER and EAKINS (1976), and updated for the gut by BENNETT (1976a); all the work described concerns PGE and PGF compounds. So far there is no PG antagonist available with a potency comparable to that of other substances such as ACh, and there are no antagonists of PGE-induced relaxation of circular muscle. The actions of the available PG blockers show considerable species differences, and some are agonists in certain tissues.

We recently examined several drugs as antagonists of various prostanoids in the gut, partly to characterise the types of prostanoid receptors present (BENNETT et al. 1980b, c; SANGER and BENNETT 1980a, b). These results on rat gastric fundus longitudinal muscle, and human and guinea-pig gastrointestinal longitudinal or circular muscle, are summarised below.

In the rat fundus, all the prostanoids studied caused contraction (see Sect. C). The PG antagonist SC-19220 (SANNER 1969) reduced contractions to PGE_2 or PGI_2 and, to a lesser extent, $PGF_{2\alpha}$, 6-keto-$PGF_{1\alpha}$ or 6,15-diketo-$PGF_{1\alpha}$. In contrast, contractions to PGD_2, TxB_2, PGH_2 or its epoxymethano analogues were reduced to about the same small extent as ACh (BENNETT and POSNER 1971; BENNETT et al. 1978, 1980b).

The β-adrenoceptor stimulant trimethoquinol was reported to antagonise PGH_2-induced platelet aggregation and rabbit aorta contraction; with TxA_2 trimethoquinol was a less effective antagonist in platelets and was ineffective against aortic contractions (MACINTYRE and WILLIS 1978). We found that contractions of rat gastric fundus to PGE_1 and to all primary prostanoids derived from arachidonic acid except PGE_2, were antagonised more than contractions to ACh (BENNETT and SANGER 1979; BENNETT et al. 1980b; LACEY and SANGER 1980). PGE_1, $PGF_{2\alpha}$, and PGI_2 were also studied in the presence of propranolol which reduced the inhibitory effect of trimethoquinol (LACEY and SANGER 1980). Thus in the rat fundus, at least a major part of the antagonism by trimethoquinol seems likely to result from β-adrenoceptor stimulation. The failure of the drug to affect PGE_2 may mean that the relationship between β-adrenoceptors and PGE_2 receptors differs from that with other prostanoids.

The PG synthesis inhibitors sodium meclofenamate 1 or 2 µg/ml or indomethacin 1 µg/ml reduced rat stomach contractions to prostanoids more than those to ACh. The reduction by meclofenamate of contractions to epoxymethano analogues of PGH_2 was particularly striking, and was greater than the reduction by indomethacin (BENNETT et al. 1980b).

We concluded that the different spectra of blocking activity with SC-19220, trimethoquinol or sodium meclofenamate in the longitudinal muscle of rat gastric fundus might be explained by the presence of different types of prostanoid receptor. In particular, none of the drugs antagonised contractions to both PGE_2 and the PGH_2 analogues, and trimethoquinol reduced contractions to PGE_1 but not PGE_2. Perhaps these results indicate separate receptors for PGE_1, PGE_2, and epoxymethano analogues of PGH_2. However, trimethoquinol and meclofenamate have other well-defined actions which may be important in reducing prostanoid responses, for example β-adrenceptor stimulation and inhibition of PG synthesis respectively.

In the longitudinal muscle of guinea-pig ileum, PGE_1, PGE_2, and $PGF_{2\alpha}$ may activate similar receptors (BENNETT and POSNER 1971; ILLÉS and KNOLL 1975). However, in gastrointestinal circular muscle, receptors for PGE and PGF compounds seem to differ, since PGF compounds usually contract the circular muscle whereas PGE compounds usually cause relaxation (BENNETT and POSNER 1971). Furthermore, these authors found that PGE-induced relaxation of guinea-pig or human gastrointestinal circular muscle could not be blocked by drugs which antagonised contraction of the longitudinal muscle by PGE or PGF compounds.

In the circular muscle of guinea-pig intestine there seem to be regional differences in the distribution of prostanoid receptors (SANGER and BENNETT 1980a; see Sect. C). In the ileum there are predominantly inhibitory receptors which can be activated by PGD_2, PGE_2, PGI_2 or sometimes by U-46619. In the colon, only PGE_2 caused relaxation when no PG antagonist was used to block excitatory responses. However, in the presence of SC-19220, excitation by PGD_2, U-46619 or PGI_2 was converted to an inhibitory effect.

A regional difference in guinea-pig intestine receptors was further indicated by experiments with sodium meclofenamate (BENNETT et al. 1980c). In the ileum longitudinal muscle, contractions to PGD_2, PGE_2 or $PGF_{2\alpha}$ were antagonised with low concentrations of meclofenamate which had little effect on contractions to ACh. Only contractions of colonic longitudinal muscle to PGE_2 were substantially reduced by meclofenamate, and then only with higher concentrations of the drug: the contractions to PGD_2 or $PGF_{2\alpha}$ in either muscle layer of the colon were even less effectively inhibited. Receptors for these prostanoids which contract guinea-pig colon therefore seem less sensitive to antagonism by meclofenamate than are receptors in the ileal longitudinal muscle. If such regional differences occur in humans it may be possible to develop prostanoid antagonists which affect only a particular gastrointestinal region.

With regard to human tissue, PGI_2 relaxed gastric and colonic longitudinal and circular muscle. Receptors for PGI_2 (and PGE_2 in the circular muscle) therefore differ from those for prostanoids which cause contraction. In addition, PGI_2 antagonised gastric longitudinal muscle contractions to PGE_2 or $PGF_{2\alpha}$, without greatly affecting those to ACh or U-46619 (BENNETT and SANGER 1980; see Sect. C). This may indicate a difference between receptors for PGE_2 and $PGF_{2\alpha}$ and those for U-46619.

We have also studied the actions of fenamates on human isolated gastrointestinal muscle (BENNETT et al. 1980c). Sodium meclofenamate or flufenamate potently inhibited contraction to $PGF_{2\alpha}$,but not to PGE_2 or ACh. However, sodium mefenamate or mefenamic acid, even in high concentrations, had little effect on contractions to $PGF_{2\alpha}$ or ACh, but tended to inhibit PGE_2-induced contractions.

Thus, there are differential effects of fenamates on responses to these PGs, and the evidence indicates a difference between PGE_2 and $PGF_{2\alpha}$ receptors in human gut. However, meclofenamate shows clear species differences in its effect on rat, guinea-pig and human gastrointestinal muscle, so that the types of receptor for a particular prostanoid may vary between species. Data on other antagonists are consistent with this view (BENNETT and POSNER 1971; COLEMAN et al. 1980 b, c, d).

Recently, COLEMAN et al. (1980 b, c, d) have characterised prostanoid receptors by determining the orders of agonist potency and their sensitivity to antagonism by SC-19220. In the longitudinal muscle of guinea-pig ileum and gastric fundus, the order of potency for prostanoid-mediated contraction is PGE_2 > PGE_1 > $PGF_{2\alpha}$ > U-46619 > ICI 81008, a selective leutolytic $PGF_{2\alpha}$ analogue (COLEMAN et al. 1980 b). SC-19220 antagonised contraction of these tissues to PGE_2 or $PGF_{2\alpha}$ without greatly affecting that to ACh or histamine; for both tissues the pA_2 values for PGE_2 or $PGF_{2\alpha}$ antagonism were similar (COLEMAN et al. 1980 c), supporting the results of BENNETT and POSNER (1971) for guinea-pig ileum and suggesting similar receptors. Since in the longitudinal muscle of guinea-pig ileum receptors for PGE_1 and PGE_2 seem similar (ILLÉS and KNOLL 1975), perhaps PGE_1, PGE_2, and $PGF_{2\alpha}$ activate the same receptor. However, responses to PGD_2, PGE_2 or $PGF_{2\alpha}$ in guinea-pig ileal and colonic longitudinal muscle differ in their sensitivity to antagonism by sodium meclofenamate (BENNETT et al. 1980; see discussion earlier in this section).

In the longitudinal muscle of chick isolated ileum (COLEMAN et al. 1980 d) the pharmacological profile of prostanoid receptors differed from that in the guinea-pig, since the order of potency was PGE_1 > PGE_2 > $PGF_{2\alpha}$, and these contractions were unaffected by SC-19220. It is not known whether tissues with the same excitatory prostanoid potency order as guinea-pig or chick ileum are, respectively, sensitive or insensitive to antagonism by SC-19220. In rat stomach, the potency order is $PGE_1 \sim PGE_2 > PGF_{2\alpha} > PGF_{1\alpha}$ (HONG 1974). Contractions to PGE_2 or $PGF_{2\alpha}$ are antagonised by SC-19220 (BENNETT and POSNER 1971; BENNETT et al. 1980 b), but contractions to PGE_2 differ from those to PGE_1 or $PGF_{2\alpha}$ in their sensitivity to antagonism by trimethoquinol (LACEY and SANGER 1980; see discussion earlier in this section). Thus two prostanoids may be antagonised similarly by one drug but differently by another. It should be stressed that an antagonist need not act at receptors for PGs, and with all the drugs discussed there is not sufficient evidence to prove that receptors are the site of action.

F. Prostanoids and Peristalsis In Vitro

Serosal, but not mucosal, application of PGE_1 or PGE_2 to guinea-pig isolated ileum enhanced the peristaltic activity of the longitudinal muscle (BENNETT et al. 1968 b; RADMANOVIĆ 1972; TAKAI et al. 1974; SANGER and WATT 1978). Low concentrations of PGE_1 or PGE_2 applied serosally can increase circular muscle peristaltic activity (RADMANOVIĆ 1972; TAKAI et al. 1974; SANGER and WATT 1978), but this contrasts with the inhibitory effect of PGE compounds on strips of circular muscle and with the finding that higher concentrations of PGE compounds inhibit circular muscle activity (BENNETT et al. 1968 b; RADMANOVIĆ 1972; FONTAINE et al. 1977). However, perhaps the type of preparation used might affect the circular muscle response to PGE compounds. ELEY et al. (1977) considered that increased circular muscle activity with PGE_1 or PGE_2 in the method of TRENDELENBURG (1917) might be secondary to an increased intraluminal pressure within the closed system owing to marked longitudinal muscle contraction; the propulsion of fluid in an open system would avoid such a build-up of pressure. SANGER and WATT (1978) found increased circular muscle activity to PGE_1 in a closed peristaltic system using isotonic or isometric longitudinal muscle recording conditions. Large changes in longitudinal muscle length cannot occur in the latter case, but perhaps alterations in longitudinal muscle tension or electrical activity affect the circular muscle.

In guinea-pig colon, ELEY et al. (1977) found that PGE_1 or PGE_2 increased both longitudinal and circular muscle contractions during peristalsis elicited by raising the intraluminal pressure, but did not significantly affect the propulsion of intraluminal fluid. The use of fluid is probably relevant to diarrhoea but a more physiological stimulus would be a semisolid bolus (FRIGO and LECCHINI 1970). Using a small plastic ball to elicit muscle activity in guinea-pig isolated colon ISHIZAWA and MIYAZAKI (1973 a) found that serosally applied PGE_1 or PGE_2 increased its propulsion.

$PGF_{1\alpha}$ or $PGF_{2\alpha}$ increased longitudinal and circular muscle peristaltic activity when applied serosally to the guinea-pig ileum (RADMANOVIĆ 1974; ELEY et al. 1977), although RADMANOVIĆ (1974) found that a long-lasting inhibition occurred after washout. PGF_{α} compounds also stimulate propulsive activity in guinea-pig colon, where they may be more potent than in the ileum (ISHIZAWA and MIYAZAKI 1973 a, b, 1975; ELEY et al. 1977).

Indomethacin 1–4 μg/ml or aspirin 20–200 μg/ml bathing the serosal surface of guinea-pig isolated ileum or colon reduced all aspects of peristalsis (BENNETT et al. 1976). Indomethacin was more consistently effective in the ileum than in the colon and the effect of aspirin was sometimes temporary, despite its continued presence. FONTAINE et al. (1977) found similar results in guinea-pig ileum except that 0.6–2.5 μg/ml indomethacin did not affect the initial (preparatory) contraction of the longitudinal muscle. PGs therefore seem unlikely to be essential for peristalsis in guinea-pig intestine, but may play a part in maintaining or allowing full activity. This is supported by the observations that PGE_1 or PGE_2 produced stronger, more regular peristaltic waves during weak and poorly coordinated peristaltic activity in guinea-pig ileum than during well-coordinated or maximal peristaltic activity (FONTAINE et al. 1977; SANGER and WATT 1978).

Apart from PGE or PGF_{α} compounds, there have been no reports concerning the effects of other prostanoids on peristalsis, although high concentrations of PGD_2 seem to have little or no effect in guinea-pig ileum (K. G. ELEY, A. BENNETT, unpublished work). In muscle strips from guinea-pig ileum or colon, PGD_2 and other prostanoids do not show activity with a potency comparable to PGE_2 or $PGF_{2\alpha}$ (see Sect. C), and to this extent they would be expected to have little action on the peristaltic reflex.

G. Prostanoids and Motility In Vivo

Most investigations on the actions of prostanoids on gastrointestinal motility in vivo have been in humans. HORTON et al. (1968) reported sensations of increased intestinal motility and passage of loose faeces after oral administration of PGE_1. DILAWARI et al. (1975) infused $PGF_{2\alpha}$ 0.05–0.8 μg kg^{-1} min^{-1} intravenously, and found increased lower oesophageal sphincter pressure but no significant change in oesophageal peristalsis or gastric fundus motility. Infusions of PGE_2 0.08 μg

kg^{-1} min^{-1} inhibited sphincter contractions to bolus injections of pentagastrin, whereas indomethacin administered rectally increased sphincter pressure. The human lower oesophageal sphincter tone may therefore normally be influenced by inhibitory prostanoids, one of which might be PGE_2. In the opossum, PGE_2 reduced the lower oesophageal sphincter pressure (GOYAL et al. 1973), but indomethacin had no effect (DANIEL et al. 1979). In the cat, PGE_2 or PGI_2 reduced lower oesophageal sphincter pressure (SINAR et al. 1979), but in the dog PGE_2 caused an increase (MAHER et al. 1978).

In other studies on the human stomach, NEWMAN et al. (1975) found that $PGF_{2\alpha}$, infused at the rate and the concentration used by DILAWARI et al. (1975), increased antral contractions. CLASSEN et al. (1973) reported that PGE_1 given intravenously inhibited antral contractions. PGE_1 given orally increased the transit through the human small intestine and colon, but this was probably due at least partly to intestinal fluid secretion which reflexly increased propulsive activity (MISIEWICZ et al. 1969).

As in the stomach, intravenously infused PGE_2 inhibited colonic segmental activity. This may have facilitated propulsion of contents and so contributed to the diarrhoea (HUNT et al. 1975). Colonic motility is low in diarrhoea, normal or high in patients below the age of 40 years with constipation, and low in patients above the age of 40 years with constipation (CONNELL 1962). Suggested explanations were that the watery stools in diarrhoea offer less resistance and therefore evoke less colonic muscle activity, and that the intraluminal contents may even move under the influence of gravity. Perhaps increased amounts of PGE_2 or PGI_2 are synthesised which relax the colonic circular muscle (see Sect. C), and so contribute to the hypoactivity.

Although intravenous $PGF_{2\alpha}$ increased net fluid secretion in the human jejunum it had no significant effect on intestinal transit time, despite the reduction in the frequency of segmental pressure waves which sometimes occurred (CUMMINGS et al. 1973). Similar results for net fluid secretion and motility occurred in the ileum, which was slightly more sensitive to $PGF_{2\alpha}$ than the jejunum. The inhibition of intestinal segmental pressure waves by $PGF_{2\alpha}$ occurred sooner and at lower doses than the increased fluid secretion, but the relative importance of motor changes to the diarrhoea caused by infusion of $PGF_{2\alpha}$ into the subjects is not clear.

No other prostanoid has been examined for an action on human gastrointestinal motility in vivo. Recently PGI_2 has been infused in humans, but apart from a report of colicky, central abdominal discomfort in one of five subjects receiving a high dose of PGI_2 (O'GRADY et al. 1979), there have been no recorded effects of PGI_2 on the gut in man.

Many PG analogues have been given to humans, mostly for an effect on the gastric mucosa or the myometrium. All the analogues tend to affect gut motility and secretion. For example 140 μg 16,16-dimethyl PGE_2 administered orally increased gastric emptying, dilated the duodenum and jejunum, and increased intestinal transit time (NYLANDER and MATTSSON 1975; JOHANSSON and EKELUND 1977). The extent to which diarrhoea with these analogues is due to a primary action on motility or on secretion remains to be determined (see Sect. H).

In laboratory animals, the effects of PGs on intestinal motility in vivo are essentially similar to those in humans. BENNETT et al. (1968 b) and ELEY and BENNETT

(1979) reported that PGE_1 and PGE_2 infused into anaesthetised rats increased ileal longitudinal muscle activity and intraluminal pressure, and contracted colonic circular muscle. Similar, but more variable, results were found for guinea-pig ileum (BENNETT et al. 1968b).

In anaesthetised dogs, $PGF_{2\alpha}{}^{1}/\mu g/kg \cdot min^{1}$ i.v. increased jejunal intraluminal pressure and duodenal and ileal circular muscle activity but reduced the longitudinal muscle tone; colonic motility was not affected (SHEHADEH et al. 1969; DAJANI et al. 1979). The increased ileal motility caused by $PGF_{2\alpha}$ in the experiments of DAJANI et al. (1979) occurred almost immediately after starting the infusion of $PGF_{2\alpha}$, whereas diarrhoea occurred only near the end of infusion (1 h). PGE_2 increased myoelectric activity in the canine small intestine (MUKHOPADHYAY et al. 1974) particularly in fasting dogs. In rats, PGI_2 inhibited gastric emptying (ROBERT et al. 1979), and in rhesus monkeys, PGI_2 inhibited basal and water-load stimulation of gastric emptying by a mechanism unrelated to inhibition of acid secretion (SHEA-DONOHUE et al. 1980).

H. Prostanoids as Factors in Disordered Gastrointestinal Motility

I. Gastro-Oesophageal Reflux

DILAWARI et al. (1975) showed that in humans, PGE_2 inhibited the pentagastrin-contracted lower oesophageal sphincter, whereas indomethacin increased sphincter tone. BENNETT (1978) also suggested that PGE_2 released in the inflamed lower oesophagus might cause sphincter relaxation and aid reflux of gastric contents. Thus, relief of "upset stomach" by Alka Seltzer, a highly buffered form of sodium acetylsalicylate, may involve a reduction of PG-aided gastro-oesophageal reflux.

II. Gastrointestinal Disturbances

COLLIER et al. (1975, 1976) found that low concentrations of several emetic, purgative or irritant compounds (such as capsaicin) could stimulate PG synthesis. The authors suggested that this could account for unpleasant side effects of such substances. ASSOULINE et al. (1977) and KNAPP et al. (1977, 1978) found that hypertonic solutions increase PG synthesis in rat stomach, and they suggested a link between PGs and the hyperosmolar dumping syndrome which can occur after partial gastrectomy.

III. Diarrhoea

The involvement of PGs in diarrhoea has been reviewed recently by RASK-MADSEN and BUKHAVE (1979). PGs cause diarrhoea in humans mainly by stimulating fluid secretion by the small intestine. The extra intraluminal volume probably increases propulsive activity, aided by direct PG stimulation of the muscle (see Sect. G), and is thought to cause diarrhoea by overloading the absorptive capacity of the colon.

PGs have been implicated as factors in diarrhoea or gastrointestinal disturbances caused by many types of disease. The evidence for this often includes the high levels of PG-lm in the blood or in faeces. Since in rat stomach or guinea-pig ileum, passive distension releases PG-lm (BENNETT et al. 1967; TAKAI et al. 1974; YAGASAKI et al. 1974), prostanoids might be released within the gut, partly as a result of hyperactivity, therefore contributing to the diarrhoea. However, peripheral blood PGE levels, determined by radioimmunoassay, are not raised in all types of diarrhoea (JAFFE and CONDON 1976), so that other prostanoids may contribute to the diarrhoea, and/or PGE released by gut hyperactivity does not reach the peripheral venous blood. At least part of the explanation may be the inactivation of PGE in the pulmonary circulation (FERREIRA and VANE 1967). Since prostanoids occur within the gut wall, and some presumably contribute to gut activity, treatment with inhibitors of PG synthesis might therefore reduce all types of diarrhoea. However, where the diarrhoea serves to expel potentially toxic or infectious material from the gut, treatment to delay the diarrhoea may be disadvantageous.

PGs have been implicated in the following types of diarrhoea, but the importance of a primary effect on gut motility has not been established.

1. Bacterial Endotoxins

PGs can be released by bacterial endotoxins at various sites. *Salmonella enteritidis* endotoxin injected intravenously into mice caused diarrhoea which was prevented with indomethacin (HARPER and SKARNES 1972). *Escherichia coli* endotoxin injected intravenously into rabbits increased PG output from the subsequently excised intestine, but endotoxin incubated with normal intestine in vitro did not increase PG release (HERMAN and VANE 1975); the authors suggested that a blood component, possibly complement, may be necessary for PG release. DUPONT et al. (1977) described successful treatment of diarrhoea with bismuth subsalicylate in patients whose stools contained high amounts of *E. coli*, but it is not known whether the bismuth or the salicylate contributed to the effect or whether prostanoid synthesis was reduced.

2. Cholera Exotoxin

BENNETT (1971) suggested that the diarrhoea of cholera exotoxin might involve PGs, and some evidence in various animals and in humans supports this hypothesis (FINCK and KATZ 1972; JACOBY and MARSHALL 1972; VALIULIS and LONG 1973; OKPAKO 1975; POWELL and FARRIS 1975; HUDSON et al. 1974; FARRIS et al. 1976; TOTHILL 1976; WALD et al. 1977). Although others claimed no relationship between cholera toxin and PGs (DE et al. 1974; DLUGLECKA 1974; GOTS et al. 1974; KIMBERG et al. 1974; HUDSON et al. 1975), BENNETT (1976c) thought that all these publications contained dubious aspects. In some there were gross errors of interpretation due to incorrect analysis of data, and in others the methods or toxin used might have been inappropriate. BENNETT and CHARLIER (1977) pointed out that although pure cholera toxin did not affect the release of PG-lm from guinea-pig ileum or human intestinal mucosa incubated in vitro, this may not be relevant; the vibrios release crude material, and purification may reduce the diarrhoeogenic activity. Data by BEDWANI and OKPAKO (1975) is consistent with this view. As described above, HERMAN and VANE (1975) showed that *E. coli* endotoxin injected in vivo increased PG output from rabbit isolated intestine, but had no effect when incubated with normal intestine in vitro. Experiments with cholera toxin in vitro may also be inappropriate for another reason: cholera toxin seems to have a systemic component contributing to diarrhoea in rabbits, since material which stimulates intestinal secretion occurs in the bloodstream (VAUGHAN-WILLIAMS and DOHADWALLA 1969). BENNETT (1976c) concluded that although PGs are not the only factor involved in the response to cholera toxin (which stimulates adenylate cyclase directly), PGs produced within the intestinal mucosa probably make some contribution to the accumulation of intraluminal fluid.

Most of the experiments with cholera toxin have concerned the measurement of PG release, or the effects of PG synthesis inhibitors on fluid transport by the proximal small intestine. However, MATHIAS et al. (1977) found that in rabbit distal ileal loops, cholera toxin caused a highly organised myoelectric pattern which the authors defined as the migrating action potential complex. Indomethacin 5 mg/kg i.v. abolished this migrating complex, but 1.5 mg/kg only reduced its velocity of propagation. However, the extent to which these concentrations of indomethacin inhibited PG synthase or other enzymes in the rabbit intestine is not known.

Finally, ROBERT et al. (1979) studied the accumulation of fluid in rat small intestine (enteropooling) with cholera toxin. Enteropooling occurred when the toxin was injected in the upper jejunum of anaesthetised rats but not when it was injected into the stomach, duodenum or terminal ileum. Indomethacin 15–250 μg/kg s.c. or PGI_2 reduced the enteropooling after intrajejunal injection of toxin, and PGI_2 or, less potently, PGD_2 antagonised the enteropooling caused by injected analogues of PGE_2 or $PGF_{2\alpha}$.

3. Irradiation

Irradiation for cancer of the cervix can cause diarrhoea which is often resistant to conventional forms of treatment. However, the diarrhoea usually responds well to aspirin (MENNIE and DALLEY 1973; MENNIE et al. 1975), suggesting a contribution from PGs released by incidental radiation damage to the gut. Irradiation in mice produced a subsequent increase in small intestinal motility and release of PG-lm (BOROWSKA et al. 1979), both of which were reduced by indomethacin. EISEN and WALKER (1976) extracted raised amounts of PG-lm from several tissues after whole-body irradiation of mice. The increase may have been due, at least partly, to reduced PG-15-hydroxydehydrogenase activity which EISEN and WALKER (1978) found in the jejunum and other tissues.

4. Tumours

Many tumours synthesise increased amounts of PG-lm (see BENNETT 1979), including human colonic cancers (JAFFE 1974; BENNETT et al. 1977a). The roles of PGs produced by tumours, and their effects on the gut are not fully elucidated. Diarrhoea is common with many endocrine tumours (for reviews see BENNETT 1976b, 1978, 1979; JAFFE and CONDON 1976; RASK-MADSEN and BUKHAVE 1979), and might be due to release of PGs into the bloodstream. However, many PGs are substantially inactivated on passage through the pulmonary circulation and the amounts reaching the gut may be small. Nevertheless, although inactivation of PGE and PGF_{α} compounds is high in dogs and rabbits (FERREIRA and VANE 1967) only about 70% of a dose of PGE_1 was inactivated in one passage though the lung (GOLUB et al. 1975) and prostacyclin is not destroyed in the pulmonary circulation (MONCADA et al. 1978a). However, it is not known whether PGI_2 is released from endocrine tumours. Various nonendocrine tumours are associated with raised blood levels of 6-keto-$PGF_{1\alpha}$ (DEMERS et al. 1979; KHAN et al. 1981) but diarrhoea is not usually a feature of the disease.

Endocrine tumours produce many substances other than PGs, and some of these could contribute to diarrhoea by stimulating PG synthesis in the gut (see RASK-MADSEN and BUKHAVE 1979). Examples may include calcitonin, vasoactive intestinal peptide (VIP) and human pancreatic polypeptide, but the evidence that these compounds increase PG synthesis is not conclusive. In rats, VIP-induced intestinal fluid secretion was inhibited by indomethacin 5 mg/kg, but a selective effect of indomethacin on prostanoid synthesis was questioned (ALBUQUERQUE et al. 1979). Furthermore, as discussed in Sect. H.III, endogenous prostanoids may contribute to the diarrhoea merely because they are produced by distended gastrointestinal tissues, and inhibitors of PG synthesis may reduce all types of diarrhoea.

It also seems feasible that increased amounts of PGs synthesised by gut tumours can affect gastrointestinal motility locally, in addition to the obstruction caused by the tumour mass. However, the location and type of tumour, and the types of PGs and other substances which they produce might affect the overall response. Mild diarrhoea is common in undifferentiated carcinomas of the caecum, whereas in the rectum, disruption of the myenteric plexus occurs and constipation is more common (GOLIGHER 1967). The latter types of tumour often yield an increased amount of PG-lm on extraction (BENNETT et al. 1977a). However, in the one specimen of caecal carcinoid studied, the amount of extracted PG-lm was unusually low. Enkephalins can affect gut motility, and it may be relevant that the amount of met-enkephalin extracted from rectal tumours, but not undifferentiated carcinomas of the caecum, is high (DAVIS et al. 1979).

5. Irritable Colon Syndrome

Diarrhoea is a common feature of the irritable colon syndrome. RASK-MADSEN and BUKHAVE (1978) found increased amounts of PGE_2 in jejunal secretions of two fasting patients with this condition. Indomethacin given orally for 14 days, "solidified" the stools, reducing their volume and frequency; relapse occurred after treatment with indomethacin was stopped.

6. Food Intolerance

BUISSERET et al. (1978) studied six patients with gastrointestinal disturbances after eating certain foods (pork chops, mussels, sweet corn, eggs, bananas, shellfish, wine, beer, citrus fruit, dairy products). Blood plasma and stool concentrations of PGs were usually raised after challenge with the appropriate food, and in five of the six patients treatment with PG synthesis inhibitors prevented the symptoms. Similarly, in experiments on himself, LIEB (1978) found that aspirin prevented gastrointestinal disturbances associated with his lactose intolerance after ingestion of dairy products. LIEB (1980) found that aspirin prevented abdominal cramps and diarrhoea evoked in a woman by black coffee.

7. Idiopathic Intestinal Pseudo-obstruction

In one patient suffering from idiopathic intestinal pseudoobstruction for several years, diarrhoea stopped and stool formation normalised after administration of indomethacin, and remained so after the 6 months of treatment was stopped (LUDERER et al. 1976). In another patient, blood plasma levels of PGE_2 and $PGF_{2\alpha}$ (measured by radioimmunoassay) increased markedly during diarrhoea associated with this condition (CHOUSETERMAN et al. 1977).

8. Dysmenorrhoea

Menstruation is associated with increased gastrointestinal motility (FOCHEM 1955) and defaecation (McCANCE and PICKLES 1960), and breast-fed babies can suffer diarrhoea during menstruation of the lactating mother (NAISH 1952). Nausea and/or vomiting occurred in 89% of patients with dysmenorrhoea, and diarrhoea occurred in 60% (KAUPPILA and YLIKORKALA 1977). Menstruation and, in particular, dysmenorrhoea are associated with increased PG synthesis by the endometrium (see COLLINS and WILLMAN 1978). In dysmenorrhoea, PG synthesis inhibitors relieve both uterine pain and gastrointestinal disturbances (KAPADIA and ELDER 1978; LUNDSTRÖM 1978), suggesting that PGs either reach the gut from the uterus, or that they are synthesised locally in increased amounts (see SANGER and BENNETT 1979).

9. Idiopathic Postural Hypotension

This condition is characterised by a partial or complete denervation of the sympathetic and especially the parasympathetic system. In one such patient treated conventionally there was recurrent, profuse diarrhoea which improved during treatment with aspirin (SMYTHIES and RUSSELL 1974).

10. Treatment of Diarrhoea with Nutmeg

This topic has been discussed by BENNETT (1978). In parts of the world such as India the spice is used widely for treatment of diarrhoea in humans. FAWELL and THOMPSON (1973) reported that nutmeg treated otherwise-resistant diarrhoea in a man with medullary carcinoma of the thyroid, and BARROWMAN et al. (1975) also obtained a good effect in this disease. SHAFRAN et al. (1977) used nutmeg to treat diarrhoea associated with Crohn's disease, and STAMFORD et al. (1978, 1980) have obtained excellent prevention or treatment of scouring in calves and bowel oedema in piglets. Results by BENNETT et al. (1974) and SHAFRAN et al. (1977) indicate that nutmeg may act by inhibiting PG synthesis.

J. Beneficial Effects of Prostanoids in Disorders of Gastrointestinal Motility

I. Worm Expulsion

KELLY et al. (1974) injected several different PGs intraduodenally into rats infected with the intestinal worms *Nippostrongylus brasiliensis*. PGE, A or B compounds caused some expulsion of worms, but PGF_α compounds were ineffective. The authors did not mention the diarrhoeagenic activity of PGs as a mechanism for expulsion (see BENNETT 1976a). KASSAI et al. (1979) did not obtain worm expulsion with PGE compounds in a similar model.

II. Postoperative Ileus

Gastrointestinal motility may be severely reduced after major abdominal surgery. Various remedies have been tried (e.g. see NEELEY and CATCHPOLE 1971), and recently PGs have been successfully used in humans. FUKUNISHI et al. (1977) infused $PGF_{2\alpha}$ (0.3–0.5 $\mu g\ kg^{-1}\ min^{-1}$) for 2 h and restored gut mechanical and electrical activity. They concluded that $PGF_{2\alpha}$ was most effective and without appreciable side effects when infused i.v. 0.5 $\mu g\ kg^{-1}\ min^{-1}$ for 2 h, 3 times daily for 3 days after surgery. Postoperative ileus has also been effectively treated with $PGF_{2\alpha}$ in rabbits (FIEDLER 1979), and with 16,16-dimethyl PGE_2 in rats and guinea-pigs (RUWART et al. 1980).

III. Laxatives

Some laxatives may act, at least in part, by stimulating PG synthesis. The effects of the diphenolic laxatives bisacodyl and phenolphthalein are associated with increased synthesis of PGE-lm in rat colon and can be reduced with indomethacin (BEUBLER and JUAN 1978a, b). However, these laxatives did not stimulate PG-lm synthesis in bull seminal vesicles (COLLIER et al. 1976). In a later study, BEUBLER and JUAN (1979) showed that many other drugs used in the treatment of constipation, including ricinoleic acid, oleic acid, dioctyl sodium sulphosuccinate, deoxycholic acid, and sennosides A and B, may act in the rat colon by stimulating PG synthesis. Notable exceptions were osmotic laxatives. Similarly, LUDERER et al. (1980) found that sodium ricinoleate stimulated synthesis of PGE and PGF compounds in rat jejunum, and that indomethacin delayed castor oil-induced diarrhoea in the rat.

K. Conclusions

Various biologically active prostanoids formed from arachidonic acid may play roles in some gastrointestinal functions and diseases. Future work should involve further elucidation of which prostanoid precursors and metabolites are formed, including lipoxygenase products and leukotrienes, and the actions of these substances on the tissues in vitro and in vivo. Since different prostanoids can have opposing actions on the same tissue, it is important to know how they interact and under what conditions a particular compound may be synthesised in preference to others. Such studies should lead to a greater understanding of physiology and pathophysiology, and to the development of more effective medicines. For example, drugs may be developed which selectively alter the synthesis or actions of prostanoids; in conditions where prostanoids have opposing actions, such as on muscle activity, it may therefore be possible to alter the balance of excitatory and inhibitory prostanoids, either to increase gut activity (e.g. in ileus) or decrease activity (e.g. spasm).

References

Abdel-Aziz A (1974) Blockade by prostaglandins E_1 and $F_{1\alpha}$ of the responses of the rabbit ileum to stimulation of sympathetic nerve and its reversal by some anti-histamines, dexamphetamine, and methylphenidate.Eur J Pharmacol 25:226

Aboulafia J, Medes GB, Miyamoto ME, Paiva ACM, Paiva TB (1976) Effect of indomethacin and prostaglandins on the smooth muscle contracting activity of angiotensin and other agonists. Br J Pharmacol 58:223–228

Akanuma M (1970) Modes of the stimulating action of prostaglandin E_1 on the gastrointestinal tract from the guinea-pig. Sapporo Igakukai Zasshi 38:41–52

Albuquerque RH, Owens CWI, Bloom SR (1979) Study of vasoactive intestinal polypeptide (VIP) stimulated intestinal fluid secretion in rat and its inhibition by indomethacin. Experientia 35:1496–1497

Ali M, Zamecnik J, Cerskus AL, Stoessl AJ, Barnett WH, McDonald JWD (1977) Synthesis of thromboxane B_2 and prostaglandins by bovine gastric mucosal microsomes. Prostaglandins 14:819–827

Al Timimi KS, Bedwani JR, Stanton AWB (1978) Effects of prostaglandin E_2 and a prostaglandin endoperoxide analogue on neuroeffector transmission in rat anococcygeus muscle. Br J Pharmacol 63:167–176

Assouline G, Leibson V, Danon A (1977) Stimulation of prostaglandin output from rat stomach by hypertonic solution. Eur J Pharmacol 44:271–273

Barrowman JA, Bennett A, Hillenbrand P, Rolles K, Pollock DJ, Wright JT (1975) Diarrhoea in medullary carcinoma of the thyroid: evidence for the role of prostaglandins and the therapeutic effect of nutmeg. Br Med J 3:11–12

Bedwani JR, Okpako DT (1975) Effects of crude pure cholera toxin on prostaglandin release from the rabbit ileum. Prostaglandins 10:117–127

Bennett A (1971) Cholera and prostaglandins. Nature 231:536

Bennett A (1972) Effects of prostaglandins on the gastrointestinal tract. In: Karim SSM (ed) The prostaglandins: progress in research. Medical and Technical, Oxford, pp 205–221

Bennett A (1973) Prostaglandins and the gut. In: Truelove SC, Jewell DP (eds) Topics in gastroenterology. Blackwell Scientific, Oxford, pp 281–293

Bennett A (1974) Prostaglandin antagonists. Adv Drug Res 8:83–118

Bennett A (1976a) Prostaglandins and the gut. Annu Res Rev, Eden Press, Montreal

Bennett A (1976b) Prostaglandins as factors in diseases of the alimentary tract. Adv Prostaglandin Thromboxane Res 2:547–555

Bennett A (1976c) The relationship of prostaglandins to cholera. Prostaglandins 11:425–430

Bennett A (1977) The role of prostaglandins in gastrointestinal tone and motility. In Berti F, Samuelsson B, Velo GP (Eds) Prostaglandins and Thromboxanes. Plenum Press, New York. pp 275–285

Bennett A (1978) Prostaglandins. In: Turner P, Shand DG (eds) Recent advances in clinical pharmacology. Churchill Livingstone, Edinburgh, pp 17–30

Bennett A (1979) Prostaglandins and cancer. In: Karim SSM (ed) Practical applications of prostaglandins and their synthesis inhibitors. MTP Press, Lancaster, pp 149–188

Bennett A, Charlier EM (1977) Evidence against the release of prostaglandin-like material from isolated intestinal tissue by pure cholera toxin. Prostaglandins 13:431–436

Bennett A, Del Tacca M, Stamford IF, Zebro T (1977a) Prostaglandins from tumours of human large bowel. Br J Cancer 35:881–884

Bennett A, Eley KG, Scholes GB (1968a) Effects of prostaglandins E_1 and E_2 on human, guinea-pig, and rat isolated small intestine. Br J Pharmacol 34:630–638

Bennett A, Eley KG, Scholes GB (1968b) Effect of prostaglandins E_1 and E_2 on intestinal motility in the guinea-pig and rat. Br J Pharmacol 34:639–647

Bennett A, Eley KG, Stockley HL (1975a) The effects of prostaglandins on guinea-pig isolated intestine and their possible contribution to muscle activity and tone. Br J Pharmacol 54:197–204

Bennett A, Eley KG, Stockley HL (1975b) Modulation by prostaglandins of contractions in the guinea-pig ileum. Prostaglandins 9:377–384

Bennett A, Eley KG, Stockley HL (1976) Inhibition of peristalsis in guinea-pig isolated ileum and colon by drugs that block prostaglandin synthesis. Br J Pharmacol 57:335–340
Bennett A, Fleshler B (1969) Action of prostaglandin E_1 on longitudinal muscle of the guinea-pig isolated colon. Br J Pharmacol 35:351–352P
Bennett A, Fleshler B (1970) Prostaglandins and the gastrointestinal tract. Gastroenterology 59:790–800
Bennett A, Friedmann CA, Vane JR (1967) Release of prostaglandin E_1 from the rat stomach. Nature 216:873–876
Bennett A, Gradidge CF, Stamford IF (1974) Prostaglandins, nutmeg and diarrhoea. N Engl J Med 290:110–111
Bennett A, Hensby CN, Sanger GJ, Stamford IF (1980a) Identification and distribution of arachidonic acid metabolites in the human gastrointestinal tract, and the ways in which some of these affect the longitudinal muscle. In: Velo GP, Berti F (eds). The Prostaglandin System. Plenum Press, New York. pp 365–375
Bennett A, Hensby CN, Sanger GJ, Stanford IF (1981) Metabolites of arachidonic acid formed, by human gastrointestinal tissues and their actions on the muscle layers. Br J Pharmacol 74:435–444
Bennett A, Jarosik C, Sanger GJ, Wilson DE (1980b) Antagonism of prostanoid-induced contractions of rat gastric fundus muscle by SC-19220, sodium meclofenamate, indomethacin or trimethoquinol. Br J Pharmacol 71:169–175
Bennett A, Jarosik C, Wilson DE (1978) A study of receptors activated by analogues of prostaglandin H_2. Br J Pharmacol 63:358P
Bennett A, Murray JG, Wyllie JH (1968c) Occurrence of prostaglandin E_2 in human stomach and a study of its effects on human isolated gastric muscle. Br J Pharmacol Chemother 32:339–349
Bennett A, Posner J (1971) Studies on prostaglandin antagonists. Br J Pharmacol 42:584–594
Bennett A, Pratt D, Sanger GJ (1980c) Antagonism by fenamates of prostaglandin action in guinea-pig and human alimentary muscle. Br J Pharmacol 68:357–362
Bennett A, Sanger GJ (1978) The effects of prostaglandin D_2 on the circular muscle of guinea-pig isolated ileum and colon. Br J Pharmacol 63:357–358P
Bennett A, Sanger GJ (1979) Trimethoquinol selectively antagonises longitudinal muscle contractions of rat isolated gastric fundus to thromboxane B_2 and epoxymethano analogues of PGH_2. Br J Pharmacol 66:450P
Bennett A, Sanger GJ (1980) Prostacyclin relaxes the longitudinal muscle of human isolated stomach and antagonizes contractions to some prostanoids. J Physiol (Lond) 298:45–46P
Bennett A, Stamford IF, Stockley HL (1977b) Estimation and characterization of prostaglandins in the human gastrointestinal tract. Br J Pharmacol 61:579–586
Bennett A, Stockley HL (1977) The contribution of prostaglandins in the muscle of human isolated small intestine to neurogenic responses. Br J Pharmacol 61:573–578
Benz M, Salzmann R (1974) The effects of PGE_1, PGE_2, $PGF_{2\alpha}$ on the parasympathetic transmission. Arch Pharmacol [Suppl] 282:R7
Beubler E, Juan H (1978a) Is the effect of diphenolic laxatives mediated via release of prostaglandin E? Experientia 34:386–387
Beubler E, Juan H (1978b) PGE-mediated laxative effect of diphenolic laxatives. Naunyn-Schmiedebergs Arch Pharmacol 305:241–246
Beubler E, Juan H (1979) Effect of ricinoleic acid and other laxatives on net water flux and prostaglandin E release by the rat colon. J Pharm Pharmacol 31:681–685
Boot JR, Dawson W, Cockerill AF, Mallen DNB, Osborne DJ (1977) The pharmacology of prostaglandin-like substances released from guinea-pig lungs during anaphylaxis. Prostaglandins 13:927–932
Borowska A, Sierakowski J, Mackowiak J, Wisniewski K (1979) A prostaglandin-like activity in small intestinal and postirradiation gastrointestinal syndrome. Experientia 35:1368–1370
Botting JH (1977) The mechanism of the release of prostaglandin-like activity from guinea-pig ileum. J Pharm Pharmacol 29:708–709

Botting JH, Salzmann R (1974) The effect of indomethacin on the release of PGE_2 and acetylcholine from guinea-pig isolated ileum at rest and during field stimulation. Br J Pharmacol 50:119–124

Buisseret PD, Youlten LJF, Heinzelmann DI, Lessof MH (1978) Prostaglandin-synthesis inhibitors in prophylaxis of food intolerance. Lancet 1:906–908

Bundy GL (1975) The synthesis of prostaglandin endoperoxide analogs. Tetrahedron Lett 24:1957–1960

Bunting S, Moncada S, Vane JR (1976) The effects of prostaglandin endoperoxides and thromboxane A_2 on strips of rabbit coeliac artery and other smooth muscle preparations. Br J Pharmacol 57:462P

Burleigh DE (1977) The effects of indomethacin on the tone and spontaneous activity of the human small intestine in vitro. Arch Int Pharmacodyn Ther 225:240–245

Burleigh DE, D'Mello A, Parks AG (1979) Responses of isolated human internal anal sphincter to drugs and electrical field stimulation. Gastroenterology 77:484–490

Burnstock G, Cocks T, Paddle B, Staszewska-Barczak J (1975) Evidence that prostaglandin is responsible for the "rebound contraction" following stimulation of non-adrenergic, non-cholinergic ("purinergic") inhibitory nerves. Eur J Pharmacol 31:360–362

Chijimatsu Y, Nguyen TV, Said SI (1977) Effects of prostaglandin endoperoxide analogues on contractile elements in lung and gastrointestinal tract. Prostaglandins 13:909–916

Chouseterman M, Petite JP, Housset E, Hornych A (1977) Prostaglandins and acute intestinal pseudo-obstruction. Lancet 2:138–139

Classen M, Sturzenhofecker P, Koch H, Demling L (1973) The effect of prostaglandin E_1 on the secretion and motility of the human stomach. Acta Hepatogastroenterol (Stuttg) 20:159–162

Coceani F, Pace-Asciak C, Volta F, Wolfe LS (1967) Effect of nerve stimulation on prostaglandin formation and release from the rat stomach. Am J Physiol 213:1056–1064

Coleman RA, Humphrey PPA, Kennedy I, Levy GP, Lumley P (1980a) U-46619, a selective thromboxane A_2-like agonist? Br J Pharmacol 68:127–128P

Coleman RA, Humphrey PPA, Kennedy I, Levy GP, Lumley P (1980b) Preliminary characterisation of three types of prostanoid receptor. Br J Pharmacol 69:265P–266P

Coleman RA, Kennedy I, Levy GP (1980c) SC-19220, a selective prostanoid receptor antagonist. Br J Pharmacol 69:266P–267P

Coleman RA, Kennedy I, Levy GP, Penning C (1980d) An analysis of the prostanoid receptors mediating contraction of chick isolated ileum. Br J Pharmacol 70:89P–90P

Coleman RA, Kennedy I, Sheldrick RLG (1980e) A simple method for generating thromboxane A_2. Br J Pharmacol 69:341P–342P

Collier HOJ (1974) Prostaglandin synthetase inhibitors and the gut. In: Robinson HJ, Vane JR (eds) Prostaglandin synthetase inhibitors. Raven, New York, pp 121–133

Collier HOJ, McDonald-Gibson WJ, Saeed SA (1975) Stimulation of prostaglandin biosynthesis by capsaicin, ethanol, and tyramine. Lancer 1:702

Collier HOJ, McDonald-Gibson WJ, Saeed SA (1976) Stimulation of prostaglandin biosynthesis by drugs: effects in vitro of some drugs affecting gut function. Br J Pharmacol 58:193–199

Collins WP, Willman EA (1978) Prostaglandins and uterine function. Top Horm Chem, pp 180–215

Connell AM (1962) The motility of the pelvic colon. II. Paradoxical motility in diarrhoea and constipation. Gut 3:342–348

Cook HW, Lands WEM (1976) Mechanism for suppression of cellular biosynthesis of prostaglandins. Nature 260:630–632

Crofts TJ, Stockley HL, Johnson AG (1979) Failure of prostaglandin E_2 to inhibit contraction of taenia coli from patients with diverticular disease. Gut 20:A444

Cummings JH, Newman A, Misiewicz JJ, Milton-Thompson GJ, Billings JA (1973) Effect of intravenous prostaglandin $F_{2\alpha}$ on small intestinal function in man. Nature 243:169–171

Dajani EZ, Bertermann RE, Roge EAW, Schweingruber FL, Woods EM (1979) Canine gastrointestinal motility effects of prostaglandin $F_{2\alpha}$ in vivo. Arch Int Pharmacodyn Ther 237:16–24

Daniel EE, Sarna S, Waterfall W, Crankshaw J (1979) Role of endogenous prostaglandins in regulating the tone of opossum lower esophageal sphincter in vivo. Prostaglandins 17:641–648
Davis WG, Tormey WP, Delaney PV (1979) Enkephalins in large bowel malignancy and in acute appendicitis. Gut 20:865–867
Davison P, Ramwell PW, Willis AL (1972) Inhibition of intestinal tone and prostaglandin synthesis by 5,8,11,14-tetraynoic acid. Br J Pharmacol 46:547–548P
De S, Sicar BK, Sasmal D, De SP, Mondal A (1974) Ibuprofen (Brufen) in cholera and other diarrhoeas. Indian J Med Res 62:756–764
Demers LM, Schweitzer J, Lipton A, Harvey H (1979) Blood 6-keto-$PGF_{1\alpha}$ levels as potential tumour marker. Poster demonstration in: First International Congress on Hormones and Cancer, Rome, Italy
Dilawari JD, Newman A, Poleo J, Misiewicz JJ (1975) Response of the human cardiac sphincter to circulating prostaglandins $F_{2\alpha}$ and E_2 and to anti-inflammatory drugs. Gut 16:137–143
Dluglecka MJ (1974) The failure of indomethacin to modify the response of cat intestine to cholera enterotoxin. Pol J Pharmacol Pharm 26:93–100
Dupont HL, Sullivan P, Pickering LK, Haynes G, Ackerman PB (1977) Symptomatic treatment of diarrhoea with bismuth subsalicylate among students attending a Mexican university. Gastroenterology 73:715–718
Dupont J, Maydani S, Lewis L, Case G, Ewens-Luby S, Mathias MM (1978) Prostaglandins and metabolites in the gastrointestinal tract. Prostaglandins 15:710
Eakins KE, Sanner JH (1972) Prostaglandin antagonists. In: Karim SMM (ed) The prostaglandins: progress in research. Wiley Interscience, New York, pp 263–292
Eisen V, Walker DI (1976) Effect of ionizing radiation on prostaglandin-like activity in tissues. Br J Pharmacol 57:527–532
Eisen V, Walker DI (1978) Effect of ionizing radiation on prostaglandin 15-OH-dehydrogenase (PGDH). Br J Pharmacol 62:461P
Elde R, Hökfelt T, Johansson O, Terenius L (1976) Immuno-histochemical studies using antibodies to leucine-enkephalin: initial observations on the nervous system of the rat. Neuroscience 1:349–351
Eley KG, Bennett A (1979) Rat colonic circular muscle: PGE_2 causes contraction in vivo but relaxes isolated strips. Abstracts 4th International Prostaglandin Conference, Washington, DC, p 30
Eley KG, Bennett A, Stockley HL (1977) The effects of prostaglandins E_1, E_2, $F_{1\alpha}$, and $F_{2\alpha}$ on the guinea-pig ileal and colonic peristalsis. J Pharm Pharmacol 29:280–296
Farris RK, Tapper EJ, Powell DW, Morris SM (1976) Effect of aspirin on normal and cholera toxin-stimulated intestinal electrolyte transport. J Clin Invest 57:916–924
Fawell WN, Thompson G (1973) Nutmeg for diarrhoea of medullary carcinoma of the thyroid. N Engl J Med 289:108–109
Ferreira SH, Herman A, Vane JR (1972) Prostaglandin generation maintains the smooth muscle tone of the rabbit isolated jejunum. Br J Pharmacol 44:328P
Ferreira SH, Herman A, Vane JR (1976) Prostaglandin production by rabbit isolated jejunum and its relationship to the inherent tone of the preparation. Br J Pharmacol 56:469–477
Ferreira SH, Vane JR (1967) Prostaglandins, their disappearance from, and release into the circulation. Nature 216:868–873
Fiedler L (1979) $PGF_{2\alpha}$ – a new therapy for paralytic ileus? Abstracts 4th International Prostaglandin Conference, Washington, DC, p 33
Fink AD, Katz RL (1972) Prevention of cholera-induced intestinal secretion in the cat by aspirin. Nature 238:273–274
Fleshler B, Bennett A (1969) Responses of human, guinea-pig, and rat colonic circular muscle to prostaglandins. J Lab Clin Med 74:872
Fochem K (1955) Über den Einfluß der Menstruation auf die Motilität des Magens. Med Klin 40:2028
Fontaine J, Van Nueten JM, Reuse JJ (1977) Effects of prostaglandins on the peristaltic reflex of the guinea-pig ileum. Arch Int Pharmacodyn Ther 226:341–343

Frankhuijzen AL, Bonta IL (1975) Role of prostaglandins in tone and effect on reactivity of the isolated rat stomach preparation. Eur J Pharmacol 31:44–52
Frigo GM, Lecchini S (1970) An improved method for studying the peristaltic reflex in the isolated colon. Br J Pharmacol 39:346–356
Fukunishi S, Amano S, Saijo H, Matsumoto K, Iriyama K, Fujino T (1977) The effect of intravenous prostaglandin $F_{2\alpha}$ on the motility of the gastrointestinal tracts after major abdominal surgery. Jpn J Smooth Muscle Res 13:141–152
Ganesan PA, Karim SMM (1973) Polyphloretin phosphate temporarily potentiates prostaglandin E_2 on the rat fundus, probably by inhibiting PG 15-hydroxy-dehydrogenase. J Pharm Pharmacol 25:229–233
Gershon MD, Ross LL (1966) Location of sites of 5-hydroxytryptamine storage and metabolism by autoradiography. J Physiol (Lond) 186:477–492
Gintzler AR, Musacchio JM (1974) Failure of prostaglandins to participate in the inhibitory response of the guinea-pig ileum to morphine. Fed Proc 33:502
Goligher JC (1967) Surgery of the anus, rectum, and colon, 2nd edn. Bailliere Tindall & Cassell, London, pp 500–503
Golub M, Zia P, Matsumo M, Horton R (1975) Metabolism of prostaglandins A_1 and E_1 in man. J Clin Invest 56:1404–1410
Gorman RR, Sun FF, Miller OV, Johnson RA (1977) Prostaglandin H_1 and prostaglandin H_2 – convenient biochemical synthesis and isolation – further biological and spectroscopic characterization. Prostaglandins 13:1043–1054
Gots RE, Formal SB, Giannella RA (1974) Indomethacin inhibition of salmonella typhimurium, shigella flexneri, and cholera-mediated rabbit ileal secretion. J Infect Dis 130:280–284
Goyal RK, Rattan S, Hersh T (1973) Comparison of the effects of prostaglandins E_1, E_2, and A_2, and of hypovolmic hypotension on the lower esophageal sphincter. Gastroenterology 65:608
Grbovic L, Radmanović BZ (1978) A modulating role of prostaglandins in responses of guinea-pig isolated ileum to various agonists. Arch Int Pharmacodyn Ther 235:230–237
Grubb MN, Burks TF (1974) Modification of intestinal stimulatory effects of 5-hydroxytryptamine by adrenergic amines, prostaglandin E_1 and theophylline. J Pharmacol Exp Ther 189:476–483
Hadházy P, Illés P, Knoll J (1973) The effects of PGE_1 on responses to cardiac vagus nerve stimulation and acetylcholine release. Eur J Pharmacol 23:251–255
Hall WJ, O'Neill P, Sheehan JD (1975) The role of prostaglandins in cholinergic neurotransmission in the guinea-pig. Eur J Pharmacol 34:39–47
Hamberg M, Hedqvist P, Strandberg K, Svensson J, Samuelsson B (1975) Prostaglandin endoperoxides. IV. Effects on smooth muscle. Life Sci 16:451–462
Harper MJK, Skarnes RC (1972) Inhibition of abortion and fetal death produced by endotoxin or prostaglandin $F_{2\alpha}$. Prostaglandins 2:295–309
Harry JD (1968) The action of prostaglandin E_1 on the guinea-pig isolated intestine. Br J Pharmacol 33:213P
Hart SL (1974) The actions of prostaglandins E_2 and $F_{2\alpha}$ on human foetal intestine. Br J Pharmacol 50:159–160
Hazra J (1975) Evidence against prostaglandin E having a physiological role in acetylcholine liberation from Auerbach's plexus of guinea-pig ileum. Experientia 31:565–566
Hedqvist P, Gustafsson L, Hiemdahl P, Svanborg K (1980) Aspects of prostaglandin action on autonomic neuroeffector transmission. Adv Prostaglandin Thromboxane Res:1245–1248
Hedqvist P, Persson N-Å (1975) Prostaglandin action on adrenergic and cholinergic responses in the rabbit and guinea-pig intestine. In: Almgen O, Carlsson A, Engel J (eds) Chemical tools in catecholamine research II. North Holland, New York, pp 211–218
Herman AG, Vane JR (1975) Endotoxin and production of prostaglandins by the isolated rabbit jejunum. Influence of indomethacin. Arch Int Pharmacodyn Ther 213:328–329
Hökfelt T, Johansson O, Ljungdahl Å, Lundberg JM, Schultzberg M (1980) Peptidergic neurones. Nature 284:515–521
Hong E (1974) Differential pattern of activity of some prostaglandins on diverse superfused tissues. Prostaglandins 8:213–220

Horton EW (1973) Prostaglandins at adrenergic nerve endings. Br Med Bull 29:148–151
Horton EW, Jones RL (1974) Biological activity of prostaglandin D_2 on smooth muscle. Br J Pharmacol 52:110–111P
Horton EW, Main IHM, Thompson CJ, Wright PM (1968) Effect of orally administered prostaglandin E_1 on gastric secretion and gastrointestinal motility in man. Gut 9:655–658
Hoult JRS, Moore PK (1980) Adaptive changes in activity of prostaglandin synthesising and metabolising enzymes are coupled. Br J Pharmacol 69:272P–273P
Hudson N, Hindi ES, Wilson DE, Poppe L (1975) Prostaglandin E in cholera toxin-induced intestinal secretion. Lack of an intermediatory role. Dig Dis 20:1035–1039
Hudson N, Poppe L, Wilson DE (1974) Role of prostaglandin E (PGE) in experimental cholera. Clin Res 22:604A
Hughes J, Kosterlitz HW, Smith TW (1977) The distribution of methionine-enkephalin and leucine-enkephalin in the brain and peripheral tissues. Br J Pharmacol 61:639–648
Hunt RH, Dilawari JB, Misiewicz JJ (1975) The effect of intravenous prostaglandin $F_{2\alpha}$ and E_2 on the motility of the sigmoid colon. Gut 16:47–49
Illés P, Hadházy P, Torma A, Vizi ES, Knoll J (1973) The effect of number of stimuli and rate of stimulation on the inhibition by PGE_1 of adrenergic transmission. Eur J Pharmacol 24:29–36
Illés P, Knoll J (1975) Specific densensitization to PGE_1 and PGE_2 in guinea-pig ileum: evidence for a common receptor site. Pharmacol Res Commun 7:37–47
Illés P, Vizi EW, Knoll J (1974) Adrenergic neuroeffector junctions sensitive and insensitive to the effect of PGE_1. Pol J Pharmacol Pharm 26:127–136
Ishii T, Sakato M, Shimo Y (1977) Effects of prostaglandin E_1 and indomethacin on the stimulation-evoked overflow of ^{3}H-noradrenaline from guinea-pig taenia caecum. Eur J Pharmacol 45:381–384
Ishizawa M, Miyazaki E (1973a) Action of prostaglandins on gastrointestinal motility. Sapporo Med J 42:366–373
Ishizawa M, Miyazaki E (1973b) Effect of prostaglandins on the movement of guinea-pig isolated intestine. Jpn J Smooth Muscle Res 9:235–237
Ishizawa M, Miyazaki E (1975) Effect of prostaglandin $F_{2\alpha}$ on propulsive activity of the isolated segmental colon of the guinea-pig. Prostaglandins 10:759–768
Jacoby HI, Marshall CH (1972) Antagonism of cholera enterotoxin by anti-inflammatory agents in the rat. Nature 235:163–165
Jaffe BM (1974) Prostaglandins and cancer: an update. Prostaglandins 6:453–461
Jaffe BM, Condon S (1976) Prostaglandins E and F in endocrine diarrheagenic syndromes. Ann Surg 184:516–523
Jaques R (1977) Inhibition effect of methionine-enkephalin and leucine-enkephalin on contractions of guinea pig ileum elicited by PGE_1. Experientia 33:374–375
Johansson C, Ekelund K (1977) Effects of 16,16-dimethyl prostaglandin E_2 on the integrated response to a meal. In: Duthie HL (ed) Gastrointestinal motility in health and disease. Proc 6th Int Symp Gastrointest Motility, Edinburgh. MTP Press, Lancaster, pp 195–202
Kadlec O, Mašek K, Šeferna I (1974) A modulating role of prostaglandins in contractions of the guinea-pig ileum. Br J Pharmacol 51:565–570
Kadlec O, Mašek K, Šeferna I (1975) The role of prostaglandins in the output of neurotransmitters from the isolated guinea-pig ileum. Abstracts 6th International Congress on Pharmacology, p 156
Kadlec O, Mašek K, Šeferna I (1978) Modulation by prostaglandins of the release of acetylcholine and noradrenaline in guinea-pig isolated ileum. J Pharmacol Exp Ther 205:635–645
Kapadia L, Elder MG (1978) Flufenamic acid in treatment of primary spasmodic dysmenorrhoea. Lancet 1:348–350
Karim SMM, Ganesan PA (1974) Prostaglandins and the digestive system. Ann Acad Med Singapore 3:286–293
Kassai T, Redl P, Balla É, Jécsay GY, Harangoźo E (1979) Nippostrongylus brasiliensis in the rat: failure to induce worm rejection by prostaglandins. Abstracts 4th International Prostaglandin Conference, Washington, DC, p 58

Kauppila A, Ylikorkala O (1977) Indomethacin and tolfenamic acid in primary dysmenorrhoea. Eur J Obstet Gynaecol Reprod Biol 7:59–64
Kelly JD, Dineen JK, Goodrich BS, Smith ID (1974) Expulsion of Nippostrongylus brasiliensis from the intestine of rats. Int Arch Allergy Appl Immunol 47:458–465
Khan O, Hensby CN, Williams G (1981) Prostacyclin in Prostatic disease. In: Lewis PG, O'Grady J (eds) Clinical pharmacology of prostacyclin. Raven Press, New York, pp 49–52
Kimberg DV, Field M, Gershon E, Henderson A (1974) Effects of prostaglandins and cholera enterotoxin on intestinal mucosal cyclic AMP accumulation. Evidence against an essential role for prostaglandins in the action of toxin. J Clin Invest 53:941–949
Kirk D, Duthie HL (1977) In vitro studies of the electrical activity of the longitudinal and circular muscle layers of the human colon. In: Duthie HL (ed) Gastrointestinal motility in health and disease. Proc 6th Int Symp Gastrointest Motility, Edinburgh. MTP Press, Lancaster, pp 327–332
Knapp HR, Oelz O, Oates JA (1977) Effects of hyperosmolarity on prostaglandin release by the rat stomach in vitro. Fed Proc 36:1020
Knapp HR, Oelz O, Sweetman BJ, Oates JA (1978) Synthesis and metabolism of prostaglandins E_2, $F_{2\alpha}$, and D_2 by the rat gastrointestinal tract. Stimulation by a hypertonic environment in vitro. Prostaglandins 15:751–757
Kowalewski K, Kotedej A (1975) Effect of prostaglandin E_2 on myoelectric and mechanical activity of total isolated, ex-vivo-perfused, canine stomach. Pharmacology 13:325
Lacey SM, Sanger GJ (1980) Antagonism of prostanoid-induced contractions of rat stomach muscle by trimethoquinol or isoxsuprine. Br J Pharmacol 70:88P–89P
Laekeman GM, Herman AG (1978) Prostaglandins restore the hyoscine-induced inhibition of the guinea-pig ileum. Prostaglandins 15:829–837
Le Duc LE, Needlemann P (1980) Prostaglandin synthesis by dog gastrointestinal tract. Adv Prostaglandin Thromboxane Res 8:1515–1517
Lieb J (1978) Prostaglandin synthesis inhibitors in prophylaxis of food intolerance. Lancet 2:157
Lieb J (1980) Prostaglandin synthesis inhibitors and prophylaxis of coffee intolerance. JAMA 243:32
Luderer JR, Demers LM, Bonnem EM, Saleem A, Jeffries GH (1976) Elevated prostaglandin E in idiopathic intestinal pseudo obstruction. N Engl J Med 295:1179
Luderer JR, Demers LM, Nomides CT, Hayes AH Jr (1980) Mechanism of action of castor oil: a biochemical link to the prostaglandins. Adv Prostaglandin Thromboxane Res 8:1633–1635
Lundström V (1978) Treatment of primary dysmenorrhoea with prostaglandin synthetase inhibitors – a promising alternative. Acta Obstet Gynecol Scand 57:421–428
MacIntyre DE, Willis AL (1978) Trimethoquinol is a potent prostaglandin endoperoxide antagonist. Br J Pharmacol 63:361P
Maher JW, Hollenbeck JI, Crandall V, McGuigan J, Woodward ER (1978) Prostaglandin E_2 effect on lower oesophageal sphincter pressure and serum gastrin. J Surg Res 24:87–91
Main IHM (1973) Prostaglandins and the gastrointestinal tract. In: Cuthbert MF (ed) The prostaglandins. Pharmacological and therapeutic advances. Heinemann, London, pp 287–323
Malmsten C (1977) Some biological effects of prostaglandin endoperoxide analogues. Life Sci 18:169–176
Mathias JR, Carlson GM, Bertiger G, Martin JL, Cohen S (1977) Migrating action potential complex of cholera: a possible prostaglandin-induced response. Am J Physiol 232:E529–E534
McCance RA, Pickles VR (1960) Cyclical variations in intestinal activity in women. J Endocrinol 20:XXVII
Mennie AT, Dalley V (1973) Aspirin in radiation-induced diarrhoea. Lancet 1:1131
Mennie AT, Dalley VM, Dineen LC, Collier HOJ (1975) Treatment of radiation-induced gastro-intestinal distress with acetylsalicylate. Lancet 2:942–943
Misiewicz JJ, Waller SL, Kiley N, Horton EW (1969) Effect of oral prostaglandin E_1 on intestinal transit in man. Lancet 1:648–651

Miyazaki E, Ishizawa M, Sunano S, Synto B, Sakagami T (1967) Stimulating action of prostaglandin on the rabbit duodenal muscle. In: Bergstrom S, Samuelsson B (eds) Proceedings of the 2nd Nobel Symposium, Stockholm. Wiley Interscience, New York, pp 277–281

Moncada S, Korbut R, Bunting S, Vane JR (1978 a) Prostacyclin is a circulating hormone. Nature 273:767–768

Moncada S, Salmon JA, Vane JR, Whittle BJR (1978 b) Formation of prostacyclin and its product 6-oxo-$PGF_{1\alpha}$ by the gastric mucosa of several species. J Physiol (Lond) 275:4P

Morris HR, Taylor GW, Piper PJ, Tippins JR (1980) Structure of slow-reacting substance of anaphylaxis from guinea-pig lung. Nature 285:104–106

Mukhopadhyay AK, Weisbrodt NW, Copeland ED (1974) Effect of prostaglandin E_2 infusion on patterns of intestinal myoelectric activity. Gastroenterology 66:A-98/752

Naish FC (1952) Breast feeding. In: Moncrieff A, Thompson WAR (eds) Child health. Eyre & Spottiswoode, London, p 218

Nakahata N, Nakanishi H, Suzuki TA (1980) A possible feedback control of excitatory transmission via prostaglandins in canine small intestine. Br J Pharmacol 68:393–398

Neeley J, Catchpole B (1971) Ileus: the restoration of alimentary tract motility by pharmacological means: Br J Surg 58:21–28

Newman A, De Moraes-Filho JPP, Philippakos D, Misiewicz JJ (1975) The effect of intravenous infusions of prostaglandins E_2 and $F_{2\alpha}$ on human gastric function. Gut 16:272–276

Nylander B, Mattsson O (1975) Effect of 16,16-dimethyl PGE_2 on gastric emptying and intestinal transit of a barium-food test meal in man. Scand J Gastroenterol 10:289–292

O'Grady J, Warrington S, Moti MJ et al. (1979) Effects of intravenous prostacyclin infusions in healthy volunteers – some preliminary observations. In: Vane JR, Bergstrom S (eds) Prostacyclin. Raven, New York, pp 409–417

Okpako DT (1975) Prostaglandins and cholera: the occurrence of prostaglandin-like smooth muscle contraction substances in cholera diarrhoea. Prostaglandins 10:769–777

Pace-Asciak C (1972) Prostaglandin synthetase activity in the rat stomach fundus. Activation by L-norepinephrine and related compounds. Biochim Biophys Acta 280:161–171

Pace-Asciak C (1976) Isolation, structure, and biosynthesis of 6-keto-prostaglandin-$F_{1\alpha}$ in the rat stomach. Am Chem Soc 98:2348–2349

Pace-Asciak C, Wolfe LS (1971) A novel prostaglandin derivative formed from arachidonic acid by rat stomach homogenates. Biochemistry 10:3657–3664

Persson N-Å, Hedqvist P (1973) Reduced intestinal muscular response to adrenergic nerve stimulation after the administration of prostaglandins. Acta Physiol Scand [Suppl] 396:108

Peskar BM (1978) Regional distribution of prostaglandin-metabolizing enzymes in the mucosa of the human upper gastrointestinal tract. Acta Hepato-gastroenterol (Stuttg) 25:49–51

Peskar BM, Peskar BA (1976) On the metabolism of prostaglandins by human gastric fundus mucosa. Biochim Biophys Acta 424:430–438

Peskar BM, Seyberth HW, Peskar BA (1980) Synthesis and metabolism of endogenous prostaglandins by human gastric mucosa. Adv Prostaglandin Thromboxane Res 8:1511–1514

Piper PJ, Seale JP (1978) Release of slow-reacting substance from guinea-pig and human lung by calcium ionophore A23187. Br J Pharmacol 63:364–365P

Powell DW, Farris RK (1975) Effect of aspirin on cholera toxin stimulated intestinal electrolyte transport. Gastroenterology 68:968

Radmanović B̌ (1968) Prostaglandins in perfusate of the rat small intestine after vagal stimulation. Jugosl Physiol Pharmacol Acta 4:123–124

Radmanović B̌ (1972) The effect of PGE_1 on the peristaltic activity of the guinea-pig isolated ileum. Arch Int Pharmacodyn Ther 200:396–404

Radmanović B̌ (1974) The effect of prostaglandins F and inderal on the peristaltic activity of the guinea-pig isolated ileum. Naunyn Schmiedebergs Arch Pharmacol 285:R.65

Rask-Madsen J, Bukhave K (1978) Indomethacin-responsive diarrhoea in irritable bowel syndrome. Gut 19:A448

Rask-Madsen J, Bukhave K (1979) Prostaglandins and chronic diarrhoea: clinical aspects. Scand J Gastroenterol [Suppl 53] 14:73–78
Robert A (1974) Effects of prostaglandins on the stomach and the intestine. Prostaglandins 6:523–532
Robert A, Hancher AJ, Lancaster C, Nezamis JE (1979) Prostacyclin inhibits enteropooling and diarrhoea. In: Vane JR, Bergstrom S (eds) Prostacyclin. Raven, New York, pp 147–158
Ruwart MJ, Klepper MS, Rush BD (1980) Prostaglandin stimulation of gastrointestinal transit in post-operative ileus rats. Prostaglandins 19:415–426
Saeed SA, McDonald-Gibson WJ, Cuthbert J et al. (1977) Endogenous inhibitor of prostaglandin synthetase. Nature 270:32–36
Sakato M (1975) Studies on the physiological role of prostaglandins in adrenergic and non-adrenergic inhibitory neurotransmission in the guinea-pig taenia coli. Folia Pharmacol Jpn 71:445–455
Sakato M, Shimo Y (1976) Possible role of prostaglandin E_1 on adrenergic neurotransmission in the guinea-pig taenia coli. Eur J Pharmacol 40:209–214
Samuelsson B, Borgeat P, Hammarström S, Murphy RC (1979) Introduction of a nomenclature: leukotrienes. Prostaglandins 17:785–787
Sanger GJ (1977) Modulation by prostaglandins of the autonomic control of motility in guinea-pig isolated ileum. PhD thesis, University of Manchester
Sanger GJ, Bennett A (1979) Fenamates may antagonise the actions of prostaglandin endoperoxides in human myometrium. Br J Clin Pharmacol 8:479–482
Sanger GJ, Bennett A (1980a) Regional differences in the responses to prostanoids of circular muscle from guinea-pig isolated intestine. J Pharm Pharmacol 32:705–708
Sanger GJ, Bennett A (1980b) Prostanoid agonists and antagonists: differentiation of prostanoid receptors in the gut. In: Velo GP, Berti F (eds) The Prostaglandin System. Plenum Press, New York, pp 377–391
Sanger GJ, Hensby CN, Stamford IF, Bennett A (1981) Identification of arachidonic acid metabolites extracted from human uterus, and their effects on the isolated myometrium, J Pharm Pharmacol 33:607–610
Sanger GJ, Watt AJ (1978) The effect of PGE_1 on peristalsis and on perivascular nerve inhibition of peristaltic activity in guinea-pig isolated ileum. J Pharm Pharmacol 30:762–765
Sanger GJ, Watt AJ (1980) Some mechanisms which may modulate noradrenaline release in guinea-pig isolated ileum. J Pharm Pharmacol 32:188–191
Sanner JH (1969) Antagonism of prostaglandin E_2 by 1-acetyl-2-(8-chloro-10,11-dihydrobenz(b,f)(1,4)oxazepine-10-carbonyl) hydrazine(SC-19220). Arch Int Pharmacodyn Ther 180:45–56
Sanner JH (1974) Substances that inhibit the actions of prostaglandins. Arch Intern Med 133:133–145
Sanner JH, Eakins KE (1976) Prostaglandin antagonists. In: Karim SMM (ed) Prostaglandins: chemical and biochemical aspects. MTP Press, Lancaster, pp 139–190
Schulz R, Cartwright C (1976) Sensitization of the smooth muscle by prostaglandin E_1 contributes to reversal of drug-induced inhibition of the guinea-pig ileum. Naunyn Schmiedebergs Arch Pharmacol 294:257–260
Shafran I, Maurer W, Thomas FD (1977) Prostaglandins and Crohn's disease. N Engl J Med 296:694
Shea-Donohue PT, Myers L, Castell DO, Dubois A (1980) The effect of prostacyclin on gastric emptying and secretion in Rhesus monkeys. Adv Prostaglandin Thromboxane Res 8:1557–1558
Shehadeh Z, Price WE, Jacobson ED (1969) Effects of vasoactive agents on intestinal blood flow and motility in the dog. Am J Physiol 216:386–392
Sinar DR, Fletcher JR, Castell DO (1979)Comparison of the effect of continuous intravenous infusion of prostaglandins E_1, E_2, I_2 or 6-keto-$F_{1\alpha}$ on lower esophageal sphincter pressure. Abstracts 4th International Prostaglandin Conference, Washington, DC, p 107
Sinzinger H, Silberbauer K, Winter M, Seyfried H (1978)Human rectal mucosa generates prostacyclin. Lancet 2:1253

Smith JB, Dawkins PD (1971) Salicylate and enzymes. J Pharm Pharmacol 23:729–744
Smythies JR, Russell RO (1974) Possible role of prostaglandins in idiopathic postural hypotension. Lancet 2:963
Spenney JG (1979) Prostaglandin-15-hydroxy-dehydrogenase and Δ^{13} reductase: differential content in rabbit fundic and antral mucosa and muscle. Gastroenterology 76:1254A
Spruegel W, Mitznegg P, Domschke W, Domschke S, Wuensch E, Moroder L, Demling L (1977) Direct inhibitory effects of enkephalins on contractile responses in the guinea-pig ileum. Gastroenterology 72:1135
Stamford IF, Bennett A, Greenhalf J (1978) Treatment of diarrhoea in cattle and pigs with nutmeg. Vet Rec 103:14–15
Stamford IF, Bennett A, Greenhalf J (1980) Treatment of diarrhoea in calves with nutmeg. Vet Rec 106:389
Stockley HL, Bennett A (1976) Modulation of activity by prostaglandins in human gastrointestinal muscle. In: Vantrappen G (ed) Fifth International Symposium on Gastrointestinal Motility. Typoff, Herentals, pp 31–36
Sun FF, Chapman JP, McGuire JC (1977) Metabolism of prostaglandin endoperoxide in animal tissues. Prostaglandins 14:1055–1074
Suzuki T, Hashikawa T, Takano S, Hayashi A (1975) Effects of prostaglandin E_1 (PGE_1) on isolated stomach, small intestine, bronchus, and uterus of experimental animals, and the intestinal effects of the agent in vivo. Folia Pharmacol Jpn 71:109–122
Tafuri WL, Raick A (1964) Presence of 5-hydroxytryptamine in the intramural nervous system of guinea-pig's intestine. Z Naturforsch [C] 19b:1130–1132
Takai M, Matsuyama S, Yagasaki O (1974) Prostaglandin release during extension of the small intestine of the guinea-pig. Jpn J Smooth Muscle Res 10:187–189
Takai M, Yagasaki O (1976) Effect of prostaglandin E_1 on the acetylcholine release from the myenteric plexus of guinea-pig ileum. Jpn J Pharmacol [Suppl] 26:146P
Thompson JH, Angulo M (1968) Prostaglandin-induced serotonin release. Experientia 25:721–722
Tonnesen MG, Jubiz W, Moore JG, Frailey J (1974) Circadian variation of prostaglandin E production in human gastric juice. Am J Dig Dis 19:644–648
Tothill A (1976) Prostaglandin E_2: a factor in the pathogenesis of cholera. Prostaglandins 11:925–933
Trendelenburg P (1917) Physiologische und pharmakologische Versuche über die Dünndarmperistaltik. Naunyn Schmiedebergs Arch Exp Pathol Pharmakol 81:55–129
Valiulis E, Long JF (1973) Effects of drugs on intestinal water secretion following cholera toxin in guinea-pigs and rabbits. Physiologist 16:475
Vanasin B, Greenough W, Schuster MM (1970) Effect of prostaglandin (PG) on electrical and motor activity of isolated colonic muscle. Gastroenterology 58:1004
Vaughan-Williams EM, Dohadwalla AN (1969) Diarrhoea and intestinal fluid accumulation in uninfected rabbits cross perfused with blood from donar rabbits intra-intestinally infected with cholera. Nature 222:586–587
Wald A, Gotterer GS, Rajendra NA, Turjman NA, Hendrix TR (1977) Effect of indomethacin on cholera-induced fluid movement, unidirectional sodium fluxes, and intestinal cAMP. Gastroenterology 72:106–110
Waller SL (1973) Prostaglandins and the gastrointestinal tract. Gut 14:402–417
Whittle BJR, Boughton-Smith NK, Moncada S, Vane JR (1978) The relative activity of prostacyclin (PGI_2) and a stable analogue 6β-PGI_2 on the gastrointestinal and cardiovascular systems. J Pharm Pharmacol 30:597–598
Willis AL, Davison P, Ramwell PW (1974) Inhibition of intestinal tone, motility and prostaglandin biosynthesis by 5,8,11,14-eicosatetraynoic acid (TYA). Prostaglandins 5:355–368
Wilson DE (1972) Prostaglandins and the gastrointestinal tract. Prostaglandins 1:281–293
Wolfe LS, Coceani F, Pace-Asciak C (1967) The relationship between nerve stimulation and the formation and release of prostaglandins. Pharmacologist 9:171–172
Yagasaki O, Matsuyama S, Takai M (1974) The release of prostaglandins from the passively distended wall of guinea-pig intestine. Jpn J Pharmacol [Suppl] 24:31

CHAPTER 5

Pharmacology of Adrenergic, Cholinergic, and Drugs Acting on Other Receptors in Gastrointestinal Muscle

E. E. DANIEL

A. General Principles

I. Myogenic Activity of Gastrointestinal Muscle

The smooth muscle of the gastrointestinal (GI) tract is universally capable of myogenic electrical and mechanical activity (DANIEL et al. 1960; DANIEL and SARNA 1978). In a few instances, e.g., esophageal smooth muscle in some species (CHRISTENSEN and DANIEL 1966, 1968; CHAN and DIAMANT 1976; SARNA et al. 1977) and guinea-pig small intestine (see BOLTON 1979), its oscillations are not spontaneous but can be initiated by acetylcholine acting on muscarinic receptors in smooth muscle. Sphincteric regions which exert continuous tension may spike continuously, unrelated to myogenic oscillatory activity or acetylcholine release (ASOH and GOYAL 1975). Elsewhere, atropine or other antagonists at muscarinic receptors or tetrodotoxin acting to prevent Na-dependent action potentials of nerves do not affect this myogenic activity. Myogenic activity in most regions consists of periodic membrane oscillations, called slow waves, electrical control activity (ECA) or pacemaker activity, on which are superimposed spikes or action potentials. Slow waves or ECA without spikes are not accompanied by contractile activity. Contractions are usually but not always accompanied by spikes; there may be massive depolarisation leading to inactivation of spike mechanisms or contraction from release of Ca^{2+} stores. In vitro, canine stomach circular muscle from some regions responds to acetylcholine by an increase in amplitude and duration of the plateau phase of the myogenic oscillation exclusive of any spikes; these effects are accompanied by contractions (DANIEL 1965; SZURSZWESKI 1975; EL-SHARKAWY et al. 1978; MORGAN et al. 1978; EL-SHARKAWY and SZURSZEWSKI 1978). In some regions, especially near the pylorus, spikes[1] are usually seen (DANIEL 1965, 1966a; DANIEL and IRWIN 1968). In vivo spikes can be recorded from all oscillating areas (nonfundal) in some preparations (DANIEL and IRWIN 1968; DANIEL and CHAPMAN 1966; S. K. SARNA and E. E. DANIEL unpublished work), but whether these derive from longitudinal or circular muscle is unclear.

The ECA is coupled electrically, so that oscillations in both layers near any one point are nearly synchronous; also good coupling within circular muscle allows ac-

1 We will use "spikes" in this discussion to avoid confusion. SZURSZEWSKI (1975) referring to canine stomach, prefers to call the total oscillation (initial depolarisation plus plateau with or without spikes) an action potential even though after administration of atropine no recordable contractions accompany the oscillations in vivo or in more cases in vitro. We will refer to this residual atropine-insensitive activity, as ECA or pacemaker activity

tivity to spread circumferentially nearly synchronously except in the distal bowel (ileum and colon). In the stomach and upper intestine, proximal oscillators have the highest intrinsic (i.e. with no input) frequency and normally pull up the frequency of distal oscillators, usually to the same frequency as the proximal oscillators (3 and 12 cycles/min in the human stomach and duodenum). In the lower jejunum and ileum, the distal oscillators have much lower intrinsic frequencies than proximal ones and cannot follow the frequency of the duodenal oscillators; they are, however, pulled up in frequency above their intrinsic frequencies (see Daniel and Sarna 1978 for details). The large bowel system of oscillators in the human (or indeed any species) has not been adequately characterised. Analysis of recording of electrical oscillators is difficult as the signal-to-noise ratio is low, multiple frequencies appear to be present when computer-based (fast Fourier transform or FFT) analysis is carried out and no frequency gradient can be discerned (Sarna et al. 1980). Coupling to the extent of phase locking of frequencies is not the rule in any dimension and experiments to define intrinsic frequencies and coupling in the human intestine have not been reported (Sarna et al. 1980). In vivo recordings of dog large intestine are similar in their general features to those of human large bowel (Bowes et al. 1978; El-Sharkawy 1978) but in vitro recordings show a regular ECA of 5 cycles/min (El-Sharkawy 1978). This paradox has not been satisfactorily explained. It may be related to disparate oscillation frequencies of circular (5 cycles/min) and longitudinal (0–20 cycles/min) muscle (El-Sharkawy et al. 1980).

The structural and functional basis for electrical coupling among intestinal muscle cells is unclear. Gap junctions, assumed to be sites of low resistance contracts between cells, are present in large numbers in circular muscle of most regions (Henderson et al. 1971; Daniel et al. 1976; Gabella 1972a, 1979). The large bowel may be an exception in lacking gap junctions between circular muscle cells (Daniel et al. 1975). The arrangement may account for the tight coupling (nearly simultaneous occurrence of myogenic electrical events) around the gut circumference and provide for ring-like contractions (see Daniel and Sarna 1978) in regions other than the large bowel. In contrast, few or no gap junctions are found in longitudinal muscle of the stomach and intestine (Henderson et al. 1971; Daniel et al. 1976). A few small particle assemblies resembling gap junctions are reported to exist in cell membranes of guinea-pig taenia coli by freeze fracture (Gabella and Blundell 1978; Fry et al. 1977); but the efficacy of these structures in cell-to-cell coupling remains to be established. Despite the near absence of gap junctions, longitudinal muscle of the intestine and stomach shows good coupling although less tight than circular muscle; space constants measured by the technique of Abe and Tomita (1968) are 1–2 mm, well over the length of one cell (~ 100 μm). Perhaps coupling is capacitative rather than resistive. Also, although there appears to be synchrony of oscillation between longitudinal and circular muscle layers of the stomach and intestine, no structural basis for this in terms of frequent contacts between muscle layers exists (E. E. Daniel unpublished work). One report suggests that other cells provide for such coupling, e.g., interstitial cells (Taylor et al. 1977), but I have been unable to confirm this as a general explanation (E. E. Daniel unpublished work).

II. Nervous Control of Gastrointestinal Muscle

Nerves rarely make close apposition contacts with smooth muscle in the bowel (RICHARDSON 1958; BENNETT and ROGERS 1967; GABELLA 1972c)[2]. Thus with some exceptions, release of mediators is into general extracellular space between muscle cells and diffusion over distance guarantees a diffuse rather than discrete action of mediators. Also, in well-coupled regions, junction potentials from release of mediator in effective concentrations at one point will spread electrotonically to many other areas. The chief role of nerves thus appears to be modulation of myogenic activity e.g. cholinergic nerves produce local and transmitted excitatory junction potentials which on the depolarised phase of the slow wave or ECA, initiate spikes; nonadrenergic inhibitory nerves hyperpolarise the membrane and prevent spikes. Most sympathetic nerves innervate intrinsic intestinal neurones and noradrenaline released from them modulates cholinergic nerve activity, inhibiting release of acetylcholine by an action on α_2-receptors on nerves (see Sect. B.I). In some regions sympathetic nerves directly innervate gut muscle and noradrenaline acts on α- or β-receptors in smooth muscle to hyperpolarise or inhibit muscle depolarisation (COSTA and GABELLA 1968, 1971; GABELLA and COSTA 1969; FURNESS and COSTA 1974; GILLESPIE and MAXWELL 1971; GABELLA 1972c). The localisation and functions of peptide as neurotransmitters and neuromodulators are considered elsewhere in this volume. In general, all nerve mediators or modulators function ultimately to enhance (bring to spiking or contraction threshold) or inhibit (hyperpolarise below spiking threshold) myogenic oscillations of the intestine; some by acting on receptors in smooth muscle, some by acting on receptors in the nervous system.

Insofar as action potentials are propagated by electrical coupling between cells, the result is an amplification of nerve- or drug-initiated responses. Thus attempts to relate number of mediator or agonist molecules, degree of receptor, receptor occupancy and muscle response may be confounded when action potentials propagate. However, it is highly probable that action potential propagation is in turn limited by the myogenic oscillations, i.e. an action potential or spike can propagate only into regions in which the membrane potential has been brought near threshold by myogenic oscillation, normally only during the depolarised phase of the membrane slow wave or ECA (DANIEL and SARNA 1978). Thus coupling of ECA and the resultant propagation or phase lag of slow waves or ECA probably determine the area available for spread of spikes in most intestinal tissues.

What has become apparent over the last few years is that the complexity of neuronal control may be at least on order of magnitude more than previously realised. Presynaptic receptors to the synaptic mediator and to other endogenous substances may enhance or inhibit the release of mediator. Thus feedback controls are exerted on the nerves, but the physiological role of these is so far unclear. A variety of peptides are contained in intrinsic nerves or endocrine cells exist within

2 The statement is sometimes made (READ and BURNSTOCK 1969; ROGERS and BURNSTOCK 1966) that such contacts are frequent in circular muscle, but this seems to be based on studies in the toad intestine. It is not true of large bowel of humans (DANIEL et al. 1975; E. E. DANIEL unpublished work) or circular muscle of small intestine of dogs, rabbits or humans (RICHARDSON 1958; DANIEL et al. 1975)

the gut; their function is not understood. Their release can probably be affected by nerves, and they may act on nerves or muscle when released. Afferent intrinsic neurones exist within the gut and allow integration within the intrinsic nervous system, at peripheral ganglia and centrally.

Clearly great caution must be exerted in analysing the sites and mechanisms of drug actions on the intestine in vivo since receptors of similar chemical affinities may be on smooth muscle, intrinsic neurones or their processes, extrinsic neurones or their processes, or even in endocrine cells of the gut or elsewhere. Relatively few studies have been made about mechanisms of drug–receptor interaction in nerves in vivo.

Analysis of sites of drug actions in vitro is slightly simpler than in vivo, at least in theory, because often only smooth muscle and axons of intrinsic neurones are present. In some preparations, functioning processes of extrinsic nerves, cell bodies of intrinsic neurones and active endocrine cells are also present. An added complication in vitro is the enhanced production of prostaglandins, especially PGE_2 and PGI_2 (usually excitatory to longitudinal muscle and inhibitory to circular muscle) or thromboxanes (excitatory), which may accompany dissection and in vitro preparation of tissues for study (FERREIRA et al. 1976). Interpretation of in vitro data may be difficult, owing to loss of various myogenic and neuronal control systems on dissection of the gut and to the failure over time at varying rates, of the remaining control processes, owing to the inadequacy of in vitro conditions for maintenance of metabolism of all cells in isolated gut wall. Access of drugs to receptors may well be different when the agent is delivered by perfusion, superfusion or immersion compared with delivery via the bloodstream or release from nerves. Thus it is dangerous to conclude that a drug action observed or absent in vitro will be observed similarly in vivo or vice versa. Nevertheless the use of in vitro studies, which provide a simpler set of control systems affecting responses and allow the possibility of more rigorously controlling relevant variables, has provided much valuable information.

The regions of the gut differ in their innervation and in their receptor populations. For example, the lower oesophageal sphincter is more sensitive to a variety of agonists than circular muscle of the oesophageal body 1–2 cm proximally (CHRISTENSEN and DONS 1968) and possesses receptors to excitatory prostaglandins ($PGF_{2\alpha}$, TxA_2, TxB_2) which are virtually absent in the body (DANIEL et al. 1979). These quantitative and qualitative distinctions may be characteristic of sphincteric circular muscle compared with other such muscle, e.g. these regions have receptors to peptides which are absent or nearly absent elsewhere (see GOYAL and RATTAN 1978). However, there also seem to be similarities in receptor populations throughout the gastrointestinal tract; all muscle layers contain muscarinic cholinergic receptors, β-adrenoceptors, and nonadrenergic noncholinergic inhibitory receptors. The extent of distribution of α-adrenergic inhibitory receptors on intestinal muscle is not known. They exist in guinea-pig taenia coli (see Sect. B.I). There are quantitative differences in the distribution of these receptor populations between muscle layers, corresponding to differences in innervation. Thus field stimulation in vitro usually produces more prominent cholinergic excitatory junction potentials in longitudinal muscle than in circular muscle and predominantly nonadrenergic inhibitory junction potentials in circular muscle (HIRST and

McKirdy 1974; Cheung and Daniel 1981). Correspondingly more muscarinic receptors may occur in longitudinal muscle than in circular muscle or they may be more readily activated, but this has not been fully studied. Since neither the mediator nor useful selective antagonists of nonadrenergic inhibitory (NAI) nerves are conclusively known and it is not certain if purines act on the same receptor as the NAI mediator, it is uncertain whether there are more receptors for it or denser inhibitory innervation in the circular muscle. The generalisation is that the outcome of experiments in which drugs acting only on muscle are applied will depend upon whether activity of longitudinal or circular muscle is being recorded. When drugs are applied which act on both nerve and muscle, the outcome will depend on the layer from which activity is recorded and the nature of the innervation of that layer (see this Handbook, Vol. 59/I, Chaps. 5, 9, 10 for further discussion of nervous control).

III. Receptors and Receptor Mechanisms

Receptors (usually located in cell membranes) are sites of selective chemical recognition in all membranes for nerve mediators or modulators, hormones and autocoids. Receptors for the same naturally occurring substance often differ in their chemistry as demonstrated by their ability to distinguish other agonists and antagonists; e.g. nicotinic and muscarinic receptors for acetylcholine. Interaction of receptors having a similar chemistry with their agonists often leads to different outcomes (e.g. acetylcholine hyperpolarises vertebrate cardiac muscle by increasing the conductance to K^+ but depolarises skeletal muscle endplates by increasing both Na^+ and K^+ conductances). This is presumably because the receptor is coupled in different tissues to different ionophores or permeability channels in cell membrane, making different conductance channels available for activation. The conclusions is that drugs acting on the same receptor in nerve, muscle or endocrine cells in the gut may have different effects on membrane electrogenesis. The ultimate effects of a drug acting on different receptors in different cells may be difficult to predict; e.g. muscarinic agonists may act on excitatory receptors in muscle and also on excitatory neural receptors in some cholinergic and nonadrenergic inhibitory neurones as well as on inhibitory receptors on sympathetic nerves (decreasing release of noradrenaline see Sect. B.I).

Since the gut is supplied with an intrinsic nervous system with inputs from mechanoreceptors and chemoreceptors, any activation of motility or secretion may initiate secondary responses involving other receptors, nerve or hormone pathways, mediators and outcome. Again the conclusion is that the use of a net contractile response to assess receptor mechanisms may be naive.

In sum, the intact intestine and even the isolated intestinal strip are not simple systems in which drug action can easily be related to occupancy of a set of receptors on muscle. Structure–activity relationships for agonists or antagonists of receptors in the intestine have been reported in great number, but it is difficult to know whether we can accept the interpretation of such studies in terms of actions at a single receptor. Even if the assumption of action at a single receptor is valid in a particular experiment, we must still determine how to relate interaction of receptor and agonist and antagonists with motor responses.

When drugs are added to the bath in vitro, it is often assumed that the bath concentration is the same as the drug concentration in the biophase near the receptor. This may be the case for some drugs. However, there are several reasons for doubting this assumption in most cases. (1) There are highly active drug uptake and inactivation sites near most receptors (only agents which are not taken up or inactivated, are likely to be in equilibrium at the receptor with drug in the bath); (2) there is an unstirred fluid layer near cell surfaces which will affect (usually lower) the drug concentration near the receptor; (3) there are diffusion barriers between the bath fluid and some cell surfaces which may limit the access of a drug to its sites of action (when this effect is combined with rapid inactivation inside the diffusion barrier, an active agent may appear to be inactive).

Furthermore, to relate receptor occupancy by an excitant agent to contractile responses, we must make assumptions about fractional receptor occupancy and response. Usually, it is assumed that fractional receptor occupancy is directly and linearly related to contractile response; and maximum contractile response occurs only when all receptors are occupied. This is inherently unlikely to be the case in gut smooth muscle under ordinary conditions of myogenic control of excitability in vivo or in vitro.

First, occupancy of receptors effects changes in permeability, usually depolarising for excitatory transmitters like acetylcholine and analogues. The effect of these membrane potential changes for contraction will depend upon the extent to which the initial membrane potential of the cells effecting contraction (say in a segment of gut) is above or below the membrane potential threshold for opening of voltage-dependent Ca^{2+} channels and initiation of spiking. This in turn will depend upon the magnitude of the electrical control oscillations in the segment and the degree of synchrony of these. Only in certain regions (stomach, upper small intestine) are there circumferential segments in which the membrane oscillations are in phase. Elsewhere occupancy of a given fraction of receptors will have variable effects related to the degree of synchrony of myogenic control activity. Even in those areas where ECA can be considered phase-locked and synchronous the response of occupancy of a given fraction of receptors will depend on the mean level of the membrane potential during oscillation. If action potentials can be propagated within the area of synchronous oscillation, this will amplify the response so that full receptor occupancy may not be required for a maximal response.

Second, permeability changes usually affect membrane potential by allowing one or more ions to pass through the membrane more freely. Since none of the ions in smooth muscle cells is in equilibrium at a membrane potential of -50 to -60 mV there will be a net flow of ions into or our of cells, tending to move the membrane potential closer to equilibrium. K^+ reaches equilibrium at -80 to -90 mV; Cl^- at -25 to -35 mV; Na^+ at $+20$ to $+40a^{2+}$ at $+50$ mV. The approach to the equilibrium potential for a given ion with receptor occupancy is not linear, but hyperbolic. So the occupancy of the first 25% of receptors would have a much bigger effect on membrane potential than the occupancy of the last 25%.

Third, receptor occupancy is unlikely to be uniform throughout the gut wall either after release of mediator from the nerve endings or after perfusion or superfusion of an active agent. Nerve release of mediator necessarily implies gradients or released material in the tissue and gradients of a different type must occur during diffusion of active agents from blood vessel or bath fluid. Thus, fractional receptor occupancy may vary dramatically in different regions of the gut wall.

As occupancy increases and occurs during the appropriate phase of ECA, the resultant excitatory junction potential (e.j.p.) reaches threshold and initiates spiking and contraction. These are usually Ca^{2+} spikes, and the resultant Ca^{2+} entry often initiates an increase in K^+ permeability (leading to afterhyperpolarisation – see MEECH 1978; PUTNEY 1979; BOLTON 1979). This afterhyperpolarisation limits spike trains, shortens slow waves and limits contractions. As further and more widespread receptor occupancy occurs, the membrane potential between spikes will not return to the values determined by the electrogenic ion pump, the prevailing electrochemical potential, and the ECA. The ECA then becomes smaller, faster, uncoupled, and asynchronous as Ca^{2+} entry becomes large. It is probable, too, that some drugs (e.g. those for which efficient inactivation mechanisms are lacking) will produce persistent baseline changes in membrane potential rather than transient potential changes. Others may release intracellular Ca^{2+} for initiation of contraction without affecting membrane potential. Thus the net effect of a drug to produce contraction will depend upon its interaction with the ECA, to modify its rate, amplitude, coupling, and relation to spike threshold and upon the ability of the drug to release sequestered Ca^{2+} by mechanisms that do not depend on the membrane potential. Unfortunately neither excitatory nor inhibitory drugs have been studied in vivo or in vitro with regard to the nature of these changes.

All the remarks about excitatory agents apply to inhibitory ones. There is the additional complication that inhibition must be measured by depression of active contraction. The degree to which a given fractional occupancy of receptors by an inhibitory agent depresses the active tension must vary with the mechanisms initiating that tension (extent and nature of permeability changes and depolarisation to open Ca^{2+} channels or actions to release sequestered Ca^{2+}), upon the site of action and distribution of the excitatory agent (plexus, nerve axons, smooth muscle of one or other layer) and upon the processes which propagate excitation (spread of action potentials) diffusion of chemicals, activation of neurones).

Also in vivo, the intestine response to variations in contractile activity by both excitants and inhibitors includes initiation of various intrinsic and extrinsic reflexes. Contraction initiates distal inhibition by intrinsic nerves and may initiate local and distant inhibition by reflexes transmitted from afferent nerves in the wall to the coeliac and other mesenteric ganglia and activating sympathetic efferents to local and distal regions (WEEMS and SZURSZEWSKI 1977). Furthermore, many drugs acting on the gastrointestinal tract directly also affect the cardiovascular system and initiate sympathetic and vagal reflexes which alter gut function. Thus, the outcome of administration of a drug in vivo is usually the net result of direct and indirect responses.

The pharmacologist studying isolated muscle strips seeks to minimise the myogenic and neurogenic activity which necessarily causes variations in the relationship between receptor occupancy and contractile responses in vivo. Strips or segments recording activity of the longitudinal muscle of ileum of guinea-pig are often studied. The guinea-pig intestine alone among common laboratory animals, differs from that of human and other mammals in having no significant myogenic ECA and spontaneous activity; also the longitudinal muscle of this species may contain almost no nerves (GABELLA 1972c). Thus it is a valuable tool for the study of drug-receptor interactions but may be of little relevance to drug effects in vivo or in vitro in other species showing ECA. Guinea-pig taenia coli is another popular tool for study, but it too is usually stretched to the point that any ECA is absent. When intestinal strips of species other than guinea-pig are studied, longitudinal strips containing few nerves are often used after being subjected to experimental conditions minimising ECA and spontaneous activity.

At present we can utilise the data from such studies to give limited insight into receptor occupancy, but must use a simpler approach, consistent with our limited knowledge, to analyses of drug actions on intact intestine or on strips and segments of most species. The approach will be to depend on pharmacological tools verified as selective by studies of receptor occupancy in simple systems, such as the guinea-pig ileum.

B. Drugs Acting on Adrenoceptors

Two types of adrenoceptors,α and β, have been recognised since the classical studies of AHLQUIST and LEVY (1959). It has become conventional to devide beta receptors into β_1 and β_2 on the basis of presumed differences in selectivity for agonists and antagonists. The validity of this concept for the intestine will be discussed in Sect. B.III. Recently, it has been proposed that α-receptors should also be subdivided into α_1 and α_2. Furthermore, in some neurones, the main catecholamine is not noradrenaline, but its precursor, dopamine. In some systems dopamine appears to act on α-receptors, in others on β-receptors and in the central nervous system, kidney vasculature and a few other places including some gut systems, a receptor for dopamine itself is found (see Sect. B.III and this Handbook, Vol. 59/I, Chaps. 10, 11).

I. Alpha-Receptors

The gut is a peculiarly unfavourable tissue for study of adrenergic receptors. It has all adrenergic receptor types localised at various sites. Also, the relationship between adrenergic innervation and gut muscle is variable; in most cases there are no intrinsic adrenergic neurones (but see FURNESS 1971) and the primary innervation is of blood vessels and intrinsic neurones (NORBERG 1964; READ and BURNSTOCK 1969; GABELLA 1972c), but sometimes, e.g. sphincters (COSTA and GABELLA 1968, 1971; FURNESS and COSTA 1973; GILLESPIE and MAXWELL 1971; BAUMGARTEN and LANGE 1969), circular muscle of ileum (SILVA et al. 1971; ABERG and ERANKO 1967), and taenia coli (GABELLA and COSTA 1969; READ and BURNSTOCK 1969; GABELLA 1972), the smooth muscle itself is innervated. There have been, as a consequence, relatively few quantitative or semiquantitative studies of adrenergic pharmacology of the gut. Recently, WIKBERG (1979) has reviewed a variety of studies including his own of α-receptor mechanisms in the small intestine.

The separation of α_1- and α_2-adrenoceptors is based on the selectivity of both agonists and antagonists, and it is claimed that this distinguishes presynaptic (α_2) from postsynaptic (α_1) receptors. In the study of the selectivity of drugs for adrenoceptors, it is necessary to: (1) rule out indirect effects (release of catecholamines or inhibition of acetylcholine release); (2) inhibit both neuronal and extraneural uptake and metabolism, and in systems with much collagen, binding to this constituent must also be eliminated or considered; (3) block any other classes of adrenergic receptors present than the one under study.

AHLQUIST and LEVY (1959) demonstrated that adrenergic relaxation of the canine gut was produced by agonists acting on both α- and β-receptors; it could not be prevented except by combined blockade of both receptors. This was verified in other gut preparations (e.g. see FURCHGOTT 1967, 1972; BUCKNELL and WHITNEY 1964; BOWMAN and HALL 1970). ANDERSSON and MOHME-LUNDHOLM (1969, 1970) reported that the relaxation by α-receptor occupancy was followed by different metabolic changes (phosphorylase activity, hexosephosphate, lactate, cyclic AMP, ATP, and creatine PO_4 decreased) from those following relaxation on β-receptor occupancy (cyclic AMP, hexosephosphate, lactate, ATP, CP increased). Also the α-effects followed and appeared to be a consequence of relaxation while β-effects accompanied or preceded relaxation. Whether cyclic AMP elevation by β-receptor stimulation is an essential component of the mechanism of smooth muscle relaxation is still debated (ANDERSSON 1972; DANIEL and JANIS 1975; BÄR 1974). Certainly, there are instances in which dissociation of relaxation from increase in cyclic AMP can be demonstrated (see BÄR 1974). In any case, agonists like phenylephrine were considered to act primarily α-receptors while isopropylnoradrenaline was considered to act primarily on β-receptors. Similar selectivity was found for antagonists, e.g. phentolamine and dibenamine were thought to be selective for α-receptors and pronethalol and propranolol for β-receptors.

In taenia coli, BÜLBRING and TOMITA (1969a, b, c, 1977a, b) showed that the relaxation from α-receptor occupation was accompanied by hyperpolarisation which inhibited spiking. They found that this hyperpolarisation depended on the gradient for K^+ and probably Cl^-, so they suggested that activation of α-receptors enhanced membrane conductance for K^+ and Cl^-. This was in partial agreement with the increased efflux of K^+ noted earlier by JENKINSON and MORTON (1967a, b) in taenia coli. These actions from receptor occupation were directly on smooth muscle as they were unaffected by TTX.

However, PATON and VIZI (1969) and KOSTERLITZ et al. (1970) showed that agonists at α-receptors could inhibit spontaneous or field-stimulated release of acetylcholine from guinea-pig longitudinal muscle strips containing the myenteric plexus. This inhibition was especially effective at low physiological frequencies of field stimulation. KOSTERLITZ et al. (1970) also showed that contractions caused by acetylcholine release from nerves were more readily blocked by agents acting on α-receptors while contractions related to addition of acetylcholine to the bath were more readily blocked by agents acting on β-receptors. They postulated that innervated α-receptors were on intrinsic nerves and β-receptors on muscle cells were affected mainly by circulating catecholamines. Not all authors were subsequently able to confirm this arrangement, and clearly in some systems (e.g. taenia coli of guinea-pigs) inhibitory α-receptors are present on muscle and noradrenaline released by nerve stimulation sometimes reaches these receptors.

Further insight about presynaptic α-adrenergic receptors is from the in vitro work of STARKE and co-workers (STARKE and MONTELL 1974; STARKE et al. 1974, 1975a, b, c, 1978; and reviewed by STARKE 1977) on both adrenergic neurones and smooth muscle of rabbit pulmonary artery. α-Receptors on neurones caused inhibition of field-stimulated contraction while activation of those in muscle initiated contractions. They concluded that α-receptors on the two loci had different affinities for agonists. Methoxamine and phenylephrine preferentially acted postsynaptically while clonidine was a partial agonist at such sites and a full agonist at presynaptic sites. Other agonists (oxymetazoline, α-methylnoradrenaline, and tramazoline) also acted preferentially presynaptically. In some cases (methoxamine and tramazoline) preferential actions were in the ratio of 500:1 for a particular site. DREW (1977) showed that contraction from field-stimulated release of noradrenaline from rat vas deferens was inhibited by clonidine, oxymetazoline, naphazoline, and xylazine but phenylephrine and methoxamine were ineffective and initiated contractions by acting on postsynaptic α-receptors.

However, in these studies there was not uniform attention to: (1) blockade of concomitant actions at β-adrenoceptors; (2) inhibition of noradrenaline or other agonist uptake or metabolism. Also since noradrenaline is released from neurones and acts presynaptically at α-receptors to inhibit its own release,the exogenous addition of agents acting at these receptors will disturb this relationship and also there will be competition between endogenous and exogenous agonists. Results may be quantitatively in error for these receptors (indicating a less than correct potency). Nevertheless, these studies suggest that agents like clonidine have a higher affinity for presynaptic α-receptors while phenylephrine and methoxamine have a higher affinity for postsynaptic α-receptors, being almost inactive at presynaptic receptors (see Table 1).

Studies with antagonists also support a pharmacological difference in pre- and postsynaptic α-receptors. DUBOCOVICH and LANGER (1974) proposed that phenoxybenzamine was more effective at inhibiting contractions to endogenous or exogenous noradrenaline in cat spleen than in increasing overflow of noradrenaline following nerve stimulation (withdrawal of presynaptic inhibition) because it preferentially inhibited postsynaptic receptors. DOXEY et al. (1977) found that yohimbine and phentolamine, but not phenoxybenzamine or prazosine could selectively block clonidine-induced inhibition of field-stimulated contractions of rat vas deferens without inhibiting contractile response to field stimulation. In rat anococcygeus muscle, yohimbine was much more effective on presynaptic receptors and prazosin and phenoxybenzamine on postsynaptic receptors. Similar results were obtained by DREW (1977) on rat vas deferens. Not all tissues nor all authors have found the same selectivity for phentolamine. In fact the only consistently and clearly selective antagonists in intestine (WIKBERG 1979) seem to be yohimbine for the presynaptic α-receptor, prazosin for the postsynaptic receptor and possibly piperoxane for the presynaptic receptor. In summary, there seems to be evidence from selectivity of both agonists and antagonists that presynaptic α-receptors (hereafter α_2) differ from postsynaptic α-receptors (hereafter α_1).

WIKBERG (1977a, 1978a, b, 1979) has studied the differentiation of α_1 and α_2 receptors in guinea-pig ileum longitudinal muscle and in rabbit jejunum. In the guinea-pig ileum he used sotalol to block β-receptors, cocaine and corticosterone to block uptakes 1 and 2 respectively and pretreatment with reserpine to block noradrenaline release (see GILLESPIE 1976; GILLIS 1976; ROSS 1976; TRENDELENBURG 1976). The relative potencies of agonists in inhibiting contractions from field stim-

Table 1. Potencies relative to noradrenaline (WIKBERG 1979)

	Guinea-pig aorta α_1	Guinea-pig ileum cholinergic neurone α_2	Quotient α_2/α_1
Clonidine	0.016	9.1	569.0
Adrenaline	1.2	3.4	2.83
Methylnoradrenaline	0.23	3.2	13.9
Tramazoline	0.054	2.9	53.7
Naphazoline	0.20	2.2	11.0
Oxymetazoline	0.2	1.7	8.5
Noradrenaline	1.0	1.0	
Xylazine	0.0035	0.5	142.9
Phenylephrine	0.12	0.0089	0.074
Norphenylephrine	0.063	0.0077	0.122
Methoxamine	0.010	0.0044	0.044

ulation at low frequencies (from release of acetylcholine from cholinergic neurones) are shown in Table 1 in comparison with values for contractile responses of guinea-pig aorta (postsynaptic α-receptors). From this he concluded that clonidine, xylazine, and tramazoline were highly selective for α-receptors on neurones (α_2) and methoxamine, phenylephrine and norphenylephrine were selective for α-receptors in smooth muscle (α_1).

He also found phentolamine to be selective in blocking postsynaptic receptors in guinea-pig terminal ileum (mediating contraction) and rabbit aorta ($pA_2 = 7.1$ and 7.6 respectively) compared with presynaptic receptors in guinea-pig ileum ($pA_2 = 6.0$). DREW (1978) has found yohimbine to be selective for blockade of presynaptic receptors in guinea-pig ileum ($pA_2 = 7.8$) compared with values reported by others for postsynaptic receptors [e.g. HARPER et al. (1978) for rabbit ileum $pA_2 = 5.6$]. Prazosin has apparently not been tested on α-receptors on cholinergic neurones, but DOXEY et al. (1977) found it to be selective for postsynaptic α-receptors on rat anococcygeal muscle ($pA_2 = 8.2$) compared with presynaptic α-receptors in rat vas deferens ($pA_2 = 6.6$). Thus in addition to selectivity of agonists, presynaptic receptors in the gut should be differentiable from those in postsynaptic gut smooth muscle by selectivity of adrenergic antagonists: yohimbine for presynaptic; phentolamine or prazosin for postsynaptic receptors. Direct evidence that release of acetylcholine from nerves of the guinea-pig ileum can be inhibited by noradrenaline, has been obtained by a number of authors. Acetylcholine stores were partially labelled with choline H^3 and spontaneous and field-stimulated release of radioactivity determined (PATON and VIZI 1969; KOSTERLITZ et al. 1970). WIKBERG (1977b) recently carried out similar studies with the refinement of separating emergent radioactivity into acetylcholine, choline, and other metabolites.

There is little evidence of α-receptors on guinea-pig ileal longitudinal muscle mediating relaxation. Thus WIKBERG (1977a, 1978a, b) found noradrenaline to be ineffective in relaxing carbachol-induced contractions after blockade of β-receptors, except in high, nonspecific doses not blocked by dibenamine or phentolamine.

Phenylephrine in concentrations up to 5×10^{-4} *M* was also ineffective. Terminal ileum sometimes possesses excitatory α-receptors (see FURCHGOTT 1972).

The pharmacological selectivity of adrenergic receptors on pre- and postsynaptic sites in other gastrointestinal preparations requires elucidation. There is evidence that in longitudinal and circular muscle lower of oesophageal sphincter of the cat (CHRISTENSEN and DANIEL 1966, 1968; GONELLA et al. 1977, 1979) there are presynaptic α-receptors mediating contraction by increased acetylcholine release. Whether they are similar pharmacologically to those mediating inhibition of acetylcholine release, remains to be determined.

In rabbit jejunum, which had prominent α-inhibitor responses associated with receptors in smooth muscle, WIKBERG (1979) found some, unconvincing evidence of additional presynaptic receptors. Adrenaline and phenylephrine were slightly more effective in inhibiting a jejunum strip contracted by field stimulation than when it was contracted by acetylcholine. On the other hand, GILLESPIE and KHOYI (1977) found in rabbit colon that there was clear evidence of presynaptic α-receptors inhibiting contractile responses to pelvic nerve stimulation (predominantly parasympathetic) when noradrenaline was released by stimulation of sympathetic nerves. Phentolamine was an effective antagonist. However, when noradrenaline was added exogenously, propranolol as well as phentolamine was required to inhibit the depression of contractions from pelvic nerve stimulation. Isopropylnoradrenaline was virtually ineffective against contractions induced by release of acetylcholine from nerves, but it and noradrenaline were highly effective against contractions induced by exogenous acetylcholine, and this inhibiting effect was nearly completely blocked by propranolol. The authors concluded that presynaptic α-receptors account for most of the response to sympathetic nerve activity but that β-receptors are predominant in the smooth muscle and contribute to inhibition of responses when noradrenaline released in the plexus spills over to the muscle.

One paradox which remains unexplained is why isopropylnoradrenaline is highly effective against exogenously added but largely ineffective against nerve-released acetylcholine. Perhaps β-adrenoceptors are not present near sites of release of acetylcholine from nerves which then initiate propagated electrical activity. If this is the case, it would also account for the greater dependence on α-receptors of inhibition by noradrenaline released in the plexus compared with noradrenaline added exogenously. Inhibition of noradrenaline reuptake, which might have increased its diffusion to β-receptors when released in the plexus, was not tested.

In summary, α-receptors in intestinal muscle usually inhibit contractions but may be located either on intrinsic neurones (and operate by inhibition of acetylcholine release) or on smooth muscle (and operate by hyperpolarising the membrane owing to increased K^+ Cl^- permeability). The relative importance of these two types of receptors on various preparations is unknown.

II. Beta-Receptors

Almost every smooth muscle possesses inhibitory β-adrenoceptors, apparently unrelated to the presence of adrenergic innervation. Perhaps this reflects the ubiquitous exposure of muscles to circulating catecholamines. The relaxation of guinea-pig taenia coli mediated by β-receptors is not accompanied by prominent membrane hyperpolarisation (BÜLBRING and TOMITA 1969a, b, c, 1977a, b) or by changes in transmembrane resistance as measured by the double sucrose gap method. Thus changes in conductance of the major current-carrying ions during β-receptor stimulation is unlikely unless there is a balance of increased conductance for some and decreased conductance for other ions. However, selective removal of ions from the external medium does not unmask a conductance change. BÜLBRING and TOMITA (1977a, b) have suggested that there is a decrease in pacemaker activity, possibly mediated by altered Ca^{2+} fluxes or binding.

More recently, BÜLBRING and DEN HERTOG (1977) have reported some hyperpolarisation of guinea-pig taenia coli on β-receptor occupation and an accompanying decrease in the membrane resistance as measured by the decrease in electrotonic potential in the sucrose gap. Also the hyperpolarisation was increased by removal of external Cl^- and decreased by elevation of external K^+, as expected if potassium permeability was increased. K-free solution did not have the expected effect of enhancing hyperpolarisation, but this may reflect effects of K removal to decrease electrogenic ion pumping as well as to decrease the K gradient. An unanswered question is whether there was complete inhibition of α-adrenoceptors in this case so that the effects could not have been related to the increase in K conductance from α-receptor occupation. It should be noted (see BOLTON 1979 for review) that in general the effects of β-receptor stimulation on myometrium usually involve hyperpolarisation and require the presence of Ca^{2+}. However, relaxation still occurs and depends on $[Ca^{2+}]$ when the membrane potential has been eliminated by high external $[K^+]$. Detailed analysis of the mechanisms of β-receptor-mediated relaxation in other gut muscles is desirable. All intestinal muscle seems to possess β-receptors but the mechanism of these inhibitory effects is mostly unknown.

III. Possible Distinction Between Beta$_1$- and Beta$_2$-Adrenoceptors

It has become commonplace to accept that there are two subclasses of β-adrenergic receptors. β_1-Receptors in the heart and intestine are defined as having less selectivity for isopropylnoradrenaline (INA) and adrenaline (A) relative to noradrenaline (NA), almost no affinity for phenylephrine (PE) and to be relatively unaffected by certain β_2-selective agonists (e.g. salbutamol, orciprenaline, soterenol); to be readily blocked by nonselective antagonists such as propranolol, but to have low affinity for certain antagonists such as practolol. However, the situation, as summarised recently by several authors and reviewed by TRIGGLE and TRIGGLE (1976), may not be so simple. FURCHGOTT (1967, 1972) has assembled data quoted by TRIGGLE and TRIGGLE (Table 2) which suggest there may be three types of β-receptor, based on apparent values of K_B, the equilibrium constants for agonist–receptor binding.

There are also inconsistencies when agonists are considered (see FURCHGOTT 1972). For example, orciprenaline is much less effective than INA on β_1-receptors affecting contractile force and rate in guinea-pig and rabbit atria (24–125 times more is required for equivalent effects) while only 4 times as much is required for equivalent inhibition of rat myometrium (β_2-receptors). Thus it appears to be selective for β_2-receptors. On guinea-pig trachea and vas deferens,also supposedly β_2-receptors, 144 and 20 times more are required. Soterenol is almost ineffective

Table 2. Selectivity for β-adrenoceptors

Tissue	Relative activities[a]				K_B Apparent ($M \times 10^8$) Pronethalol	Receptor class
	INA	A	NA	PE		
Rabbit aorta	130	64	1	0.1	3.4	1
Guinea-pig trachea	47	12	1	0.06	3.1	
Guinea-pig atria force	3	0.5	1	<0.01	7.4	
Rabbit atria force	3.5	0.5	1		7.5	2
Guinea-pig duodenum	3	0.5	1		9.5	
Rabbit duodenum	1.5	0.2	1	<0.01	49.1	3
Rabbit stomach	2.5	1.2	1		56	

[a] INA isopropylnoradrenaline; A adrenaline; NA noradrenaline; PE phenylephrine

Table 3. Apparent K_B in rabbit tissues

Tissue	Presumed receptor	Propranolol ($M \times 10^9$)	Practolol ($M \times 10^7$)
Atrium	β_1	1.3	1.7
Aorta	β_1	1.1	1100
Stomach	β_1	180	Inactive
Trachea	β_2	[a]	26.4

[a] K_B could not be determined; slope of dose – ratio plot $\neq 1$

on rat atria rate and force responses but only 1–5 times the concentration of INA is required to activate most β_2-receptors. Thus it too appears selective for β_2-receptors. For β_1-receptors of guinea-pig atria, this compound increases force equivalently to INA at only 3 times its dose. Trimethquinol has similar potency on β_2-receptors in guinea-pig trachea and vas deferens and in rat atrium force but is inactive on guinea-pig atrium.

With β-receptor antagonists, the situation is also unclear. BRISTOW et al. (1970) compared several antagonists on rabbit atrium, aorta, and stomach (β_1-receptors) against rabbit trachea (β_2-receptors). The data for propranolol (supposedly nonselective) and practolol (supposedly β_1-selective) are given in Table 3. Thus β-receptors in rabbit stomach were like neither β_1- nor β_2-receptors. The inconsistency extended to other gastrointestinal tissues (Table 4). Again the gastrointestinal tissue (rat ileum) behaved more as if it possessed β_2-receptors, defined as having a low affinity for practolol. Clearly, it would be unwise to assume that β-receptors in gastrointestinal tissues are uniform in their pharmacological behaviour and correspond to β_1-receptors in the heart. These data are inconsistent with any simple classification of these receptors. Perhaps the problem arises from the usual focus on classifying β-receptors on the heart (β_1) and lung (β_2). Gastrointestinal recep-

Table 4. Selectivity of antagonists for β-receptors

Tissue	Presumed receptor	pA_2	
		Propranolol	Practolol
Guinea-pig atria	β_1	8.7	7.3
Rat ileum	β_1	8.7	5.9
Guinea-pig trachea	β_2	8.7	5.4
Guinea-pig vas deferens	β_2	8.9	6.8
Rat uterus	β_2	8.5	5.0

Table 5. Dopamine agonists (GOLDBERG 1978)

Active agonists	Potency	Inactive compounds
Dopamine	1.0	α-Methyl dopamine
Epinine	1.0	*N*,*N*-Dimethyl dopamine
A-6,7-DTN	1.0	A-5,6-DTN
N-methyl-A-6,7-DTN	0.5–1.0	Bromocryptine
N,*N*-Di-*n*-propyl dopamine	0.03	
6-*N*-*n*-Propylnorapomorphine	0.02	
Apomorphine (partial agonist)	0.01	

tors may not fit either classification. There may be more than two classes of β-adrenoceptors. In addition, it may be that apparent differences arose from insufficient attention to blocking α-receptors also present or blocking uptake and metabolism of catecholamines.

IV. Dopamine Receptors

Dopamine is a precursor of noradrenaline. In several brain neuronal systems it is the major catecholamine mediator. However, in no gastrointestinal system have neurones (identifiable as containing or capable of producing dopamine in significant quantities) been found (see FURNESS and COSTA 1974, 1978; also COSTA et al. 1976; FURNESS et al. 1979). Dopamine receptors have been found and several postulates of functional roles for dopamine have been made, but until a source of transmitter dopamine has been identified, they cannot be more than speculation.

That dopamine receptors, distinct from α- and β-receptors, exist has been established in brain and renal blood vessels by showing that distinct agonist and antagonist selectivities exist for these receptors. This has recently been reviewed by GOLDBERG (1972, 1978). Furthermore, there may be some distinctions between dopamine receptors in the central nervous system and the periphery (GOLDBERG et al. 1978). On the renal vasculature (studied after blockade of α-adrenoceptors) among phenylethylamines, besides dopamine only *N*-methyldopamine (epinine) was a potent relaxant agonist, roughly equivalent in potency to dopamine, while all others tested have been found to be inactive with the exception of *N*,*N*-di-*n*-propyldopamine, 30 times less potent than dopamine (Table 5). Unlike dopamine and

Table 6. Dopamine antagonists: renal vasculature (GOLDBERG 1978)

Antagonist	Dose shifting dose – response curve 3-fold	Range of selectivity
Haloperidol	1.4×10^{-7}	< 2
Chlorpromazine	2.5×10^{-7}	< 2
Prochlorperazine	2.5×10^{-7}	< 2
Bulbocapnine	1.5×10^{-8}	~ 8
Metoclopramide	1.5×10^{-6}	> 10
Sulpiride	2.9×10^{-8}	> 10

epinine, it lacks β_1-receptor activity. Apomorphine, an active non-phenylethylamine, is related structurally to dopamine and both can be viewed as α-rotamers. Tetrahydronaphthalene derivatives also act on dopamine receptors, but those in α-rotamer configuration are inactive (active on β_2-receptors) while the β-rotamer is active on dopamine but not β_2-receptors. Dopamine receptors have also been demonstrated in sympathetic ganglia but there apomorphine is equipotent with dopamine, so they may not be identical to renal vascular dopamine receptors.

Antagonists for dopamine receptors (Table 6) are quite distinct from those for α- or β-adrenoceptors. They include phenothiazines, (e.g. chlorpromazine), butyrophenones (e.g. haloperidol), pimizide, and metaclopramide. Recently domperidone has been synthesised as a dopamine antagonist. Most antagonists are selective for dopamine receptors over only a very narrow concentration range; so must be used cautiously as tools to study dopamine-mediated actions. Also dopamine receptors in the central nervous system (CNS) differ from receptors on renal blood vessels in their susceptability to antagonists but not in their responses to agonists. For example, in the CNS, metoclopramide and sulpiride were vitually inactive as antagonists, in contrast to their effectiveness in the periphery. However, it should be kept in mind that metoclopramide has other actions in the periphery than blockade of dopamine receptors (see the following paragraphs), and this probably applies to all antagonists.

Recently, specific dopamine receptors have been demonstrated in the gastrointestinal tract. DE CARLE and CHRISTENSEN (1976) showed, during in vitro studies, that the lower oesophageal sphincter (LES) of the North American opossum was relaxed and the "off" contraction after field stimulation of the body was inhibited by dopamine and epinine. These effects were not abolished by doses of propranolol which abolished the relaxant effects of INA and NA, but were reduced by haloperidol (10^{-5} *M*) or abolished by bulbocapnine (10^{-5} *M*). Phenoxybenzamine (10^{-5} *M*) had no effect. Since tetrodotoxin was also ineffective, it was suggested that the receptors were on smooth muscle.

Similar results were obtained by RATTAN and GOYAL (1976) giving dopamine intravenously in vivo to the same organ. Basal active tension of the LES was nearly abolished but there were delayed contractions of oesophageal body muscle. These effects were abolished by 3 mg/kg haloperidol. Phentolamine (1 mg/kg) abolished the contractile effects of phenylephrine in LES but did not affect responses to dopamine. Neither did 1 mg/kg proparanolol, cervical vagotomy or infiltration of

TTX. The authors considered the possibility that dopamine might mediate LES relaxation induced by vagal stimulation but rejected the hypothesis since haloperidol in dopamine-blocking doses failed to affect these responses. Since these responses were TTX insensitive, they presumably did not involve dopamine receptors in ganglia extrinsic to the gut.

VALENZUELA (1976) showed that dopamine (i.v. infusion; 10 μg kg^{-1} min^{-1}) reduced the fundus pressure observed when a flaccid balloon was inserted via a gastric fistula in dogs and filled with 500 ml H_2O. A similar effect of 2 μg kg^{-1} min^{-1} infusion of noradrenaline was nearly blocked by a combination of phenoxybenzamine and propranolol (each 1 mg/kg). The response to dopamine was unaffected by propranolol alone and reduced only 33% by phenoxybenzamine alone. It was abolished by 0.1 mg/kg pimozide or by 0.25 mg/kg of metoclopramide. Furthermore, each of these two agents increased the fundus pressure generated by stepwise elevation of balloon volume. Metoclopramide also decreased the duration of fundus relaxation. However, while the results provide some preliminary evidence for dopamine receptors in canine gastric fundus, they do not provide strong evidence that dopamine is the mediator of the relaxation. Evidence was not provided that dopamine was acting on smooth muscle rather than ganglia, and neither the selectivity of antagonists used nor their ability to block the intended receptors completely was demonstrated. The fact that nobody has demonstrated dopamine-containing neurones or substantial quantities of dopamine in any gut tissue, needs to be kept in mind (see also this Handbook, Vol. 59/I, Chaps. 10, 11).

LANFRANCHI et al. (1978b) have shown that dopamine in a dose of 5 μg kg^{-1} min^{-1} inhibited gastric antral mechanical activity and accelerated or made ECA irregular in normal subjects. These effects, but not the accelerated heart rate which accompanied dopamine infusion, were blocked by 100 mg sulpiride. This same group has also studied dopamine effects in distal colon of a mixed group of normal subjects and these with irritable bowel, idiopathic constipation and ulcerative colitis (LANFRANCHI et al. 1978a). All responded similarly to 5–20 μg kg^{-1} min^{-1} dopamine. In contrast to its gastric inhibitory effects, dopamine caused increased frequency amplitude and persistence of motility of the distal bowel. This effect diminished after about 5 min, despite continued dopamine infusion. Neither phentolamine nor propranolol (1 mg/kg) inhibited these effects but propranolol inhibited the accompanying acceleration of heart rate. Atropine (1 mg i.v.) potentiated dopamine responses; use of dopamine-blocking agents was not reported. Thus there is preliminary evidence that dopamine receptors also exist in the human, affecting motility of the oesophagus, fundus, antrum, and colon. However, it should be stressed that in vivo studies involving intravenous infusions do not localise these receptors to the bowel; dopamine might affect motility by actions on the peripheral ganglia or on other sites. Presumably dopamine does not cross the blood–brain barrier in sufficient amounts to act on dopamine receptors inside the blood–brain barrier.

V. Metoclopramide and Domperidone

1. Possible Role as Dopamine Antagonists

Metoclopramide (2-methoxy-5-chloroprocainamide) has been shown to be an antagonist to dopamine and other agents acting at dopamine receptors in renal blood

Table 7. Effects of metoclopramide in vivo

Organ	Effect	References[a]
Oesophagus	Increased LES pressure in vivo	HEITMANN and MOLLER (1970) McCALLUM et al. (1977)
	Increased peristaltic contractions	BIHAR and BIANCANI (1976)
Stomach	Fundus, none established	
	Increased phasic activity of corpus and antrum	JOHNSON (1971) JACOBY and BRODIE (1967) JOHNSON (1969) FOX and BEHAR (1980)
	Increased transit and accelerated gastric emptying (even after vagotomy)	RAMSBOTTOM and HUNT (1970) CONNELL and GEORGE (1969) METZGER et al. (1976) SHEINER and CATCHPOLE (1976) MALAGELADA et al. (1980) PERKEL et al. (1979)
	Pylorus: increase antroduodenal coordination	JOHNSON (1971)
Intestine	Increased phasic activity of upper intestine	JACOBY and BRODY (1967) JOHNSON (1971)
	Increased transit to ileoaecal valve	EISNER (1971)
	Increased spiking in phases II and III of interdigestive migrating myoelectric complex of shortened phase I	WINGATE et al. (1980)
Large bowel	None established	
Biliary tract	No effect	LIPTON and KNAUER (1977)

[a] For further references see review by SCHULZE-DELRIEU (1979)

vessels, the brain and oesophageal and gastric smooth muscle (see Sect. B.IV). In addition (PINDER et al. 1976), it has a number of effects on gastrointestinal motility (Tables 7 and 8).

The major question regarding its affects on motility that remains unanswered is – by what mechanism (or mechanisms)? Do any of these involve dopamine receptors, since dopaminergic control of gut function remains to be demonstrated? In vitro in different gastrointestinal smooth muscles a variety of findings have been made (Table 8). A number of studies have shown that cholinergic mechanisms are involved; either potentiation of the effects of added released acetylcholine (OKWUASABA and HAMILTON 1975, 1976; HAY 1977; BEANI et al. 1970, 1971; BURY and MASHFORD 1976), or (less established) enhanced release of acetylcholine (HAY 1977; HAY and MANN 1979). Clearly in some tissues, e.g. guinea-pig stomach, responses to metoclopramide in vitro depend upon stores of releasable acetylcholine (HAY and MANN 1979). In the canine stomach and intestine, atropine partially blocks stimulation by metoclopramide (e.g. JACOBY and BRODIE 1967). Additional effects demonstrated include decreased inhibiting effects of 5-HT in guinea-pig colon and other tissues (BEANI et al. 1970 a, b) decreased nonadrenergic inhibitory responses in a variety of intestinal preparations and selective inhibition of depression

Table 8. Effects of metoclopramide in vitro

Organ	Effect	References
Oesophagus	Increased LES myogenic tension (not confirmed)	COHEN and DIMARINO (1976)
Stomach	Increased contractile actions of antrum in presence of acetylcholine	JUSTIN-BESANCON and LAVILLE (1964)
	Increased spontaneous contraction responses to field stimulation and acetylcholine (both prevented by atropine) only field-stimulated effects blocked by TTX and dependent on acetylcholine stores	EISNER (1968) JACOBY and BRODIE (1967) BURY and MASHFORD (1976) HAY (1977) HAY and MAN (1979) OKWUASABA and HAMILTON (1975)
Intestine	Increased tone and phasic responses to acetylcholine, carbachol and nicotine (not histamine, PGE_1 or KCl); partly inhibited by atropine methysergide, morphine, TTX or these combined (hexamethonium, mepyramine or indomethacin; no effect)	OKWUASABA and HAMILTON (1975) BURY and MASHFORD (1976)
	Decreased inhibition by purine nucleotides (not noradrenaline, theophylline) on intestinal contractions and peristalsis	OKWUASABA and HAMILTON (1976)
	Potentiation of the peristaltic reflex and lowered threshold, restored response after fatigue; no effect on inhibition of reflex by morphine, hexamethonium, methysergide or high concentrations of 5-HT	OKWUASABA and HAMILTON (1976)
Colon	Enhanced effects to acetylcholine and nicotine; opposed inhibitory effects of 5-HT	BEANI et al. (1970, 1971)

of motility by purine nucleotides (OKWUASABA and HAMILTON 1975a, b), and enhanced peristaltic reflexes in isolated gut (OKWUASABA and HAMILTON 1976; BIRTLEY and BAINES 1973). No study demonstrates the ability of metoclopramide to interfere competitively with dopamine effects on gastrointestinal muscle. BAUMAN et al. (1979) showed in human volunteers that oral or intravenous L-dopa (500 or 1,000 mg) antagonised the effects of metoclopramide on LES pressure without affecting responses to bethanechol. The lower dose had no effect on LES pressure but the higher dose significantly decreased it. L-dopa, a precursor of dopamine used to increase dopamine in brain neurones may have acted to raise local or circulating dopamine levels. COHEN and DI MARINO (1976) reported that metoclopramide increased the tone of opossum LES in vitro by a myogenic mechanism unrelated to known receptors. In the high concentration used, it is a nonspecific depressant of muscle function in most other preparations of GI muscle, possibly because of its structural resemblance to local anaesthetics. Thus its myogenic stimulant action requires confirmation.

The lack of agreement as to mechanism may result in part from using inappropriate tissues: the guinea-pig ileum and colon have not been demonstrated to be major sites of metoclopramide actions in vivo. In other species the upper GI tract is more involved. This raises the question of the relevance of in vitro investigations of metoclopramide to its actions in vivo. In general, effects of metoclopramide in vitro on muscle from the upper GI tract require acetylcholine stores or the presence of acetylcholine while these on ileum or colon do not (see SCHULZE-DELRIEU 1979). The absence of established effects on the lower bowel in vivo may reflect its difficulty of access for measurement or the lack of understanding of how its motility is controlled and should be studied (see Sects. A.I, II). Also, the activity of the distal bowel may be affected by nervous and hormonal mechanisms initiated in the proximal bowel. These may obscure direct effects of the drug.

Similarly, the effects of metoclopramide on LES tone in vivo have not been studied mechanistically, except for the antagonism by L-dopa; do they depend, for example, on cholinergic mechanisms? It is unlikely that the myogenic action of higher doses in vitro in opossum LES (COHEN and DIMARINO 1976) provides an explanation.

Thus, we are forced to conclude that the basis of the in vivo actions of metoclopramide is obscure. No evidence exists of dopamine-containing neurones in the gut or of a dopamine control over gut function. No critical evidence is available that action of metoclopramide depends on dopaminergic receptor blockade. The drug has several other actions which may or may not be relevant, especially enhancement of acetylcholine release or effects or antagonism to inhibitory mechanism. Perhaps a more specific dopamine antagonist might provide further insight.

Recently, a synthetic compound, domperidone, has been reported to be more selective as a dopamine antagonist. In the isolated guinea-pig stomach VAN NUETEN and JANSSEN (1978) showed that it inhibited dopamine-induced relaxation (presumably involving the fundus), in doses that did not affect relaxation induced by sympathetic nerve stimulation or by vagal stimulation (after atropine). Doses approximately ten times higher were required to affect these functions. In contrast to domperidone, metoclopramide showed little selectivity in these experiments and inhibited all relaxant responses at approximately equal doses. Domperidone has also been shown to be a selective ligand for dopamine receptors (BAUDRY et al. 1979).

Additional studies with domperidone on the isolated, vascularly perfused guinea-pig stomach were carried out by VAN NUETEN et al. (1976, 1978), again recording volume (reflecting mainly fundal receptive relaxation). In this preparation, intra-arterial dopamine (0.1 or 0.2 ml, 0.25 μg/ml) increased gastric volume and inhibited phasic activity. Domperidone (0.25 μg/ml bath) and haloperidol (0.16 μg/ml bath) prevented these effects. This paper also reports the puzzling observation that secretin (0.1 or 0.2 ml; 6.7 mU/ml) inhibited vagally induced gastric relaxation and that domperidone (0.04–0.16 μg/ml bath; effective against dopamine) prevented this effect. Whether this implied that domperidone is a selective secretin antagonist or that secretin acts through dopamine release was not clarified. A recent extension of this work (VAN NUETEN and JANSSEN 1980) confirmed the effects of domperidone on secretin-induced interference with vagal relaxation of the fundus but not the relaxation itself or that from ATP or noradrenaline. Substance P and serotonin-induced relaxation were inhibited at higher domperidone concentrations (1–3 μg/ml). Obviously the mode of action of domperidone requires further analysis. Definitive studies of its interaction with gut dopamine receptors or its mode of action on gut motility remain to be done.

2. Clinical Applications

Despite uncertainties about the mode of action of domperidone and metoclopramide in the gastrointestinal tract (arising because they are supposed to be dopamine antagonists, but dopamine has no known functions in the tract), they have been shown to be active in a variety of clinical conditions involving disordered gastrointestinal motility (compare Tables 7 and 9).

The site of action of domperidone, in most circumstances, must be peripheral to the central nervous system since it apparently crosses the blood–brain barrier poorly (REYNTTENS et al. 1978; HEYKANTS et al. 1979; LAUDRON and LEYSEN 1979). Also it does not exacerbate extrapyramidal symptoms from neuroleptics in dyspeptic schizophrenic patients (DEBERDT 1979). However, it is reported to antagonise apomorphine-induced slowing of gastric emptying (BROCKAERT 1979); since apomorphine is usually considered to act centrally, the site of its antagonism by domperidone is conjectural. Domperidone, like metoclopramide, increases the amplitude of oesophageal peristalsis, lowers oesophageal pressure, antral, and duodenal motility (frequency, duration, and amplitude of contractions) and reduces gastroesophageal reflux symptoms and signs and accelerates gastric emptying (see Tables 7 and 9). It is not clear as yet whether any effects on gastroesophageal reflux are due to improved clearing of refluxed material (more effective peristalsis) or reduction of refluxed material (higher LES pressure). Neither is it clear how increased gastric emptying is produced, since duodenal contractions (which impede gastric emptying) are increased in number, amplitude, and duration. Perhaps an increase in antroduodenal coordination is involved, but this has not been studied.

Enhanced duodenal contraction together with increased pyloric diameter during emptying has been reported (PLATTEBORSE et al. 1979) when domperidone is given (Table 9), and this raises the question of whether, together with increased gastric emptying, this drug causes increased gastroduodenal reflux. This has not been studied, but it is interesting that acid regurgitation and nausea were hardly improved over placebo levels in one double-blind trial (HAARMANN et al. 1979) although belching, sense of fullness, inability to finish a meal, abdominal distention, epigastric burning, and heartburn were apparently relieved. Domperidone was also effective in treating nausea and vomiting in a variety of circumstances. Few comparisons with metoclopramide have been made (e.g. VAN OUTRYVE et al. 1979; VAN EYGEN et al. 1979) and in these there was no evidence that an optimal dose of each had been chosen. On the basis of the doses used, domperidone was claimed to be more effective and freer of side effects, but it is clear that better designed trials are required to establish these claims.

Table 9. Effect of domperidone in vivo

Region studied	Contractile activity	References
Oesophagus		
Peristaltic contractions, lower oesophageal sphincter pressure	Increased (less in reflux patients)	WEIHRAUCH et al. (1979)
Stomach		
Fundus	Increased	PLATTEBORSE et al. (1979)
Corpus	Increased	BROCKAERT (1979)
Antrum–duration of contraction	Increased	BAEYENS et al. (1979)
Pylorus diameter	Increased	BAEYENS et al. (1979)
Emptying rate of H_2O	Increased	BAEYENS et al. (1979)
Duodenum		
Frequency of contractions	Increased	WEIHRAUCH et al. (1979)
Amplitude of contractions	Increased	WEIHRAUCH et al. (1979)
Duration of contractions	Increased	WEIHRAUCH et al. (1979)
Antroduodenal coordination	?	
Disease states	Effect of domperidone	
Reflux oesophagitis	Improved	HAARMANN et al. (1979)
Chronic postprandial dyspepsia	Improved	LIENARD et al. (1978)
Gastroparesis of diabetics and (after vagotomy)	Improved	VAN GANSE et al. (1978) ENGLERT and SCHLICK (1979) BEKHTI and RUTGEERTS (1979)
Postprandial nausea (and vomiting)	Improved	VAN OUTRYVE et al. (1979) VAN EYGEN et al. (1979)

Metoclopramide seems to have essentially similar actions on human gastrointestinal motility and clinical disorders to domperidone (compare Tables 7 and 9). There is, however, evidence that it crosses the blood–brain barrier and, together with other dopamine antagonists, can initiate or exacerbate extrapyramidal symptoms (see Sect. B.V.I).

C. Cholinergic Receptors in the Gastrointestinal Tract

This section deals with muscarinic receptors, presynaptic cholinergic receptors and nicotinic receptors. Futher details are given in this Handbook, Vol. 59/I, Chaps. 10 and 11.

I. Muscarinic Receptors

Acetylcholine is released from preganglionic nerves in the ganglia of the myenteric plexus. Some of it acts on postganglionic neurones or their processes. In the guinea-pig intestine, some nerve varicosities with the appearance of cholinergic terminals occur at the surface of the ganglia not too far distant from smooth muscle (GABELLA 1972b, c). Acetylcholine apparently leaks from these endings in these ganglia.

Its release into the interstitial space and ultimately into the bath in vitro is increased by field stimulation (PATON and ZAR 1968; PATON and VIZI 1969). In some species, such as the guinea-pig, few nerves innervate longitudinal smooth muscle, and it seems possible that the contractions of this layer observed on field stimulation occur in large part by diffusion of acetylcholine from the plexus (PATON and VIZI 1969; GABELLA 1972b, c) to the muscle.

In circular muscle, the innervation is more dense, and in many species there is a dense nerve plexus (although devoid of neurone cell bodies) between the inner (dense) and outer (less dense) layer of circular muscles. This dense layer plexus contains many varicosities, appearing to be cholinergic. Also in the submucous plexus there are many axon varicosities with the same appearance. There has been no study of the release of acetylcholine from these plexuses. The predominant response of the circular muscle of guinea-pig (HIRST and MCKIRDY 1974), rabbit intestine (DANIEL and TAYLOR 1975; CHEUNG and DANIEL 1980) and lower oesophageal sphincter (EL-SHARKAWY et al. 1976) to field stimulation is hyperpolarisation and inhibition from activation of nonadrenergic inhibitory neurones. There is, however, evidence that acetylcholine is also released in circular muscle of rabbit intestine (CHEUNG and DANIEL 1980).

Receptors for acetylcholine on smooth muscle of both layers throughout the GI tract are clearly muscarinic. This has been most thoroughly studied in guinea-pig ileum, guinea-pig stomach, rabbit small intestine, and rat small intestine (see TRIGGLE and TRIGGLE 1976 for review). Moreover in all areas, in all species, responses are antagonised by atropine or hyoscine and provoked by methacholine and bethanechol as well as other muscarinic agonists. Some data for better studied systems regarding both agonists and antagonists are assembled from the analysis and reviewed by TRIGGLE and TRIGGLE (Tables 10 and 11). The muscarinic receptor is much more discriminating in its requirements for agonist actions than nicotinic receptors. It accepts only very limited substitution other than a methyl group on the quarternary amine or on the carboxy group of the acetyl component. It also shows chirality, favouring among the structurally rigid muscarinic derivatives, the L(+) form, 2S, 3R, 5S, over the D(−) form and DL over DL-*epi*, DL-*allo*, and DL-*epallo* forms (Table 12). Also, a rather puzzling aspect is the opposite configuration (see TRIGGLE and TRIGGLE 1976) favoured in the muscarone series of compounds. In derivatives of acetyl-β-methylcholine there is also an inversion of stereoselectivity; the dioxolone derivatives on the other hand are like the muscarinic derivatives. TRIGGLE and TRIGGLE (1976) suggested that L(+) muscarine, S(+)acetyl β-methylcholine, and 2S, 4R(+)*cis*-2-methyldimethylaminomethyl-1,3-dioxolone methiodide all fit the same structure. Other data are interpreted as suggesting at least two binding sites for agonists at the muscarinic receptor: a polar region of high stereoselectivity and a nonpolar region with little stereoselectivity. Studies of the muscarinic receptor by the binding properties of ligands such as the antagonist, quinuclidinyl benzilate ^{3}H have not yet been as detailed as those with contraction; they show one class of stereospecific binding sites with properties generally consistent with those already summarised (RIMELE et al. 1979).

The mode of action of muscarinic agonists on gut smooth muscle has recently been reviewed by BOLTON (1979). In all intestinal muscle, they depolarise. There

Table 10. Structural requirements for cholinergic receptors equiactive molar ratios: acetylcholine = 1 (TRIGGLE and TRIGGLE 1976)

Compounds of RN^+Me_3	R	Nicotine receptors in frog rectus	Nicotine receptors in ganglia	Muscarinic receptors in rabbit intestine
	H	700		~ 500
	CH_3	1	1	1
	CH_3CH_2	0.6	0.65	33
	$CH_3(CH_2)_2$	1	0.47	400
	$CH_3(CH_2)_3$	0.95		500
	$(CH_3)_3$–C	5.0	0.10	Inactive
	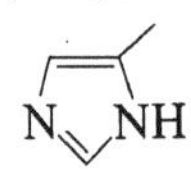	1,000	1.2	Inactive
	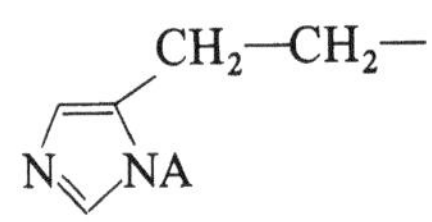	1.4	0.12	Inactive
	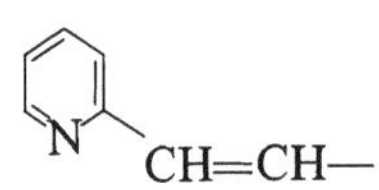	1.2	0.17	Inactive
	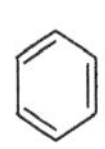	100	0.88	~1,000

is an excitatory junction potential (e.j.p.) in some cells when acetylcholine is released from intrinsic cholinergic neurones (presumably those cells near axon varicosities). The e.j.p. characteristically has a long latency, about 100 ms or more, too long to be attributed to diffusion delay. PURVES (1974) has shown that this long latency occurs even when acetylcholine is applied iontophoretically on cultured smooth muscle cells where diffusion delays are irrelevant. Presumably it is a property of receptor agonist kinetics or of the subsequent events; e.g. activation on ion channels. There is also a long duration of the e.j.p. from acetylcholine acting on muscarinic receptors. PURVES (1976) suggests that this slow kinetic property of muscarinic receptors is a property that has evolved to allow summation of responses.

In different GI smooth muscles, there are somewhat different responses to release of acetylcholine. Perhaps the most common (though not the best studied) is exemplified by rabbit large and small intestine; it is initiation of a spike by the e.j.p. (evoked by field stimulation) or by the e.j.p. when it coincides with the depolarised phase of a slow wave (plateau of ECA). The number or frequency of spikes may be increased in some cells without detectable e.j.p. (possibly owing to propagation from cells with e.j.p.). Slow waves (or ECA) are essentially unchanged in size (GILLESPIE 1968; DANIEL et al. 1975; CHEUNG and DANIEL 1980). Larger e.j.p. may be produced by release of acetylcholine during the repolarised phase of the ECA be-

Table 11. Requirements for muscarinic agonist activities[a] (TRIGGLE and TRIGGLE 1976)

Compounds of $RCOOCH_2CH_2N^+Me_3$ R	Intrinsic activity	pD_2	pA_2
H	1	5.2	
CH_3	1	7.6	
CH_3CH_2	0.9	5.0	
$(CH_3)_2CH_2$	0.4	4.1	
$CH_3(CH_2)_2$	0.3	3.8	
$CH_3(CH_2)_4$	0		4.0
$CH_3(CH_2)_{10}$	0		5.2

[a] All these modifications leave action at nicotine receptors nearly unchanged

Table 12. Chirality requirements for combination of muscarines with muscarinic receptors (TRIGGLE and TRIGGLE 1976). Equiactive molar ratios (acetylcholine = 1)

Compound	Cat blood pressure	Frog heart	Rabbit ileum	Frog rectus	Intrinsic activity	pD_2^e
DL	0.75	10	1.0	> 50	1	6.8
L(+)[a]	0.32	5	0.33	> 50		
D(−)	350		130	> 50		
DL-*epi*-[b]	230	>1000	230	>100	1	3.9
DL-*allo*[c]	130	>1000	150	>200	1	4.4
DL-*epiallo*[d]	75	>1000	220	>100	1	5.0

[a] L(+)= 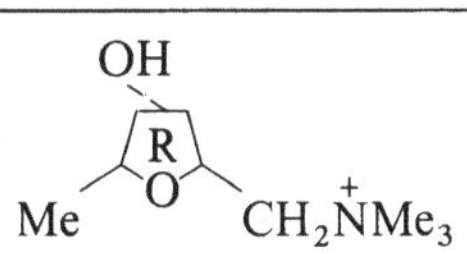

(2S, 3R, 5S);

[b] *epi*= 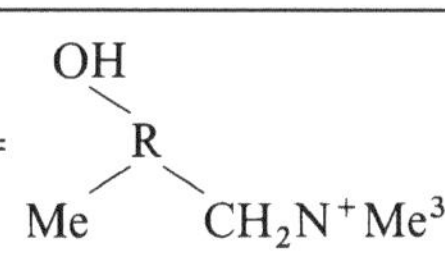

(2S, 3S, 5S);

[c] *allo*= 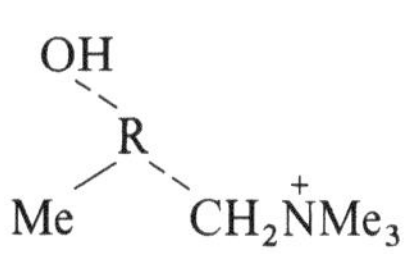

(2S, 3R, 5R);

[d] *epiallo*= 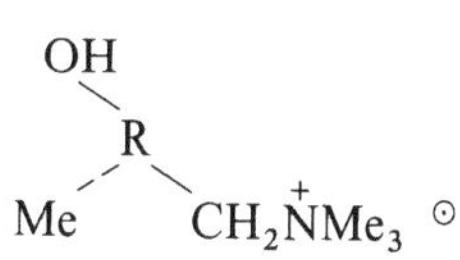

(2S, 3S, 5R)

[e] For acetylcholine $pD_2 = 7.1$.

cause of the greater difference between the resting potential and the equilibrium potential for acetylcholine, but they fail to reach threshold for spiking. This interaction between e.j.p. and ECA probably occurs in the small intestine and large intestine of most mammals other than the guinea-pig (DANIEL and SARNA 1978; BOLTON 1979).

In contrast to the intestine, acetylcholine added exogenously to canine antrum longitudinal or circular muscle, increases the duration and amplitude of the plateau portion of the periodic ECA (DANIEL 1965, 1966a; SZURSZEWSKI 1975; EL-SHARKAWY et al. 1978; EL-SHARKAWY and SZURSZEWSKI 1978). Effects of acetylcholine released from nerves in the antrum have not been reported. In guinea-pig ileum in vitro, exogenous acetylcholine induces an oscillating slow wave component or, if a small one is already present, enhances it. Action potentials are usually associated with the depolarised phase of these slow waves.

When guinea-pig intestinal muscles were studied (see BOLTON 1979), with attempts to produce a voltage clamped region in the double sucrose gap, a region of inward current and negative resistance was found at potentials from -10 to -40 mV; in this voltage range in the absence of acetylcholine there was only outward current. By applying slowly rising ramp potentials to avoid activating the action potential mechanism, BOLTON felt that he had demonstrated that agonist occupation of muscarinic receptors opened ion channels whose conductance increased from -10 to -40 mV, initiating flow of inward current, carried mainly by Na^+. This mechanism would explain the action potentials generated by acetylcholine on slow waves (ECA) since, like the action potentials of nerve and skeletal muscle, those in intestinal muscle would be regenerative. As an additional mechanism to explain the actions of acetylcholine on other muscles, it was suggested that muscarinic receptor activation changed the current–voltage characteristics of channels carrying a slow inward current (Na^+ or Ca^{2+}) responsible for agonist-induced slow waves in the guinea-pig intestine and for the plateau of the ECA in the dog antrum. Depolarisation in either case would be limited by inactivation of the current-carrying channels, by approach to equilibrium potential (since conductance to ions other than sodium was increased this was considerably more negative than $V_{Na} = +35$; see following discussion), or by activation of channels carrying outward current, most likely potassium ions.

The oscillatory slow wave system induced by muscarinic agonists occurs in few gut systems; e.g. guinea-pig intestine. Stomach muscle of most species and the intestines of all other mammals studied have slow waves or ECA which are independent of activation of muscarinic receptors (i.e. occur in the presence of atropine, etc; GILLESPIE 1968; SZURSZEWSKI 1975; EL-SHARKAWY and SZURSZEWSKI 1978; CHEUNG and DANIEL 1980). In the oesophagus of the cat (CHRISTENSEN and DANIEL 1966, 1968; EL-SHARKAWY and DIAMANT 1970; EL-SHARKAWY et al. 1976) a mechanism similar to that in guinea-pig intestine may operate, since oscillatory membrane electrical activity can be induced by muscarinic agonists, although normally absent.

The equilibrium potential for effects of muscarinic agonists has been approximated (-10 mV) only for guinea-pig ileum (see the review by BOLTON 1979). He used a large dose of carbachol to produce a large conductance change, intended to drive the membrane potential near the equilibrium potential. BOLTON has pointed out the limitations to this technique, especially the occurrence of altered ionic gradients consequent to the increased conductance but estimated the value is in error by 10 mV or less. As expected, if Na^+ channels are activated by muscarinic agonists, reduction in extracellular sodium by replacement with this cation reduced the depolarisation by acetylcholine. Hyperpolarisation to acetylcholine resulted when Ca^{2+} was also removed. Sucrose replacement of NaCl was more effective than $Tris^+$ replacement of Na^+ and the hyperpolarisation produced in Na-free sucrose was reversed by replacing it with K-benzenesulphonate. Chloride-deficient solutions had no effect on the depolarisation. Muscarinic receptor stimulation increases ^{24}Na influx and total Na content, but an increase in Na^+ efflux has not been consistently observed, even when efflux via the Na^+ pump or via Na^+–Na^+ exchange has been minimised. This may reflect difficulties in the technique of measuring efflux of intracellular Na^+ from smooth muscle, the occurrence of a limitation on Na^+ efflux into the bath at a site other than the membrane or some rectification in the Na^+ channel.

Potassium conductance is also increased by activation of muscarinic receptors: ^{42}K or ^{86}Rb efflux are increased, less in depolarised muscle (see BOLTON 1979). ^{42}K influx is accelerated by acetylcholine in depolarised muscle; presumably in polarised muscle the depolarisation induced by the agonists diminishes the influx by decreasing the inward electrochemical gradient for K^+. Changing the electrochemical gradient for potassium, however, had few of the expected effects. In the absence of external Ca^{2+} or Na^+, elevation of potassium reversed the hyperpolarisation produced by carbachol to depolarisation. The changes in the depolarisation produced by lowering external potassium were small and in the wrong direction (increased). These anomalous results may relate to effects of external K^+ on the electrogenic Na^+ pump or to effects of intracellular Ca^{2+} changes accompanying altered Na^+ or K^+ gradients on K^+ conductance.

Calcium influx is also somewhat increased by muscarinic agonists, especially clearly in depolarised muscle (see BOLTON 1979). Effects on Ca^{2+} efflux are small and variable, as might be expected if most of the Ca^{2+} efflux does not directly reflect transmembrane passive transport of this ion but rather extracellular exchanges, back flux and active extrusion.

Chloride fluxes are increased by acetylcholine in taenia coli but depolarisation produced in guinea-pig taenia coli, guinea-pig ileum or canine antrum are unaffected by chloride removal. Whether chloride flux changes reflect movements of other ions or whether chloride redistribution is so rapid that V_{Cl} remains unchanged, has not been studied.

BURGEN and SPERO (1968) noted that much higher concentrations of carbachol and acetylcholine were required to produce half-maximal or full activation of ^{86}Rb efflux (as K^+ tracer) than to produce half-maximal contractions. Later they found (BURGEN and SPERO 1970) that partial agonists, such as tetramethylammonium produced similar responses of contraction and Rb efflux at various concentrations. They considered spare receptors for acetylcholine in relation to initiation of contraction as an explanation; although an irreversible antagonist shifted the dose – response curve to the right, it also flattened the efflux dose – response curve.

This anomaly may depend merely on the fact that maximal contractile response required only partial depolarisation of cell membranes and therefore partial occupation of receptors, while full activation of muscarinic receptor-coupled ion channels required full occupation of all receptors and complete depolarisation. Alternatively, it may be that doses submaximal for receptor occupancy of these agents initiate propagated action potentials which activate a higher proportion of muscle cells than would be activated directly by receptor occupation. Elevation of medium calcium and reduction of medium magnesium brought contraction and efflux dose – response curves together by shifting the contraction curve (BURGEN and SPERO

1970). This may be a result of uncoupling of cells and inhibition of propagation of action potentials. BOLTON (1979) has suggested that there are two receptor sites for muscarinic agonists, one of high and one of low affinity.

OHASHI et al. (1974, 1975), SHIBATA et al. (1978), and CASTEELS and RAEYMAKERS (1979) have shown that high concentrations (10^{-5} *M*) but not low ones (10^{-7} *M*) of carbachol can initiate contractions in Ca^{2+}-free (2 m*M* EGTA) solutions when the muscle is unresponsive to high [K^+]. This response disappears in about 6–10 min and is enhanced and prolonged by prior exposure to high [K^+] solutions. These brief contractions are further enhanced in amplitude by having β-adrenergic agonists present during the high [K^+] exposure. β-Adrenergic agonists added during brief exposure to Ca^{2+}-free EGTA solution also enhance them. Presumably β-adrenergic agonists enhance uptake of Ca^{2+} into internal stores. Responsiveness to carbachol in Ca^{2+}-free EGTA solution can be restored by brief exposure to Ca^{2+}, but this effect is prevented if Ca^{2+} antagonists are used to inhibit Ca^{2+} influx during exposure to Ca^{2+}.

These results may suggest that there are two sites of action (and two receptors?) for carbachol or acetylcholine; one, activated by low concentrations, increases Ca^{2+}-dependent action potentials and Ca^{2+} influx, the other, activated by higher concentrations, releases Ca^{2+} from internal stores in the plasma membrane or endoplasmic reticulum. It is well known that Ca^{2+} entrance or injection into a variety of cells enhances K^+ conductance (see MEECH 1978; PUTNEY 1979); this may be a property of a resultant Ca^{2+} redistribution and binding in the membrane rather than of the concentration of free Ca^{2+} inside the membrane. Low concentrations of carbachol may induce some increase in K^+ conductance by increasing Ca^{2+} entrance into cells, but full activation as in the experiments of BURGEN and SPERO (1968) may require release of additional Ca^{2+} from internal membrane binding sites. Clearly the cellular mode of action of acetylcholine on muscarinic receptors remains to be fully elucidated.

1. Molecular Mode of Action of Cholinergic Agonists

That cholinergic agonists acting on muscarinic receptors (together with some other excitatory stimulants) increased phospholipid (phosphoinositol and phosphatidic acid) turnover in smooth muscle and exocrine cell membranes, has been realised since the work of MITCHELL and of HOKIN (both reviewed by MITCHELL 1975). Although clearly associated with agonist activation of muscarinic receptors as well as with some other stimulants, net breakdown of phosphoinositol leading to formation of phosphatidic acid followed by resynthesis of labelled phosphoinositol, has been considered irrelevant to the events associated with receptor activation: i.e. opening of receptor operated ion channels, depolarisation, activation of voltage-sensitive Ca^{2+} channels, release of sequestered Ca^{2+} in some systems and contractions or secretion. This was because the time course was relatively slow and the first increase in labelling could not be detected until contraction was underway.

Recently, however, SALMON and HONEYMAN (1980), using isolated muscle cells from frog stomach, showed that the increased ^{32}P incorporation (presumably from phosphinositol) into phosphatidate followed a time course resembling that of contraction in response to carbachol. The increased ^{32}P incorporation into phosphoinositol was delayed relative to these events, as found previously by others. Phosphatidate (10^{-8} *M*) itself added to the bath caused contraction within 10 s.

One problem about the work in isolated stomach cells is that the membrane events associated with Ca^{2+} entrance or release undoubtedly precede contraction, and the study showed only that contraction and elevated phosphatidate had a similar time course. Thus both may be secondary to membrane events initiated by occupation of muscarinic receptors and phosphatidate formation may not be involved in the initial events by serving as a Ca gate as proposed.

2. Transmission at Gastrointestinal Neuronal Synapses

A substantial body of evidence supports the hypothesis that sympathetic ganglia innervating the heart in dogs (e.g. the stellate ganglia) have functional involvement of muscarinic receptors in ganglionic transmission. The evidence so far does not include direct recording from neurones but depends on the finding that eliminating the contribution of nicotinic transmission does not prevent preganglionic stimulation from accelerating heart rate, especially at higher frequencies (FLACKE and GILLIS 1968). Inhibitors of muscarinic receptors alone have little effect, but combined antagonists of muscarinic and nicotinic receptors markedly inhibit transmission, much more than a nicotinic antagonist alone[3]. Evidence that, under certain circumstances, acetylcholine or other agonists acting at muscarinic receptors can provide for transmission is available from neuronal recording for other ganglia; e.g. superior cervical ganglia in cats or rabbits (LIBET and TOSAKA 1969; LIBET 1970; LIBET and KOBAYASHI 1974; ERANKÖ 1978; VOLLE 1966; VOLLE and HANCOCK 1970; TRENDELENBURG 1966, 1967); but usually partial depolarisation of some ganglion structures, presumably neurones, is required; e.g. by perfusion with elevated [K^+] solutions or conditioning with repetitive stimuli. A slow e.j.p., however, can be recorded on preganglionic stimulation which is blocked by atropine.

Muscarinic transmission at parasympathetic ganglia is not so well established, but circumstantial evidence exists for such transmission at ganglia in canine bladder (e.g. see TAIRA et al. 1971). In the gut, the evidence for a role of muscarinic receptors in transmission between vagal preganglionic and intrinsic postganglionic neurones is incomplete. HIRST and MCKIRDY (1974) have found in studies of intracellular activity of neurones in the myenteric plexus of guinea-pig intestine, that preganglionic stimulation leads to an excitatory junction potential blocked by hexamethonium or curare alone. GOYAL and RATTAN (1975), studying relaxation of the lower oesophageal sphincter of the opossum on vagal stimulation, obtained findings similar to those in stellate ganglia. In this case neither atropine nor hexamethonium alone was very effective in shifting the stimulus frequency–response curve to the right, but a combination of the two antagonists was effective.

It is difficult to analyse this problem by other than intracellular recording from intrinsic neurones when dealing with transmission to cholinergic neurones, since

3 The finding that inhibitory muscarinic receptors exist on cardiac sympathetic nerves raises the question whether the role of muscarinic transmission in sympathetic ganglia supplying the heart may have been underestimated; muscarinic antagonists inhibit the effects of preganglionic sympathetic stimulation by blocking transmission, but enhance these effects by withdrawing inhibition of release of noradrenaline from postganglionic nerves

antagonists to muscarinic receptors on ganglia will also interfere with contractile responses mediated by similar receptors on smooth muscle. Conceivably a pharmacological analysis could be carried out for transmission to nonadrenergic inhibitory neurones in regions, such as the LES, where noncholinergic myogenic activity allows the demonstration of inhibitory responses to preganglionic stimulation. Unfortunately it is usually necessary to use atropine or hyoscine to block muscarinic and unmask nonadrenergic inhibitory responses to nerve stimulation. This precludes any possibility of discovering muscarinic transmission at intestinal ganglia. Use of muscarinic antagonists may have prevented such findings by PATON and VANE (1963), by BEANI et al. (1971) and by others. This was confirmed in a recent report (DOWNING and MORRIS 1979) in which a vagally stimulated guinea-pig stomach preparation (like that of PATON and VANE), was initially studied without a muscarinic antagonist. Either hexamethonium or hyoscine reversed the contractile response to vagal stimulation to a relaxation. Furthermore, hyoscine after administration of hexamethonium reduced the relaxation response more than 50%. The implication is that nicotinic receptors are primarily responsible for transmission to cholinergic gut neurones while both nicotinic and muscarinic receptors function in transmission to nonadrenergic inhibitory neurones. CREMA et al. (1970) made similar findings in the guinea-pig colon; descending inhibition was blocked by hyoscine.

The question whether muscarinic ganglionic transmission occurs to nonadrenergic inhibitory neurones obviously deserves further study. For example, there is no clear evidence that ganglionic muscarinic receptors differ from those on smooth muscle in drug selectivity. Some agents, such as McNeill A343 [or 4-(*m*-chlorophenylcarbamoyloxy)-2-butynyltrimethylamonium chloride] act on muscarinic receptors in sympathetic ganglia in lower concentrations than are required to activate muscarinic receptors on smooth muscle (see ROSZKOWSKI 1961; GOYAL and RATTAN 1978). However, no systematic study of structure–activity relationships for actions at the receptors located in nerves, has been carried out.

II. Presynaptic Cholinergic Receptors

The importance of presynaptic α-adrenoceptors, which operate a negative feedback control of release of noradrenaline from sympathetic nerves and usually inhibit release of acetylcholine from cholinergic nerves, has been mentioned earlier. In some systems there is also evidence of cholinergic receptors which affect release of mediators from cholinergic and adrenergic nerves. Nicotinic receptors exist on sympathetic nerves, and BURN and RAND (1965) provoked a mass of publications by proposing an essential role for release of acetylcholine to act on these in sympathetic transmission. While it is clear that such receptors do exist, they have not been shown to play any essential role in transmission (e.g. FERRY 1963, 1966). In motor nerves innervating skeletal muscle, a recent review (MIYAMOTO 1977) concluded that there was clear evidence of nicotinic presynaptic receptors which were capable of enhancing acetylcholine output. It also concluded that such receptors played no primary role in release of acetylcholine, i.e. were not a necessary amplifying step in neuromuscular transmission and, although possibly active at levels of acetylcholine accumulating in the synaptic cleft, were not important for transmission.

Potent nicotinic agonists may act at receptors on nerve fibres of all types in pharmacological experiments. Identification of such a mode of action is difficult, and the importance of presynaptic nicotinic receptors in the physiology and pharmacology of GI motor function has not been analysed. The major impediment is the existence of nicotinic receptors directly involved in transmission from preganglionic vagal to postganglionic neurones (see Sect. C.III). Any nicotinic agonist or antagonist would have its major actions on motor function at these receptors. Conceivably, the presynaptic receptors could be studied by analysis of effects of nicotinic agents on release of acetylcholine or noradrenaline. However, the early studies of acetylcholine release by PATON and ZAR (1968) during transmural field stimulation of nerves of guinea-pig ileum or guinea-pig longitudinal muscle strips revealed that hexamethonium only diminished acetylcholine release. In a preparation of longitudinal muscle and myenteric plexus, there are relatively few postsynaptic terminals (GABELLA 1972b, c). The minor effect of hexamethonium implies that positive feedback from action of released acetylcholine on nicotinic receptors is not important to the overall release from ganglionic presynaptic terminals. Nicotinic agonists also cause activation of nonadrenergic inhibitory nerves. This is probably a result of an action of postsynaptic receptors on the nonadrenergic inhibitory neurone; not a presynaptic action (see Sect. C.III). Studies measuring release of noradrenaline or nonadrenergic mediator by nicotinic agonists in the gut are not available.

Recently, a substantial body of evidence has been accumulated that presynaptic muscarinic receptors exist which when occupied inhibit release of noradrenaline. The evidence is strongest in heart and vas deferens (see WESTFALL 1977). Evidence also exists in blood vessels (VASE and VANHOUTTE 1974; ALLEN et al. 1975; VAN HEE et al. 1978; VANHOUTTE et al. 1980). In the heart, there is close proximity of cholinergic to adrenergic nerve varicosities (HIGGINS et al. 1973; WESTFALL 1977) and the structural basis for inhibition of sympathetic activity by vagal, cholinergic activity exists. A recent review (WESTFALL 1977) concludes that this interrelation is probably physiologically relevant. A similar anatomical basis for interaction, – cholinergic nerve varicosities near adrenergic ones – is widespread in the gut and also provides the basis for adrenergic inhibition of acetylcholine output, as discussed previously. The question is: does a reciprocal relation exist with acetylcholine inhibiting noradrenaline release as well as noradrenaline inhibiting acetylcholine release? This could easily be tested, but so far the outcome has not been reported.

However, there is good evidence for presynaptic muscarinic receptors on cholinergic intrinsic neurones, chiefly from studies of guinea-pig ileum. Their existence has been shown by measuring acetylcholine output in preparations of longitudinal muscle and plexus of the type introduced by PATON and ZAR (1968) and PATON and VIZI (1969). In these preparations, muscarinic agonists, for example oxotremorine, decrease acetylcholine output (SZERB 1975, 1976, 1980; WATERFIELD and KOSTERLITZ 1973; FOSBRAEY and JOHNSON 1980) and muscarinic antagonists potentiate it (COWIE et al. 1978). When this preparation is studied by means of physostigmine or another anticholinesterase to inhibit acetylcholine breakdown, the resultant accumulation of acetylcholine, either leaking spontaneously from neurones or released by field stimulation, is apparently sufficient to provide a negative feedback brake on acetylcholine release since muscarinic antagonists enhance release (SZERB 1980; COWIE et al. 1978; FOSBRAEY and JOHNSON 1980). Whether such negative feedback plays any role in limiting excitation of intestine by cholinergic nerves under physiological conditions, is uncertain.

SZERB (1975, 1976) has shown that acetylcholine release from the field-stimulated guinea-pig ileal muscle preparation is kinetically divisible into fast and slow components. He stimulated at 0.1 Hz and attributed the fast release to spontaneously active myenteric plexus neurones, as described by NORTH and WILLIAMS (1976, 1977). He attributes the slower phase of release to silent neurones activated only by field stimulation. Morphine decreased the acetylcholine pool size for both fast and slowly emergent acetylcholine and decreased the rate of fast efflux. This was suggested to be a consequence of the hyperpolarisation by morphine (NORTH 1977; NORTH et al. 1976; NORTH and TONINI 1977) which decreases the firing rate for spontaneously active neurones and decreases the number of neurones in the silent group responding to field stimulation.

The muscarinic agonist, oxotremorine, on the other hand, decreased rates of release as well as pool sizes for both fast and slow components of acetylcholine release. $MnCl_2$ (0.5 mM) eliminated the fast component of acetylcholine release, decreased evoked acetylcholine release and prevented the contraction by oxotremorine. In the presence of $MnCl_2$, oxotremorine or decreased medium [Ca^{2+}] diminished the rate of acetylcholine release without affecting pool size. These effects of the muscarinic agonist were prevented by atropine. The effects of occupation of presynaptic muscarinic receptors on release rates were attributed to decreased Ca^{2+} influx into nerve varicosities, and those on pool size in the absence of $MnCl_2$ to altered efficacy of field stimulation in the shortened, contracted state. In any case, oxotremorine apeared to affect acetylcholine release like lowered Ca^{2+} rather than like morphine. The interpretation by SZERB of fast and slow components of acetylcholine release seems to imply that the kinetics of release of mediator differ when it is evoked by a spontaneous action potential (fast kinetics) from that when evoked by a stimulated action potential (slow kinetics). Why this should be so, is not clear.

III. Nicotinic Receptors

Nicotinic receptors in the GI tract have not been thoroughly studied since these are not readily isolated or accessible. None have been found on smooth muscle (see DANIEL 1968). They seem to be located on both cholinergic and nonadrenergic inhibitory neurones. In regions such as gastric fundus or lower oesophageal sphincter, both cholinergic excitatory responses and nonadrenergic inhibitory responses can be elicited by stimulation of vagal preganglionic fibres or by intra-arterial injection of nicotine, or dimethylphenylpiperazinium (DMPP; GOYAL and RATTAN 1978). Acetylcholine is not very effective when similarly administered (e.g. after administration of atropine in the lower oesophageal sphincter). This may be a consequence of its destruction by cholinesterase.

In the canine gastric corpus and antrum (DANIEL and SARNA 1976), the response to intra-arterial DMPP is excitatory. Lack of inhibition may relate to lack of nonadrenergic inhibitory nerves or to lack of nicotinic receptors on them.

Throughout the GI tract, including regions like the distal small intestine with poor vagal motor innervation, the neurones of the nonadrenergic inhibitory system apparently contain nicotinic receptors. Exposure to nicotine or DMPP leads to relaxation (e.g. DANIEL 1966a, 1968; BURLEIGH et al. 1979) and hexamethonium or curare decrease or block descending inhibition (HIRST and MCKIRDY 1974), although this could be a result of blockade of transmission at an interneurone. It is clear that cholinergic motor and nonadrenergic inhibitory neurones with nicotinic receptors are located in the myenteric plexus (HIRST and MCKIRDY 1974, 1975), but the evidence about nicotinic receptors on neurones in the submucous plexus which may exert motor control over the intestine is minimal.

D. Morphine and Drugs Acting on Opiate Receptors

I. Endogenous Opiates

The existence of receptors for morphine-like agonists with highly specific site requirements, including stereospecificity, implies the existence of endogenous hormones or transmitters which act on these receptors (see BEAUMONT and HUGHES 1979 for review). Subsequently, the pentapeptides leucine enkephalin and methionine enkephalin, which interact with opiate receptors, were found in the gut (HUGHES et al. 1977; SMITH et al. 1976). They are synthesised in and released from the gut (SOSA et al. 1977) as well as the brain (HUGHES et al. 1975, 1977). Nearly simultaneously, it was discovered that β-endorphin exists as a brain and anterior pituitary peptide (GOLDSTEIN 1976), derived from amino acids 61–91 of the 91 amino acid protein, β-lipoprotein and containing the enkephalin sequence. These findings have radically changed our perceptions of the physiology and pharmacology of opiates affecting gut motility. Endogenous opiates must be seriously considered as neurotransmitters and neuromodulators. Immunocytochemical evidence shows that the endogenous pentapeptides are located in axons innervating the myenteric plexus and in neurones (ELDE et al. 1976; SCHULTZBERG et al. 1980). The cell bodies of opiates containing nerves are located almost exclusively in this plexus (FURNESS and COSTA 1980; SCHULTZBERG et al. 1980). Axons containing enkephalins are also present in circular muscle and the deep muscular plexus (dense layer plexus); although no direct action of enkephalins on smooth muscle has been established. Enkephalins are released, apparently by axon varicosities innervating cholinergic neurones of the myenteric plexus (MCKNIGHT et al. 1978; WATERFIELD et al. 1977; SCHULZ et al. 1977; PUIG et al. 1978), by a Ca^{2+}-dependent process (OKA and SAWA 1979).

II. Mode of Opiate Action in Guinea-Pig Intestine

In the guinea-pig ileum where most work has been carried out, enkephalins, like morphine, inhibit release of acetylcholine (COX and WEINSTOCK 1966; GREENBERG et al. 1970; WATERFIELD and KOSTERLITZ 1973, 1975; WATERFIELD et al. 1977; PATON 1957; HENDERSON et al. 1975; SZERB 1980; DOWN and SZERB 1980). They may act to inhibit release of a variety of mediators, e.g. noradrenaline from mouse vas deferens (see BEAUMONT and HUGHES 1979 for review). In this function, like α_2-

adrenergic agonists, they are much more effective at low frequencies and submaximal strengths of field stimulation (PATON 1957; HENDERSON et al. 1975; WATERFIELD et al. 1977), and their actions require no secondary transmitter function, since they still occur when zero [Ca^{2+}] or hexamethonium has inhibited transmission (GREENBERG et al. 1970; DINGLEDINE et al. 1974; DINGLEDINE and GOLDSTEIN 1976; HENDERSON et al. 1975). NORTH (1977), NORTH and TONINI (1977), and NORTH et al. (1976) have shown that about 60% of type 1 myenteric neurones in the myenteric plexus of guinea-pig ileum (apparently corresponding to intrinsic cholinergic nerves[4] were hyperpolarised by opioids perfused over the plexus, usually but not always associated with decreased input resistance (increased soma membrane conductance). Usually excitability was decreased and the sizes of e.p.s.p. on focal stimulations of ganglia were decreased. However, iontophoretic application of enkephalin to the soma of myenteric neurones uniformly failed to hyperpolarise them (NORTH et al. 1978). NORTH (1979) has suggested that the opiates act on sites (cell processes) other than the soma of the neurone, thus failing to be effective on iontophoretic application and may hyperpolarise without affecting somal resistance. KARRAS and NORTH (1979) have shown that cyclic AMP is not an intermediate in the hyperpolarising action of opiates on neurones. SATO et al. (1973), DINGLEDINE et al. (1974), DINGLEDINE and GOLDSTEIN (1975, 1976), NORTH and WILLIAMS (1976, 1977), and EHRENPREIS et al. (1976) have also shown that there is a population of spontaneously active neural elements in the myenteric plexus in this tissue, which can be recorded by extracellular electrodes. Their activity is suppressed by morphine or enkephalins, independent of ganglionic transmission (in Ca^{2+}-free solution).

NORTH et al. (1976) have postulated that the hyperpolarisation and decreased excitability related to increased permeability in cell processes result in decreased acetylcholine output and activity of myenteric neurones. All these effects are reversed stereospecifically by opiate antagonists. The effects of opiates on contractile twitches of guinea-pig ileum have been carefully studied in response to field stimulation by KOSTERLITZ and co-workers (see KOSTERLITZ and WATERFIELD 1975) and by others (PATON and ZAR 1968); thus the hyperpolarisation and decreased acetylcholine release can be correlated with contractile effects. This hyperpolarisation could account for the decrease in acetylcholine release observed from these neurones in vitro, both those spontaneously active and those stimulated electrically to activity (NORTH 1979; DOWN and SZERB 1980; SZERB 1980). However, a portion of the acetylcholine release on field stimulation is from preganglionic terminals, and it is not clear how hyperpolarisation of the neuronal soma or its processes would account for a decreased release from presynaptic axons. If the action of morphine on the guinea-pig ileum is confined to intrinsic cholinergic neurones and their processes, there should be morphine or opiate resistant fractions of acetylcholine release. Perhaps preganglionic cell processes are also affected, but this point has not been specifically examined.

The nature of spontaneously active neuronal elements is also uncertain. Nearly all cells penetrated with microelectrodes by NORTH and NISHI (1973) or by HIRST et al. (1974) were not sponanteously active. In a review article, WOOD (1975) finds

4 Type 1 neurones also probably include intrinsic nonadrenergic inhibitory nerves; no action of morphine in this system is established

that there are spontaneously active as well as inactive neurones whose soma can be penetrated by microelectrodes. Studies of opiate actions by intracellular recordings from spontaneously active neurones are not available. DOWN and SZERB (1980) have suggested that the elements from which acetylcholine release is suppressed by opiates are axonal elements. However, the class or classes of neurones associated with these axonal elements is uncertain.

Other changes in function of guinea-pig ileum in the presence of opiate agonists or antagonists have been observed, consistent with decreased release of acetylcholine. These include decreased peristalsis on distention, decreased transit of fluid, decreased action in response to other agents which release acetylcholine; e.g. DMPP, 5-HT. Nearly all these studies on guinea-pig ileum have been carried out in vitro; and a recent study of the guinea-pig ileum in situ (ALDUNATE et al. 1975) suggests that the inhibitory motor effects of morphine observed by PRUITT et al. (1974) are mediated by release of noradrenaline. The pressure increment to induce peristalsis was increased by morphine. This action was prevented or reduced by reserpinisation, guanethidine or phentolamine (not by propranolol); these drugs reduced the pressure increment required in the absence of morphine. DL-dopa infusion reestablished the effect of morphine in reserpinised animals. Conceivably, noradrenaline is released in vivo by morphine to cause inhibition of cholinergic neurones by an action on α-adrenoceptors (see Sect. B.I). This hypothesis is inconsistent with reports already mentioned, that morphine inhibits release of noradrenaline from a number of sites. Further study of the mode of action of opiates on guinea-pig intestine in vivo is warranted.

In intestine of species other than the guinea-pig, there is evidence that serotonin (5-HT) and acetylcholine release are involved in mediating excitatory actions of morphine (see Sect. D.IV). Interestingly, in isolated ileum from morphine-tolerant guinea-pigs, naloxone appears to excite contractions by releasing 5-HT and acetylcholine (GINTZLER 1979) or substance P, and acetylcholine (GINTZLER 1980) tolerance to morphine is accompanied by hypersensitivity to 5-HT (SCHULZ and GOLDSTEIN 1973; TAKAYANAGI et al. 1974; WARD and TAKEMORI 1976). Hyposensitivity to noradrenaline has also been associated with morphine tolerance (SCHULZ and GOLDSTEIN 1973; GOLDSTEIN and SCHULZ 1973), but this finding was not confirmed by WARD and TAKEMORI (1976). How these findings relate, if they do, to the mechanism of morphine effect on ileum of normal guinea-pigs is not clear.

III. A Physiological Role for Endogenous Opiates in Guinea-Pig Intestine

The argument for a physiological role for endogenous opiates is best developed by in vitro studies of guinea-pig ileum but is incomplete. It has been shown that the enkephalins are present in nerve cells of the myenteric plexus (SCHULTZBERG et al. 1980; FURNESS and COSTA 1980) and in axons innervating muscles, synthesised in the myenteric plexus in this organ (MCKNIGHT et al. 1978), and released on field stimulation from the plexus (MCKNIGHT et al. 1978; SCHULZ et al. 1977). After a period of 10 Hz field stimulation, contractions to slower frequencies of field stimulation were depressed, an effect relieved by naloxone (PUIG et al. 1978). Also (−)-naloxone stereospecifically increased acetylcholine release by field stimulation from the plexus, but contractions were not increased (WATERFIELD and KOSTERLITZ 1975). VAN NUETEN et al. (1976) reported that, in ileal segments fatigued by maintained distention, the peristaltic contractions gradually fail because an inhibitory, naloxone-antagonisable substance accumulates in the bath. However, similar inhibition of peristalsis by added adenine nucleotides (ATP, ADP, AMP, and adenosine) was also antagonised by naloxone. This might cast doubt on the specificity of naloxone-antagonist effects in identifying actions originating from occupation of opiate receptors. However, it should be kept in mind that there is a potential multitude of controls over acetylcholine release (α-adrenergic agonists, muscarinic cholinergic agonists, purinergic agonists, prostaglandins etc.) so that naloxone may relieve a depression caused by the sum of action of several negative systems by inhibiting the contribution resulting from occupation by opiate receptors. As in any system with a variety of controls operating on a common pathway, physiological and receptor-specific interactions may be difficult to untangle.

In this particular case, KROMER and PRETZLAFF (1979) reported that they are unable to duplicate the result of VAN NUETEN et al. (1976) but that the naloxone stereospecifically increased the frequency of distension-induced peristalsis in ileal segments and decreased the duration and number of peristalsis-free periods. This was observed in ileum from foetal or adult pigs, in ileum from pregnant guinea-pigs and in fatigued ileum. The phenomenon was not observed in duodenum or jejunum. Acceptance of this as evidence for a physiological role of endogenous opiates in guinea-pig intestine requires acceptance of the assumption that the isolated Trendelenburg preparation of ileum is in a physiological state. This is uncertain at best, and the extent of damage probably varies with the particular experimental techniques used.

Convincing evidence for a physiological role of endogenous opiates requires demonstration of a stereospecific effect of naloxone in vivo under something close to physiological conditions. This might also allow demonstration of physiological affects originating from opiates in the central nervous system. Surprisingly, the guinea-pig is almost never studied in vivo. In other species there is a dearth of evidence to date for any such effect of naloxone on gut function. Alternative approaches (to be use of naloxone) might be inhibition of synthesis or degradation of endogenous opiates, but there is so far insufficient information about the metabolic pathways of enkephalins and controls over it.

IV. Mode of Opiate Action in Other Species

The guinea-pig small intestine is clearly not a universal model for drug effects on motility. In most species, including humans, there is no evidence that morphine or other opiates act by inhibiting acetylcholine release (DANIEL and BOGOCH 1959; DANIEL et al. 1959). The most thoroughly studied species other than the guinea-pig, is the dog. In this species, BURKS and LONG (1967) and BURKS (1973, 1976) have demonstrated that the direct excitant action of morphine and related agents on the gut wall observed after intra-arterial injection (DANIEL 1965) is due mainly to release of serotonin (5-HT) which then acts indirectly to release acetylcholine and directly to contract intestinal circular and longitudinal muscle. We (DANIEL et al. 1981) have recently found that methionine enkephalin also contracts in part by releasing acetylcholine (atropine- or TTX-sensitive) and in part by an atropine- and TTX-insensitive mechanism when given intra-arterially in dog intestine. However, 5-HT did not contract the ileum when given intra-arterially after atropine and TTX, and doses of 5-HT sufficient to produce tachyphylaxis did not affect the residual response to enkephalins after administration of atropine. Thus, the role of 5-HT in the action of methionine enkephalin may require further study.

In contrast to guinea-pig intestine, where morphine inhibits tone and peristaltic contractions by preventing acetylcholine release, the occupation of opiate receptors in dog intestine leads to increased nonpropulsive segmental contraction. Excitation of nonpropulsive contractions is also observed in small intestine of human, cat, horse, and many other species (see WEINSTOCK 1971; DANIEL 1966a, 1968). In humans, morphine initially causes phasic and tonic contractions of intestine, colon, rectum, internal anal sphincter, gallbladder, and biliary tract muscle, and possibly lower oesophageal sphincter (DANIEL and BOGOCH 1959, 1968; AMBINDER and SCHUSTER 1979). The duration of these initial contractions may not be as long in humans as the constipating effect of morphine, but this needs further study. Morphine inhibits gastric peristaltic contractions, but this may be an induced or reflex consequence of its pronounced effects to contract duodenum. The colon of other species (e.g. dog) is also excited to initiate nonpropulsive segmental contractions (DANIEL 1968; AMBINDER and SCHUSTER 1979), and there is increased resistance to transit of a bolus through the small and large intestines (GOODMAN and GILMAN 1980). In contrast, the contractions of stomach in the dog (DANIEL 1966a) are inhibited by intra-arterial opiate agonists.

Recently, it has been reported (UDDMAN et al. 1980) that many nerves with enkephalin-like immunoreactivity exist in the distal oesophagus of the cat, although there was no special accumulation of these in the most distal oesophagus. UDDMAN et al. (1980) reported also that both leucine enkephalin and methionine enkephalin caused dose-dependent inhibition of both "on" and "off" contractions to field stimulation. Contractions to acetylcholine and noradrenaline were unaffected. They concluded that enkephalins might inhibit field-stimulated noradrenaline release since "on" and "off" contractions of cat oesophageal circular muscle in vitro were abolished by prior reserpinisation or by adding phentolamine but not by adding atropine or TTX. These findings are in partial contrast to earlier work by CHRISTENSEN and DANIEL (1966, 1968) or GONELLA et al. (1979), that sympathetic agonists and noradrenaline, released by field stimulation, act on α-adrenoceptors to release acetylcholine from nerves in both longitudinal and circular muscle of the cat distal oesophagus.

EDIN et al. (1980) reported that intravenous morphine or enkephalinamide caused increased gastric tone and inhibited flow through the pylorus in the cat. Naloxone blocked these responses and a similar inhibition of transpyloric flow by vagal stimulation. Effects on vagal stimulation were insensitive to atropine and guanethidine. Since enkephalin-like immunoreactivity was present in the pyloric regions, these authors postulated a direct effect of enkephalins, either exogenous or released from nerves, on the pyloric muscle. A site of action outside gut was not excluded.

In the isolated segments of rat intestine, morphine (KAYMAKCALAN and TEMELLI 1964; WEINSTOCK 1971) and opiate endorphins (NIJKAMP and VAN REE 1980) were spasmogenic. Colon and rectum responded similarly in the latter study; naloxone reversed the effects of endorphins. Also, in the rat rectum, atropine, hexamethonium, burinamide, mepyramine, propranolol, and indomethacin failed to affect the responses to methionine enkephalin. In doses antagonising actions of 5-HT selectively, methysergide, and cyproheptadine reduced rectal responses to methionine enkephalin in a noncompetitive manner while phentolamine potentiated them. TTX decreased sensitivity to methionine enkephalin up to 20-fold but increased the maximum response. NIJKAMP and VAN REE suggested that endorphin actions might involve 5-HT (excitatory) but not by direct release. The potentiating effects of TTX and phentolamine on maximal contractions may imply a tonic inhibition by noradrenaline release. This shift to the right of the endorphin dose-response curve by TTX suggests nerve mediation of the effects.

In intact rats, BURKS (1976) found a dose-related, naloxone-sensitive, tonic and phasic increase in intestinal motility in response to morphine, which did not involve central receptors since intravenous administration was at least as effective as intracerebral administration. The response was atropine insensitive, but antagonised by methysergide (which also antagonised responses to 5-HT but not to cholecystokinin CCK). Cyproheptadine and cinanserin were ineffective against morphine and 5-HT contractions. He suggested that 5-HT was involved in the response. Surprisingly, the same laboratory (WEISBRODT et al. 1980) has now reported that morphine, given subcutaneously to fasting rats, inhibited spikes on the ECA (slow waves).

GILLAN and POLLOCK (1980) found that rat colon was excited by morphine and opiate peptides and these responses were unaffected by 5-HT desensitisation or adrenergic blockade, and potentiated by lysergic acid diethylamide (LSD), TTX, atropine, hexamethonium, and (+)-tubocurarine. Excitatory effects of opiates were inhibited by field stimulation, catecholamines, purines, and phosphodiesterase inhibitors. These authors suggested either a direct excitatory action of opiates on rat colon muscle or a presynaptic inhibitory action on a nonadrenergic inhibitory system. The mode of the spasmogenic action of opiates in rat gut obviously requires further study.

In any case, it is clear that morphine effects mammalian gut to produce constipation by a variety of mechanisms; some on the guinea-pig intestine involve inhibition of motility and inhibition of acetylcholine release, and others in a variety of species involve enhanced nonpropulsive motility and increased release of serotonin and/or acetylcholine or perhaps a direct excitatory action on smooth muscle. No unifying hypothesis is apparent at the moment.

V. Central and Peripheral Sites of Action of Opiate Agonists

Since endogenous opiates and their receptors have been shown to exist in brain, in pituitary and in gut, the question arises as to the site of opiates, given systemically, in affecting intestinal motility. MARGOLIN and PLEKSO (1965) showed that morphine injected into the central ventricle of rats was about 50 times more potent than morphine injected systemically. Other experiments led him to argue against a nervous pathway for the effects of intracerebroventricular (i.c.v.) morphine and to postulate release of a humoral agent from the isolated head which affects motility. PAROLARO et al. (1977) showed that the effects on motility of morphine given in this manner were reversed by naloxone. SCHULZ et al. (1979) recently considered whether this humoral substance was β-endorphin released from the pituitary. However, hypophysectomy in rats did not affect the potency of i.c.v. morphine. It was also shown, however, that morphine was 40–60 times more potent when given i.c.v. than when given intravenously or intraperitonically in rats, mice, and guinea-pigs. Furthermore, opiate receptor antagonists which could not cross the blood–brain barrier (quarternary naloxone) were relatively and equally ineffective against i.c.v. or systemic morphine in rats, but inhibited gut effects of loperimide as well as of stabilised enkephalin (FK33-824) which neither cross the blood–brain barrier nor cause analgesia. These studies were interpreted as indicating that the constipating action of systemic morphine in rats, like that of i.c.v. morphine, was on opiate receptors in the brain and involved some nervous pathway, but that gut transit was also capable of being inhibited by opiate agonists acting directly on the intestine. In these experiments, gut transit was assessed by giving a charcoal meal by stomach tube. This technique may reflect opiate effects on gastric emptying more than those on small intestinal transit.

However, STEWART et al. (1978) have used a technique in rats in which transit of a $^{51}CrO_4$-labelled meal given by an intraduodenal cannula was measured and diarrhoea and weight changes were also assessed. They found that i.c.v. morphine was more potent than systemic subcutaneous morphine (only 15–60 µg required compared with 2.5 mg/kg) and that its effects could be blocked by subdiaphragmatic vagotomy or 5 µg i.c.v. naltrexone. Even after vagotomy, 5 mg/kg subcutaneous morphine caused inhibition of intestinal transit. These authors concluded that morphine could possibly produce its effects by actions on either central or peripheral opiate receptors but in the usual dose acted on central opiate receptors. Their experiments do not clarify whether systemic morphine acts exclusively centrally or at both sets of receptors.

Earlier experiments in the dog (DANIEL 1966b) showed that intra-arterial morphine in low doses (10–100 µg = 0.5–2 µg/kg) had local effects causing duodenal spasm. Recently we have observed that 2 ng or more of methionine enkephalin given intra-arterially into the dog ileum, causes spikes on electrical activity and contractions which are reduced by atropine or TTX pretreatment (E. E. DANIEL et al. unpublished work 1981). KONTUREK and SIEBERS (1980) reported that this agent, when infused intravenously, acts to inhibit spiking and to decrease the frequency of migrating myoelectric complexes; this probably reflects a different response of the intestine to an action on opiate receptors at another site.

VI. Opiate Receptor Types

There appears to be more than one type of opiate receptor. When potencies of opiate receptor agonists in the guinea-pig longitudinal muscle plexus preparation from the ileum are compared with those in mouse vas deferens, there are different rank orders (LORD et al. 1976, 1977; WATERFIELD et al. 1977, 1979; KOSTERLITZ and HENDERSON 1977; SIMNANTOV et al. 1976; KOSTERLITZ et al. 1980). Typical morphine-like agents were relatively more potent in the ileal preparation compared with enkephalins and the reverse was true in the vas deferens preparation. Thus,

Table 13. Affinity (K_d) for opiate ligands: brain opiate receptors

	K_d (mM)			
	Morphine (μ) receptor		Enkephalin (δ) receptor	
	−Na	+Na	−Na	+Na
Morphine	0.3	6	36	130
Leu-enkephalin	8.5	57	0.5	1.7
Naloxone	0.6	0.6	16	15
Diprenorphine	0.2	0.2	0.25	0.23

enkephalins, enkephalin analogues, and extended fragments of β-lipoprotein (containing more amino acids than Met-enkephalin itself) were more potent relative to morphine-like drugs in vas deferens in contrast to their relative potencies in the ileum. β-Endorphin was equipotent in the two test systems. The ability of these agents to displace labelled ligand showed corresponding differences. In the vas deferens, enkephalins were more potent in displacing ^{3}H-labelled enkephalins and less effective in displacing naloxone ^{3}H and related ligands. Typical morphine-like agonists were effectively antagonized by naloxone in both ileum and vas deferens and were more effective in displacing naloxone ^{3}H, naltrexine ^{3}H, and related antagonists, than ^{3}H-labelled enkephalins. The receptors with higher affinity for morphine-like agonists and naloxone-like antagonists were tentatively designated μ receptors; they predominate in the ileum. These with higher affinity for enkephalins and from which enkephalins are less readily displaced by naloxone (and vice versa) were designated δ receptors). β-Endorphin appears to act on both receptors.

This classification of opiate receptors based on ligand binding studies in guinea-pig ileum myenteric plexus corresponds to that proposed for the types of opiate receptor in the brain (see CHANG et al. 1980 a, b). CHANG et al. point out that for both μ and δ receptors in the brain and plexus, Na^+ or guanosine 5′-triphosphate decreases the affinity of agonists but not antagonists. This effect of Na^+ was more pronounced in morphine (μ) receptors than in enkephalin (δ) receptors (see Table 13).

Some relative potencies of agonists for *morphine* receptors are morphine > Tyr-DAla-Gly-N(Me)-Phe-Met(O)ol (Sandoz FK33824) ≃ (DAla^{2}Met^5)enkephalinamide ≃ (Dmet^{2}Pro^5 enkephalin > (DAla^{2}DLeu^5)enkephalin and for *enkephalin* receptors (DAla^2-DLeu^5)enkephalin > (DAla^{2}Met^5)enkephalinamide (DMet^{2}Pro^5)enkephalin > Sandoz FK33824 ≧ morphine (see also KOSTERLITZ et al. 1980). Whether different receptors subserve different functions remains to be determined for the gut.

The low affinity of enkephalins for morphine receptors suggests that another endogenous substance exists to interact with these receptors. For this role dynorphin – (1,13), discovered in brain, has been suggested (GOLDSTEIN et al. 1979). It can be considered as a COOH-terminal extension of Leu-enkephalin. In guinea-pig ileum, it was 700 times more potent than Leu-enkephalin, but in mouse vas deferens, it was only 3 times more potent. WÜSTER et al. (1980) suggest that in the mouse vas deferens, this substance acts on a separate (neither μ nor δ) class of opiate receptor. Obviously elucidation of receptor types for opiates is incomplete, and present hypotheses will be revised in the light of future experiments.

VII. Opiate Agonists Selective for Gut Receptors

Recently a number of synthetic opiate agonists have been studied and reported to be selective for opiate receptors in the gut, i.e. to have little or no analgesic or euphoric effects in doses much larger than required to produce constipation. These include diphenoxylate (JANSSEN et al. 1959; DAZANI et al. 1975), loperamide (VAN NUETEN et al. 1974; NIEMEGEERS et al. 1974a, b), SC-27166 or 2-(3-5-methyl-1,3,4-oxadiazol-2-DL)3,3-diphenylpropyl)-2-azabicyclo- (2,2,2)octane (MACKERER et al. 1977; DAZANI et al. 1977). While differential sensitivity of brain and gut opiate receptors of these agents after systemic or oral administration was convincingly demonstrated, later studies showed that these agents all readily displace naloxone H^3 from opiate receptors in homogenates of guinea-pig brain (MACKERER et al. 1976; CLAY et al. 1977). Clearly, most of the inability of these agonists to active brain opiate receptors is related to their inability to cross the blood–brain barrier. Differential affinity for δ over μ receptors has not been established for any of these agents.

VIII. Clinical Applications of Opiate Antidiarrhoeal Agents

Diphenoxylate and loperamide are both congeners of domperidone. Diphenoxylate has much less effect on opiate receptors in the CNS than in the periphery because it does not readily cross the blood–brain barrier (see Sect. D.VI; NIEMEGEERS et al. 1974a, b). However, it certainly can reach central opiate receptors and serious, sometimes fatal, poisonings have resulted, especially in children (PENFOLD and VOLANS 1977; SMITH and CHAMBERS 1978; CURTIS and GOEL 1979; CUTLER et al. 1980). Diphenoxylate is supplied in tablets containing 2.5 mg mixed with 0.025 mg atropine sulphate, under the name Lomotil, and the recommended daily dose for diarrhoea is 20 mg (8 tablets). However, at doses of 40–60 mg, it produces typical opiate effects, including euphoria and can suppress signs and symptoms of morphine withdrawal (JAFFE and MARTIN 1980). In poisoning from accidental ingestion of Lomotil by children, the serious symptoms are usually of opiate excess effect on the central nervous system. They include respiratory depression, coma and other changes which are usually naloxone reversible (PENFOLD and VOLANS 1977; SMITH and CHAMBERS 1978; CUTLER et al. 1980; CURTIS and GOEL 1979). Atropine effects are said to be mild in these cases of poisoning and to disappear after a few hours, to be replaced by opiate effects. Gastric lavage or emesis is essential in poisoning cases because Lomotil arrests gastrointestinal transit function and leaves the drug to be absorbed. Diphenoxylate potentiates the hypnotic effects of ethanol in animals (MCGUIRE et al. 1978), is abused by addicts or addiction-prone persons (RUBINSTEIN 1979) and can prevent the withdrawal syndrome during methadone detoxification (KLEINMAN and ARNON 1971). Difenoxin, a metabolite of diphenoxylate, has actions similar to the parent compound (JAFFE and MARTIN 1980).

In contrast to diphenoxylate, loperamide is reported to have much less ability to cross the blood–brain barrier (NIEMEGEERS et al. 1974 a, b; HEYKANTS et al. 1974). It does not produce analgesia, except in near fatal doses (NIEMEGEERS et al. 1974 a, b). So far no reports of its causing poisoning nor of its abuse are available. Abuse of loperamide is unlikely because its poor water solubility makes its parenteral injection difficult or impossible. However, JAFFE and MARTIN (1980) pointed out that it can suppress morphine withdrawal symptoms in addicted monkeys when given in sufficient doses, so poisoning and abuse may occur.

Loperamide and diphenoxylate have been demonstrated to be nearly equally effective in diarrhoea with a wide variety of causes: e.g. ulcerative colitis, ulcerative colitis with cholostomy, Crohn's disease, short bowel syndrome, subtotal colectomy, postvagotomy, following administration of PGE, in cholera (SCHEURMANS et al. 1974; ENGBACK et al. 1975; DEMEULENAERE et al. 1974; AMERY et al. 1975; PELEMANS and VANTRAPPEN 1976; GALAMBOS et al. 1976; MAINGUET and FIASSE 1977; LANGE et al. 1977; BINNIE et al. 1979). As expected, from their relative abilities to cross the blood–brain barrier, more undesirable effects have usually been reported to diphenoxylate than to loperamide in comparative trials. Loperamide is also longer acting than diphenoxylate (HEYKANTS et al. 1974). The rationale for the use of constipating agents in treating diarrhoeas caused by enterotoxins acting on the gut wall to increase electrolyte and water secretion into the lumen (see Sect. E) is obscure, and there is evidence that their use may be ineffective and prolong the diarrhoea (e.g. DUPONT and HORNICK 1973; NOVAK et al. 1976).

The relative importance in the antidiarrhoeal effects of these agents of altered motility and decreased secretion of intestinal electrolytes and water remains to be determined; recently HARFORD et al. (1980) found that diphenoxylate plus atropine (Lomotil) decreased faecal frequency and stool weight and diminished faecal incontinence, without affecting rectal or anal sphincter pressures, continence to a rectal infusion of saline, or ability to retain small spheres placed in the rectum. In these patients with chronic diarrhoea and faecal incontinence, an important action on colonic fluid and electrolyte movement may have been involved as well as a primary effect on motility (see Sect. D).

E. Laxatives and Constipating Agents

Laxatives cannot yet be classified by their mechanism of action (see Sect. E) in most cases. One diverse group, *osmotic laxatives*, does seem to have a known mode of action. Some are saline cathartics ($MgSO_4$, $Mg(OH)_2$, magnesium citrate, sodium phosphates, sodium sulphate); others are indigestible carbohydrates; e.g. lactulose (digested only in the colon to oscmotically active fragments), mannitol and lactose (in patients lacking lactose). All are claimed to act by increasing luminal fluid by setting up an osmotic gradient. However, it has been pointed out that these agents, notably Mg salts and various sulphates, are effective in doses too low to be explained by an osmotic effect on fluid distribution and act too rapidly for this to be a feasible explanation (HARVEY and READ 1973). They decrease net Na absorption, cause secretion of an enzyme-rich pancreatic juice, evacuate the gallbladder and in general duplicate the effects of CCK. Thus, it has been proposed by HARVEY and READ that in whole or in part they act to release CCK. What is lacking is direct evidence for such a release of CCK by these salts; no accepted radioimmunoassay for CCK is available.

Other laxatives have to be grouped by their chemical and hopefully mechanistic similarity: e.g. phenolphthalein, bisacodyl, and oxyphenisatin are *diphenylmethane derivatives;* senna, sennosides A and B, cascara sargrada, and danthron are all *anthroquinones;* ricinoleic acid (the active ingredients produced from castor oil by hydrolysis in the intestine) is a *hydroxy fatty acid* and deoxycholic acid and chenodeoxycholic acid are *dihydroxy bile acids.* Many textbooks of pharmacology still approach the laxative actions of these drugs as primarily involving alterations in intestinal motility. In diarrhoea, there are certainly motility changes, e.g. in the colon there is a marked reduction in motility (KERN et al. 1951; CONNELL 1962; WALLER et al. 1972; WALLER 1975). In experimental animals, laxatives produce diarrhoea associated with decreased contractile function of the small and large intestine (STEWART and BASS 1976a, b). In both the fasting and the fed state, decreased spike myoelectric activity occurred in the small and large intestine (GARCIA-VILLAR et al. 1980). In a patient with bacterial overgrowth and diarrhoea, the migrating myoelectric complex was absent (VANTRAPPEN et al. 1977). Thus, decreased motility and myoelectric spiking is associated with diarrhoea produced by disease or laxation. The functional consequence has been postulated by CONNELL (1962) to be decreased resistance to flow and more rapid transit.

However, both pathological and experimental diarrhoea (or laxation) invariably involve changes in net salt and electrolyte movement into the gut lumen. HENDRIX and BAYLESS (1970) and BINDER (1977, 1980) have summarised the evidence that diarrhoea from a wide variety of causes (lactase deficiency, coeliac and tropical sprue, Crohn's disease ulcerative colitis, intestinal obstruction, carcinoid syndrome, watery diarrhoea syndrome, cholera, acute undifferentiated diarrhoea, and medullary carcinoma of the thyroid) involves increased net salt and water movement into the lumen of the small and large intestine. In some cases, this is related to increased cyclic AMP production, leading to increased active transport of Cl^- followed by Na^+ and water into the gut lumen (possibly occurring in crypt epithelial cells) and to decreased active absorption of NaCl via a neutral transport system (possibly occurring in villous epithelial cells); see FRIZZELL et al. 1979; BINDER 1980. This has been postulated to be the mode of the diarrhoeal action of cholera enterotoxin, heat labile enterotoxin of *Escherichia coli*, vasoactive intestinal polypeptide (VIP), prostaglandins (PGE), deoxycholic acid, and ricinoleic acid (FELDMAN and GIBALDI 1969; FIELD et al. 1972; BANWELL and SHEER 1973; BRIGHT-ASARE and BINDER 1973; WILD and BAKER 1974; BINDER and RAWLINS 1973; AMMON and PHILLIPS 1973, 1974; AMMON et al. 1974; COYNE et al. 1977; TAUB et al. 1977; BINDER 1979, 1980; WANITSCHKE et al. 1977). A so-called wetting agent, dioctylsulphosyccinate, may also act in this way (DONOWITZ and BINDER 1975). Heat stable enterotoxin of *E. coli* increases cyclic GMP, not cyclic AMP in intestinal mucosa; but the function of cyclic GMP in promoting net luminal fluid accumulation is not certain. Enterotoxins of *Shigella dysenteriae* I and *Stapholoccus* spp. damage intestinal mucosa and inhibit net fluid absorption. Hormones which appear to cause diarrhoea and net accumulation of intestinal fluid when present in large amounts include calcitonin, serotonin, gastric inhibitory polypeptide and cholecystokinin. They act via cyclic AMP-independent, unknown mechanisms (see BINDER 1977, 1980).

Other laxatives, like the dihydroxy bile acids (e.g. deoxycholic acid or chenodeoxycholic acid) or the hydroxy fatty acids (ricinoleic acid), also cause net fluid accumulation (see BINDER 1979, 1980; FORTH et al. 1963, 1966). Proposed mechanisms for the effects of other laxatives on fluid transport are diverse: osmotic attraction of water, inhibition of mucosal Na^+, K^+-ATPase or increased leakiness of mucosa membranes. Mannitol, lactose, lactulose, and indigestible high molecular weight polysaccharides, Mg salts, various sulphates etc. all reach the colon without absorption and cause an osmotically driven net flow of water into the lumen. This is presumed to cause laxation, but these agents may act by other means (e.g. CCK release). Phenolphthalein and bisacodyl can *increase* PGE production and cyclic AMP levels as a consequence (BEUBLER and JUAN 1978). Inhibition of the Na^+, K^+-ATPase of the intestinal epithelium by cardiac glycosides which are excreted in the bile predominantly (e.g. proscillaridin or its methyl derivatives) causes conversion of net water, Na^+ and Cl^- absorption to net secretion in the jejunum and increased the loss of K^+; active K^+ secretion in the colon was increased (WANITSCHKE and EWE 1978; EWE 1980a). Phenolphthalein, bisocodyl, emodin, danthron, rhein, and deoxycholate all have been reported to *inhibit* Na^+, K^+-ATPase in the intestinal mucosa (PHILLIPS et al. 1965; PAPE et al. 1966; CHIGNELL 1968; WANITSCHKE 1980; EWE 1980a). However, such studies do not establish that Na^+, K^+-ATPase inhibition is either contributing to or exclusively causing the laxative effect in vivo.

Bile salts (deoxycholate) and oxyphenisation *increased the hydraulic conductivity* of intestinal membrane in vitro (FELDMAN and GIBALDI 1969; BINDER and RAWLINS 1973; WALL and BAKER 1974; SCHWIETER et al. 1975; NELL et al. 1976; WANITSCHKE et al. 1977). This decreases electrolyte and water absorption from the gut. It is not clear in the case of deoxycholate whether its effects on active transport or on hydraulic conductivity are paramount in the resultant net fluid accumulation it causes in the gut. Rhein, the oxidised product of sennosides (anthroquinine), may also increase hydraulic conductivity of intestinal mucosa but the evidence is so far indirect (EWE 1980b). Impure oxidised sennosides (LENG-PESCHLOW 1980) reduced net Na^+, Cl^-, and H_2O absorption from isolated intestine of rats; but increased hydraulic conductivity and other mechanisms have not been examined.

Motility changes definitely also occur after taking laxatives. Most early studies of such effects were carried out in vitro and were characterised by BINDER and DONOWITZ (1975) as having "merely demonstrated an in vitro effect of the agent on smooth muscle." It is also just to state that most of the studies of the effects of laxatives on intestinal active ion transport and hydraulic permeability can be characterised as having merely demonstrated an in vitro effect of the agent on gut mucosa. There are, however, several reports of laxative effects on intestinal absorption in vivo, including studies in humans (see EWE 1980a, b). Only a few studies have been made of the motility changes induced by laxatives in vivo. In nearly all cases, they demonstrated decreased motility during laxation or diarrhoea (STEWART et al. 1975; STEWART and BASS 1976a, b; GARCÍA-VILLAR et al. 1980). MATHIAS et al. (1977) report that cholera toxin initiates periodic migrating action potential complexes in rabbit intestine; but the lack of demonstrated generality or relevance to diarrhoea of such a motility change make the significance of this finding obscure. Ricinoleic acid, but not oleic acid, has been shown to disrupt the organisation of myogenic electrical activity of the cat colon (CHRISTENSEN and FREEMAN 1972) but these findings have not been extended to other laxatives nor connected to either motility or fluid movement changes in vivo.

The most detailed study is that of GARCÍA-VILLAR et al. (1980) who demonstrated that there were effects of various senna preparations on fasting or fed dogs studied under chronic, conscious conditions. Sennosides are believed to be hydrolised to sennidins which are then reduced (rhein anthrone) and oxidised (rhein) by bacteria in the large bowel (LEMLI and LEMMENS 1980). The oxidised forms like rhein are believed to be active. Oxidised sennosides administered into the colon decreased motility there and also disorganised the migrating myoelectric complex (MMC) pattern in the ileum in fasted dogs, even though none of the active material presumably reached the ileal lumen. Unoxidised Ca-sennosides administered by mouth decreased colonic motility in fed dogs and in fasted animals, disorganised MMC patterns throughout the gastrointestinal tract and decreased colonic activity within 2 h of administration. They caused diarrhoea in about 6 h in both fed and fasted animals. These effects on motility of the upper intestine and colon occurred prior to any possible passage of sennosides to and hydrolysis in the colon[5]. Purified sennosides given by mouth had similar motility effects only after 6–8 h while oxidised sennosides had similar effects within 1 h. Presumably some oxidised sennosides were present as impurities in the unoxidised sennosides and acted directly to disorganise motility in the stomach and small intestine: these events also led to decreased colon motility.

In parallel experiments on Na^+, Cl^- and fluid absorption from intestine of anaesthetised rats (LENG-PESCHLOW 1980), pure sennosides had no effect, but all others decreased net Na^+, Cl^-, and H_2O absorption in the ileum and colon and the intensity of the effects was proportional to the amount of oxidised sennoside used. In these studies, it is hard to attribute the motility effects of sennosides solely to their effects on intestinal absorption and/or secretion. There was little or no effect of the unoxidised sennosides (which probably contain small quantities of oxidised impurities) on absorption and secretion but this mixture, or its very low levels of oxidised material, markedly affected upper gastrointestinal motility prior to its arrival in the large bowel. Also oxidised sennosides applied locally in the colon affected motility in the ileum and disruption of upper bowel motility by unoxidised sennosides was immediately accompanied by inhibition of colonic activity.

These time and space relations of senna effects suggest transmission of sennoside action by nerve or hormonal mechanisms. Also insufficient systemic absorption of sennosides occurs to account for these effects. It is impossible to explain them in terms of effects on absorption or secretion alone, although these undoubtedly contribute to the overall laxation. Possibly they were mediated by release of gastrointestinal hormones or by gastrointestinal reflexes.

5 There is no evidence that sufficient anthroquinines are absorbed to be effective systemically; moreover, only hydrolysed and oxidised products are known to be absorbed. On the other hand, once absorbed, less than 10% of a given dose has been accounted for (LEMLI and LEMMENS 1980)

Future clarification of the mode of laxative action will require answers to the following questions. (1) What motility changes and changes in absorption and secretion actually occur during laxation in vivo? (2) Could these motility changes be entirely secondary to increased lumen content of fluids? (3) Could these changes in luminal fluid content be entirely secondary to motility changes? As the answers to questions (2) and (3) are almost certainly "no" in each case, since motility is normally increased by increased luminal fluid but it is apparently decreased and fluid transit is increased during laxation, we must also ask a further question. (4) What additional mechanisms (hormone release, gastrointestinal reflex activity, alteration in myogenic activity) are involved in the chain of events leading from laxative administration to altered motility, absorption, secretion and transit?

Not only do laxative effects inhibit net transfer of intestinal electrolytes on fluid from lumen to blood, antidiarrhoeal agents acting on opiate receptors inhibit the increased secretion and decreased absorption of salt and water caused by PGE_1 and VIP (presumably acting via cyclic AMP increase) in experimental models by a naloxone-sensitive, stereospecific mechanism (COUPAR 1978; WÜSTER and HERZ 1978; BEUBLER and LEMBECK 1979; LEMBECK and BEUBLER 1979). Since loperamide, which cannot cross the blood–brain barrier, shared this action in vivo as well as in vitro (WÜSTER and HERZ 1978), it appears that intestinal rather than CNS opiate receptors are involved. It is tempting to postulate a role for endogenous endorphins in regulation of salt and electrolyte movements; but in vitro naloxone had no effect on basal fluid volume. However, it did enhance the effects of PGI_1 and VIP to increase intestinal fluid. Thus, it appears that the endogenous endorphins may modulate increased salt and fluid movement into the intestine. The question that these results raise but do not answer, is: does the constipating effect of opiates involve altered motility or decreased fluid movement, or both?

F. Direct and Indirect Actions

To test whether agents affecting intestinal motility are acting directly or indirectly, a variety of approaches have been made. None of them is without pitfalls; these have been discussed in detail (DANIEL 1968). In addition to limitations to the pharmacological tools used (e.g. TTX-insensitive nerves or release of mediator), there are limitations based on the experimental system studied.

First of all, the use of in vitro preparation may be misleading with respect to agents with a mixed action in vivo on both smooth muscle and nerves. Many substances of interest (substance P, gastrin, motilin) have actions on nervous structures in some (not all) regions of the gut in some species (COOK et al. 1974). Yet there are studies in vitro in which the action of the agents (all of which release acetylcholine in vivo in some regions) were unaffected by atropine (or other muscarinic blocking agents), TTX and other nerve inhibitors (STRUNZ et al. 1975; MORGAN et al. 1978). There are several reasons for these discrepancies. One is that nerves may not be functioning or receiving appropriate inputs in vitro or the site of action of a substance may be eliminated by the dissection (e.g. removal of all but longitudinal muscle and plexus). Another is that substances or field stimulation may act directly on nerve varicosities to affect mediator release by a mechanism not involving Na channels. They also may release acetylcholine in high concentrations locally – in a region not accessible to atropine or other pharmacological tools administered into the bath. If the motor action of an agonist is produced by release of a noncholinergic mediator by a TTX-insensitive mechanism, we would probably end by classifying it as direct action, unless we happened to possess and test an antagonist selective for the mediator in question. Rebound excitation after stimulation of nonadrenergic inhibitory nerves by an indirect acting substance is a case in point. If the preparation was studied in vitro or in vivo and lacked tone or regular phasic activity, the preliminary inhibition might easily be missed and the response would be resistant to atropine and conceivably to TTX, for reasons already discussed. Another possible cause of difficulty is the tendency for dissection procedures, in preparations for in vitro experiments, to increase the output of prostaglandins (often PGE_2 or PGI_2) enormously. These may act by increased or decreased motor function, or both, and may variably affect nerve release mechanisms. Accumulation of the metabolites may affect muscle or nerve function in vitro.

In addition, an indirect site of action may not involve structures in the gut. Morphine, as discussed in Sect. D.V, probably has its gut propulsion inhibiting action on opiate receptors in the central nervous system and another action, with similar outcome, on gut opiate receptors, but at higher doses. It would be impossible to learn about the central action of morphine on gut motility from in vitro experiments. This particular situation has been discovered by applying morphine or related agents and antagonists locally in brain receptors inside the blood–brain barrier and comparing potencies by various routes of both agonists and antagonists. It should be kept in mind, whenever agents are administered systemically, that the site of observed response may not be the site of initial action. In the case of morphine, actions of low doses in rats, mice, and guinea-pigs appear to be central. It is still uncertain whether systemic morphine acts primarily centrally in those species in which it does not act by inhibiting acetylcholine release; e.g. dog, cat, human.

These remarks make it obvious that adrenergic and cholinergic agonists already discussed have indirect, neuronal sites of action as well as direct actions on intestinal muscle. Thus the presynaptic α_2 actions of noradrenaline and other agonists should be considered indirect, as should the presynaptic actions of β_2-adrenergic and dopamine-like agonists and of muscarinic and nicotinic cholinergic agonists. Opiates, at present, seem to have most, if not all, their actions at neuronal sites; no direct action on smooth muscle has been proved.

Although not discussed in this chapter, gastrointestinal peptides acting both as hormones and as neuromodulators or transmitters all seem to have neural sites of action as well as in most cases, direct actions on smooth muscle. If classical or recent putative neurotransmitters can affect the release of these peptides from endocrine cells and/or nerves, a new order of complexity of drug action may exist (see Chaps. 2a–2e). The judicious use of tools like TTX, scorpion venom and others that selectively act on Na channels of nerves, is very valuable. What is still needed is a technique to obliterate nerve function completely but selectively, to rule out actions of drugs on Ca^{2+}-dependent processes leading to mediator release. An alternative approach is the study of single, isolated gastrointestinal muscle cells, but so far this has had very limited utilisation.

G. Serotonin Receptors and Antagonists

I. Early Studies

In an earlier review (DANIEL 1968) it was pointed out that serotonin (5-hydroxytryptamine, 5-HT) has both direct and indirect actions. Evidence was summarised that, at low doses, 5-HT had mainly a direct action in vitro and in vivo on human small intestine and in vitro on human stomach, guinea-pig terminal ileum, rat colon, isolated stomach of mice, rats, and kittens. Methysergide, bromolysergic acid, phenothiazines, phenoxybenzamine, and related compounds were competitive antagonists at such sites. However, the caution already mentioned that damage to nervous structure during and after isolation may have eliminated indirect actions of 5-HT in vitro, should be borne in mind.

In the guinea-pig ileum in vitro, especially circular muscle, the canine antrum in vivo, the perfused canine small intestine and the rat colon in vitro, 5-HT was known in 1968 to have prominent indirect as well as direct excitatory actions. Indirect actions were inhibited by atropine, hyoscine, morphine, local anaesthetics, botulinus toxins, large antagonistic doses of nicotine or DMPP, and sometimes (not always) by hexamethonium. None of these inhibitory agents acted directly on neural 5-HT receptors, and they presumably interfered with the activation of intrinsic cholinergic neurones by 5-HT or the effects of the acetylcholine released thereby. Hexamethonium insensitivity on several tissues was taken to imply a postsynaptic site of action directly on the cholinergic neurone instead of its presynaptic input. A locus for 5-HT receptors on myenteric neurones also provided one explanation for the ability of 5-HT to inhibit contractions in preparations such as isolated human taenia coli and distal colon by a mechanism insensitive to hexamethonium, procaine or β-adrenergic blockade, i.e. a site of action on nonadrenergic inhibitory neurones.

Thus in 1968 there was evidence that 5-HT excited the intestine by acting on cholinergic neurones or elsewhere to release acetylcholine and directly on smooth muscle. It had inhibitory actions in some preparations which also seemed to be indirect. Although 5-HT competitive antagonists (e.g. methysergide) were available for receptors on smooth muscle, none was established for 5-HT receptors on nerves. A considerable amount of confusion has arisen because of the assumption without adequate evidence that methysergide was such an antagonist. Chapter 3 and this Handbook, Vol. 59/I, Chap. 11 give further details of early work.

II. Neuronal Receptors

Study of nerve and muscle 5-HT receptors in the guinea-pig ileum is the most thoroughly investigated aspect of the work reported here. Early work established that part of the excitatory action was directly on smooth muscle and could be blocked by agents like methysergide or dibenamine and another part involved an action on nerves and could be blocked by morphine or atropine (LEWIS 1960; DAY and VANE 1963; GADDUM and PICARELLI 1967; COSTA and FURNESS 1976). Neither morphine nor atropine acts directly on the serotonin receptors but instead inhibits the release or action of acetylcholine from neurones stimulated by 5-HT (LEWIS 1960; KOSTERLITZ and ROBINSON 1958; see DANIEL 1968 for review). Direct evidence was recently obtained that 5-HT excited myenteric neurones (SATO et al. 1974; DINGLEDINE and GOLDSTEIN 1976; HIRST and SILINSKY 1975) and released acetylcholine (ADAM-VIZI and VIZI 1978; HIRST and SILINSKY 1975). DINGLEDINE and GOLDSTEIN (1976) presented evidence that morphine inhibited this action by raising the threshold of processes of myenteric neurones so that substances like 5-HT could no longer initiate impulses or these impulses could no longer invade nerve varicosities.

Recently it has been suggested that this neuronal excitatory action of 5-HT in the guinea-pig ileum myenteric plexus may be related to a slow excitatory postsynaptic potential (slow e.p.s.p) of type 2 or H cells which can be induced by repetitive focal stimulation of nerve tracts in the myenteric plexus (WOOD and MAYER 1979a, b). 5-HT mimics this response and this effect of 5-HT was blocked by 30 μM methysergide as was the slow e.p.s.p. However, substance P also imitates the slow e.p.s.p (see MORITA et al. 1980), and evidence for its role as mediator of that potential has also been obtained. Furthermore, methysergide is not effective in blocking neuronal excitatory action of 5-HT in the small intestine (DRAKONTIDES and GERSHON 1968; FURNESS and COSTA 1979; FOZARD and MOBAROK ALI 1978; FOZARD et al. 1979). Methysergide is an effective antagonist against excitatory effects of 5-HT on smooth muscle (see Sects. C.II, III), but its action on 5-HT receptors in nerves is probably nonspecific, since it is reported to be equally effective against the depression of the myenteric neurone e.p.s.p which is caused by noradrenaline (R. A. NORTH and HENDERSON unpublished work; see NORTH et al. 1980). On midbrain and forebrain neurones, methysergide fails to antagonise the depressant effects of 5-HT; it does prevent excitatory effects of 5-HT in the facial nucleus and reticulum formation (MCCALL and AGHAJANIAN 1979; see also JACOBY 1978). COSTA and FURNESS (1979) concluded that bromolysergic acid, phenyldiguanide and tryptamine were nonspecific antagonists at neural 5-HT receptors in the guinea-pig intestine. FOZARD et al. (1979) have shown that (−)-cocaine can competitively inhibit 5-HT actions at neuronal receptors in rabbit heart and in guinea-pig ileum; in the latter case higher concentrations of cocaine also reduced maximal responses as well as shifting the dose–response curve to the right.

RATTAN and GOYAL (1977, 1978b) have shown that serotonin acts by exciting inhibitory myenteric neurones in the lower oesophageal sphincter muscle of the opossum studied in vivo. Relaxation to vagal stimulation was partly inhibited by hexamethonium and atropine (see Sect. G.I); 5-methoxydimethyltryptamine (5-MDT) eliminated any residual responses to vagal stimulation after administration of hexamethonium and atropine. Alone 5-MDT had no effects but made relaxation to vagal stimulation capable of abolition by subsequent administration of hexamethonium and atropine. Treatment with *P*-chlorphenylalanine, to eliminate 5-HT stores, likewise made relaxation to vagal stimulation susceptible to cholinergic blockade. Since neural (TTX-sensitive) effects of 5-HT which caused LES relaxation were also blocked by 5-MDT (RATTAN and GOYAL 1977), these data suggested that there was an interneurone innervated by vagal fibres (apparently with a noncholinergic mediator) which released 5-HT; the 5-HT in turn activated noncholinergic, nonadrenergic inhibitory neurones. Nobody has apparently tested the effect of 5-MDT on 5-HT activation of cholinergic neurones of the guinea-pig ileum.

COSTA and FURNESS (1976) found that distension contracted the isolated colon or rectum of the guinea-pig. There was a methysergide-sensitive (inhibition of direct action of released 5-HT) as well as a hyoscine-sensitive (inhibition of action of released acetylcholine) component in the peristaltic contraction of the colon. The rectum relaxed on distension and lacked a methysergide-sensitive component. COSTA and FURNESS therefore concluded, in contrast of DRAKONTIDES and GERSHON (1972) from studies of the mouse intestine, that 5-HT might be involved in the excitatory pathway to cholinergic neurones, but not in any inhibitory pathway. Consistent with such a conclusion, VERMILLION et al. (1979) found no effect of 5-HT on inhibition or rebound from field stimulation of guinea-pig taenia coli or of ileal circular muscle. However, the experiments of COSTA and FURNESS as well as VERMILLION et al. were carried out in vitro (so that the interneuronal sites postulated by RATTAN and GOYAL or another neural site of action may have been nonfunctional). No antagonists of 5-HT at neural receptors were tested (so that a neural pathway involving noncholinergic mediation might have been missed). Thus, any conclusion ruling out 5-HT receptors on inhibitory neurones seems premature.

Serotonin has an additional action on the neurones of the myenteric plexus of the guinea-pig ileum. It causes presynaptic inhibition of acetylcholine release (NORTH et al. 1980). In type 1 or S neurones, 5-HT inhibited the fast cholinergic e.p.s.p whether applied by iontophoresis or by perfusion. It did not affect e.p.s.p evoked by acetylcholine iontophoretically applied to the ganglion. This action accounts for the inhibition of the peristaltic reflex observed in this preparation when 5-HT was applied to the serosal surface (KOSTERLITZ and ROBINSON 1957; BÜLBRING and CREMA 1958). The neural presynaptic receptor for 5-HT was, like the receptor on type 2 cells, nonspecifically depressed by methysergide (NORTH et al. 1980). This agent also depressed the fast e.p.s.p, prevented the depression of this e.p.s.p by noradrenaline and inhibited the slow e.p.s.p (see earlier in this section). Cyproheptadine prevented the 5-HT-induced depression of the fast e.p.s.p in some, but not all neurones. Lysergic acid diethylamide (LSD) acted like 5-HT itself in depressing the fast e.p.s.p. The possibility that 5-HT acts on presynaptic α_2-adrenergic receptors like noradrenaline (HIRST and MCKIRDY 1974) has not yet been excluded.

III. Muscle Receptors

Understanding of the interaction of 5-HT with receptors on intestinal smooth muscle has not advanced much since 1968 (e.g. no clarifying studies using the approach of ligand binding are available). Interaction of 5-HT with such receptors occurs in the mouse duodenum (DRAKONTIDES and GERSHON 1968), guinea-pig ileum (FOZARD and MOBAROK ALI 1978; FOZARD et al. 1979; COSTA and FURNESS 1979 and many others), dog small intestine (BURKS 1973), human small intestine (see DANIEL 1968), lower oesophageal sphincter of the opossum (RATTAN and GOYAL 1977, 1978 b), guinea-pig colon and rectum (COSTA and FURNESS 1976), and in many other intestinal muscle preparations (perhaps in all; see DANIEL 1968 for review of earlier studies). Lysergic acid derivatives such as methysergide, bromolysergic acid are usually effective, competitive antagonists at smooth muscle 5-HT receptors. Dibenamine, phenoxybenzamine and other haloalkylamines, at somewhat higher concentrations than at α-adrenergic receptors, inhibit 5-HT receptors on smooth muscle by a competitive, irreversible interaction (see DANIEL 1968).

Recent evidence from other smooth muscle systems (e.g. dog vascular smooth muscle) suggests that there may be subtypes of smooth muscle 5-HT receptors. FENIUK et al. (1977) showed that, in the femoral artery, 5-HT effects were blocked by cyproheptadine ($pA_2 = 8.7$) while in dog saphenous veins, methysergide as well as 5-HT caused contraction and neither was blocked by cyproheptadine. It is also possible that subtypes of 5-HT receptors exist in various intestinal smooth muscles. BURLEIGH (1977) reported that in addition to the usual excitatory effects of 5-HT in human colonic longitudinal muscle (partly neurally medicated, partly direct muscle action) there was a 5-HT-induced relaxation of circular muscle which was reduced about 50% by TTX but not affected by methysergide, phentolamine or propranolol. Thus the TTX-insensitive (presumably muscle – located) receptor which mediates relaxation seems to be different from most 5-HT receptors and so 5-HT receptors on intestinal muscle may also prove to be heterogenous.

In 1968 no conclusive evidence existed that 5-HT was playing a physiological role in peristalsis. As is still the case for dopamine, there was no evidence at that time for a neurone which released 5-HT as a mediator. Evidence for the existence of such an enteric 5-HT neurone is now available, but there is puzzling negative evidence. A variety of workers have failed to find any 5-HT-containing intrinsic neurones in the intestine of the guinea-pig and other species, despite the application of a variety of techniques, including labelling by materials giving a fluorescence specific for 5-HT and localisation by immunological or histochemical methods of 5-HT synthesising enzymes (FURNESS 1970; FURNESS and COSTA 1974, 1975; COSTA and FURNESS 1973; JUORIO and GABELLA 1974; AHLMAN and ENERBACK 1974; DUBOIS and JACOBOWITZ 1974). In contrast, evidence was presented by JONAKAIT et al. (1979a) that neurones in the myenteric plexus of guinea-pig ileum contain tryptophan hydroxylase, take up 5-HT and have 5-HT-binding protein. Also the 5-HT taken up was released by field stimulation by a Ca^{2+}-dependent, TTX-sensitive and Mg-sensitive process; 5-HT-binding protein of synaptosomes was also released (but over a longer time period), K^+ and a Ca^{2+}-ionophore (X537A) also induced 5-HT release. Synaptosomes containing labelled 5-HT and its binding protein has also been isolated from this tissue (JONAKAIT et al. 1979b). Thus there is strong evidence for 5-HT intrinsic neurones in this case. However, the 5-HT released in these studies was the radioactive material taken up from an exogenous source. Release of endogenous 5-HT from neurones remains to be proved and since storage of endogenous 5-HT in gut neurones has not been demonstrated, this might be an important point. This question was recently reviewed by FURNESS and COSTA (1979).

H. Histamine Receptors and Antagonists

Histamine location, release and sites of action have been discussed elsewhere in this volume (see Chap. 3 and this Handbook, Vol. 59/I, Chap. 11). Histamine receptors have recently been shown to consist of at least two types. H_1-receptors, as we now know them, have been known for many years and classical antihistamines are antagonists on these sites (see GOODMAN and GILMAN 1980). The classical work of

Table 14. Characteristics of histamine receptor ligands

Agonists	Potencies relative to histamine	
	H_1-receptors	H_2-receptors
Histamine	100	100
2-Methylhistamine	17	5
2-Thiazolylhistamine	26	3
4-Methylhistamine	0.2	43
Dimaprit	0.0001	70
Impromidine	0.0001	4,800
Antagonists	$K_\beta(M)$	
Mepyramine	0.5×10^{-9}	
Burinamide	3×10^{-3}	7.8×10^{-6}
Metiamide	$>10^{-3}$	0.9×10^{-6}
Cimetidine	45×10^{-3}	0.8×10^{-6}

BLACK and his colleagues, recently reviewed by BERTACCINI (1978) and by HIRSCHOWITZ (1979) revealed that receptors for histamine mediating gastric secretion and some cardiac effects in vitro involved H_2-receptors. This work has led to discovery of selective H_1- as well as H_2-receptor agonists as well as antagonists. SCHWARTZ (1979) has recently reviewed the characteristics of agonists and antagonists binding to H_1- and H_2-receptors in the brain (see Table 14).

I. H_1-Receptors

Histamine receptors of the H_1 or classical type on intestinal muscles and nerves have been documented many times (see DANIEL 1968 for review). These are usually excitatory in their effect and are probably found in every gastrointestinal smooth muscle (BERTACCINI et al. 1980). In the 1968 review, evidence that histamine acted indirectly to release acetylcholine as well as directly in a variety of tissues, was reviewed. In guinea-pig ileal longitudinal muscle histamine produced an initial transient contraction by acting on a neural site and a secondary sustained contraction by a direct action on smooth muscle. In isolated guinea-pig ileum, the indirect action was independent of neural 5-HT receptors and apparently did not involve nicotinic receptors (insensitive to hexamethonium or DMPP). The receptor was postulated to be on postganglionic cholinergic neurones. In isolated rabbit intestine, histamine also had a major indirect action was but it was inhibited by nicotinic receptor antagonists. Indirect excitatory action of histamine less completely analysed at that time were reported in dog antrum and duodenum in vivo, in strips of rat fundus, in stomach of cats and guinea-pig in vitro, in isolated guinea-pig stomach (even after vagotomy). Many of these responses were reported sensitive to hexamethonium, and it was inferred that the receptors were presynaptic in relation to the intrinsic cholinergic neurone.

In nearly all cases, a direct action of histamine to excite smooth muscle was also evident and in a few cases, sometimes only after administration of atropine, a direct inhibitory action of histamine was observed, i.e. guinea-pig fundus, human ileal and colon circular muscle, and taenia coli. Excitatory action of histamine on H_1-receptors of intestinal muscle was competitively inhibited by classical antihistamines: dephenhydramine, chlorpheniramine, and mepyramine. Tritiated mepyramine has recently been introduced as a ligand for H_1-receptors using homogenates of guinea-pig ileum (HILL et al. 1977).

H_1-receptors in the guinea-pig ileum (CHANG and CUATRECASAS 1979) were concentrated in homogenates of longitudinal muscle compared with those of circular muscle (3.0 compared with 0.6 pmol mepyramine H^3 bound/g wet weight). Some receptors may have been located in the myenteric plexus (4.1 pmol/g wet weight in longitudinal muscle plus plexus compared with 3.0 pmol/g in longitudinal muscle alone). The dissociation constant of the histamine–receptor complex $K_d = 1.4$ nM; the maximum number of binding sites $B_{max} = 1.8$ pmol/g (from Scatchard plots showing a single class of binding sites); the dissociation constants of the antagonist (inhibitor)–receptor complexes K_i were as follows: for (+)-chlorpheniramine $K_i = 2.4$ μM (compared with 190 μM for the (−) stereoisomer); for mepyramine $K_i = 1.3$ μM. For histamine $K_i = 12{,}000$ μM; but only 120 μM was required for 50% of maximum contraction. This suggested a large receptor reserve or slowly interconverting agonist and antagonist receptor configurations.

The existence of H_1-receptors on nerves is also well established (see DANIEL 1968 for review); their activation usually promotes postsynaptic excitation by acetylcholine release. SAKAI (1979) has recently shown that isolated blood-perfused rat small intestine was contracted by histamine. These responses were blocked by TTX, hexamethonium, morphine, and mepyramine but not by atropine. In contrast, SAKAI et al. (1979) found no effect of histamine on isolated rat ileum strips. SAKAI suggests that histamine may act on the plexus in blood-perfused rat small intestine to activate noncholinergic excitatory nerves; rebound excitation was not ruled out. These nerves may not be functional in strips isolated in vitro. Recently, RATTAN and GOYAL (1978a) showed that intravenous or close intra-arterial injection of histamine or selective H_1-receptor agonists(2-methylhistamine) caused brief contraction of the lower oesophageal sphincter of the opossum, followed by prolonged relaxation. Only the relaxation was abolished by TTX, leaving a potentiated excitatory response. Pyrilamine or diphenhydramine abolished both inhibitory and excitatory responses to 2-methylhistamine, a selective H_1-receptor agonist, but left a residual relaxation in response to histamine. A selective H_2-receptor agonist, 4-methylhistamine, caused a TTX-insensitive relaxation, which, together with the H_1-receptor-antagonist-insensitive relaxation to histamine was abolished by metiamide. Neither H_1- nor H_2-receptor antagonists alone affected LES function significantly or selectively. These authors concluded there were excitatory H_1-receptors on, or presynaptic to, inhibitory neurones causing TTX-sensitive relaxation as well as on LES muscle (causing TTX-insensitive contraction). There were also inhibitory H_2-receptors on LES muscle. However, histamine apparently played no physiological role in LES function since antagonists alone had no effect.

According to recent studies (BERTACCINI and CORUZZI, to be published; BERTACCINI and DOBRILLA, to be published) some new H_2-blockers are able to modify LES tension in isolated preparations from different species including humans. Ranitidine increases LES tension (1–10 μg/ml are necessary) whereas oxmetidine

(SKF 92994) has a biphasic effect (stimulation with 0.5–3 μg/ml and relaxation with 10–100 μg/ml). It seems obvious that these effects are independent of H_2-receptor blockade.

II. H_2-Receptors

Since the elucidation of the existence of H_2-receptors and the availability of selective H_2-receptor agonists and antagonists, there has been examination in various gastrointestinal muscles of the possible existence of H_2- as well as H_1-receptors. Relaxation or inhibition of contraction by H_2-agonists prevented by H_2-antagonists, potentiation of contraction by histamine after administration of H_2-antagonists as well as other approaches have been used. WALDMAN et al. (1977) and IMPICCIATORE (1978) found such inhibitory H_2-receptors together with excitatory H_1-receptors, in guinea-pig gallbladder muscle; DE CARLE et al. (1976) as well as RATTAN and GOYAL (1977) found them together with H_1-receptors in opossum LES; OHGA and TANEIKE (1978) found such H_2-receptors as well as excitatory H_1-receptors in bovine reticulum and rumen; CHAND and DEROTH (1978) found inhibitory H_2-receptors as well as excitatory H_1-receptors in chicken ileum muscle. However, not all muscles have H_2-receptors; BERTACCINI (1979) failed to find them in strips of guinea-pig ileal longitudinal muscle and plexus or in whole segments. In apparent contradiction FJALLAND (1979) found that, in the presence of 10^{-6} M mepyramine, histamine reduced twitches of the coaxially stimulated guinea-pig ileum to field stimulation. This effect was reversed by 5×10^{-6} M burimamide or 10^{-4} M cimetidine; methysergide, propranolol, and naloxone had no effect. However, the concentrations of H_2-antagonists were rather high and not demonstrated to be competitive; their actions may be nonspecific since they also prevented inhibition of field-stimulation-induced twitches by clonidine in similar or lower doses. If these effects are the result of histamine actions on H_2-receptors, there may still be no contradiction with BERTACCINI's finding since H_2-receptors in nerves may have been involved. KONTUREK and SIEBERS (1980) reported that neither dimaprit nor metiamide affected the fasted (MMC) or the fed pattern of motility in the dog. Histamine or 2-methylhistamine increased the frequency and propagation velocity of MMC during fasting; tripelennamine abolished these effects. Effects of this H_1-antagonist alone were probably nonspecific, involving action on muscarinic cholinergic receptors. In any case, it was clear that observable exogenous or endogenous effects of histamine on motility of intact dog intestine involved H_1- rather than H_2-receptors.

III. Problems of Classification

The relationship between H_1- and H_2-receptors has been suggested by studies of KENAKIN et al. (1974). They found that after incubation at 12 °C excitatory responses to histamine in guinea-pig ileum were shifted to the right by metiamide. The H_2-receptor antagonist had no effect on segments kept at 37 °C. They suggest that the excitatory H_1-receptors had been converted to receptors chemically resembling H_2-receptors. Since excitation still resulted from occupation of these modified receptors, they may have remained coupled to the same membrane ionophores or enzymes, despite any conversion.

Some confusion has arisen because of reports (CASTELL and HARRIS 1970; FARRELL et al. 1973) that betazole, an agent selective but not specific for H_2-receptors, increased LES pressure in normal subjects, although it had no effects on patients with pernicious anaemia. The HCl secretion, which is also induced by betazole, lowers LES pressure and cannot explain these results. They can probably be explained by the fact that betazole has actions at H_1- as well as H_2-receptors, and those on H_1-receptors tend to predominate (RATTAN and GOYAL 1979) in the absence of an H_1-antagonist. KRAVITZ et al. (1978) reported that in low doses histamine increased but at higher doses inhibited LES pressure; both these effects were inhibited by cimetidine. Perhaps patients with pernicious anaemia fail to respond to activation of H_1-receptors because their LES is less capable of contraction; it is in fact less responsive to a variety of excitatory agents including pentagastrin and edrophonium (FARRELL et al. 1973), but the antagonism of excitatory effects of low doses of histamine by cimetidine is difficult to explain.

COHEN and SNAPE (1975) found, as did others, that the opossum LES muscle had both inhibitory H_1-receptors and excitatory H_2-receptors. They also noted that metiamide potentiated responses to gastrin I, both in vivo and in vitro. This they attributed to blockade by metiamide of an inhibiting effect of gastrin I which was normally overwhelmed by the excitation. The effect of gastrin could be unmasked by raising LES pressure in vitro with KCl. A similar inhibitory effect was produced by histamine in the presence of KCl and diphenhydramine and was also blocked by metiamide. Since excitatory effects of gastrin I could be elicited in the presence of diphenhydramine, COHEN and SNAPE (1975) considered that it probably did not act by release of histamine. Also nonspecific inhibition by metiamide was ruled out by showing that relaxations to isoprenaline and field stimulation were not blocked. They concluded that gastrin I did not act by histamine release or by direct activation of the H_2-receptor. Rather they suggested some association between the gastrin and histamine receptors, i.e. action of gastrin at its receptor activated histamine H_2-receptors in some fashion.

WALDMAN et al. (1977), in studies of guinea-pig gallbladder muscle in vitro, found that metiamide potentiated responses to CCK; its effects were consistent with an increase in affinity of CCK for its receptors. They, too, postulated an interaction between histamine H_2-receptors and hormone receptors. In guinea-pig fundus recorded in vitro with a balloon, GERNER et al. (1979) reported that 3.2×10^{-5} *M* mepyramine reduced spontaneous contractions and contractile responses to histamine, gastrin, and CCK PZ without affecting responses to acetylcholine. They suggested an interaction between histamine and hormone receptors. That inhibition by mepyramine was nonspecific remains a possibility even though previous work (GERNER and HAFFNER 1977) showed that, in contrast to the antrum, CCK did not act by activation of cholinergic nerves. DE CARLE and GLOVER (1974) found no relationship between gastrin and histamine receptors in the LES of Australian opossums and of monkeys. Cimetidine did not affect LES responses to gastrin in normal subjects (OSBORNE et al. 1977; see also FREELAND et al. 1977). Obviously the nature of the possible interaction between histamine and hormone receptors requires further analysis. Resolution of whether an interaction between histamine and hormone receptors occurs, will probably require study of displacement of ligands binding to H_1- or H_2-receptors by gastrin or CCK and displacement of ligands binding to gastrin or CCK receptors by agonists and antagonists at H_1- or H_2-receptors.

No evidence is available that effective doses of either H_1- or H_2-antagonists have significant effects on gastrointestinal function in vivo. There is thus no convincing evidence that histamine plays any physiological role in controlling gastrointestinal motility.

J. Projections for the Future

During the last decade, there has been rapid advance in our understanding of control of gastrointestinal motor function. The role of *myogenic electrical control*, especially of stomach and small intestine, has been elucidated at least partially; similar understanding of the myogenic control of the large intestine may emerge in the next few years. Application of techniques for recording electrical activities of single cells, in vitro, and from multicellular preparations in vivo and in vitro and sophisticated analysis of the resultant data have contributed. Any future investigator should be prepared to apply these, if appropriate.

There has been a similar advance in our understanding of *neural controls* of gastrointestinal motor function and their interaction with myogenic controls. Morphological, physiological, and pharmacological techniques have clarified how sympathetic and parasympathetic controls are exerted. For example, we are now aware of the importance of sympathetic control by modulation of intrinsic cholinergic neurones, of the existence of both neural and muscle sites of action of these mediators with different receptors, of the existence of a diverse group of neural peptides, such as the enkephalins, in extrinsic and intrinsic nerves supplying intestinal muscle.

A major problem for the future is to clarify the mediation of intrinsic intestinal inhibitory nerves: Are they purinergic, peptidergic, serotonergic or something else? Another problem is to define the function of neural peptides. Some tools are in hand to resolve these problems, e.g. a variety of analogues of purines and peptides, immunological techniques to localise and assay many of these compounds. Electrophysiological study of intrinsic intestinal neurones combined with pharmacological analysis has contributed to resolution of neural control mechanisms and may be essential to understanding the function of peptides and to elucidating the wiring systems and signals of intestinal nerves. Only a few laboratories throughout the world are capable of applying these techniques. Conditions for their successful application limit the repertoire of responses which can be obtained. Hopefully there will be an expansion and simplification of the conditions of use of such techniques. However, a major deficiency in our tool-kit is lack of selective antagonists to purines and to most peptides. The existence of naloxone has enabled us to push ahead in understanding the function of opiate-like peptides; similar antagonists to other neural peptides and to purines would be invaluable.

Endogenous chemicals released from non-nerve cells (histamine, prostaglandins, serotonin, etc.) may act on nerve or on muscle. Much of their modes and sites of action has been elucidated in a pharmacological sense, but their physiological functions, if any, remain mostly obscure. Here the pharmacological tools to determine these functions (selective antagonists, a range of agonists, inhibitors of formation and degradation) are available, but have to be applied with pharmacological insight.

I expect the next decade to yield even greater understanding of myogenic and neural control of intestinal function. We are coming to the time when understanding of control of gastrointestinal motor function will have a rational basis so that treatment of disorders can be directed toward correcting pathophysiology or toward modifying function toward normal at appropriate control points. Selective interventions such as I envisage, will require new pharmacological tools. Thus there is the challenge both to understand and to develop rational interventions.

References

Abe Y, Tomita T (1968) Cable properties of smooth muscle. J Physiol (Lond) 196:87–100

Aberg G, Eranko O (1967) Localization of noradrenaline and acetylcholinesterase in the taenia of the guinea-pig cecum. Acta Physiol Scand 69:383–384

Adam-Vizi V, Vizi ES (1978) Direct evidence for acetylcholine release effect of serotonin in the Auerbach's plexus. J Neural Transm 42:127–138

Ahlman H, Enerbäck L (1974) A cytofluorometric study of the myenteric plexus in the guinea pig. Cell Tiss Res 153:419–434

Ahlquist RP, Levy B (1959) Adrenergic receptor mechanism of canine ileum. J Pharmacol Exp Ther 127:146–149

Aldunate J, Yojay L, Mardones J (1975) Studies on the mechanism of action of morphine on the peristalsis of guinea pig ileum. Naunyn Schmiedeberg Arch Pharmacol 291:395–403

Allen GS, Glover AB, McCulloch WW, Rand JJ, Story DF (1975) Modulation by acetylcholine of adrenergic transmission in the rabbit ear artery. Br J Pharmacol 54:49–53

Ambinder RJ, Schuster MM (1979) Endorphins: new gut peptides with a familiar face. Gastroenterology 77:1132–1140

Amery W, Duyck F, Polak J (1975) A multicentre double-blind study in acute diarrhea comparing loperamide (R18553) with two common antidiarrhocal agents and a placebo. Curr Ther Res Clin 17:263–270

Ammon HV, Phillips SF (1973) Inhibition of colonic water and electrolyte absorption by fatty acids in man. Gastroenterology 65:744–749

Ammon HV, Phillips SF (1974) Inhibition of ileal water absorption by intraluminal fatty acids. Influence of chain length, hydroxylation, and conjugation of fatty acids. J Clin Invest 53:205–210

Ammon HV, Thomas PJ, Phillips SF (1974) Effects of oleic and ricinoleic acids on net jejunal water and electrolyte movement. J Clin Invest 53:374–379

Andersson RGG (1972) Cyclic AMP and calcium ions in mechanical and metabolic responses of smooth muscles; influence of some hormones and drugs. Acta Physiol Scand [Suppl] 382:1–59

Andersson RGG, Mohme-Lundholm E (1969) Studies on the relaxing actions mediated by stimulation of adrenergic α- and β-receptors in taenia coli of the rabbit and guinea pig. Acta Physiol Scand 77:372–384

Andersson RGG, Mohme-Lundholm E (1970) Metabolic actions in intestinal smooth muscle associated with relaxation mediated by adrenergic α- and β-receptors. Acta Physiol Scand 79:244–261

Asoh R, Goyal RK (1975) Electrical activity of the opossum lower esophageal sphincter in vivo: its role in the basal sphincter pressure. Gastroenterology 74:835–840

Bär HP (1974) Cyclic nucleotides and smooth muscle. Adv Cyclic Nucleotide Res 4:195–237

Bär HP, Drummond GI (eds) (1979) Physiological and regulatory functions of adenosine and adenine nucleotides. Raven, New York

Baeyens R, Van de Velde E, De Schepper A, Wollaert F, Reyntjens A (1979) Effects of intravenous and oral domperidone on the motor function of the stomach and small intestine. Postgrad Med J [Suppl] 55:19–23
Banwell JG, Sheer H (1973) Effect of bacterial enterotoxins on the gastrointestinal tract. Gastroenterology 56:467–497
Baudry M, Martres MP, Schwartz JP (1979) ^{3}H-Domperidone: A selective ligand for dopamine receptors. Naunyn Schmiedeberg Arch Pharmacol 308:231–237
Baumann HW, Sturdevant RAL, McCallum RW (1979) L-dopa inhibits metoclopramide stimulation of the lower esophageal sphincter in man. Dig Dis Sci 24:289–295
Baumgarten HG, Lange W (1969) Adrenergic innervation of the oesophagus in the cat (Felis domestica) and rhesus monkey (Macaca rhesus). Z Zellforsch Mikrosk Anat 95:529–545
Beani L, Bianchi P, Crema C (1970) Effects of metoclopramide on isolated guinea pig colon. 1) Peripheral sensitization of acetylcholine. Eur J Pharmacol 12:320–331
Beani L, Bianchi L, Crema A (1971) Vagal non-adrenergic inhibition of guinea pig stomach. J Physiol (Lond) 217:259–279
Beaumont A, Hughes J (1979) Biology of opioid receptors. Annu Rev Pharmacol Toxicol 19:245–268
Bekhti A, Rutgeerts L (1979) Domperidone in the treatment of functional dyspensia in patients with delayed gastric emptying. Postgrad Med J [Suppl 1] 55:30–32
Bennett MR, Rogers DC (1967) A study of the innervation of the taenia coli. J Cell Biol 33:573–596
Bertaccini G (1978) Histamine H_2-receptors and gastric secretion. Adv Exp Med Biol 106:69–74
Bertaccini G (1979) Histamine receptors in the guinea pig ileum. Naunyn Schmiedeberg Arch Pharmacol 309:65–68
Bertaccini G, Coruzzi G Azione dei bloccanti dei recettori istaminici H_2 sullo sfintere esofageo inferiore (LES) isolato del ratto. Il Farmaco (to be published)
Bertaccini G, Dobrilla (to be published) Histamine H_2-receptor antagonists: old and new generation. Pharmacology and clinical use. Ital J Gastroenterol
Bertaccini G, Scarpignato C, Coruzzi G (1980) Histamine receptors and gastrointestinal motility: an overview. In: Torsoli A, Lucchelli P, Brimblecombe RW (eds) H_2-Antagonists. Excerpta Medica, Amsterdam
Beubler E, Juan H (1978) PGE-mediated laxative effect of diphenolic laxatives. Naunyn Schmiedeberg Arch Pharmacol 305:241–246
Beubler E, Lembeck F (1979) Inhibition of stimulated fluid secretion in the rat small and large intestine by opiate agonist. Naunyn-Schmiedeberg Arch Pharmacol 306:113–118
Bihar J, Biancani P (1976) Effects of oral metoclopramide on gastroesophageal reflux in the post state. Gastroenterology 70:331–335
Binder HJ, Donowitz M (1975) A new look at laxative action. Gastroenterology 69:1001–1005
Binder HJ (1977) Pharmacology of laxatives. Annu Rev Pharmacol Toxicol Toxicol 17:355–367
Binder HJ (1980) Net fluid and electrolyte secretion: the pathological basis of diarrhea. Viewpoints Dig Dis 12(2):1–4
Binder HJ, Rawlins CL (1973) Effect of conjugated dihydroxyl bile salts on electrolyte transport in rat colon. J Clin Invest 52:1460–1466
Binnie JS et al. (1979) Multicentre general practice comparison of loperamide and diphenoxylate with atropine in the treatment of acute diarrhea in adults. Br J Clin Pract 33:77–79
Birtley RDN, Baines MW (1973) The effects of metoclopramide on some isolated intestinal preparations. Postgrad Med J [Suppl 4] 49:13
Bolton TB (1979) Mechanisms of action of transmitters and other substances on smooth muscle. Physiol Rev 59:606–718
Bowes KL, Shearin NL, Kingma YJ, Koles ZJ (1978) Frequency analysis of electrical activity in dog colon. In: Duthie HL (ed) Gastrointestinal motility in health and disease. MTP Press, Lancaster, pp 251–270
Bowman WC, Hall MT (1970) Inhibition of rabbit intestine mediators by α- and β-adrenoceptors. Br J Pharmacol 38:399–415

Bright-Asare P, Binder HJ (1973) Stimulation of colonic secretion of water and electrolytes by hydroxy fatty acids. Gastroenterology 64:81–88

Bristow M, Sherrod TR, Green RD (1970) Analysis of beta-receptor drug interactions in isolated rabbit atrium, aorta, stomach, and trachea. J Pharmacol Exp Ther 171:52–61

Brockaert A (1979) Effect of domperidone on gastric emptying and secretion. Postgrad Med J [Suppl 1] 55:11–14

Brown FC, Castell DO (1976) Histamine receptors in primate lower esophageal sphincter(-LES) smooth muscle (Abstr). Clin Res 24:533A

Bucknell A, Whitney B (1964) A preliminary investigation of the pharmacology of the human isolated taenia coli preparation. Br J Pharmacol 23:164–175

Bülbring E, Crema A (1958) Observations concerning the action of 5-hydroxytryptamine on the peristaltic reflex. Br J Pharmacol 13:444–457

Bülbring E, Den Hertog A (1977) The beta action of catecholamines on the smooth muscle of guinea-pig taenia coli. J Physiol (Lond) 268:29–30

Bülbring E, Tomita T (1969a) Increase of membrane conductance by adrenaline in the smooth muscle of guinea-pig taenia coli. Proc R Soc Lond [Biol] 172:89–102

Bülbring E, Tomita T (1969b) Suppresion of spontaneous spike generation by catecholamines in the smooth muscle of the guinea-pig taenia coli. Proc R Soc Lond [Biol] 172:103–119

Bülbring E, Tomita T (1969c) Effect of calcium, barium, and manganese on the action of adrenaline in the smooth muscle of the guinea-pig taenia coli. Proc R Soc Lond [Biol] 172:121–136

Bülbring E, Tomita A (1977a) The alpha-action of catecholamines on the guinea-pig taenia coli in K-free and Na-free solution and in the presence of ouabain. Proc R Soc Lond [Biol] 197:255–269

Bülbring E, Tomita T (1977b) Calcium requirement for the alpha-action of catecholamines on guinea-pig taenia coli. Proc R Soc Lond [Biol] 197:271–1284

Burgen ASV, Spero L (1968) The action of acetylcholine and other drugs on the efflux of potassium and rubidium from smooth muscle of the guinea-pig intestine. Br J Pharmacol 34:99–115

Burgen ASV, Spero L (1970) The effects of calcium and magnesium on the response of intestinal muscle to drugs. B J Pharmacol 40:492–500

Burks TF (1973) Mediation by 5-hydroxytryptamine of morphine stimulant actions in dog intestine. J Pharmacol Exp Ther 185:530–539

Burks TF (1976) Acute effects of morphine in rat intestinal motility. Eur J Pharmacol 40:279–283

Burks TF, Long JP (1967) Responses of isolated dog small intestine to analgesic agents. J Pharmacol Exp Ther 158:264–271

Burleigh DE (1977) Evidence for more than one type of 5-hydroxytryptamine receptors in the human colon. J Pharm Pharmacol 29:538–541

Burleigh DE, D'Mello A, Parks AJ (1979) Responses of isolated human intestinal and sphincter to drugs and electrical field stimulation. Gastroenterology 77:484–490

Burn JH, Rand MJ (1965) Acetylcholine in adrenergic transmission. Annu Rev Pharmacol Toxicol 5:163–182

Bury RW, Mashford ML (1976) The effects of metoclopramide in modifying the response of isolated guinea pig ileum to various agonists. J Pharmacol Exp Ther 197:641–646

Casteels R, Raeymaekers L (1979) The action of acetylcholine and catecholamines on an intracellular calcium store in the smooth muscle cells of the guinea-pig taenia coli. J Physiol (Lond) 294:51–68

Castell DO, Harris LD (1970) Hormonal control of gastro-esophageal sphincter strength. N Engl J Med 282:886–889

Chan WWL, Diamant NE (1976) Electrical off response of cat esophageal smooth muscle: an analog simulation. Am J Physiol 230:233–238

Chand N, De Roth L (1978) Occurrence of H_2-inhibitory histamine receptors in chicken ileum. Eur J Pharmacol 57:143–145

Chang K-J, Cuatrecasas P (1979) Multiple opiate receptors enkephalins and morphine kind to receptors of different specificity. J Biol Chem 254:2610–2618

Chang K-J, Hazum E, Cuatrecasas P (1980a) Multiple opiate receptors. Trends Neurosci 3:160–162
Chang KJ, Muller RJ, Cuatrecasas P (1980b) Interaction with opiate receptors in intact cultured cells. Mol Pharmacol 14:961–970
Cheung D, Daniel EE (1980) Comparative study of the smooth muscle layers of the rabbit duodenum. J Physiol (Lond) 309:13–27
Chignell CF (1968) The effect of phenolphthalein and other purgative drugs on rat intestinal (Na^{+} + K^{+}) adenosine triphatase. Biochem Pharmacol 17:1207–1212
Christensen J, Daniel EE (1966) Electric and motor effects of autonomic drugs on longitudinal esophageal smooth muscle. Am J Physiol 211:387–394
Christensen J, Daniel EE (1968) Effects of some autonomic drugs on circular esophageal smooth muscle. J Pharmacol Exp Ther 159:243–249
Christensen J, Dons RF (1968) Regional variations in response of cat esophageal muscle to stimulation with drugs. J Pharmacol Exp Ther 161:55–58
Christensen J, Freeman BW (1972) Circular muscle electromyogram in the cat colon: local effect of sodium ricinoleate. Gastroenterology 63:1011–1015
Clay GA, Mackerer CR, Lin TK (1977) Interaction of loperamide with ^{3}H-naloxone binding sites in guinea pig brain and myenteric plexus. Mol Pharmacol 13:533–540
Cohen S, Dimarino AJ (1976) Mechanism of action of metoclopramide on opossum lower esophageal pressure. Gastroenterology 71:996–998
Cohen S, Snape WJ Jr (1975) Action of metiamide on the lower esophageal sphincter. Gastroenterology 69:911–919
Connell AM (1962) The motility of the pelvic colon. II. Paradoxical motility in diarrhea and constipation. Gut 3:342–348
Connell AM, George JD (1969) Effect of metoclopramide on gastric function in man. Gut 10:678–680
Cook MA, Kowalewski K, Daniel EE (1974) Electrical and mechanical activity recorded from the isolated, perfused canine stomach: the effects of some GI polypeptides. In: Daniel EE (ed) 4th International Symposium on Gastrointestinal Motility. Mitchell, Vancouver, pp 233–242
Costa M, Furness JB (1973) The origins of the adrenergic fibers which innervated the internal anal sphincter, the rectum and other tissues of the pelvic region in the guinea pig. Z Anat Entwickl Gesch 140:129–142
Costa M, Furness JB (1976) The peristaltic reflex – an analysis of the nerve pathways and their pharmacology. Naunyn-Schmiedeberg Arch Pharmacol 294:47–60
Costa M, Furness JB (1979) The sites of action of 5-hydroxytryptamine in nerve-muscle preparations from the guinea pig small intestine and colon. Br J Pharmacol 65:237–248
Costa M, Gabella G (1968) L'innervation adrenergique des sphincters digestifs. C R Ass Anat 53:884–888
Costa M, Gabella G (1971) Adrenergic innervation of the alimentary canal. Z Zellforsch 122:357–377
Costa M, Furness JB, McLean JR (1976) The presence of aromatic 1-aminoacid decarboxylase in certain intestinal nerve cells. Histochemistry 48:120–143
Coupar JM (1978) Inhibition by morphine of prostaglandin-stimulated fluid secretion in rat jejunum. Br J Pharmacol 63:57–63
Cowie AL, Kosterlitz HW, Waterfield AA (1978) Factors influencing the release of acetylcholine from the myenteric plexus of the ileum of the guinea pig and rabbit. Br J Pharmacol 64:565–580
Cox BM, Weinstock M (1966) The effects of analgesic drugs on the release of acetylcholine from electrically stimulated guinea-pig ileum. Br J Pharmacol 27:81–92
Coyne MJ, Bonnoris GG, Chung A, Conley D, Schoenfield LJ (1977) Propranolol inhibits bile acid and fatty acid stimulation of cyclic AMP in human colon. Gastroenterology 73:971–974
Crema A, Frigo GM, Lecchini S (1970) A pharmacological analysis of the peristaltic reflex in the isolated colon of the guinea pig or cat. Br J Pharmacol 39:334–345
Curtis JA, Goel KM (1979) Lomotil poisoning in children. Arch Dis Child 54:222–225
Cutler EA, Barrett GA, Craven PW, Cramblatt HG (1980) Delayed cardiopulmonary arrest after lomotil ingestion. Pediatrics 65:157–158

Daniel EE (1965) The electrical and contractile activity of the pyloric region in dogs and the effects of drugs. Gastroenterology 49:403–418
Daniel EE, (1966a) Electrical and contractile responses of the pyloric region to adrenergic and cholinergic drugs. Can J Physiol Pharmacol 44:951–979
Daniel EE (1966b) Further studies of the pharmacology of the pyloric region. Can J Physiol Pharmacol 44:981–1019
Daniel EE (1968) Pharmacology of the gastrointestinal tract. In: Code CF (ed) Alimentary canal. Williams & Wilkins, Baltimore (Handbook of physiology, vol IV, chap 108, pp 2267–2324)
Daniel EE, Bogoch A (1959) The mechanism of the spasmogenic action of morphine on the small intestine of man and dog. Proc World Congr Gastroenterol 1958. Williams & Wilkins, Baltimore
Daniel EE, Janis R (1975) Calcium regulation in the uterus. Pharmacol Therap 1:695–729
Daniel EE, Sarna SK (1976) Distribution of excitatory vagal fibers in canine gastric wall to control motility. Gastroenterology 71:608–613
Daniel EE, Sarna SK (1978) The generation and conduction of activity in smooth muscle. In: Annual Review of Pharmacology and Toxicology 18:145–166
Daniel EE, Chapman KM (1963) Electrical activity of the gastrointestinal tract as an indication of mechanical activity. Am J Dig Dis 8:54–102
Daniel EE, Irwin J (1968) The electrical activity of the gastric musculature. In: Handbook of Physiology: Alimentary canal. IV. Motility, ed CF Code. Williams & Wilkins, Baltimore, Maryland, USA, chap 96, pp 1969–1984
Daniel EE, Taylor GS (1975) Junctional potentials and control of motility of the small intestine. In: Vantrappen G (ed) 5th International Symposium on Gastrointestinal Motility. Typoff, Herentals, pp 213–218
Daniel EE, Sutherland WH, Bogoch A (1959) Effects of morphine and other drugs on motility of the terminal ileum. Gastroenterology 36:510–523
Daniel EE, Wachter B, Honour AJ, Bogoch A (1960) The relationship between electrical and mechanical activity of the small intestine of dog and man. Can J Biochem Physiol 38:777–791
Daniel EE, Duchon G, Bowes KL (1975) The structural bases for control of human gastrointestinal motility. In: Vantrappen G (ed) 5th International Symposium on Gastrointestinal Motility. Typoff, Herentals, pp 190–197
Daniel EE, Gonda T, Domoto T, Oki M, Yanaihara N (1981) Effects of substance P in dog ileum: Relation of enkephalins (Abstr). Gastroenterology 80:1131
Daniel EE, Daniel VP, Duchon G, Garfield RE, Nichols M, Malhotra SK, Oki M (1976) Is the nexus necessary for cell-to-cell coupling of smooth muscle? J Membrane Biol 28:207–239
Daniel EE, Crankshaw J, Sarna S (1979) Prostaglandins and myogenic control of tension in lower esophageal sphincter in vitro. Prostaglandins 17:629–639
Day M, Vane JR (1963) An analysis of the direct and indirect actions of drugs on the isolated guinea pig ileum. Br J Pharmacol 20:150
Dazani EZ, Roge EA, Bertermann RE (1975) Effects of E-prostaglandins, diphenoxylate, and morphine on intestinal motility in vivo. Eur J Pharmacol 34:105–113
Dazani EZ, Bianchi RG, East PF, Blass JL, Adelstein GW, Yen CH (1977) The pharmacology of SC-27166: a novel antidiarrheal agent. J Pharmacol Exp Ther 203:512–526
Deberdt R (1979) Compatibility of high doses of both oral domperidone and neuroleptics in chronic psychotics. Postgrad Med J [Suppl] 55:48–49
De Carle DJ, Christensen J (1976) A dopamine receptor in esophageal smooth muscle of the opossum. Gastroenterology 70:216–219
De Carle DJ, Glover WE (1974) Independence of gastrin and histamine receptors in the lower esophageal sphincter of the monkey and opossum. J Physiol (Lond) 245:78P–79P
De Carle DJ, Brody MJ, Christensen J (1976) Histamine receptors in esophageal smooth muscle of the opossum. Gastroenterology 70:1071–1075
Demeuleanaere L, Verbeke S, Muls M, Reyntjens AA (1974) Loperamide: an open multicenter trial and a double-blind cross-over comparison with placebo in patients with chronic diarrhea. Curr Ther Res Clin Exp 16:32–39

Dingledine R, Goldstein A (1975) Single neurone studies of opiate action in the guinea pig myenteric plexus. Life Sci 17:57–62
Dingledine R, Goldstein A (1976) Effect of synaptic transmission blockage on morphine action in guinea-pig myenteric plexus. J Pharmacol Exp Ther 196:97–106
Dingledine R, Goldstein A, Kendig J (1974) Effects of narcotic opiates and serotonin in the electrical behaviour of neurones in the guinea pig myenteric plexus. Life Sci 14:2299–2309
Donowitz M, Binder HJ (1975) Effect of diotyl sodium sulfosuccinate on colonic fluid and electrolyte movement. Gastroenterology 69:941–950
Down J, Szerb JC (1980) Kinetics of morphine-sensitive [^{3}H] acetylcholine release from the guinea pig myenteric plexus. Br J Pharmacol 68:47–56
Downing OA, Morris JS (1979) A hyosine sensitive component of vagal gastric relaxation. Br J Pharmacol 66:457p
Doxey JC, Smith CFC, Walker TM (1977) Selectivity of blocking agents for pre- and postsynaptic α-adrenoceptors. Br J Pharmacol 60:91–96
Drakontides AB, Gershon MD (1968) 5-hydroxytryptamine receptors in the mouse duodenum. Br J Pharmacol Chemother 33:480–492
Drakontides AB, Gershon MD (1972) Studies of the interaction of 5-hydroxytryptamine and the perivascular innervation of the guinea pig caecum. Br J Pharmacol 45:417–434
Drew GM (1977) Pharmacological characterization of the presynaptic α-adrenoceptor in the rat vas deferens. Eur J Pharmacol 42:123–130
Drew GM (1978) Pharmacological characterization of the presynaptic α-adrenoceptors, regulating cholinergic activity in the guinea pig ileum. Br J Pharmacol 614:293–300
Dubocovich ML, Langer SZ (1974) Negative feedback regulation of noradrenaline release by nerve stimulation in the perfused cat's spleen: differences in potency of phenoxybenzamine in blocking the pre- and postsynaptic adrenergic receptors. J Physiol (Lond) 237:505–519
Dubois A, Jacobowitz DM (1974) Failure to demonstrate serotoninergic neurones in the myenteric plexus of the cat. Cell Tiss Res 150:493–496
Dupont HL, Hornick RB (1973) Adverse effect of lomotil therapy in shigellosis. JAMA 226:1525–1528
Edin R, Lundberg J, Terenius L, Dahlström A, Hökfelt T, Kewenter J, Ahlman H (1980) Evidence for vagal enkehalinergic neural control of the feline pylorus. Gastroenterology 78:492–497
Ehrenpreis J, Sato T, Takayanagi I, Comaty JE, Takagi K (1976) Mechanism of morphine block of electrical activity in ganglia of Auerbach's plexus. Eur J Pharmacol 40:303–309
Eisner M (1971) Effect of metoclopramide on gastro-intestinal motility in man. Am J Dig Dis 16:409
Eisner M (1968) Gastro-intestinal effects of metoclopramide in man. In vitro experiments with human smooth muscle preparations. Br Med J 4:679
Elde R, Hökfelt T, Johansson O, Terenius L (1976) Immunohistochemical studies using antibodies to leucine-enkephalin: initial observations in the nervous system of the rat. Neuroscience 1:349–351
El-Sharkawy TY (1978) Electrophysiological control of motility in canine colon. In: Duthie HL (ed) Gastrointestinal motility in health and disease. MTP Press, Lancaster, pp 387–398
El-Sharkawy TY, Diamant NE (1970) Contraction patterns of esophageal circular smooth muscle induced by cholinergic excitation. Gastroenterology 70:969
El-Sharkawy TY, MacDonald WM, Diamant NE (1980) Electrophysiological control of motility in longitudinal and circular muscle layers of canine colon (Abstr). Gastroenterology 78:1162
El-Sharkawy TY, Szurszewski JH (1978) Modulation of canine antral circular smooth muscle by acetylcholine, noradrenaline, and pentagastrin. J Physiol (Lond) 279:309–320
El-Sharkawy TY, Chan WW-L, Diamant NE (1976) Neural mechanisms of lower esophageal sphincter relaxation: a pharmacological analysis. In: Vantrappen G (ed) 5th International Symposium on Gastrointestinal Motility. Typoff, Herentals, pp 178–180
El-Sharkawy TY, Morgan KG, Szurszewski JH (1978) Intracellular electrical activity of canine and human gastric smooth muscle. J Physiol (Lond) 279:291–307

Engback J, Ersböll J, Fairby V, Riis P (1975) The constipating effect of dephinoxylate (Retardius) in ulcerative colitis. A double blind controlled trial. Scand J Gastroenterol 10:695–698

Englert W, Schlick D (1979) A double-blind crossover trial of domperidone in chronic postprandial dyspepsia. Postgrad Med J [Suppl 1] 55:28–29

Eränko O (1978)Small intensely fluorescent (SIF) cells and nervous transmission in sympathetic ganglia. Ann Rev Pharmacol Toxicol 18:417–430

Ewe K (1980a) The physiological basis of laxative action. Pharmacology [Suppl 1] 20:2–20

Ewe K (1980b) Effects of rhein on the transport of electrolytes, water, and carbohydrates in the human jejunum and colon. Pharmacology [Suppl 1] 20:27–35

Farrell RL, Nebel OT, McGuire AT, Castell DO (1973) The abnormal lower esophageal sphincter in pernicious anemia. Gut 14:767–777

Feldman S, Gibaldi M (1969) Bile salt-induced permeability changes in the isolated rat intestine. Proc Soc Exp Biol Med 132:1031–1034

Feniuk W, Humphrey PPA, Levy GP (1977) Further evidence for two types of excitatory receptor for 5-hydroxytryptamine in dog vasculature. Br J Pharmacol 61:466

Ferreira SH, Herman AG, Vane JR (1976) Prostaglandin production by rabbit isolated jejunum and its relationship to the inherent tone of the preparation. Br J Pharmacol 56:469–477

Ferry CB (1963) The sympathomimetic effect of acetylcholine on the spleen of the cat. J Physiol (Lond) 167:487–504

Ferry CB (1966) Cholinergic link hypothesis in adrenergic neuroeffector transmission. Physiol Rev 46:420–456

Field M, Fromm D, Al-Awqati Q (1972) Effect of cholera enterotoxin upon ion transport across isolated ileal mucosa. J Clin Invest 51:796–804

Fjalland B (1979) Evidence for the existence of another type of histamine H_2-receptor in guinea pig ileum. J Pharm Pharmacol 31:50–51

Flacke W, Gillis RA (1968) Impulse transmission via nicotinic and muscarinic pathways in the stellate ganglion of the dog. J Pharmacol Exp Ther 163:266–276

Forth W, Baldauf J, Rummel W (1963) Ein Beitrag zur Klärung des Wirkungsmechanismus einiger Laxantien. Naunyn-Schmiedebergs Arch Exp Pathol Pharmakol 246:91–92

Forth W, Rummel W, Baldauf J (1966) Wasser and Electrolytbewegung am Dünn- und Dickdarm unter dem Einfluß von Laxantien; ein Beitrag zur Klärung ihres Wirkungsmechanismus. Arch Pharmakol Exp Pathol 254:18–32

Fosbraey P, Johnson ES (1980) Release-modulatory acetylcholine receptors on cholinergic neurones of the guinea pig ileum. Br J Pharmacol 68:289–310

Fox J, Behar J (1980) Pathogenesis of diabetic gastroparesis: a pharmacologic study. Gastroenterology 78:757–763

Fozard JR, Mobarok Ali ATM (1978) Receptors for 5-hydroxytryptamine on the sympathetic nerves of the rabbit heart. Naunyn-Schmiedeberg Arch Pharmacol 301:223–235

Fozard JR, Mobarok Ali ATM, Newgrosh G (1979) Blockade of serotonin receptors on autonomic neurones by (−)-cocaine and some related compounds. Eur J Pharmacol 59:195–210

Freeland GR, Higgs RN, Castell DO (1977) Lower esophageal sphincter response to oral administration of cimetidine in normal subjects. Gastroenterology 72:28–30

Frizzell RA, Field M, Schultz SG (1979) Sodium-coupled chloride transport by epithelial tissues. Am J Physiol 236 (5/1):Fl-F8

Fry GN, Devine CE, Burnstock G (1977) Freeze-fracture studies of nexuses between smooth muscle cells. J Cell Biol 72:26–34

Furchgott RF (1967) The pharmacological differentiation of adrenergic receptors. Ann NY Acad Sci 139:553–570

Furchgott RF (1972) Classification of adrenoceptors (adrenergic receptors). An evaluation from the standpoint of receptor theory. In: Blaschko H, Muscholl E (eds) Catecholamines. Springer, Berlin Heidelberg New York (Handbook of experimental pharmacology, vol 33, pp 283–335)

Furness JB (1970) The origin and distribution of adrenergic nerve fibers in the guinea pig colon. Histochemie 21:295–306

Furness JB (1971) Morphology and distribution of intrinsic adrenergic neurones in the proximal colon of the guinea pig. Z Zellforsch 120:346–363
Furness JB, Costa M (1973) The ramifications of adrenergic nerve terminals in the rectum, anal sphincter, and anal acessory muscles of the guinea pig. Z Anat Entw Gesch 140:109–128
Furness JB, Costa M (1974) The adrenergic innervation of the gastrointestinal tract. Ergeb Physiol 69:1–51
Furness JB, Costa M (1975) The use of glyoxylic acid for the fluorescence histochemical demonstration of peripheral stores or noradrenaline and 5-hydroxytryptamine in whole mounts. Histochemistry 41:335–353
Furness JB, Costa M (1978) Distribution of intrinsic nerve cell bodies and axons which take up aromatic amines and their precursors in the small intestine of the guinea pig. Cell Tissue Res 188:527–543
Furness JB, Costa M (1979) On the possibility that an indoleamines is a neurotransmitter in the gastro-intestinal tract. Biochem Pharmacol 28:565–572
Furness JB, Costa M (1980) Types of nerves in the enteric nervous system. Neuroscience 5:1–20
Furness JB, Costa M, Freeman CG (1979) Absence of tyrosine hydroxylase activity and dopamine β-hydroxylase immuno-reactivity in intrinsic nerves of the guinea pig ileum. Neuroscience 4:305–310
Gabella G (1972a) Intercellular junctions between circular and longitudinal intestinal muscle layer. Z Zellforsch 125:191–199
Gabella g (1972b) Fine structure of the myenteric plexus in the guinea pig ileum. J Anat 111:69–97
Gabella G (1972c) Innervation of the intestinal muscle coat. J Neurocytol 1:341–362
Gabella G (1979) Nexus between the smooth muscle cells of the guinea pig ileum. J Cell Biol 82:239–247
Gabella G, Blundell D (1978) Effects of stretch and contraction on caveolae of smooth muscle cells. Cell Tissue Res 190:255–271
Gabella G, Costa M (1969) Adrenergic innervation of the intestinal smooth musculature. Experientia 25:395–396
Gaddum JG, Picarelli ZP (1957) Two kinds of tryptamine receptors. Br J Pharmacol 12:323–328
Galambos JR, Hersh T, Schoder S, Wenger J (1976) Loperamide: a new antidiarrhea agent in the treatment of chronic diarrhea. Gastroenterology 70:1026–1029
García-Villar R, Leng-Peschlow E, Ruckebusch Y (1980) Effects of antroquinone derivatives on canine and rat intestinal motility. J Pharm Pharmacol 32:323–329
Gerner T, Haffner JFW (1977) The role of local cholinergic pathways in the motor response to cholecystokinin and gastrin in isolated guinea pig fundus and antrum. Scand J Gastroenterol 12:751–757
Gerner J, Haffner JFW, Norstein J (1979) The effects of mepyramine and cimetidine on the motor responses to histamine, cholecystokinin, and gastrin in the fundus and antrum of isolated guinea pig stomach. Scand J Gastroenterol 14:65–72
Gillan MGC, Pollock D (1980) Acute effects of morphine and opiod peptides on the motility and responses of rat colon to electrical stimulation. Br J Pharmacol 68:381–392
Gillespie JS (1968) Electrical activity in the colon. In: Code CF (ed) Alimentary canal. Williams & Wilkins, Baltimore (Handbook of physiology, vol IV, pp 2093–2120)
Gillespie JS (1976) Extraneuronal uptake of catecholamines in smooth muscle and connective tissue. In: Paton DM (ed) Mechanism of neuronal and extraneuronal transport of catecholamines. Raven, New York, pp 325–354
Gillespie JS, Khoyi MA (1977) The sites and receptors responsible for the inhibition by sympathetic nerves of intestinal smooth muscle and its parasympathetic motor nerves. J Physiol (Lond) 267:767–789
Gillespie JS, Maxwell JD (1971) Adrenergic innervation of the sphincteric and non-sphincteric smooth muscle of the rat intestine. J Histochem Cytochem 19:676–681
Gillis CN (1976) Extraneuronal transport of noradrenaline in the lung. In: Paton DM (ed) Mechanism of neuronal and extraneuronal transport of catecholamines. Raven, New York, pp 281–297

Gintzler AR (1979) Serotonin participation in gut withdrawal from opiates. J Pharmacol Exp Ther 211:7–12
Gintzler AR (1980) Substance P involvement in the expression of gut dependence on opiates. Brain Res 182:224–228
Goldberg LI (1972) Cardiovascular and renal actions of dopamine: potential chemical application. Pharmacol Rev 24:11–29
Goldberg LI (1978) Vascular dopamine receptors as a model for other dopamine receptors. Adv Biochem Psychopharmacol 19:119–129
Goldberg LI, Volkman PH, Kohli JD (1978) A comparison of the vascular dopamine receptor with other dopamine receptors. Annu Rev Pharmacol Toxicol 18:57–79
Goldstein A (1976) Opioid peptides (endorphines) in pituitary and brain. Science 193:1081–1086
Goldstein A, Schulz R (1973) Morphine tolerant longitudinal muscle from guinea pig ileum. Br J Pharmacol 48:655–666
Goldstein A, Tachibana S, Lowney LJ, Hunikapiller M, Hood L (1979) Dynorphin (1-13), an extraordinarily potent opiod peptide. Proc Natl Acad Sci USA 76:6666–6670
Gonella J, Niel JP, Roman C (1977) Vagal control of lower esophageal sphincter motility in cat. J Physiol (Lond) 273:647–664
Gonella J, Niel JP, Roman C (1979) Sympathetic control of lower esophageal sphincter motility in the cat. J Physiol (Lond) 287:177–190
Goodman LS, Gilman A (eds) (1980) The pharmacological basis of therapeutic, 5th edn. Macmillan, New York, pp 494–534
Goyal RK, Rattan S (1975) Nature of vagal inhibitory innervation to the lower esophageal sphincter. J Clin Invest 55:1119–1126
Goyal RK, Rattan S (1978) Neurohumoral hormonal and drug receptors for the lower esophageal sphincter. Gastroenterology 74:598–619
Greenberg R, Kosterlitz HW, Waterfield AA (1970) The effects of hexamethonium, morphine, and adrenaline in the output of acetylcholine from the myenteric plexus longitudinal muscle preparation of the ileum. Br J Pharmacol 40:553P
Haarmann K, Lebkuchner F, Wildmann A, Kief W, Esslinger M (1979) A double-blind study of domperidone in the symptomatic treatment of chronic post-prandial upper gastrointestinal dishes. Postgrad Med J [Suppl 1] 55:24–27
Harford WV, Kreys GJ, Santa Ana CA, Fordtran JS (1980) Acute effect of diphenoxylate with atropine (lomitol) in patients with chronic diarrhea and fecal incontinence. Gastroenterology 78:440–443
Harper B, Hughes IE, Noormokamed FH (1978) Possible differences in α-adrenoceptors in rabbit ileum and spleen. J Pharm Pharmacol 30:167–172
Harvey RF, Read AE (1973) Saline purgatives act by releasing cholecystokinin. Lanced 2:185–187
Hay AM (1977) Pharmacological analyses of the effects of metoclopramide on the guinea pig isolated stomach. Gastroenterology 72:864–869
Hay AM, Man WK (1979) Effect of metoclopramide on guinea pig stomach. Gastroenterology 76:492–496
Heitmann P, Moller N (1970) The effects of metoclopramide on the gastrooesophageal junctional zone and the distal oesophagus in man. Gastroenterology 5:621
Henderson RM, Duchon G, Daniel EE (1971) Cell contracts in duodenal smooth muscle layers. Am J Physiol 221:564–574
Henderson G, Hughes J, Kosterlitz HW (1975) The effects of morphine on the release of noradrenaline from cat isolated nictitating membrane and the guinea pig ileum myenteric plexus longitudinal muscle preparation. Br J Pharmacol 53:505–512
Hendrix JR, Bayless TM (1970) Digestion: intestinal secretion. Annu Rev Physiol Toxicol 32:139–164
Heykants J, Michiels M, Kaneps A, Brugmans J (1974) Loperamide (R18553) a novel type of antidiarrheal agent. Part 5. The pharmacokinetics of loperamide in rats and man. Arzneim Forsch 24:1649–1953
Heykants J, Meuldermans W, Michiels M, Reyntjens A (1978) Pharmacokinetics in man of domperidone, a novel gastrokinetic. In: Boissier JR, Lechat P (eds) VII th International Congress of Pharmacology. Pergamon, Oxford, p 200

Higgins CB, Vatner SF, Braunwald E (1973) Parasympathetic control of the heart. Pharmacol Rev 25:120–155
Hill SJ, Young JM, Marriau DJ (1977) Specific binding of ^{3}H-mepyramine to histamine H_1 receptors in intestinal smooth muscle. Nature 270:361–363
Hirschowitz BI (1979) H_2 histamine receptors. Annu Rev Pharmacol Toxicol 19:203–244
Hirst GDS, McKirdy HC (1974) A nervous mechanism for descending inhibition in guinea pig small intestine. J Physiol (Lond) 238:129–143
Hirst GDS, McKirdy HC (1975) Synaptic potentials recorded from neurones of the submucous plexus of guinea pig small intestine. J Physiol (Lond) 249:369–389
Hirst GDS, Silinsky EM (1975) Some effects of 5-hydroxytryptamine, dopamine, and noradrenaline on neurones in the submucous plexus of guinea pig small intestine. J Physiol (Lond) 251:817–832
Hirst GDS, Holman ME, Spence I (1974) Two types of neurons in the myenteric plexus of the duodenum in the guinea pig. J Physiol (Lond) 236:303–326
Hughes J, Smith JW, Kosterlitz HW (1975) Identification of two related pentapeptides from the brain with potent opiate agonist activity. Nature 258:577–579
Hughes J, Kosterlitz HW, Smith JW (1977) The distribution of methionine-enkephalin and leucine-enkephalin in the brain and peripheral tissue. Br J Pharmacol 61:639–647
Impicciatore M (1978) Occurrence of H_1 and H_2 histamine receptors in the guinea pig gall bladder in situ. Br J Pharmacol 64:219–222
Jacoby JH (1978) On the central anti-serotonergic actions of cyproheptadine and methysergide. Neuropharmacology 17:299–306
Jacoby HI, Brodie DA (1967) Gastro-intestinal actions of metoclopramide. An experimental study. Gastroenterology 52:676–684
Jaffe JH, Martin WR (1980) Opioid analgesics and antagonists. In: Goodman LS, Gilman A (eds) Pharmacological basis of therapeutics. Macmillan, New York, pp 494–534
Janssen PA, Jagenau AH, Huygens J (1959) Synthetic antidiarrheal agents. 1. Some pharmacological properties of R1132 and related compounds. J Med Chem 1:299–808
Jenkinson DM, Morton IKM (1967a) The effect of noradrenaline on the permeability of depolarized intestinal smooth muscle to organic ions. J Physiol (Lond) 188:373–389
Jenkinson DM, Morton IKM (1967b) The role α- and β-adrenergic receptors in some actions of catecholamines in intestinal smooth muscle. J Physiol (Lond) 188:387–402
Johnson AG (1969) The action of metoclopramide on the canine stomach, duodenum, and gall-bladder. Br J Surg 56:696
Johnson AG (1971) The action of metoclopramide on human gastroduodenal motility. Gut 12:421–426
Jonakait GM, Jamir H, Gintzler AR, Gershon MD (1979a) Release of [^{3}H] serotonin and its binding protein from enteric neurones. Brain Res 174:55–69
Jonakait GM, Gintzler AR, Gershon MD (1979b) Isolation of axinal varicosities (autonomic synaptosomes) from the enteric nervous system. J Neurochem 32:1387–1400
Juorio AV, Gabella G (1974) Noradrenaline in guinea pig alimentary canal regional distribution and sensitivity of denervation. J Neurochem 22:851–859
Justin-Besancon L, Laville C (1964) Action du metocloparamide sur le système nerveux autonome. C R Soc Biol (Paris) 158:1016
Karras PJ, North RA (1979) Inhibition of neuronal firing by opiates: evidence against the involvement of cyclic neucleotides. Br J Pharmacol 65:647–652
Kaymakcalan S, Temelli S (1964) Response of the isolated intestine of normal and morphine-tolerant rats to morphine and nalorphine. Arch Int Pharmacol 151:136–141
Kenakin TP, Kreuger CA, Cook DA (1974) Temperature-dependent interconversion of histamine H_1 and H_2 receptors in guinea pig ileum. Nature 252:54–55
Kleinman MH, Arnon D (1971) The use of diphenoxylate hydrochloride (lomotil) in the management of the minor withdrawal syndrome during methadone detoxification. Br J Addict 72:167–169
Konturek SJ, Siebers R (1980) Role of histamine H_1 and H_2 receptors in myoelectric activity of small bowel in the dog. Am J Physiol 238:G50–G56
Kosterlitz HW, Henderson G (1977) In vitro pharmacology of the opioid peptides, enkephalins, and endorphins. Eur J Pharmacol 43:107–116

Kosterlitz HW, Robinson JA (1957) Inhibition of the peristaltic reflex of the isolated guinea pig ileum. J Physiol (Lond) 136:249–262
Kosterlitz HW, Robinson JA (1958) The inhibitory action of morphine on the contraction of the longitudinal muscle coat of the isolated guinea pig ileum. Br J Pharmacol 13:296
Kosterlitz HW, Waterfield AA (1975) In vitro models in the study of structure activity relationships of narcotic analgesics. Annu Rev Pharmacol Toxicol 15:29–42
Kosterlitz HW, Lydon RJ, Watt AJ (1970) The effects of adrenaline, noradrenaline, and isoprenaline in inhibitory α and β adrenoceptors in the longitudinal muscle of the guinea pig ileum. Br J Pharmacol 39:398–413
Kosterlitz HW, Ford JAH, Paterson SJ, Waterfield AA (1980) Effects of changes in the structures of enkephalins and narcotic analgesic drugs on their interactions with μ and δ receptors. Br J Pharmacol 68:333–342
Kravitz JJ, Snape WJ Jr, Cohen S (1978) Effect of histamine and histamine antagonists on human lower esophageal sphincter function. Gastroenterology 74:435–440
Kromer W, Pretzlaff W (1979) In vitro evidence for the participation of intestinal opioids in the control of peristalsis in the guinea pig small intestine. Naunyn-Schmiedeberg Arch Pharmacol 309:153–157
Laduron PM, Leysen JE (1979) Domperidone, a specific in vitro dopamine antagonist, devoid of in vivo central dopaminergic activity. Biochem Pharmacol 28:2161–2165
Lanfrancchi GA, Marzio L, Cortini C, Asset EM (1978a) Motor effects of dopamine on human sigmoid colon. Evidence for specific receptors. Am J Dig Dis 23:257–263
Lanfrancchi GA, Marzio L, Cortini C, Trento L, Labo G (1978b) Effect of dopamine on gastric motility in man: evidence for specific receptors. In: Duthie HL (ed) Gastrointestinal motility in health and disease. MTP Press, Lancaster, pp 161–172
Lange AP, Secher NJ, Amery W (1977) Prostaglandin-induced diarrhea treated with loperamide or diphenoxylate. A double blind trial. Acta Med Scand 202:449–454
Lembeck F, Beubler E (1979) Inhibition of PGE_1 induced intestinal secretion by the synthetic enkephalin analogues FK33-824. Naunyn-Schmiedeberg Arch Pharmacol 308:261–264
Lemli J, Lemmens L (1980) Metabolism of sennosides and rhein in the rat. Pharmacology [Suppl 1] 20:50–57
Leng-Peschlow E (1980) Inhibition of intestinal water and electrolyte absorption by senna derivatives in rats. J Pharm Pharmacol 32:2330–2351
Lewis GP (1960) The inhibition by morphine of the action of smooth muscle stimulants on the guinea pig intestine. Br J Pharmacol 15:425–431
Libet B (1970) Generation of slow inhibitory and excitatory postsynaptic potentials. Fed Proc 29:1945–1956
Libet B, Kobayashi H (1974) Generation of adrenergic and cholinergic potentials in sympathetic ganglion cells. Science 164:1530–1532
Libet B, Tosaka T (1969) Slow inhibitory and excitatory post-synaptic potentials in single cells of mammalian ganglia. J Neurophysiol 32:43–50
Lienard J, Janssen J, Verhaegen H, Bourgeois E, Willcox P (1978) Oral domperidone (R33812) in the treatment of chronic dyspepsia. A multicentre evaluation. Curr Ther Res 23:529–537
Lipton AB, Knauer CM (1977) Pseudo-obstruction of the bowel. Therapeutic trial of metoclopramide. Am J Dig Dis 22:263–265
Lord JAH, Waterfield AA, Hughes J, Kosterlitz HW (1976) Multiple opiate receptors. In: Kosterlitz HW (ed) Opiates and endogenous opioid peptides. Elsevier-North-Holland, Amsterdam, pp 275–280
Lord JAH, Waterfield AA, Hughes J, Kosterlitz HW (1977) Endogenous opioid peptides: multiple agonists and receptors. Nature 267:495–499
Mackerer CR, Clay GA, Dajani EZ (1976) Loperamide binding to opiate receptor sites of brain and myenteric plexus. J Pharmacol Exp Ther 199:131–140
Mackerer CR, Brougham LR, East PF, Bloss JL, Dajani EZ, Clay GG (1977) Antidiarrheal and central nervous system activities of SC-27166 [2-C3-5-methyl-1,3,4-oxadiozol-2-YL)-3,3-diphenylpropyl)-2-azabicyclo (2.2.2)octane], a new antidiarrheal agent, resulting from binding to opiate receptor sites for brain. J Pharmacol Exp Ther 203:527–538

Mainguet P, Fiasse R (1977) Double-blind placebo-controlled study of loperamide (imodium) in chronic diarrhea caused by iteocolic disease or resection. Gut 8:575–579
Malagelada JR, Rees WDW, Mazzotta LJ, Go VLW (1980) Gastric motor abnormalities in diabetes and post vagotomy gastroparisis: effect of metoclopramide and bethanechol. Gastroenterology 78:286–293
Margolin S, Plekso VJ (1965) A neurohumoral substance discharged into blood perfusate from isolated rabbit heads by intracerebral morphine. Med Pharmacol Exp 12:1–7
Mathias JR, Carlson GM, Bertiger G, Martin JL, Cohen S (1977) Migrating action potential complex of cholera: a possible prostaglandin-induced response. Am J Physiol 232:E529–E534
McCall RB, Aghajanian GK (1979) Serotonergic facilitation of facial motoneurone excitation. Brain Res 169:11–28
McCallum R, Ippoliti AL, Cooney C (1977) A controlled trial of metoclopramide in symptomatic gastroesophageal reflux. N Engl J Med 296:354–357
McGuire JL, Awouters F, Niemegeers CJE (1978) Interaction of loperamide and diphenoxylate with ethanol and methohexitol. Arch Int Pharmacodyn Ther 236:51–59
McKnight AJ, Sosa RP, Hughes J, Kosterlitz HW (1978) Biosynthesis and release of enkephalins. In: Van Reeh CJM, Terenius L (eds) Characteristics and function of opioids. Developments in neurosciences. Elsevier-North Holland Biomedical, Amsterdam, pp 259–269
Meech RW (1978) Calcium-dependent potassium activation in nervous tissues. Annu Rev Biophys Bioeng 7:1–18
Metzger WH, Cano R, Sturdevant RAL (1976) Effects of metoclopramide in chronic gastric retention after gastric surgery. Gastroenterology 71:30–32
Mitchell RH (1975) Inositol phospholipids and cell surface receptor function. Biochim Biophys Acta 415:81–147
Miyamoto MD (1977) The actions of cholinergic nerves on motor nerve terminals. PharmacolRev 29:225–247
Morgan KG, Schmalz PF, Go VLW, Szurszewski JH (1978) Effects of pentagastrin G17 and G34 on the electrical and mechanical activities of canine antral smooth muscle. Gastroenterology 75:405–412
Morita K, North RA, Katayama Y (1980) Evidence that substance P is a neurotransmitter in the myenteric plexus. Nature 287:151–152
Nell G, Forth W, Rummel W, Wanitsche R (1976) Pathways of sodium moving from blood to intestinal lumen under the influence of oxyphenisatin and deoxycholate. Naunyn-Schmiedeberg Arch Pharmacol 293:31–37
Niemegeers CJ, Lenaerts FM, Janssen PAJ (1974a) Loperamide (R18553), a novel type of antidiarrheal agent. Part. 1. In vivo oral pharmacology and acute toxicology. Comparison with morphine, codeine, diphenoxylate, and difenoxine. Arzneim Forsch 24:1633–1636
Niemegeers GJ, Lenaerts FM, Janssen PAJ (1974b) Loperamide (R18533), a novel type of antidiarrheal agent. Part II. In vivo parenteral pharmacology and acute toxicology. Comparison with morphine, codeine, and diphenoxylate. Arzneim Forsch 24:1636–1641
Nijkamp EP, Van Ree JM (1980) Effects of endorphins on different parts of the gastro-intestinal tract of rats and guinea pig in vitro. Br J Pharmacol 68:599–606
Norberg KA (1964) Adrenergic innervation of the intestinal wall studied by fluorescence microscopy. Int J Neuropharm 3:379–382
North RA (1977) Hyperpolarization of myenteric neurones by enkephalin. Br J Pharmacol 59:504–505
North RA (1979) Opiates, opioid peptides, and single neurones. Life Sci 24:1527–1546
North RA, Nishi S (1973) Properties of the ganglion cells in the myenteric plexus of the guinea pig ileum determined by intracellular recordings. In: Daniel EE (ed) 4th International Symposium on Gastrointestinal Motility. Mitchell, Vancouver, pp 667–676
North RA, Tonini M (1977) The mechanism of action of narcotic analgesics in guinea pig ileum. Br J Pharmacol 61:541–549
North RA, Williams JT (1976) Enkephalin inhibits firing of myenteric neurones. Nature 264:460–461

North RA, Williams JT (1977) Extracellular recording from the guinea pig myenteric plexus and the action of morphine. Eur J Pharmacol 45:23–33

North RA, Katayama Y, Williams JT (1976) On the mechanism and site of action of enkephalin on single myenteric neurones. Brain Res 165:67–77

North RA, Henderson G, Katayama Y, Johnson SM (1980) Electrophysiological evidence for presynaptic inhibition of acetylcholine release by 5-hydroxytryptamine in the enteric nervous system. Neuroscience 5:581–586

Novak E, Lee JG, Seckman CE, Phillips JP, Di Santa AR (1976) Unfavourable effect of atropine-diphenoxylate (lomotil) therapy in lincomycin caused diarrhea. JAMA 235:1451–1454

Ohashi H, Takewaki T, Okada T (1974) Calcium and the contractile effect of carbachol on the depolarized guinea pig taenia caeci. Jpn J Pharmacol 24:601–611

Ohashi H, Takewaki T, Shibata N, Okada T (1975) Effects of calcium antagonists on contractile responses of guinea pig taenia caeci to carbachol in a calcium deficient, potassium rich solution. Jpn J Pharmacol 25:214–216

Ohga A, Taneike T (1978) H_1 and H_2 receptors in the smooth muscle of the ruminant stomach. Br J Pharmacol 62:333–337

Oka J (1980) Enkephalin receptor in the rabbit ileum. Br J Pharmacol 68:193–195

Oka T, Sawa A (1979) Calcium requirements for electrically induced release of an endogenous opiate receptor ligand from the guinea pig ileum. Br J Pharmacol 65:3–5

Okwuasaba F, Hamilton JT (1975) The effect of metoclopramide on inhibition of induced by purine nucleotides noradrenaline thephylline elthendimine in intestinal muscle and in peristalsis in vitro. Can J Physiol Pharmacol 53:972–977

Okwuasaba FK, Hamilton JT (1976) The effect of metoclopramide on intestinal muscle responses and the peristaltic reflex in vitro. Can J Physiol Pharmacol 54:393–404

Osborne DH, Lennon J, Henderson M, Lidgard G, Creel R, Carter DC (1977) Effect of cimetidine on the human lower esophageal sphincter. Gut 18:99–105

Parolaro O, Sala M, Gori E (1977) Effects of intracerebroventricular administration of morphine upon intestinal motility in rat and its antagonism with naloxone. Eur J Pharmacol 46:329–338

Paton WDM (1957) The action of morphine and related substance on contraction and on acetylcholine output of coaxially stimulated guinea pig ileum. Br J Pharmacol 12:119–127

Paton WDM, Vane JR (1963) An analysis of the response of the isolated stomach to electrical stimulation and to drugs. J Physiol (Lond) 165:10–46

Paton WDM, Vizi ES (1969) The inhibitory action of noradrenaline and adrenaline on acetylcholine release by guinea pig ileum longitudinal muscle strip. Br J Pharmacol 35:10–28

Paton WDM, Zar AM (1968) The origin of acetylcholine released from the guinea pig intestine and longitudinal muscle strips. J Physiol (Lond) 194:13–33

Pelemans W, Vantrappen G (1976) A double-blind crossover comparison of loperamide with diphenoxylate in the symptomatic treatment of chronic diarrhea. Gastroenterology 70:1030–1034

Penfold D, Volans GN (1977) Overdose from lomotil. Br Med J 2:1401–1402

Perkel MS, Moore C, Hersh T, Davidson EE (1979)Metoclopramide therapy in patients with delayed gastric emptying. A randomized double blind study. Dig Dis Sci 24:662–665

Phillips RA, Lowe AHG, Mitchell TG, Neptune EM Jr (1965) Cathartics and the sodium pump. Nature 206:1367–1368

Pinder RM, Bradgon RN, Sawyer PR, Speight TM, Avery GS (1976) Metoclopramide: a review of its pharmacological properties and clinical use. Drugs 12:81–131

Platteborse R, Hermans CI, Van Loon J, Smet F, Loots W, Van Gup A, Jagenau A (1979) The effect of domperidone on pyloric activity in dog and in man. Postgrad Med J [Suppl 1] 55:15–18

Priutt DB, Grubb MN, Jacquette DC, Burks TF (1974) Intestinal effects of 5-hydroxytryptamine and morphine in guinea-pigs, dogs, cats, and monkeys. Eur J Pharmacol 26:208–305

Puig MM, Gascon P, Craviso GJ, Musacchio JM (1977) Endogenous opiate receptor ligand. Electrically induced release in the guinea pig ileum. Science 195:419–420
Puig MM, Gascon P, Musacchio JM (1978) Electrically induced opiate-like inhibition of the guinea pig ileum: cross tolerance to morphine. J Pharmacol Exp Ther 206:289–302
Purves RD (1974) Muscarinic excitation: a microelectrophoretic study on cultured smooth muscle cells. Br J Pharmacol 52:77–86
Purves RD (1976) Function of muscarinic and nicotinic acetylcholine receptors. Nature 26:149–151
Putney JW (1979) Stimulus-permeability coupling: role of calcium in the receptor regulation of membrane permeability. Pharmacol Rev 30:209–245
Ramsbottom N, Hunt JN (1970) Studies of the effects of metoclopramide and apomorphine on gastric emptying and secretion in man. Gut 11:989
Rattan S, Goyal RJ (1976) Effects of dopamine on the esophageal smooth muscle. Gastroenterology 70:377–381
Rattan S, Goyal RJ (1977) Effects of 5-hydroxytryptamine on the lower esophageal sphincter in vivo: evidence for multiple sites of action. J Clin Invest 59:125–133
Rattan S, Goyal RK (1978a) Effects of histamine on the lower esophageal sphincter in vivo: evidence for action at three different sites. J Pharmacol Exp Ther 204:334–342
Rattan S, Goyal RK (1978b) Evidence of 5-HT participation in vagal inhibitory pathway in opossum LES. Am J Physiol 234:E273–E276
Read JB, Burnstock G (1969) Adrenergic innervation of the gut musculature in vertebrates. Histochemie 17:263–272
Reyntjens AJ, Niemegeers CJE, Van Nueten JM et al. (1978) Domperidone, a novel and safe gastrokinetic antinauseant for the treatment of dyspepsia and vomiting. Arzneim Forsch 28:1194–1196
Richardson KC (1958) Electromicroscopic observations on Auerbach's plexus in the rabbit, with special reference to the problem of smooth muscle innervation. Am J Anat 103:99–136
Rimele TJ, Rogers WA, Gaginella TS (1979) Characterization of muscarinic cholinergic receptors in the lower esophageal sphincter of the cat: binding of [^{3}H] quinuclidinyl benzilate. Gastroenterology 77:1225–1234
Rogers DC, Burnstock G (1966) Multiaxonal autonomic junctions in intestinal smooth muscle of the toad (Bufo marinus). J Comp Neurol 126:625
Ross SB (1976) Structural requirements for uptake into catecholamine neurones. In: Paton DM (ed) Mechanism of neuronal and extraneuronal transport of catecholamines. Raven, New York, pp 67–93
Roszkowski AP (1961) An unusual type of sympathetic ganglionic stimulant. J Pharmacol Exp Ther 137:156–170
Rubinstein JS (1978) Abuse of anticholinergic drugs (letter) N Engl J Med 299:834
Sakai K (1979) A pharmacological analysis of the contractile action of histamine upon the ileal region of the isolated blood perfused small intestine of the rat. Br J Pharmacol 67:587–598
Sakai K, Shirake Y, Tatsumi T, Tsuji K (1979) The actions of 5-hydroxytryptamine and histamine on the isolated ileum of the tree shrew (Tupaia glis) Br J Pharmacol 66:405–408
Salmon DM, Honeyman TW (1980) Proposed mechanism of cholinergic action in smooth muscle. Nature 284:344–345
Sarna S, Daniel EE, Waterfall WE (1977) Myogenic and neural control systems for esophageal motility. Gastroenterology 73:1345–1352
Sarna SK, Bardakjian BL, Waterfall WE, Lind JF (1980) Human colonic electrical control activity (ECA). Gastroenterology 78:1526–1536
Sato T, Takanyagi I, Takagi K (1973) Pharmacological properties of electrical activities obtained from neurones in Auerbach's plexus. Jpn J Pharmacol 23:665–671
Sato T, Takayanagi J, Takagi K (1974) Effects of acetylcholine release drugs on electrical activities obtained from Auerbach's plexus in the guinea pig ileum. Jpn J Pharmacol 24:447–451

Scheurmans V, Van Lemmel R, Dorn J, Brugmans J (1974) Loperamide (R18553) a novel type of antidiarrheal agent. Part 6. Clinical pharmacology. Placebo controlled comparison of the constipating activity and safety of loperamide, diphenoxylate, and codeine in normal volunteers. Arzneim Forsch 24:1653–1657
Schulz R, Goldstein A (1973) Morphine tolerance and supersensitivity to 5-hydroxytryptamine in the myenteric plexus of the guinea pig. Nature 244:168–170
Schultzberg M, Hökfelt T, Nilsson GL et al. (1980) Distribution of peptide- and catecholamine-containing neurones in the gastro-intestinal tract of rat and guinea pig: immunohistochemical studies with antisera to substance P, vasoactive intestinal polypeptide, enkephalins, somatostatin, gastrin/cholecystokinin, neurotensin, and dopamine-β-hydroxylase. Neuroscience 5:689–744
Schulz R, Wüster M, Simanto R, Snyder S, Hay A (1977) Electrically stimulated release of opiate-like material from the myenteric plexus of the guinea pig ileum. Eur J Pharmacol 41:347–348
Schulz R, Wüster M, Herz A (1979) Centrally and peripherally mediated inhibition of intestinal motility by opioids. Naunyn-Schmiedeberg Arch Pharmacol 308:256–260
Schulze-Delrieu K (1979) Metoclopramide. Gastroenterology 77:768–779
Schwartz JC (1979) Minireview: histamine receptors in brain. Life Sci 25:895–911
Schwiter EJ, Hepner GW, Rose RC (1975) Effects of bile acids on electrical properties of rat colon. Evaluation of an in vitro model for secretion. Gut 16:477–481
Sheiner HJ, Catchpole BN (1976) Drug therapy for postvagotomy gastric stasis. Br J Surg 63:608–611
Shibata N, Ohashi H, Takewaki T, Okada T (1978) Calcium source for contractile response of guinea pig taenia caeci to carbachol in a calcium deficient potassium rich solution. Jpn J Pharmacol 28:561–568
Silva DT, Ross G, Osborne LW (1971) Adrenergic innervation of the ileum of the cat. Am J Physiol 220:347–352
Simantov R, Snyder SH (1976) Morphine-like peptides in mammalian brain; isolation, structure elucidation, and interactions with the opiate receptor. Proc Natl Acad Sci USA 73:2515–2519
Smith JW, Hughes J, Kosterlitz HW, Sosa RP (1978) Enkephalins isolation, distribution, and function. In: Kosterlitz HW (ed) Opiates and endogenous opioid peptides. Elsevier-North Holland, Amsterdam, pp 57–62
Smith M, Chambers TL (1978) Overdose of lomotil. Br Med J 1:179
Sosa RP, McKnight AT, Hughes AT, Kosterlitz HW (1977) Incorporation of labelled amino acids into the enkephalins. FEBS Lett 84:195–198
Starke K (1977) Regulation of noradrenaline release by presynaptic receptor systems. Rev Physiol Biochem Pharmacol 77:124
Starke K, Montell H (1974) Influence of drugs with affinity for α-adrenoceptors on noradrenaline release by potassium, tyramine, and dimethylphenylpiperazinium. Eur J Pharmacol 27:273–280
Starke K, Montell H, Gayk W, Merker R (1974) Comparison of the effects of clonidine on pre- and postsynaptic adrenoceptors in the rabbit pulmonary artery. Naunyn-Schmiedeberg Arch Pharmacol 285:133–150
Starke K, Borowski E, Endo T (1975 a) Preferential blockade of presynaptic0 a-adrenoceptors by yohimbine. Eur J Pharmacol 34:385–388
Starke K, Endo T, Taube HD (1975 b)Pre- and postsynaptic components in effect of drugs with α-adrenoceptor affinity. Nature 254:440–441
Starke K, Endo T, Taube HD (1975 c) Relative pre- and postsynaptic potencies of α-adrenoceptor agonists in the rabbit pulmonary artery. Naunyn-Schmiedeberg Arch Pharmacol 291:55–78
Stewart JJ, Bass P (1976 a) Effect of intravenous C-terminal octapeptide of cholecystokinin and intraduodenal ricinoleic acid on contractile activity of the dog intestine. Proc Soc Exp Biol Med 152:213–217
Stewart JJ, Bass P (1976 b) Effects of ricinoleic and oleic acids on the digestive contractile activity of the canine small and large bowel. Gastroenterology 70:371–376

Stewart JJ, Gaginella TS, Olsen WA, Bass P (1975) Inhibitory actions of laxatives on motility and water and electrolyte transport in the gastrointestinal tract. J Pharmacol Exp Ther 192:458–467
Stewart JJ, Weisbrodt NW, Burks JF (1977) Centrally mediated intestinal stimulation by morphine. J Pharmacol Exp Ther 202:174–181
Stewart JJ, Weisbrodt NW, Burks JF (1978) Central and peripheral actions of morphine in intestinal transit. J Pharmacol Exp Ther 205:547–555
Strunz U, Domschke W, Mitznegg P et al. (1975) Analysis of the motor effects of 13-norleucine motilin on the rabbit, guinea pig, rat, and human alimentary tract in vitro. Gastroenterology 68:1485–1491
Szerb JC (1975) Endogenous acetylcholine release and labelled acetylcholine formation from [^{3}H] choline in the myenteric plexus of the guinea pig ileum. Can J Physiol Pharmacol 53:566–574
Szerb JC (1976) Storage and release of labelled acetylcholine in the myenteric plexus of the guinea pig ileum. Can J Physiol Pharmacol 54:566–574
Szerb JE (1980) Effects of low calcium and oxotremorine in the kinetics of the evoked release of [^{3}H]-acetylcholine from the guinea pig myenteric plexus; comparison with morphine. Naunyn-Schmiedeberg Arch Pharmacol 311:119–127
Szurszewski JH (1975) Mechanism of action of pentagastrin and acetylcholine on the longitudinal muscle of the canine antrum. J Physiol (Lond) 252:335–361
Taira N, Matsumura S, Hashimoto K (1971) Excitation of the parasympathetic ganglia of the canine urinary bladder through a muscarinic mechanism. J Pharmacol Exp Ther 176:92–100
Takayanagi I, Sato T, Takagi K (1974) Action of 5-hydroxytryptamine on electrical activity of Auerbach's plexus on the ileum of the morphine dependent guinea pig. Eur J Pharmacol 27:252–254
Taub M, Bonorres G, Chung A, Coyne MJ, Schoenfield LJ (1977) Effect of propranolol on bile acid and cholera enterotoxin-stimulated c-AMP and secretion in rabbit intestine. Gastroenterology 72:101–105
Taylor AB, Kreulen D, Prosser CL (1977) Electron microscopy of the connective tissues between longitudinal and circular muscle of small intestine of cat. Am J Anat 150:427–441
Trendelenburg U (1966) Transmission of preganglionic impulses through the muscarinic receptors of the superior cervical ganglion of the cat. J Pharmacol Exp Ther 154:426–440
Trendelenburg U (1967) Some aspects of the pharmacology of autonomic ganglion-cells. Ergebn Physiol 59:1–85
Trendelenburg U (1976) The extraneuronal uptake and metabolism of catecholamines in the heart. In: Paton DM (ed) Mechanism of neuronal and extraneuronal transport of catecholamines. Raven, New York, pp 259–280
Triggle DJ, Triggle CR (1976) Chemical pharmacology of the synapsis. Academic Press, London
Uddman R, Alumeto J, Hakanson R, Sundler F, Walles B (1980) Peptidergic (enkephalin) innvervation of the mammalian esophagus. Gastroenterology 78:732–737
Valenzuela JE (1976) Dopamine as a possible neurotransmitter in gastric relaxation. Gastroenterology 71:1019–1022
Van Canse W, Van Damme L, Van der Mierop L, Deruyttere M, Lauwers W, Coenegrachts J (1978) Chronic dyspepsia: double blind treatment with domperidone (R33812) or a placebo. A multi-centre therapeutic evaluation. Curr Ther Res 23:695–701
Van Eygen M, Dhondt F, Heck E, Ameryckx L, Van Ravensteyn H (1979) A double-blind comparison of domperidone and metoclopramide suppositories in the treatment of nausea and vomitting in children. Postgrad Med J [Suppl 1] 55:36–39
Van Hee RH, Vanhoutte PM (1978) Cholinergic inhibition of adrenergic neurotransmission in the canine gastric artery. Gastroenterology 74:1266–1270
Vanhoutte PM, Levy MN (1980) Prejunctional cholinergic modulation of adrenergic neurotransmission in the cardiovascular system. Am J Physiol 238:H275–H281
Van Nueten JM, Janssen PA (1978) Is dopamine and endogenous inhibitor of gastric emptying? In: Duthie HL (ed) Gastrointestinal motility in health and disease. MTP Press, Lancaster, pp 173–181

Van Nueten JM, Janssen PAJ (1980) Effect of domperidone on gastric relaxation caused by dopamine, secretion, 5-hydroxytryptamine, substance P, and adenosine triphosphate. In: Christensen J (ed) Gastrointestinal motility. Raven, New York, pp 225–231
Van Nueten JM, Janssen PA, Fontaine J (1974) Loperamide (R18553), a novel type of antidiarrheal agent. Part 3. In vitro studies on isolated tissue. Arzneim Forsch 24:1641–1645
Van Nueten JM, Janssen PAJ, Fontaine J (1976) Unexpected reversal effects of naloxone on the guinea pig ileum. Life Sci 18:803–810
Van Nueten JM, Ennis C, Helsen L, Lauduron PM, Janssen PAJ (1978) Inhibition of dopamine receptors in the stomach: an explanation of the gastrokinetic properties of domperidone. Life Sci 23:453–458
Van Outryve M, Lauwers W, Verbeke S (1979) Domperidone for the symptomatic treatment of chronic post-prandial nausea and vomiting. Postgrad Med J [Suppl 1] 55:33–35
Vantrappen G, Janssens J, Hellemans J, Ghoos Y (1977) The interdigestive motor complex of normal subjects and patients with bacterial overgrowth of the small intestine. J Clin Invest 59:1158–1166
Vase SM, Vanhoutee PM (1974) Inhibition by acetylcholine of adrenergic neurotransmission in vascular smooth muscle. Circ Res 34:317–326
Vermillion DL, Gillespie JP, Cooke AR, Wood JD (1979) Does 5-hydroxytryptamine influence purinergic inhibitory neurones in the intestine? Am J Physiol 237:E198–E202
Volle RL (1966) Muscarinic and nicotinic stimulant actions at autonomic ganglia. Pergamon, New York
Volle RL, Hancock JC (1970) Transmission in sympathetic ganglia. Fed Proc 29:1913–1918
Waldman DB, Zfass AM, Makhlouf GM (1977) Stimulatory (H_1) and inhibitory (H_2) histamine receptors in gall bladder muscle. Gastroenterology 72:932–936
Wall MJ, Baker RD (1974) Intestinal transmural properties. Effects of conjugated bile salts in vitro. Am J Physiol 227:499–506
Waller SL (1975) Differential measurement of small and large bowel transit times in constipation and diarrhea: a new approach. Gut 16:372–378
Waller SL, Misiewicz JJ, Kiley N (1972) Effect of eating on motility of the pelvic colon in constipation or diarrhea. Gut 13:805–811
Wanitschke R (1980) Influence of rhein on electrolyte and water transfer in the isolated rat colonic mucosa. Pharmacology [Suppl 1] 20:21–26
Wanitschke R, Ewe K (1978) Die elektrische Potentialmessung im Sigma als diagnostische Methode. Z Gastroenterol 16:206–209
Wanitschke R, Nell G, Rummel W, Specht W (1977) Transfer of sodium and water through isolated rat colonic mucosa under the influence of deoxycholate and oxyphenisatin. Naunyn-Schmiedeberg Arch Pharmacol 297:185–190
Ward A, Takemori AE (1976) Effects of 6-hydroxydopamine and 5,6-dihydroxytryptamine on the response of the coaxially stimulated guinea pig ileum to morphine. J Pharmacol Exp Ther 199:124–130
Waterfield AA, Kosterlitz HW (1973) Release of acetylcholine from the myenteric plexus of the guinea pig ileum. In: Daniel EE (ed) 4th International Symposium on Gastrointestinal Motility. Mitchell, Vancouver, pp 659–666
Waterfield AA, Kosterlitz HW (1975) Stereospecific increase by narcotic antagonists of evoked acetylcholine output in guinea pig ileum. Life Sci 16:1787–1792
Waterfield AA, Smockum RWJ, Hughes J, Kosterlitz HW, Henderson G (1977) In vitro pharmacology of the opioid peptides, enkephalins, and endophins. Eur J Pharmacol 43:107–116
Waterfield AA, Leslie FM, Lord JA, Ling N, Kosterlitz HW (1979) Opioid activities of fragments of β-endorphin and its leucine 45-analogue comparison of the binding properties methonine and leucine enkephaline. Eur J Pharmacol 58:11–18
Weems WA, Szurszewski JH (1977) Modulation of colonic motility by peripheral neural inputs to neurones of the inferior mesenteric ganglia. Gastroenterology 73:273–278
Weihrauch TR, Förster CF, Krieglstein J (1979) Evaluation of effects of domperidone on human oesophageal motility by intra-luminal manometry. Postgrad Med J [Suppl 1] 55:7–10

Weinstock M (1971) Sites of action of narcotic analgesis drugs – peripheral tissues. In: Clouet DH (ed) Narcotic drugs – biochemical pharmacology. Plenum, New York, pp 394–407

Weisbrodt NW, Sussman SE, Steward JJ, Burks TF (1980) Effect of morphine sulfare on intestinal transit and myoelectric activity of the small intestine of the rat. J Pharmacol Exp Ther 214:333–338

Westfall TC (1977) Local regulation of adrenergic neurotransmission. Physiol Rev 57:659–728

Wikberg J (1977a) Localization of adrenergic receptors in guinea pig ileum and rabbit jejunum to cholinergic neurones and to smooth muscle cells. Acta Physiol Scand 99:109–207

Wikberg J (1977b) Releases of ^{3}H-acetylcholine from isolated guinea pig ileum. A radiochemical method for studying the release of the cholinergic transmitter in the intestine. Acta Physiol Scand 101:302–317

Wikberg JCC (1978a) Pharmacological classification of adrenergic alpha-receptors in the guinea pig. Nature 273:164–166

Wikberg J (1978b) Differentiation between pre- and post-junctional α-receptors in guinea pig ileum and rabbit aorta. Acta Physiol Scand 103:225–239

Wikberg J (1979) The pharmacological classification of adrenergic α_1 and α_2 receptors and their mechanisms of action. Acta Physiol Scand 468:1–99

Wingate D, Pearce E, Hutton M, Ling A (1980) Effect of metoclopramide on interdigestive myoelectric activity in the conscious dog. Dig Dis Sci 25:15–21

Wood JD (1975) Neurophysiology of Auerbach's plexus and control of intestinal motility. Physiol Rev 55:307–324

Wood JD, Mayer CJ (1979a) Intracellular study of tonic-type enteric neurones in guinea pig small intestine. J Neurophysiol 42:569–581

Wood JD, Mayer CJ (1979b) Serotonergic activation of tonic-type enteric neurones in guinea pig small bowel. J Neurophysiol 42:582–593

Wüster M, Herz A (1978) Opiate agonist action of antidiarrheal agents in vitro and in vivo – findings in support for selective actions. Naunyn-Schmiedeberg Arch Pharmacol 301:187–194

Wüster M, Schulz R, Herz A (1980) Highly specific opiate receptors for dynorphin (1-13) in the mouse vas deferens. Eur J Pharmacol 62:235–236

CHAPTER 6

Hydrophilic Colloids in Colonic Motility

M. A. Eastwood and A. N. Smith

A. Introduction

Colonic motor activity has been shown to be of clinical importance in diverticular disease, the irritable bowel syndrome and the patient with colitis who is constipated. A decrease in colonic intraluminal pressure may be obtained by pharmacological agents but increasing stool weight may also decrease colonic pressure.

A curious paradox exists in which a relaxation of the colonic musculature is achieved by an increased bolus of stool. The easiest way to produce an increase in stool weight is by dietary fibre or hydrophilic colloids, either as cereal bran, fruit, and vegetables, or the gums developed by the pharmaceutical industry. The effect of these hydrophilic colloids both on stool weight and colonic pressure is variable. In an attempt to lay a logical basis for treatment regimes, we have discussed the different types of dietary fibre and the problems associated with identifying their physiological properties and their effects on colonic physiology, especially colonic pressure.

The treatment and the theories associated with diverticular disease changed as a result of the work of Painter (1974) who, in defiance of previous concepts, suggested that an increased bulk content of the diet and the faeces might result in a decrease in the pressure of the sigmoid colon. (His hypothesis was that, in parallel with the increase in bulk content of the diet and the decrease in the motility index, there would be an increase in stool weight.) Painter originally emphasised the role of wheat bran as possibly inducing such changes and described its effect on stool weight and intestinal transit. However, the use of dietary fibre in altering stool weight and colonic motility was extended beyond wheat bran, in part because bran is not universally acceptable. It was also recognised that fruit and vegetables can influence stool weight. However, the use of different sources of fruit and vegetables introduced unknown variables and furthermore, the shelf-life of fruit and vegetables is quite short. Therefore in order to meet the demands of contemporary marketing and culinary practice, the food industry has had to provide means of preserving fruit and vegetables, e.g. freezing, canning, and dehydration. In order to extend the shelf-life of fruit and vegetables as sources of dietary fibre it is attractive to use fibre concentrates. In making fibre concentrates, changes occur in the biological properties of the fibre. It is important therefore to develop some logic to anticipate the biological effect of these fibre concentrates along the gastrointestinal tract.

The spectrum of fibre sources is as large as the plant kingdom. There are of course chemical and physicochemical differences between fruit and vegetables. The age, species and anatomy vary; the site and the climatic conditions where the plant is grown influence the properties of the fibre. The mode of cooking and preparation may make important changes, so that even the relatively simple cereal bran is more complex than appears at first. For example, the varieties of wheat grown in North America and Europe are chemically and physically distinct, and the chemistry and physical properties of each bran are further affected by the particular milling process used and at what milling stage the bran is obtained.

The commonly used hydrophilic colloids provided by the pharmaceutical industry are a quite distinct group of plant materials. These are gums which exude from trees, often grown in arid desert areas. These plants are of immense importance in the ecology of a region, stabilising uncertain water areas. Some of the gums leak from the plant when there is injury and therefore they have a protective role. Others, e.g. ispaghula, are derived from the coats of seeds which grow in desert areas; these become hydrated and hold the available water so as to allow germination to take place.

B. The Nature of Stool Bulk and How it is Provided

There is a considerable variation in colonic function both between subjects and from day to day in healthy subjects. WYMAN et al. (1978) demonstrated the extent of the variability between individual faecal wet and dry weights, the faecal volume and the frequency of defecation. The size of individual stools varied over a ten-fold range. There was no significant difference between males and females. This variation in the weight of individual stools indicates the importance of collecting stools for several days. However, it is not known how long it is necessary to collect stools in order to measure accurately the constituents of the stool and to calculate an accurate daily output. There is little variation in the water content of the stool which has a value of $75\% \pm 4\%$.

It is possible that the variability in colonic function is a function of the segmenting activity of the colon. It is known that when the caecum contracts during a barium enema, and the barium is expressed along the colon, some barium remains in the filled caecum (MCLAREN et al. 1955). It has also been suggested in the past by ELLIOTT and BARCLAY-SMITH (1904) that antiperistaltic waves drive the fluid contents of the colon towards the caecum, the antiperistaltic waves being replaced from time to time by peristaltic waves. This type of movement, though it may occur anywhere in the colon, is usually confined to the proximal colon so that the liquid chyme newly received from the ileum is passed to and fro on the surface of the colon for absorption to occur. It is therefore possible that the nature of the contractions makes it impossible for the colon to produces tool of a regular size each day. On the other hand it is conceivable that it is the constituents of the stool, either in concentration or in daily output which dictate faecal excretion. It is also recognised that water-soluble markers of stool content, e.g. PEG 4000 and insoluble markers, e.g. chromium sesquioxide, may pass along the intestine at differing rates (MITCHELL and EASTWOOD 1976). Such stratification of flow along the intestine does not facilitate our understanding of the events which occur in the transformation of liquid ileal effluent into the normal stool.

There has long been an interest, however, in the manner in which food controls the bulk of faeces. WILLIAMS and OLMSTED in 1936 reviewed the causes of constipation. They stated that both clinicians and physiologists agreed that the indigestible carbohydrates of food have a greater effect on stool volume than protein, fat, and carbohydrate. They believed that, of the three classes of carbohydrates which most markedly increased stool weight, hemicellulose was the most efficacious and cellulose in its natural state was somewhat less effective. They suspected that the highly hygroscopic carbohydrates were the most effective. Lignin-containing residues were costive.

They thought that the effectiveness of indigestible residues was not due primarily to the mechanical stimulus of swollen fibre but rather to the chemical stimuli of compounds arising from the effect of intestinal flora on hemicelluloses and celluloses, with the generation in particular of short chain volatile fatty acids. However, it should be noted that in these experiments, as in others, concentrates of fibre isolated from widely differing sources were fed and, as will be explained later, this is not the same as feeding raw vegetables. In more recent experiments CUMMINGS et al. (1978a) showed that enhancing the fat content of the diet from 62 to 152 g/day under metabolic ward conditions did not alter stool wet or dry weight or mean transit time: however, the faecal bile acid excretion increased from 140 ± 63 mg/day on 62 g fat to 320 ± 120 mg/day on 152 g fat. The average faecal fat excretion also increased from 1.14 to 3.1 g/day. Therefore, dietary fat had no effect on overall colonic function. WILLIAMS and OLMSTED'S concept, however, of short chain fatty acids being important in determining stool weight (1936) has to be reevaluated by the demonstration by MCNEIL et al. (1978) that the colon readily absorbs short chain fatty acids. They calculated that from a daily intake of 20 g fibre, 10–15 g would be broken down with the production of at least 100 mmol short chain fatty acids. Only approximately 5–20 mmol short chain fatty acids are excreted in the faeces so that 80% of fatty acids must be absorbed. Therefore the role of short chain fatty acids in faecal bulking remains unclear.

I. Water

There is little doubt that water is the most important single component of stool, and represents approximately 75% of the stool weight. The ability of the human colon to absorb fluid is immense, but estimates of the capacity of the large intestine to absorb dietary and secretory fluids vary. The calculation of amounts absorbed depends on the method of study used; whether this be a comparison of ileostomy effluent with normal stools, a comparison of ileal content and faecal output in normal volunteers ingesting their usual diet, or studies of colonic perfusion. From these methods the estimate of absorption capacity varies from 0.5 to 3 l per day. The studies claiming to represent physiological conditions have tended to examine the absorption of water alone instead of the normal conditions of absorption of water from a gel or sludge. DEBONGNIE and PHILLIPS (1978) have calculated that the normal colon is capable of absorbing 6 l/day water and 800 mequiv./day sodium. There is a relationship between absorption, total flow and the rate at which the fluid enters the colon. These authors have speculated that the sudden arrival in the caecum of a large bolus of fluid might cause acute diarrhoea. Unabsorbed solute, e.g. bile acids, possibly fatty acids and carbohydrates, may impair the absorption of water. Notwithstanding this, the stool weight varies between 10 and 500 g in the normal subject, and therefore there must be a factor or factors altering the residual water in the stool.

II. Bacteria

Faeces are complex mixtures of microorganisms, undigested food residues, excreted organic compounds, ions, and water. Whilst there are many studies on the faecal microbial flora, the faecal chemical composition and metabolism, these studies have almost without exception considered the faecal mass as a homogeneous mixture from which chemicals and bacteria can be isolated for study. This holistic view is reasonable in the identification of pathogenic bacteria by the pathologist, but it gives little insight into the role of bacteria in the normal stool. It is perhaps important to know the manner in which particles of fibre interact with microorganisms and other faecal components. Such a study was initiated by WILLIAMS et al. (1978) when they examined several specimens of stool by light and scanning electron microscopy. The matrix of faeces contained a large number of bacteria intermingled with smaller amorphous particles of food residue. Many aleurone cells of bran appeared to be intact. In general the various bacterial types were randomly mixed. However, occasional colonies of Gram-positive bacteria and yeast cells could be seen. By scanning electron microscopy, the matrix of fibre residues apeared to be surrounded by the amorphous mass. There are plant hairs and fibres in the stools and bran residues were seen to be undigested. The mass of bacteria consisted of a densely packed mixture of bacteria of quite diverse morphology, i.e. cocci and rods. There were also yeast bodies present. Although some particles of food residues were intermingled with the bacteria, the latter appeared to comprise most of the interfibre substance. Clearly at the interface between the plant residues and bacterial mass there is contact and plant fibres have bacteria on their surfaces. Bacteria are also seen with areas of damage on the outer seed coat of bran residue and other fibre, suggesting that extra cellular bacterial enzymes may be responsible for production of changes within the fibre.

The role of bacteria in the faecal mass has been extended further by STEPHENS and CUMMINGS (1980), who have used the methods developed by ruminant physiologists to separate fibrous material and bacteria by centrifugation and filtering techniques. They have shown that the stool is made up of 50%–60% bacteria.

III. Fibre

Of the dietary constituents, it would appear that vegetable dietary fibre is a significant contributor to stool weight. From here, problems arise. Dietary fibre has yet to be adequately defined. The chemistry and biological effects of plants vary with their source, the age of the plant and the anatomy of the plant. Cooking and processing add complications to the manner in which the fibre behaves along the gastrointestinal tract.

The definition of the term "dietary fibre" has been the subject of considerable discussion (TROWELL et al. 1978). Although of crucial importance, a major stumbling block to a definition of dietary fibre is the function of dietary fibre. Once a definition has been elaborated then, to an extent, thinking becomes less flexible and future ideas on fibre immediately become hidebound by that definition. It would be more appropriate to look at the biological effects of various sources of fibre and thereafter define fibre within that scope. To an extent the term dietary fibre is ad-

Table 1. Constituents of dietary fibre

Reserve polysaccharides	Starches, e.g. amylose, amylopectin, dextrins Glycogen Fructans Galactomannans, e.g. guar gum
Structural polysaccharides	Cellulose Peptic substances Hemicelluloses
Nonstructural polysaccharides	Gums Mucilages Pectin
Algal polysaccharides	Sulphated, e.g. carrageenan, agar Unsulphated, alginate

equately covered by the term "plant cell wall material." There are those who would like the definition to include the difficult term "indigestible." In this it is implied that enzymes of the human gastrointestinal tract do not hydrolyse the major skeleton of the polysaccharide material. On the other hand, bacteria in the colon extensively digest dietary fibre in the caecum. If a physicochemical approach is adopted to explain the biological role of dietary fibre, then it must be recognised that there may well be changes in the physical properties as a result of exposure to enzymes and solutions of different osmotic pressure and pH. A working definition is that dietary fibre is the amalgam of lignin and polysaccharides that are not digested by the endogenous secretion of the human digestive tract (SOUTHGATE et al. 1978). TROWELL et al. (1978) have argued that the term dietary fibre should be applied only to structural materials of the plant cell wall and indigestible storage polysaccharides in the body of the plant cell. This may well be the best definition that is available and perhaps the most useful.

Dietary fibre is a mixture of polymers derived in the main from the plant cell walls. SOUTHGATE (1976) has done a great deal to clarify and define what had previously been a confused, even contentious, subject. The polysaccharides and lignins are intimately intermeshed within the plant anatomy, being different in the cell wall, xylem, phloem, and seed coat and this clearly will be affected by the age of the plant. Table 1 indicates some of the constituents of dietary fibre. Amylose and amylopectins, the starches, are major components of the diet, whereas dextrins, glycogen, fructans, galactomannans, pectic substances, hemicelluloses, gums, mucilages, pectins, and polysaccharides are minor or trace constituents of the diet.

The starches, i.e. the α-glucans, are hydrolysed by the mammalian digestive enzymes so that both the α (1–4) and (1–6) glycoside linkages can be hydrolysed. It is believed that there are no endogenous enzymes capable of hydrolysing cellulose β (1–3, 1–4) – glucans, pectic substances, and hemicelluloses, gums and mucopolysaccharides. These polysaccharides are present in plant structure in a variety of structural forms so that it is possible for cellulose occasionally to have a degree of polymerisation with sugars present other than glucose. By and large, cellulose is a highly ordered structure, capable of strong intermolecular hydrogen bonding. It is insoluble in water, and is resistant to chemical and enzymatic attack. It may be polymerised in a microcrystalline form which can be used in the food industry as a stable aqueous suspension to be used as an emulsifier. On the other hand, if the cellulose is made into an ether, i.e. carboxymethyl or methylcellulose, then the result is a gel which is used to control the physical properties of food.

The β-glucans have a considerable degree of branching and degree of polymerisation. These form water-soluble materials which are gummy in texture. The pectic substances are important in the immature cell wall and consist of rhamnogalacturonans which are α (1–4)-D-galacturonans, with rhamnosyl insertions, and a variable proportion of carboxyl-carrying methoxyl groups. The water-soluble pectins form gels when combined with divalent ions. The methoxyl groups on uronic acid residues affect the gelling properties. Arabinogalactans, i.e. β (1–4) or (1–3)-D-galactopyranosides with arabino side chains found in most plants are water insoluble. The hemicelluloses are classified as galactomannans, i.e. β(1–4)-D-mannopyranosides with galactose side chains. Xylans are β(1–4)-D-xylopyranodyl chains with branching (1–3) with arabino and 4-O-methylglucuron side chains and xyloglucanan, i.e. β(1–4)-D-glucans with xylo side chains. These are found in many cell walls. They may form the storage forms in many seeds.

The plant gums which are used extensively pharmaceutically are the galactan (gum arabic), glucuronomannan (gum ghatti), galactomannan (tragacanthic acid gums, sterculia gum, locust bean gum, and guar gum), xylan (sapote gum) and xyloglucan (tamarind). These consist of a core structure with side chains which give rise to the complex physical properties of these substances. Often these gums are important for giving protection to the plant or holding water in seed coats. There are also algo polysaccharides which are used in foods such as agar, carrageens, and alginates. Again these are highly complex polymers in which the intermeshing of side chains are of paramount importance (SOUTHGATE 1976).

However, there are problems associated with regarding fibre as a chemical structure. The analogy with enzyme kinetics is perhaps a useful one. Imagine the amino acid sequence of chymotrypsin and urease being elucidated before the concept of Michaelis–Menten kinetics. Clearly the structural analysis of enzymes is of great importance, in the biological sense. Similarly, the nutritional value of vitamins preceded their chemical elucidation. There should thus be merit in seeking the role of fibre along the gastrointestinal tract. One such approach is to regard fibre as a physicochemical structure, passing like a sponge along the gastrointestinal tract. Such physicochemical properties include water-holding capacity, cation-exchange capacity, adsorption, matrix provision, and gel formation (EASTWOOD and MITCHELL 1976). It is only when the biological effects of fibre are understood that the complexities of the chemical analysis can be fully realised and the work of the analysts bear full fruition.

The problems of the analysis of dietary fibre are many. SOUTHGATE (1976) has elaborated a useful procedure for the analysis of dietary fibre. However, all methods are dogged by the presence of starch. These may cause certain restrictions on the quality of the results obtained. While the importance of the chemical classification of fibre is clearly recognised, few laboratories are capable of the meticulous attention required for the analysis. It is also assumed that the cultivars of fruit and vegetables from different countries grown under different circumstances all have the same chemical constitution, but the particular plant example analysed

Table 2. Physicochemical properties and gastrointestinal effects of dietary fibre

Physiochemical properties	Type of fibre	Modifying
Gel formation	Pectin Mucilages	Gastric emptying Mouth-to-caecum transit Small intestinal absorption
Water-holding capacity	Polysaccharides Lignins	Mouth-to-rectum transit Faecal weight Intraluminal pressure Faecal electrolytes
Matrix formation		Caecal bacterial metabolism
Bile acid adsorption	Lignin Pectin	Faecal steroids Cholesterol turnover
Cation exchange	Acidic polysaccharides Lignin	Faecal minerals
Antioxidant	Lignin	Free radical formation and action

may not be typical of its type. All the fruit and vegetables which we now eat have changed through the ages (Eastwood and Robertson 1978). The carrot is a good example. Originally this was a purple tap root, first described in Afghanistan in the sixth century. It reappeared in Holland in the seventeenth century as a white carrot for cattle food and an orange or modern carrot for human consumption. Until fairly recently carrots had a hard yellow core with an orange outer layer. This has been replaced by a cultivar which has an even appearance. The carrots which are now developed are often used for canning or freezing, so that the developmental work by the horticultural industry has been directed towards the requirements of the food industry rather than the fibre content of the carrot.

Although vegetable dietary fibre may be regarded as a physicochemical bolus passing along the gastrointestinal tract, it may alter gastric emptying time and absorption from the small intestine (Eastwood and Mitchell 1976). Furthermore, vegetable dietary fibre may also function in the colon. Here it forms a supporting matrix and provides surfaces upon which bacteria and intestinal contents can react. The principal physical properties of the matrix include water absorption, cation exchange and bile acid adsorption. Table 2 summarises the various physicochemical properties of dietary fibre and the effect of these along the gastrointestinal tract (Eastwood and Kay 1979). However, such a description of fibre is deceptive in that physical properties will, in the first instance, be influenced by the origin of the fibre and how it is prepared.

The physical properties, if they are analagous to, say, chromatography material, will be dictated by the capillary structure or ability to form gels. Therefore, a fibre source which has not been dried will behave quite distinctly from one which has been dried. The manner of drying, whether this be by air, freeze-drying or heat, will also affect the collapse of the capillaries and hence the ability to rehydrate. Straightforward evaporation of water from the gel collapses the gel to a nonporous solid. Another reaction which can cause problems in the heating of fibre sources

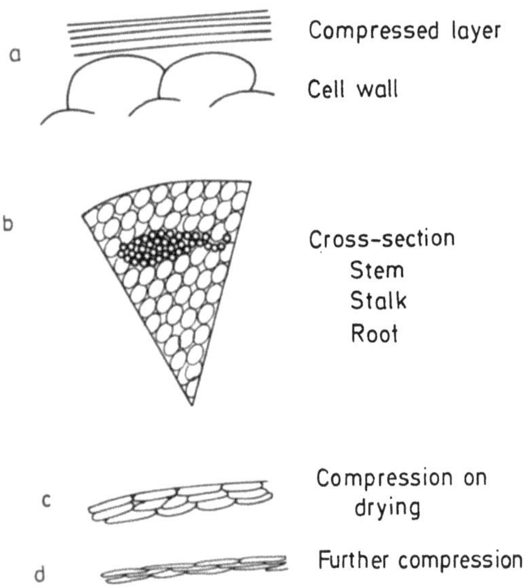

Fig. 1 a–d. Diagrammatic representations of fibre source in relationship to plant structure

in a nonenzymic browning called a Maillard reaction which alters the surface structure of the fibre. Such properties have been studied by paper industry chemists (Stone and Scallon 1968) and also by ruminant physiologists (Osbourn et al. 1976). In the conversion of wood to pulp for paper-making there is an excess of water present and the pulp production involves a constant modification of the lignocellulose gel as chemical and mechanical treatment removes materials from within the gel or ruptures the bonds which hold the matrix together. To some extent the processes of cooking or the production of fibre concentrates from fruit and vegetables are similar modifying processes. Again in the rumen, forage crops exist in the water-swollen state and the digestibility of the cellulose in the cell wall of these plants is almost certainly a function of the accessibility of the swollen wall to cellulose enzymes. A similar situation may well exist in the human colon.

Different types of structures are shown in Fig. 1 a which shows a structure of a seed coat, e.g. bran; a cross-section of a stem (Fig. 1 b); and the effect of drying that stem to a varying extent (Fig. 1 c, d). It is clear that the manner in which these fibres behave as they pass along the gastrointestinal tract will be different. The ability of water to infiltrate, expand and hence influence the sponge performance along the gut will be dictated by the space available to it within the plant cell wall.

Various sources of dietary fibre bind bile acids in vitro (Eastwood and Hamilton 1968; Birkner and Kerns 1974; Story and Kritchevsky 1976), and it has been shown that different lignins adsorb bile acids to a varying extent. Lignin is a complex polymer consisting of oxygenated phenylpropane units and obviously each polymer will have its own properties, Kay et al. (1979), have demonstrated that lignins vary in their capacity to bind bile acids. Autohydrolysis extraction conditions were maintained to produce lignins of known chemical composition, free from contaminants. The most effective lignin preparations in their studies were intermediate in their methoxyl content. This material demonstrated a preferential affinity for the unconjugated dihydroxy bile acids such as are formed by bacterial action in the colon. The possible adsorption mechanism may be through hydrophobic bonds.

IV. Gas

A further important physical phase along the length of the gastrointestinal tract is gas. Anaerobic bacteria in the gastrointestinal tract produce partially degraded low molecular weight carbon compounds, e.g. volatile fatty acids and a number of gases (PRINS 1977). Of these gases the major ones are carbon dioxide, hydrogen, and methane. The formation of hydrogen and methane is unique to anaerobic bacteria since no higher animal cells are known to produce these gases (CALLOWAY 1978; LEVITT and BOND 1970).

V. Bulking Agents

It is clear therefore that in evaluating the effects of bulking agents along the gut it is necessary to know the chemical structure, the physicochemical properties, the accessibility to bacterial degradation in the caecum and the consequence of this degradation, whether it be absorbable organic materials or volatile gases. This is not information that is readily available for any of the hydrophilic colloids either dietary or therapeutic. In discussing the effect of different fibres on colonic motility it is also important to recognise the effect of different fibre sources acting on the gastrointestinal tract. There are many contradictory experiments reported in the literature, which are often a function of the type and preparation of the fibre and the technique used to measure events along the gut rather than inherent differences between different experiments. GRIMES and GODDARD (1977) showed that there was no difference in the rate at which the solid phase of the gastric contents left the stomach after ingestion of wholemeal or white bread. Furthermore, the amount of liquid leaving the stomach unaccompanied, and therefore unbuffered by solid, was significantly greater after ingestion of white bread than wholemeal bread.

Gums and natural and synthetic particulate materials with quite different physical properties and chemical structures all affect the glucose tolerance curve. JENKINS et al. (1978) showed that the most important physical property is the viscosity and this has a considerable effect on absorption and transit time. Guar, the most viscous substance, was the most effective in decreasing postprandial glucose and insulin concentrations. Similarly, xylose excretion tended to be less than that of a control experiment. This suggests that there is slower absorption in the presence of these gels. The mouth-to-caecum transit time was related to the viscosity of the materials given. The action of viscous agents may be at two points, delaying gastric emptying and the absorption of glucose from the small intestinal lumen. The latter would result from a barrier to diffusion caused by an increased viscosity and the holding of materials within the gel.

The effect of various brans on stool weight in normal subjects and in patients with diverticular disease has been well explored. However, there are certain anomalies in the literature. For example, it was shown by FANTUS et al. (1941) that the size and shape of bran particles are factors in the laxative action of bran. They

Table 3. Effect of wheat bran on stool weight

Weight of Bran (g)	Period (weeks)	Stool weight (g)		Reference
		Initial	Final	
56	30	170 128–212	171 125–215	Hoppert and Clark (1942)
16	3	107±44	174±51	Eastwood et al. (1973)
20	4	120±18	183±22	Findlay et al. (1974)
12[a]	2	131±17	140± 9	Wyman et al. (1976)
20[a]			164±20	
12[b]			183±21	
20[b]			159±13	
17–45	3	79± 1	228±30	Cummings et al.·(1976)
23–35	3	125 (59–194)	225 (154–290)	Kay and Truswell (1977a)
38	1	93±10	166±15	Walters et al. (1975)
84	3	103±40	266±90	Fuchs et al. (1976)
20	3	140	320[c] 199[b]	Brodribb and Groves (1978)
20	3	95	197	Cummings et al. (1978b)
36	3	71± 6.2	217±12	Jenkins et al. (1975)

[a] Cooked bran; [b] raw bran; [c] coarse bran; [d] fine bran

used bran of different particle size which had previously been through the processes employed in the manufacture of a commercial bran breakfast cereal. They found that there was no correlation between the particle size of bran and the laxative action when measured by the effect on stool weight. Crude fibre prepared from bran also showed laxative effects, and so crude fibre itself appeared to be the active principle of bran. However, Brodribb and Groves (1978) showed that wheat bran, when taken as large particulate material, or after milling to small particles, had differing effects on the stool weight. After ingestion of coarse bran, the stool weight (219 g/day) was significantly greater than after ingestion of fine bran (199 g/day). The reason for the differing effect is that the coarse bran they used had a greater water-holding capacity: 7.3 g water for 1 g coarse bran, compared with 3.9 g water for 1 g fine bran.

Some important experiments by Cummings et al. (1978b) showed that fibre concentrates from different sources had a variable effect on stool weight. It must be emphasised, however, that these experiments used fibre concentrates, not fresh plant material. The concentrates represented fibre which had been dried and concentrated 20–40 times, although the fibre concentrate had a similar chemical composition to that of fresh carrot, cabbage and apple fibre. This suggested to them that processing had not altered the fibre to any extent chemically. Groups of six subjects took apple, carrot, cabbage, and bran and the increase in stool weight varied for the different concentrates. The faecal weight changes correlated with the amount of the pentose fraction of the noncellulose polysaccharides. The hexose and pentose contents of noncellulose polysaccharides are usually inversely related. There are individual variations in response to a given fibre intake, and such individual responses could not be ascribed to the intake of pentose-containing polysaccharide.

Table 4. Comparison of effects of fruit and vegetable fibre sources

Fibre source	Weight (g)	Period (days)	Stool weight (g)		Reference
			Initial	Final	
Carrot concentrate	20	21	117	189	CUMMINGS et al. (1978b)
Cabbage concentrate	20	21	88	143	
Apple concentrate	20	21	141	203	
Guar concentrate	20	21	120	139	
Plant fibre	60	28	177±40	240±35	RAYMOND et al. (1977)
Fruit and vegetable fibre	20	26	89± 9	208± 9	KELSAY et al. (1978)
Citrus pectin	15	21	140	168	KAY and TRUSWELL (1977b)
Pectin		21	150±10	186±15	DURRINGTON et al. (1976)
Carrot	6	21	142±37	177±33	ROBERTSON et al. (1979)
Fruit, vegetables 50%, bran 50%	20	21	69±50	184±75	STASSE-WOLTHUIS et al. (1979)
Cellulose	16	21	152±32	221±58	

In humans, all fractions of dietary fibre, except lignin, are digested to some extent by colonic microflora. Such digestion may alter the water-holding capacity. The extent of digestion of the fibre could determine individual responses to a given fibre. The digestion of dietary fibre fractions was underlined by HOLLOWAY et al. (1978), who compared two groups of subjects: healthy subjects with an ileostomy and normal subjects. Both groups were given a regulated diet of known cellulose, hemicellulose and lignin content. The fibre content of the faeces was measured by the acid and neutral detergent method. Some 85% of the ingested cellulose was excreted intact by the ileostomy subjects. Where the colon was intact in normal subjects only 22% of ingested cellulose was excreted, indicating that approximately 80% of the cellulose was digested in normal subjects. Of the water-insoluble hemicellulose ingested, 28% was excreted from the small bowel, 4% from normal subjects. This represents approximately 96% digestion of the hemicellulose in normal subjects.

However, the large unknown is the role of bacteria in influencing stool weight. STEPHENS and CUMMINGS (1980) take the view that a factor in changing the stool weight is an increase in the bacterial content of the stool. This is more likely to apply with fruit and vegetables than with bran which appears to pass through the gastrointestinal tract unchanged by the presence of bacteria. Tables 3 and 5 summarise a number of papers in which the effects of bran and fruit and vegetables on stool weight have been examined. It will be seen that there is a wide range of responses. Whether or not the fibre is hydrolysed by bacteria in the caecum, bran appears not to be hydrolysed and other fruit and vegetables appear to be extensively hydrolysed. Pentose-containing noncellulose polysaccharides appear to be the most resistant to hydrolysis by bacteria. However, highly hydrated fibre sources with large water-holding capacity may well be the most vulnerable to bacterial attack and therefore compression of fibre and collapse of capillary structure may be another important factor.

C. Actions of Fibre and of Operations on the Colon Muscle in Diverticular Disease

Pari passu with the fibre studies already described, fundamental advances were being achieved in the physiopathology of diverticular disease and its management. Three important advances were made. First, the recognition that the disease is characterised by marked thickening of the large bowel muscle in the region of the sigmoid colon. The muscle abnormality is often the main abnormality, rather than any inflammatory change. The diverticula are sometimes difficult to show in resected specimens and even their demonstration in radiographs may occasionally be difficult. Second, the thickened muscle produces a high intraluminal pressure, as the thickened circular muscle, plus the overlying crescent folds of mucosa, occludes the lumen, producing localised "chambers" within which the high pressure is created. These high pressures have been described by ARFWIDSSON (1964), PAINTER and TRUELOVE (1964), ATTISHA and SMITH (1969) and others, and are thought to be the principal reason for the herniation of the mucosa. The third, most recent advance has been the clinical finding that cereal fibre produced clinical improvement in patients with constipation and diverticular disease. When this was introduced as a clinical regimen there was no correlation with the other two factors. It had already been argued on epidemiological grounds that because of the low fibre content of Western diet, and perhaps with its higher content of refined absorbable products, the faeces were low in bulk and became further diminished or dehydrated as a result of prolonged transit in the large intestine. It was thus envisaged that it would be more difficult for the faecal bolus to pass through the sigmoid colon and enter the rectum. In this process the mechanical difficulties of onward transmission of pellety faecal contents were seen as leading to smooth muscle thickening. Thus the emphasis swung away from the diverticulum to the abnormal muscle function of the large bowel. It is in the alteration of this sequence that the importance of fibre lies.

Fibre has been further implicated in colonic disease by the contrasting states of Africa and Asia on the one hand and the Western World on the other: in the former there is minimal diverticular disease, a high fibre diet and bulky faeces and a fast intestinal transit – changed in each detail in the West to a high incidence of diverticular disease, a low fibre intake, pellety stools and an intestinal transit time prolonged several days more than that of the African and the Asian. Yet if this hypothesis were true the dietary abnormality must operate for a very long period of time before overt disease is produced since the incidence of the defect (colonic diverticulosis) does not become appreciable until the fifth decade of life.

In view of the clinical improvement generally recorded with cereal fibre it appeared important to document the action of this substance on the intraluminal pressure, seen according to the "pressure theory" as the established main factor. But first, proof was required that pressure was high. The operation of longitudinal colomyotomy had been introduced by REILLY in 1966 and afforded the opportunity not only to assess the efficacy of the operation in relationship to how far it is possible to lower the intraluminal pressure by this means, but also to analyse the role of the colonic muscle in this condition. If excessive intraluminal pressure were the important factor in the genesis of diverticular disease, operations for diverticular disease should be judged on their ability to reduce this. If the action of fibre were to reduce the pressure and were this a valid treatment, operations would have to withstand comparison with this. Moreover, possible beneficial effects of operations could easily lapse if patients continued to be exposed after operation to the same conditions of fibre deficiency as preoperatively, and this could be counteracted, perhaps simply by increasing the fibre content of the diet.

It therefore seemed important: (1) to define the effect of the common operations performed for diverticular disease on the muscle on the intraluminal pressure, i.e. motility terms; (2) to determine how long the effects of operation last in patients left on their original diet compared with others given bran supplements postoperatively; (3) to define the effect, compared with (1), of added dietary fibre alone; and (4) to determine the changes produced by the bulk-producing agents such as bran ispaghula, lactulose, and sterculia. (For details of methods see SMITH et al. 1974.)

I. Changes Induced by Operation

There was no difference in basal motility between normal subjects and diverticular disease patients before and after the operation of myotomy. Colonic activity was significantly increased after all forms of stimulation in diverticular disease, the effect being greatest after administration of prostigmine (ATTISHA and SMITH 1969). These responses in diverticular disease patients were reduced to normal levels by myotomy and the patients were rendered symptom free. Myotomy thus confirmed the importance of the smooth muscle and of the pressure theory in diverticular disease.

Resection of the sigmoid colon was performed in a group comparable to the myotomy patients, i.e. with local obstructive features, high intraluminal pressure and a thick bowel muscle at operation. The motility index, high initially, remained raised after operation compared with normal subjects. Thus local resection of the pelvic colon (this was all that was carried out) did not restore to normal the inherent abnormality of the large bowel muscle, which must be more generalised than in the sigmoid area. Myotomy and resection patients were then followed for more than 3 years. A fall in the mean motility index (shown for prostigmine stimulation only) occurred during the first year following myotomy but over the subsequent 3-year period there was a considerable return in the mean pressure activity, and by 5 years this had risen to the same high preoperative level. In contrast, the motility index after colonic resection rose to levels very slightly above those recorded before operation. Furthermore, many of these patients still had symptoms. All the myotomy patients had a recurrence of their original symptoms at 3–5 years but with less severity than formerly.

The mean motility indices in patients after resection and myotomy were also contrasted with a comparable group of patients who were given 20 g unprocessed bran daily postoperatively. It has already been recorded that the mean motility indices after resection rose; this level was markedly lower in resection patients maintained on bran postoperatively. The mean motility indices after myotomy fell at

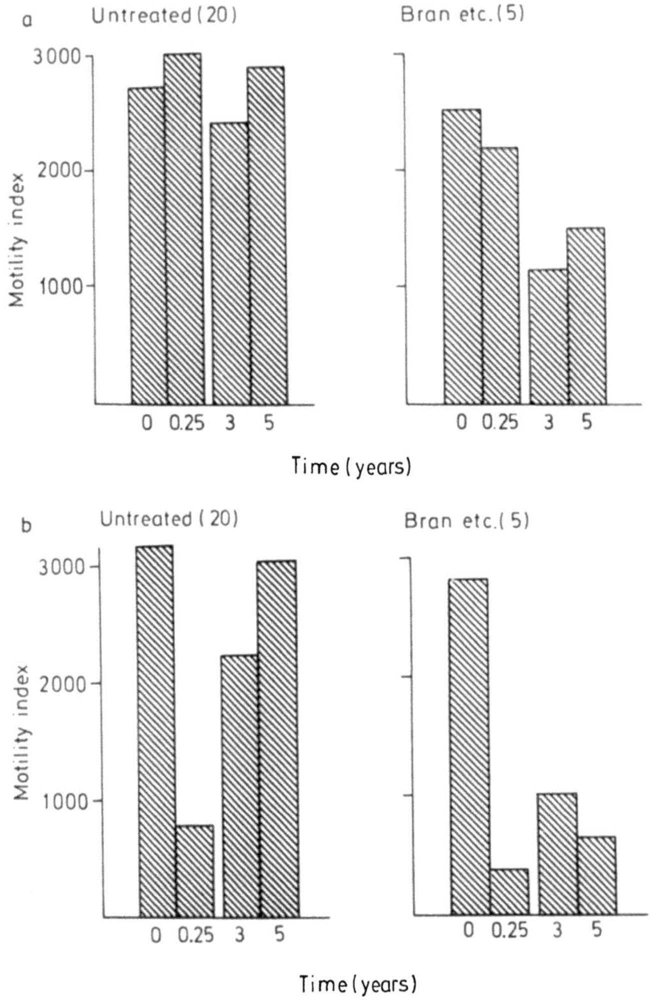

Fig. 2. a Mean motility index for 5 years after resection; lower values in patients taking bran. Numbers of patients shown in parentheses. **b** Mean motility index lowered by myotomy but partial recovery in 3 years, complete by 5 years, lower values in patients taking bran. Numbers of patients shown in parentheses (Smith et al. 1974)

first, but by 5 years this trend had reversed (Fig. 2). However, when myotomy patients took bran postoperatively they showed a fall in pressure which was held at a much lower level than in comparable patients with uncomplicated diverticular disease treated by operation without bran.

II. Changes Induced by Cereal Fibre

The weight of faeces produced by Africans has been shown in field studies by Burkitt et al. (1972) to contrast markedly with the European output. When bran was given to normal British subjects it significantly increased the stool weight and this can be shown to be due to an increase in its water content. The increase in stool

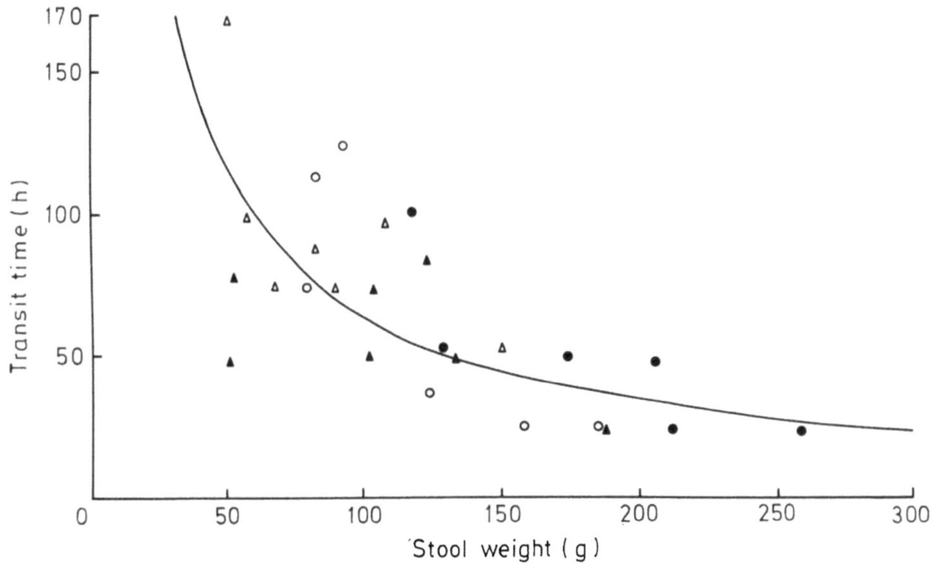

Fig. 3. Plot of transit time against daily stool weight. *Open circles* normal subjects before bran therapy; *closed circles* normal subjects after bran therapy; *open triangles* diverticular disease patients before bran therapy; *closed triangles* diverticular disease patient after bran therapy (FINDLAY et al. 1974)

weight is less apparent in diverticular disease, probably because it starts from a lower value (FINDLAY et al. 1974). Relative changes in weight can be shown by marking the liquids and solids. The intestinal liquids are marked by the water-soluble PEG 4000, the solids by chromium sesquioxide. Both are injested at the same time and mix well with their respective phases. After equilibration of markers of the two phases, both are reduced in concentration after bran consumption. This suggests that, whatever the increase in solids as a result of bran intake, dilution occurs in the colon and that the effect of bran is mainly due to water binding. This is in keeping with the observed alteration to a more gelatinous stool consistency after ingestion of bran.

Africans also have a reduced transit time. Several observations have now shown that the intestinal transit is prolonged in symptomatic diverticular disease compared with normal subjects and that it is significantly shortened by bran, more so than in normal subjects. There is an interesting reciprocal relationship apparent in the graph of Fig. 3. In normal subjects, a change in stool weight induced by bran may not be accompanied by much change in transit time, since it occurs where the curve has flattened off; whereas in symptomatic diverticular disease, transit time may be significantly accelerated with very little change in the faecal weight, since with lower faecal weights the curve is steeper. In general, therefore, little change in the output of faeces is necessary to provide an expeditious transit in diverticular disease and can thus correct both "anomalies." Slow transit was evident throughout the various segments of the colon; in both symptomatic diverticular disease and idiopathic constipation the acceleration produced by bran occurred in all segments (KIRWAN and SMITH 1977).

Table 5. Mean motility indices (±standard errors) in 13 patients with diverticular disease before and after 4 weeks treatment with coarse bran

	Basal	After food	After neostigmine
Before coarse bran	878±192	1,812±391	2,758±514
After coarse bran	335±108	733±237	1,545±355
P	<0.01	<0.01	<0.01

The motility paradox of CONNELL (1962) is well known: that raised intracolonic pressures accompany constipation and that pressures are low in diarrhoea. Partly this is explicable by the local conditions which accompany the pressure change – spasmodic contraction may produce a long "open" length of gut in which there is little measurable pressure change. The sigmoid intraluminal pressure in diverticular disease has generally been found to be raised (ARFWIDSSON 1964; PAINTER and TRUELOVE 1964; ATTISHA and SMITH 1969) but to be lowered by the administration of bran. The high pressure of diverticular disease is also lowered by severing the colonic muscle in the operation of myotomy (ATTISHA and SMITH 1969). Bran may exert its action like myotomy; both may affect the muscle by diminishing its segmenting activity, but both could also act by creating a bowel with a wider lumen which would automatically, on physical grounds, lead to a reduced pressure or tension acting on the wall.

The transit time was only significantly reduced in diverticular disease patients on bran. The stool weight was increased by an average of 63 g in normal subjects but not significantly in diverticular disease patients (17 g; FINDLAY et al. 1974).

In 13 patients with diverticular disease, basal motility was reduced by bran therapy but the response to food fell below basal levels; the response to cholinergic stimulation (prostigmine) fell by 50% after ingestion of bran (Table 5). The main findings in regard to bran and diverticular disease are thus in agreement with the hypothesis that this agent, known to be capable of relieving the symptoms, also lowers the intraluminal pressure, increases the bulk of the faeces and speeds the transit. TAYLOR and DUTHIE (1978) have also described pressure reduction and have added the observation that the rapid electrical rhythm which is characteristic of diverticular disease is abolished by bran. BRODRIBB and HUMPHREYS (1976) reinforce this by adding the finding that the counts of waves were greatly reduced in the sigmoid colon in 40 patients treated with bran for a longer period of 6 months.

The mechanism of the action of bran on the colon muscle has been further elucidated in a study of the respective actions of coarse and fine bran in diverticular diseases (KIRWAN et al. 1974). The former was much more effective than the latter in reducing the intraluminal colonic pressure and the transit time. That one bran was coarser than the other was shown by shaking the two brans for 90 min in test sieves of increasing aperture. The flour from each bran which passed through the mesh was weighed. Less of the coarse bran passed through the sieves of small pore size.

The water-binding capacity was more marked for the coarse bran. Coarse and fine bran respectively held 6.0 and 2.4 g water for 1 g bran. The acid detergent fibre

Table 6. Comparison of the effects on colonic motility of fine and coarse bran taken separately and consecutively

	Basal	After food	After neostigmine
A. Coarse and fine bran motility index taken separately			
Before coarse bran	892 ±196	1,513 ±456	2,120 ±405
After coarse bran	648.7±339	446.1±130	1,216.8±398
P	n.s.	<0.01	<0.01
Before fine bran	1,181±489	1,429±405	4,075±873
After fine bran	1,269±468	2,534±653	4,661±410
P	n.s.	n.s.	n.s.
B. Fine bran followed by coarse bran			
After fine bran	1,202±596	2,369±811	4,726±522
Followed by coarse bran	303±168	1,459±637	2,746±749
P	<0.01	<0.01	<0.05
Comparison of motility change	n.s.	<0.005	<0.05

n.s. = not significant

content was 15.1% and 9.7% with a higher lignin content for the coarse (4.1%) than the five (2.6%) bran. After milling both brans to a particle size of <1 mm in the laboratory, the water-holding capacities were approximately equal, although the fibre content remained the same. Our observations suggest that bran with coarse particles binds more water and thus provides more bulk in the stool than does bran with finer particles. The marked difference in the effect of the two brans on bowel function was unexpected. Fine bran failed completely, unlike coarse bran, to reduce the colonic motility index (Table 6) and the gastrointestinal transit time. The beneficial effect of coarse bran is probably related to its water-holding effect which gives rise to a soft bulky stool which is easily passed. The change in the motility index resulting from ingestion of bran may also depend upon the bulk provided, since intraluminal pressure depends not only on the force exerted by the colonic muscle, but also upon the diameter of the bowel lumen and the viscosity of its contents. These results indicate that particle size could be of fundamental importance in determining not only the water-holding capacity but also the clinical efficacy of bran. It is possible, however, that if fine bran were given in a large dose, there would be sufficient large particles with a water-holding capacity to improve bowel function; but fine bran also contains a considerable amount of absorbable carbohydrate and the dose used might result in unacceptable weight gain.

III. Other Agents

The symptoms of diverticular disease arise in patients who have, in the main, a small stool weight, prolonged intestinal transit and a raised intracolonic pressure (Painter 1975). The rational basis of the treatment of diverticular disease is prin-

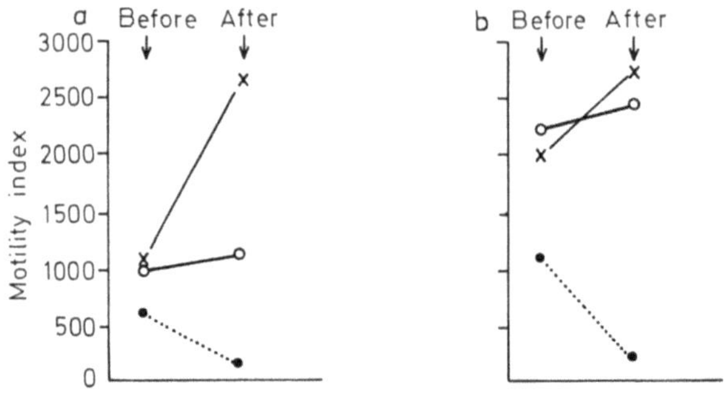

Fig. 4 a, b. Mean motility indices after treatment with bran, Fybogel and lactulose; change in the basal motility index **a** and also after food **b**, with each agent. *Open circles*, lactulose; *full circles*, bran; *crosses*, Fybogel

cipally to reduce the raised intraluminal pressure. Since the various agents used in therapy would be expected to share in promoting this, we have recently examined three compounds which can be used in the treatment of diverticular disease: wheat bran, Fybogel, whichis an ispaghula colloid (GODDING 1976), and lactulose, which is a synthesised disaccharide unabsorbed in the small intestine and hydrolysed by bacteria in the caecum.

All the agents administered were found to increase the stool weight although only in patients on Fybogel did it reach significance. All the patients expressed satisfaction at the increased stool production, but the patients on lactulose complained of excessive flatus. Cereal bran reduced the transit time from a median of 88 to 50 h. Bran lowered motility but the effect of lactulose was insignificant (Fig. 4): but, Fybogel increased the basal motility from a median of 1150 (range 284–2,034) to 2,100 (range 0–3,309). Bran also reduced the food-stimulated pressure, but there was no significant effect of Fybogel or lactulose on the food-stimulated colonic motility.

Changes in motility expressed as "motility index" could mask the nature of the underlying motor response, as this index is a product of the wave amplitude and the duration of the motor effect. For example, a common "motility" result could be arrived at by many smaller waves or less frequent large waves. Waves of greater amplitude might, however, be more damaging to the colon and responsible for some of the symptoms or of the pathology of diverticular disease. Furthermore, it could be argued that these are the ones which the effective agents should be abolishing. Counts of the waves (Fig. 5) in the amplitude range 50–80 cm H_2O were made and the average number of waves recorded per patient in each treatment group. On bran, the number of waves was reduced at each 10 cm H_2O pressure level in a 1-h period of activity examined after a food stimulus. Fybogel, on the contrary, raised the average number of waves whereas lactulose had no effect. Since the effect of Fybogel in raising the basal motility and the number of high pressure waves present after ingestion of food is contrary to what one expects of a bulk-acting agent, the experiment was repeated with four patients on a double dose of Fybogel per day. The stool weight and the basal motility were again increased but without further significant changes.

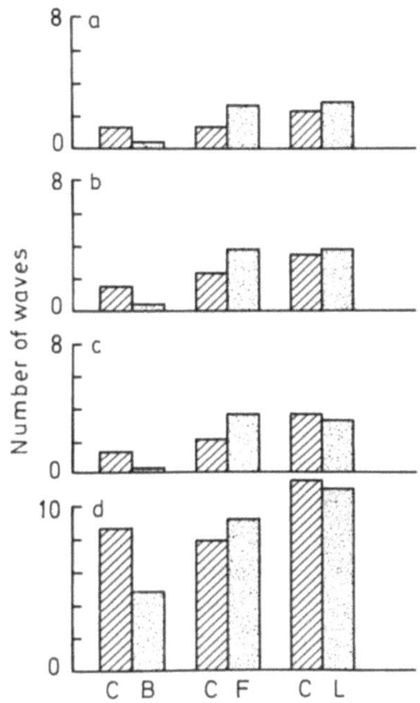

Fig. 5 a–d. Effect of bran *B*, Fybogel *F*, and Lactulose *L* on postprandial waves before *C* and after treatment *B*, *F*, *L*. Pressures (in cmH_2O) are 80 **a**; 70 **b**; 60 **c**; 50 **d**. Vertical axis shows average number of waves per patient (EASTWOOD et al. 1978)

This type of result reflects the diversity which can be obtained in the manometry of diverticular disease (EASTWOOD et al. 1978). The therapeutic agents which we tested might have been expected to decrease intracolonic pressure since they equally relieved the symptoms of diverticular disease. Given raised pretreatment pressures, a reduction would be expected after successful therapy, not, as is found for Fybogel, an increase. Coarse bran has already been shown to exert a reduction in pressure (KIRWAN et al. 1974). There is no uniform relationship between the modification of symptoms and the efficacy of the compounds in lowering pressure, in the short term at least. This raises some doubt about the overall importance of "features" of diverticular disease – low stool weight, the prolonged transit time, and the raised intraluminal pressure – normally considered to be hallmarks of this disease. Although two of the agents used here raised the intraluminal pressure or left it unchanged, both produced an equivalent symptomatic relief. The patients were mainly complaining of constipation, apart from abdominal pain and discomfort, and it is possible that part of the therapeutic effect is achieved by overcoming factors such as stasis. Yet agents which raise or leave pressure unchanged, even though they relieve symptoms, may not in the long run be entirely free of the risk of producing further damage to the bowel in diverticular disease. Thus we would have to draw a distinction between what constitutes a truly efficacious agent and what does not; and conclude that coarse bran remains the most efficacious agent, not only by reducing symptoms but by adding to the stool weight and lowering the intraluminal pressure in diverticular disease.

D. Actions in Other Colonic Diseases

The muscle abnormality in the irritable bowel syndrome has certain similarities with early diverticular disease. The main points of differentiation appear to be the increased basal pressure, probably derived from muscle spasm. In diverticular disease the resting pressure is not elevated although the muscle is thick and hypertrophic, and the intraluminal pressure is increased only after stimulation by food and cholinergic drugs. Another significant difference is the presence of fast waves in the irritable bowel of a type not seen in diverticular disease. On the basis of the raised motility index present after stimuli such as the gastrocolic reflex one could make a case for the use of cereal fibre or hydrophilic colloids in the "spastic" type of irritable bowel syndrome. Even in diverticular disease WEINRICH (1977) has suggested that a "colicky sigmoid syndrome" and diverticula might occur independently in the population. The probability of coincidence increased with age since the presence of diverticula is age dependent. The action of bulk additives might lower the incidence of the colicky sigmoid syndrome, but on this basis might not necessarily lower the incidence of diverticula. One has to differentiate between an action on the muscle which may induce relief of symptoms and actions which may influence the aetiology of the disease. Another means whereby hydrophilic colloid agents might find a role in the irritable colon syndrome is in the management of the form associated with diarrhoea rather than constipation. HEATON and his colleagues have described how bran may "normalise" the intestinal transit; paradoxically, the addition of bulking agents to the diet can influence constipation, but may just as readily by water and electrolyte absorption influence the diarrhoeal state (PAYLER et al. (1975). Clinical trials in these aspects of the irritable colon syndrome are lacking and are of course needed.

Bulk agents may be used in ulcerative colitis on similar grounds. DAVIES and RHODES (1978) attempted to study this and compared a high fibre diet and sulphasalazine to determine whether fibre could replace sulphasalazine in keeping ulcerative colitis patients in remission. Only 25% of patients with ulcerative colitis could satisfactorily take the high fibre diet instead of sulphasalazine. A greater application may be in patients liable to develop colonic stasis, the so-called constipated colitics who may occasionally have diverticular disease but who may have a condition like diverticular disease with high intraluminal pressure in the left or distal colon and who may develop dilatation of the right or proximal colon.

There is no record of patients with carcinoma of the colon having elevated intraluminal pressures in the distal colon, yet their intestinal transit is in general prolonged, as befits differences between the Western World and Africa and Asia, described so well by BURKITT et al. (1972). HILL et al. (1975) gave point to the Burkitt hypothesis by describing a mechanism whereby delayed colonic transit and the action of organisms, particularly nuclear dehydrogenating (NDH) clostridia, might conspire to allow the degradation of the bile acids to a carcinogenic form within the colon. Confirmatory evidence of this is as yet lacking. In the long term, studies are required of groups who are prepared voluntarily to speed up their own intestinal transit by fibre and other agents. They would after all only be following the example of the population of doctors, now an interesting group, who abandoned smoking 20 years ago. It would be interesting to know in the long term if the experiences of such a group would change the incidence of carcinoma of the colon in high risk countries such as Scotland.

E. Clinical Application of Fibre and Hydrophilic Colloid Additives

Experience with the therapeutic use of dietary fibre has resulted in the formulation of the following general principles (BRODRIBB 1978):

1) A precise diagnosis, with routine examination by sigmoidoscopy and barium enema, should be made before starting a high fibre diet. The use of bran as a diagnostic test is strongly deprecated.
2) Fibre intake should be increased in stages over a 3–4-week period to reduce the sensations of abdominal distension and discomfort associated with a sudden change in colonic filling.
3) It may be helpful to give an antispasmodic agent as well for the first few months.
4) It is probably best to use cereal fibre. An increase of 5–20 g/day in dietary fibre may be required. This can be given as bran or high fibre products such as wholemeal bread, bran biscuits, and high fibre breakfast cereals. The increased fibre intake should be taken regularly each day. The aim should be to establish a new dietary regime that can be maintained for a lifetime. A dietitian is usually best qualified to achieve this.
5) Patients should be warned that a maximal therapeutic response will probably take at least 3 months from the time a high fibre diet is started, and that a dramatic, rapid effect is not to be anticipated.
6) Even if a high fibre diet has been established, 10%–20% of subjects may have persistent symptoms. This may have a number of causes. Undiagnosed inflammatory complications such as chronic pericolic abscess or stricture may be present. Many patients in our studies had other diseases such as gallstones, peptic ulcers or hiatus hernias and the symptoms may be due to these. Severe neuroses may be associated with a very low pain threshold, so that normal abdominal sensations appear as symptoms. CORRY (1963) described a group of patients with diverticular disease who improved with a milk-free diet, and screening for hypolactasia should be considered. The possibility that a carcinoma of the colon or other colonic lesion had been missed initially should always be considered.

The value of dietary fibre in the treatment of uncomplicated diverticular disease has now been established. It appears to be more effective even than ablative surgery and no other treatment has been shown to give a better therapeutic response.

References

Arfwidsson S (1964) Pathogenesis of multiple diverticula of the sigmoid colon in diverticular disease. Acta Chir Scand [Suppl] 342:1–68

Attisha RP, Smith AN (1969) Pressure activity of the colon and rectum in diverticular disease before and after sigmoid myotomy. Br J Surg 56:891–894

Birkner HJ, Kerns F Jr (1974) In vitro adsorption of bile salts to food residues salicylazosulphapyridine and hemicellulose. Gastroenterology 67:237–244

Brodribb AJM (1978) The treatment of diverticular disease with dietary fibre. In: Third Kellog Nutrition Symposium. Libbey, London, pp 63–73
Brodribb AJM, Groves C (1978) Effect of bran particle size on stool weight. Gut 19:60–63
Brodribb AJM, Humphreys DM (1976) Diverticular disease – three studies. Br Med J 1:424–430
Burkitt DP, Walker ARP, Painter NS (1972) Effect of dietary fibre on stools and transit times, and its role in the causation of disease. Lancet 2:1408
Calloway DH (1978) Gas in the alimentary canal. In: Code CF (ed) Alimentary canal. American Physiological Society, Washington, DC (Handbook of physiology, vol IV, sect 6, p 2839)
Connell AM (1962) The motility of the pelvic colon. Gut 3:342–348
Corry DC (1963) Milk in diverticula of the colon. Br. Med J 1:930
Cummings JH, Hill MJ, Jenkins DJ et al. (1976) Changes in fecal composition and colonic function due to cereal fibre. Am J Clin Nutr 29:1468–1473
Cummings JH, Wiggins HS, Jenkins DJA, Houston H, Jivraj T, Drasar BS, Hill MJ (1978 a) Influence of diets high and low in animal fat on bowel habit, gastrointestinal transit time, fecal microflora, bile acid, and fat excretion. J Clin Invest 61:953–963
Cummings JH, Branch W, Jenkins DJA, Southgate DAT, Houston H, James WPT (1978 b) Colonic response to dietary fibre from carrot, cabbage, apple, bran, and guar gum. Lancet 1:5–8
Davies PS, Rhodes J (1978) Maintenance of remission in ulcerative colitis with a sulphasalazine or a high fibre diet: a clinical trial. Br Med J 1:1524–1525
Debongnie JC, Phillips SF (1978) Capacity of the human colon to absorb fluid. Gastroenterology 74:698–703
Durrington PN, Manning AP, Boston CH et al. (1976) Effects on serum lipids and lipoproteins, whole gut transit time and stool weight. Lancet 2:394–396
Eastwood MA, Hamilton D (1968) Studies on the adsorption of bile salts to non-absorbed components of diet. Biochim Biophys Acta 152:165–173
Eastwood MA, Kay RM (1979) A hypothesis for the action of dietary fibre along the gastrointestinal tract. Am J Clin Nutr 32:364–367
Eastwood MA, Mitchell WD (1976) Physical properties of fibre. In: Spiller GA, Amer RJ (eds) Fibre in human nutrition. New York, London, pp 109–129
Eastwood MA, Robertson JA (1978) The place of dietary fibre in our diet. J Human Nutr 32:53–61
Eastwood MA, Kirkpatrick JR, Mitchell WD, Bone A, Hamilton T (1973) Effects of dietary supplements of wheat bran and cellulose on faeces and bowel function. Br Med J 4:392–394
Eastwood MA, Smith AM, Brydon WG, Pritchard J (1978) Comparison of bran, ispaghula, and lactulose on colon function in diverticular disease. Gut 19:1144–1147
Elliott TR, Barclay-Smith E (1904) Antiperistalsis and other muscular activities of the colon. J Physiol (Lond) 31:272–304
Fantus B, Hirschberg N, Frankl W (1941) Mode of action of bran. Rev Gastroenterol 8:277–280
Findlay JM, Smith AN, Mitchell WD, Anderson AJB, Eastwood MA (1974) Effects of unprocessed bran on colon function in normal subjects and in diverticular disease. Lancet 1:146–149
Fuchs HM, Dorfmann S, Floch MH (1976) The effect of dietary fiber supplements in man. Alterations in fecal physiology and bacterial flora. Am J Clin Nutr 29:1443–1447
Godding EW (1976) Constipation and allied disorders, reprinted from the Pharmaceutical Journal. Pharmaceutical Press, London
Grimes DS, Goddard J (1977) Gastric emptying of wholemeal and white bread. Gut 18:723–729
Hill MJ, Drasar BS, Williams REO, Meade TW, Cox AG, Simpson DEP, Morson BC (1975) Faecal bile acids and clostridia in patients with bowel cancer. Lancet 1:535–538
Holloway WD, Tasman-Jones C, Lee SP (1978) Digestion of certain fractions of dietary fiber in humans. Am J Clin Nutr 31:927–930

Hoppert CA, Clark AJ (1942) Effect of long continued consumption of bran by normal men. J Am Diet Assoc 18:524–525
Jenkins DJA, Hill MJ, Cummings JH (1975) Effect of wheat fibre on blood lipids, fecal steroid excretion and serum iron. Am J Clin Nutr 28:1408–1411
Jenkins DJA, Wolever TMS, Leeds AR et al. (1978) Dietary fibres, fibre analogues and glucose tolerance: importance of viscosity. Br Med J 1:1392–1394
Kay RM, Truswell AS (1977a) The effect of wheat fibre on plasma lipids and faecal steroids excretion in man. Br J Nutr 37:227–235
Kay RM, Truswell AS (1977b) The effect of citrus pectins on blood lipids and fecal steroid excretion in man. Am J Clin Nutr 30:171–175
Kay RM, Strasberg SM, Petrunka CN, Wayman M (1979) Differential adsorption of bile acids by lignin. In: Inglett C, Falkehag I (eds) Dietary fibers: chemistry and nutrition. Academic Press, New York, pp 57–67
Kelsay JL, Behall KM, Prather ES (1978) Effects of fiber from fruits and vegetables on the metabolic responses of human subjects. Am J Clin Nutr 31:1149–1153
Kirwan WA, Smith AN (1977) Colonic propulsion in diverticular disease, idiopathic constipation, and the irritable colon syndrome. Scand J Gastroenterol 12:331–335
Kirwan WO, Smith AN, Mitchell WD, Anderson AJB, Eastwood MA (1974) Effects of unprocessed bran on colon function in normal subjects and in diverticular disease. Lancet 1:146–149
Levitt MD, Bond HJ Jr (1970) Volume composition and source of intestinal gas. Gastroenterology 59:921–929
McLaren JW, King JB, Copland WA (1955) Preliminary observations on veripaque and colonic actuates for use with barium enemata. Br J Radiol 28:285–294
McNeil NI, Cummings JH, James WPT (1978) Short chain fatty acid absorption by the human large intestine. Gut 19:819–822
Mitchell WD, Eastwood MA (1976) Dietary fiber and colon function. In: Spiller GA, Amen RJ (eds) Fiber in human nutrition. Plenum, New York London, p 185
Osbourn DF, Beever DE, Thomson DJ (1976) The influence of physical processing on the intake digestion and utilization of dried herbage. Proc Nutr Soc 35:191–199
Painter NS (1975) Diverticular disease of the colon. Heinemann, London
Painter NS, Truelove SC (1964) The intraluminal pressure patterns in diverticula of the colon. Gut 5:365–373
Payler DK, Pomare EW, Heaton KW, Harvey RF (1975) The effect of wheat bran on intestinal transit. Gut 16:209–213
Prins RA (1977) Biochemical activities of gut micro-organisms. In: Clark RTS, Bauchop T (eds) Microbial ecology of the gut. Academic Press, London, p 71
Raymond TL, Conner WE, Lin DS et al. (1977) The interaction of dietary fibers and cholesterol upon the plasma lipids and lipoproteins sterol balance and bowel function in human subjects. J Clin Invest 60:1429–1437
Reilly M (1966) Sigmoid myotomy. Br J Surg 53:859
Robertson J, Brydon WG, Tadesse K, Wenham P, Walls A, Eastwood MA (1979) The effect of raw carrots on lipids and colonic function. Am J Clin Nutr 32:1889–1892
Smith AN, Kirwan WO, Shariff S (1974) Motility effects of operations performed for diverticular diesease. Proc R Soc Med 67:1041–1043
Southgate DAT (1976) The chemistry of dietary fiber. In: Spiller GA, Amen RJ (eds) Fiber in human nutrition. Plenum, New York London, pp 31–72
Southgate DAT, Hudson GJ, Englyst H (1978) The analysis of dietary fibre – the choices for the analyst. J Sci Food Agric 29:979–988
Staase-Wolthuis M, Hermus RJJ, Bausch JE (1979) The effect of a natural high fibre diet on serum lipids, faecal lipids, and colonic function. Am J Clin Nutr 32:1881–1888
Stephens A, Cummings JH (1980) The microbial contribution to human faecal mass. J Med Microbiol 13:45–56
Stone JE, Scallan AM (1968) A structural model for the cell wall of water swollen wood pulp fibres based on their accessibility to macromolecules, cellulose, chemistry, and technology. 2:343–358

Story JA, Kritchevsky D (1976) Dietary fiber and lipid metabolism. In: Spiller GA, Amen RJ (eds) Fiber in human nutrition. Plenum, New York London,pp 171–184
Taylor I, Duthie HL (1978) The effect of bran on colonic myoelectrical function in diverticular disease. In: Duthie HL (ed) Gastro-intestinal motility in health and disease. MTP Press, Lancaster, pp 225–230
Trowell H, Godding E, Spiller G, Briggs G (1978) Fiber bibliography and terminology. Am J Clin Nutr 31:1489–1490
Walters RL, Baird IM, Davies PS et al. (1975) Effects of two types of dietary fibre on faecal steroid and lipid excretion. Br Med J 2:536–538
Weinrich H (1977) Fibre symposium, quoted in discussion. J Plant Foods 3:80
Williams RD, Olmsted WH (1936) The manner in which bran controls the bulk of the feces. Ann Intern Med 10:717–727
Willams AE, Eastwood MA, Cregeen R (1978) SEM and light microscope study of the matrix structure of human feces. Scan Electron Microsc 2:707–711
Wyman JB, Heaton KW, Manning AP et al. (1976) The effect on intestinal transit and the feces of raw and cooked bran in different doses. Am J Clin Nutr 29:1474–1479
Wyman JB, Heaton KW, Manning AP, Wicks ACB (1978)Variability of colonic function in healthy subjects. Gut 19:146–150

CHAPTER 7

Motility and Pressure Studies in Clinical Practice

A. TORSOLI and E. CORAZZIARI

A. The Esophagus

I. Motor Activity

The esophagus controls transit of ingesta from the hypopharynx to the stomach. It allows eructation and vomiting and opposes reflux and regurgitation into the pharynx. Esophageal function is therefore dependent on motor activity and is regulated by the anatomic and functional characteristics of the muscle walls at the level of the upper esophageal sphincter, the esophageal body, and the lower esophageal sphincter, respectively.

1. Upper Esophageal Sphincter

The upper esophageal sphincter is located between the hypopharynx and the cervical tract of the esophageal body. It separates the atmospheric pressure from the negative intrathoracic pressure. In humans, the sphincter is formed by the striated fibers of the cricopharyngeal muscle and by some adjacent pharyngeal and esophageal fibers (COHEN and WOLF 1968). Under resting conditions, intraluminal pressure recorded at the level of the pharyngoesophageal junction is higher than in the proximal and distal segments. This high pressure zone, on average 3 cm long (FYKE and CODE 1955), may vary from 2.5 to 4.5 cm (ATKINSON et al. 1957b). Intraluminal pressure is maximal for a 1 cm long tract corresponding to the cricopharyngeus muscle (SOKOL et al. 1966). During swallowing pressure falls rapidly, returning immediately afterwards to basal values (Fig. 1). The fall in pressure follows, in rapid sequence, the contraction of the muscles of the tongue and of the upper part of the pharynx. Simultaneously the pharynx and larynx move forward and cranially (SOKOL et al. 1966). Inhibition of the sphincter also occurs, at least in dog, during retching, vomiting, and eructation (MONGES et al. 1978).

2. Esophageal Body

The esophageal body extends from the upper esophageal sphincter to about 2 cm proximal to the diaphragmatic hiatus. It is formed by two muscle layers, the external longitudinal and the internal circular layer. In humans, muscle fibers are striated in the proximal 2–6 cm, striated and smooth, in variable proportion, for a few centimeters distally, then, and, exclusively smooth in the remaining part of the esophageal body. Under resting conditions, the esophageal body is a virtual cavity, in which no motor activity is present. Proper stimuli can elicit both peristaltic and nonperistaltic phasic contractions.

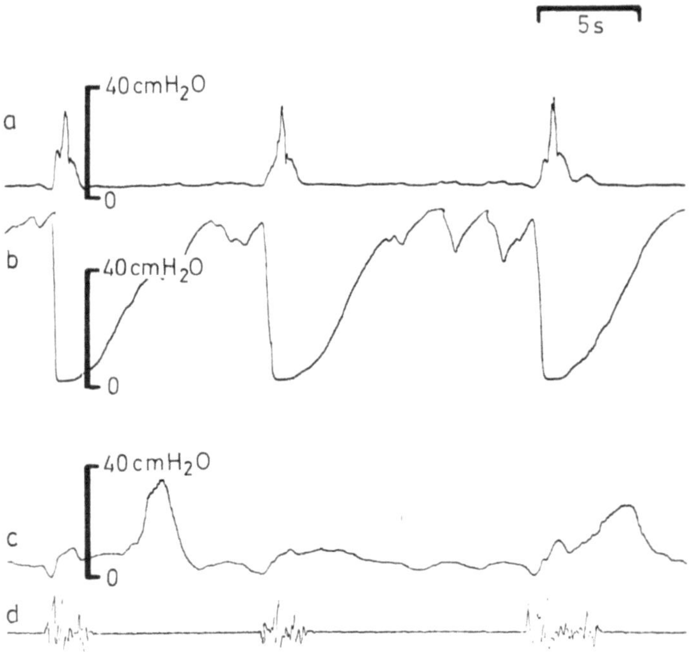

Fig. 1 a–d. Intraluminal pressure recordings from the hypopharynx **a**, upper esophageal sphincter **b**, cervical esophageal body **c**. Deglutition **d** is also shown. Relaxation of the high pressure zone during swallowing takes place at the level of the upper esophageal sphincter. Monophasic waves corresponding to wall contractions move from the hypopharynx to the cervical esophageal body after the first and the third swallow. Calibration in cmH_2O

Peristalsis is a coordinated motor activity moving in an aboral direction with a propulsive effect on the intraluminal contents. On manometric tracings, peristalsis appears as a series of positive pressure variations in coherent temporal sequence, corresponding to the progressive wall contraction (Fig. 2). Synchronized analysis of manometric recordings and cinefluorography, however, shows that the contraction is immediately preceded by a progressive relaxation of the wall (TURANO 1957). Similar analysis of the peristaltic movement at colonic and duodenal levels shows an identical sequence of motor events (TORSOLI et al. 1971 a, b).

In the esophagus, peristalsis is called primary when it follows an act of swallowing and secondary when it is not preceded by the oropharyngeal phase of deglutition. The main function of the primary peristaltic wave is to transport a swallowed bolus into the stomach; however it may vary in relation to the physical characteristics of the bolus and the posture while swallowing. In an erect position, nonviscous boluses reach the esophagogastric junction only with the aid of oropharyngeal pressure and gravity; peristaltic contraction occurs after passage of the bolus and may empty the esophageal body of any residual contents. If the bolus is viscous and swallowed in a horizontal position, esophageal transit depends entirely upon pressure gradients caused by motor propulsive activity.

Secondary peristalsis is induced by intraluminal distention of the esophageal body and this usually occurs when ingesta are not entirely emptied into the stomach after primary peristalsis or reflux takes place from the stomach into the esoph-

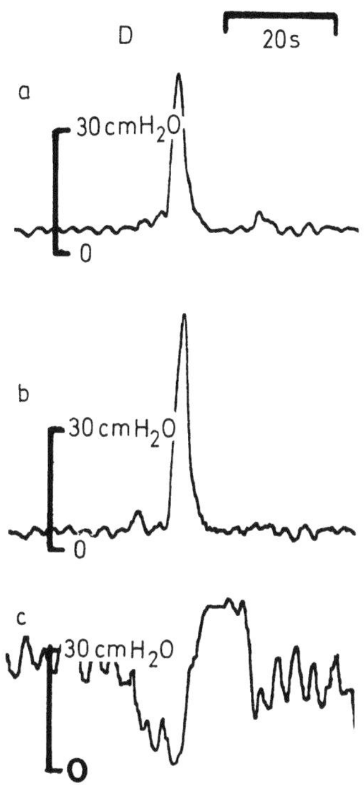

Fig. 2a–c. Intraluminal pressure recordings from the middle **a** and lower **b** esophageal body and the lower esophageal sphincter **c**. Esophageal body level at rest: transmitted respiratory activity; after swallowing *D*, peristalsis appears as monophasic pressure variations in craniocaudal temporal sequence. Lower esophageal sphincter level at rest: a high pressure zone; after swallowing: fall in pressure to fundic level followed by a contraction

agus. The threshold of intraluminal distension to elicit a peristaltic reflex is fairly constant in a given subject and can be reduced with boluses of low pH values (Corazziari et al. 1978).

A third form of mechanical activity in the esophageal body consists in the simultaneous contractions. These contractions are local, intermittent, and segmenting, appearing at the same time at different levels and usually failing to propel the contents (Donner et al. 1966). Occasionally, simultaneous contractions are compatible with normal motor activity of the esophagus.

3. Lower Esophageal Sphincter

The lower esophageal sphincter separates the negative intraesophageal pressure from the positive intragastric pressure. It is made up of smooth muscle fibers of the terminal tract of the gastric fundus. For a long time this area was considered a purely functional sphincter, but recent data show that the circular muscle layer, at this level, displays a modest but definite asymmetric thickening (Liebermann-Meffert et al. 1979).

Under resting conditions, the intraluminal pressure is higher at the esophagogastric junction than in the esophageal body and the gastric fundus. In humans, the high pressure zone is 1.5–3 cm long (Cohen and Harris 1972). During swallowing the pressure falls to the fundic pressure level and then returns to basal values after 5–20 s (Fig. 2). Inhibition of the sphincter starts immediately after deglutition and is maintained until peristaltic contraction reaches the level of the sphincter.

II. Use of Esophageal Manometry in Clinical Practice

Manometric recordings from the *pharyngoesophageal junction* do not provide reliable information; motor activity in this area is better evaluated by cinefluorography. Cinefluorographic observations, however, give only a qualitative description of the mechanical events.

Accuracy of manometric recordings from the pharyngoesophageal region is affected mainly by the high compliance of the perfused catheters which underestimate elevated and rapidly changing pressure (DODDS et al. 1976). The compliance of the manometric system can be reduced by increasing the rate of perfusion but this approach may induce fluid aspiration in the respiratory tree. A possible technical solution is the use of miniaturized intraluminal pressure transducers (STEF et al. 1974) or a hydraulic capillary infusion apparatus with very low infusion rates (ARNDORFER et al. 1977).

Also contributing to inaccuracy in this area is the asymmetric anatomy of the upper esophageal sphincter which appears as a radial pressure asymmetry (RINALDO and LEVEY 1968; WINANS 1972). Manometric recordings are therefore influenced by the orientation of the side hole of the catheter. Mobility of the pharyngoesophageal junction during swallowing may also contribute to inaccuracy. Cineflurographic observations have shown that, during swallowing, this area moves cranially for a distance equivalent to about three-quarters of one cervical vertebral body (SOKOL et al. 1966).

Until now, few manometric studies of the pharyngoesophageal junction have been performed using a low compliance recording system while simultaneously controlling the radial orientation of the recording side holes (BERLIN et al. 1977; GERHARDT et al. 1978), but in none of these studies was the influence of regional mobility evaluated during swallowing. Results of previous manometric studies cannot therefore be regarded as quantitative and repeatable. Likewise, even the description of altered inhibition of the sphincter or of motor incoordination of this region should be considered with caution. For example, the pharyngeal diverticulum and the so-called cricopharyngeal spasm or cricopharyngeal achalasia have been interpreted as an expression of a premature contraction (ELLIS et al. 1969) and/or a delayed inhibition of the cricopharyngeal muscle. However manometric evidence of the absence of sphincter inhibition during swallowing (achalasia) has not been forthcoming; furthermore, it is possible that manometric alterations reported in patients with pharyngeal diverticulum may be the effect rather than the cause of this anatomic alteration.

Manometric alterations at the level of the *esophageal body*, appear as one or more of the following: increase in resting pressure; absence of peristaltic activity; presence of uncoordinated motor activity; phasic pressure variations of either increased or decreased amplitude. At *lower esophageal sphincter* level one or more of the following manometric patterns may be recorded: increase or decrease in resting pressure; absence or insufficient inhibition during swallowing.

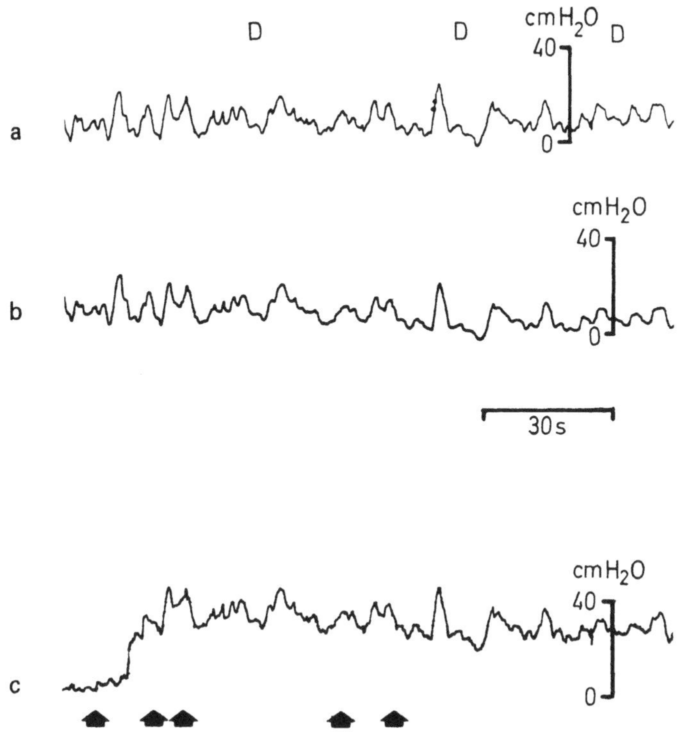

Fig. 3a–c. Achalasia. Intraluminal pressure recordings from the esophageal body **a, b** and the lower esophageal sphincter **c**. After swallowing *D*, there is a lack of peristaltic waves in the esophageal body and of relaxation in the lower esophageal sphincter. Spontaneous and simultaneous waves of low amplitude can be seen in the esophageal body. *Arrows*, 0.5 cm cranial pull-through of the catheter

Manometric investigations on the esophagogastric junction have proved to be of particular diagnostic interest. Recordings from this area, like those from the upper esophageal sphincter, may show some variability in the radial asymmetry and axial mobility of the sphincter (CHATTOPADHYAY and POPE 1979). However, unlike those encountered in the pharyngoesophageal sphincter, these limitations do not prevent satisfactory evaluation of the motor behavior of the sphincter. Moreover, within well-defined limits, pressure data are reproducible and can characterize altered motor activity (FOX et al. 1973; PÉREZ-AVILA and IRVOR 1975; HAY et al. 1979).

The primary indication for esophageal pressure studies is to investigate *dysphagia of inorganic origin*. The associated motor disorders have long been classified either as achalasia (lack of peristalsis in the esophageal body; absent or insufficient inhibition of the lower esophageal sphincter, Fig. 3; COHEN 1965; CREAMER et al. 1957) or as diffuse esophageal spasm (uncoordinated contractions which may be of increased strength and longer duration and peristalsis in the esophageal body, Fig. 4; regular inhibition of the lower esophageal sphincter; FLESHLER 1967; KRAMER 1970). However other motor patterns besides these clear-cut manometric alterations are characterized by lack of peristalsis and normal lower esophageal sphincter inhibition (Fig. 5) or by irregular presence of peristalsis and absence of or insuf-

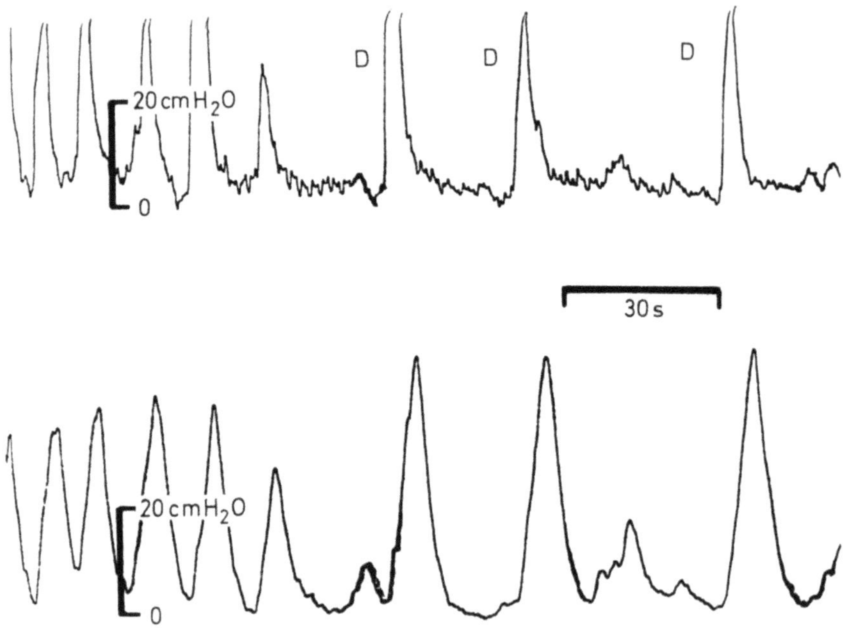

Fig. 4. Diffuse esophageal spasm. Intraluminal pressure recordings from the esophageal body. Spontaneous, simultaneous, and repetitive waves accompanied by retrosternal angina-like pain are followed by three normal peristaltic sequences. *D*, swallow

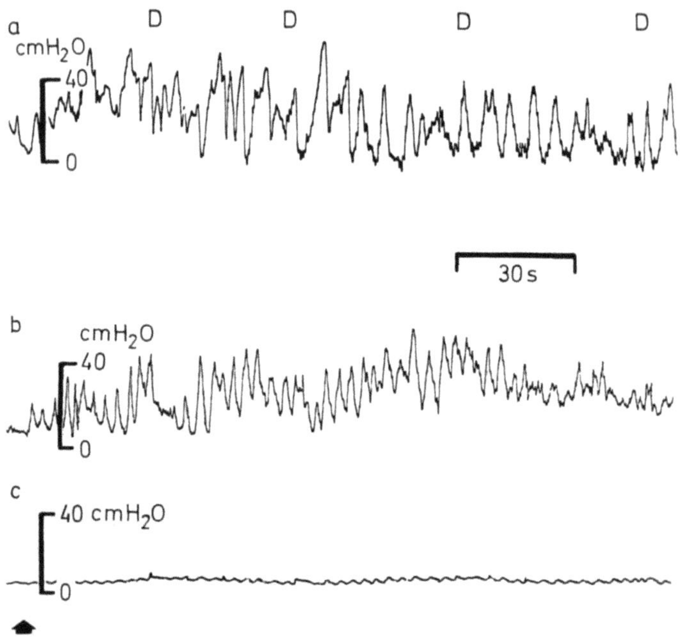

Fig. 5 a–c. Achalasia-like disorder. Intraluminal pressure recordings from the esophageal body **a**, the lower esophageal sphincter **b**, and gastric fundus **c**. Repetitive nonperistaltic waves in the esophageal body. Relaxation of the lower esophageal sphincter is complete after the first, incomplete after the second, and lacking after the third swallow *D*. *Arrow*, 0.5 cm cranial pull-through of the catheter ficient inhibition of the lower esophageal sphincter. Each of these manometric patterns can be associated with single or repetitive contractions or increased resting pressure of the lower esophageal sphincter (VANTRAPPEN et al. 1979a). Esophageal manometry is helpful in the evaluation of *chest pain* which is sometimes induced by diffuse spasm or by peristaltic contractions of increased amplitude and duration (BRAND et al. 1977).

The third, and perhaps the most frequent, indication for esophageal manometry is to evaluate *gastroesophageal reflux*. The pressure of the lower esophageal sphincter is an index of its strength (COHEN and HARRIS 1972) and is usually inversely correlated with the frequency of gastroesophageal reflux (A. TORSOLI, E. CORAZZIARI unpublished work). Pressure values of the lower esophageal sphincter in healthy subjects and patients, however, show a substantial overlap (POPE 1967; BENNETT 1973). Better evaluation of gastroesophageal reflux can be obtained from pH measurements, but manometry is essential for the exact positioning of the intraluminal glass electrode.

Esophageal manometric studies, used to evaluate patients for *antireflux surgery*, offer important information regarding the outcome of the operation. For example, demonstration of altered motor patterns are often followed by poor results (BOMBECK et al. 1972) and antireflux surgery does not appear to alleviate symptoms secondary to motor disorders which are not caused by reflux itself. Likewise in patients with altered or absent peristalsis, dysphagia may occur postoperatively (POPE 1978).

Esophageal manometry is also useful to evaluate results of *medical or surgical treatment*. This technique has in fact been used to establish the efficacy of drugs such as metoclopramide and bethanechol (McCALLUM et al. 1975), of pneumatic dilatations (VANTRAPPEN et al. 1971; HEITMANN 1971), of extramucosal myotomies and of antireflux operations (LIPSHUTZ et al. 1974; BEHAR et al. 1974). Although still open to debate, *intraoperative monitoring of the intraluminal pressure* at the level of the esophagogastric junction has been reported to be a useful guide for the surgeon to regulate pressure when performing a fundoplication in patients with reflux esophagitis or a Heller's myotomy in patients with achalasia (COOPER et al. 1977). Esophageal pressure measurements may also be useful to detect esophageal motor activities in the tract distal to the squamocolumnar junction in the *esophagus lined with columnar epithelium* (WIENBECK 1976).

Esophageal manometry should be performed in patients in whom *chronic idiopathic intestinal pseudoobstruction* is suspected. Esophageal motor activity is always altered in this syndrome, although dysphagia is not necessarily present. The manometric findings are similar to those found in primary motor abnormalities (Fig. 6) (ANURAS 1978; FAULK et al. 1978). The manometric investigation is useful to support the diagnosis of the syndrome and may avoid proceeding with useless and often dangerous surgical operations.

Manometry may also be usefully employed to evaluate motor impairments sometimes present in *neonatal and senile patients* or secondary to *collagen diseases or nervous and muscle disorders*. Motor abnormalities in these situations are rarely sufficiently severe to be symptomatic; and whenever esophageal symptoms are present, they are generally less marked than those of the primary condition. In some instances, however, manometry is useful in the identification of the primary

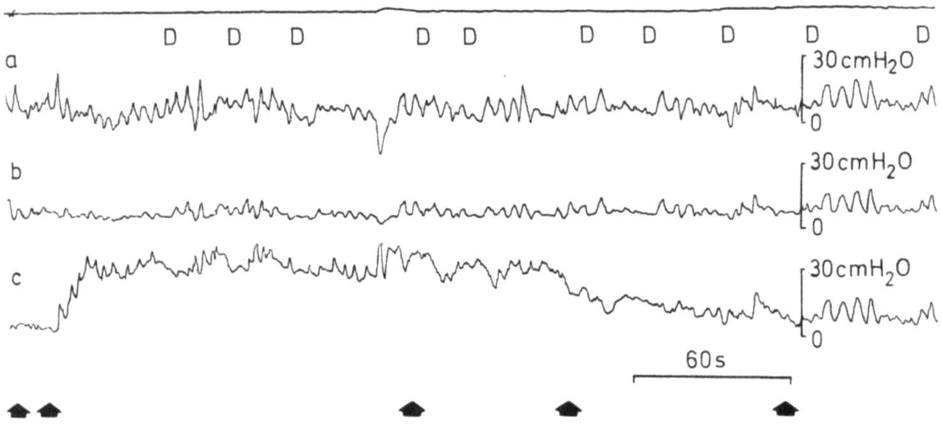

Fig. 6 a–c. Idiopathic chronic intestinal pseudoobstruction. Intraluminal pressure recordings from the esophageal body **a, b** and pressure profile of the lower esophageal sphincter **c**. No peristalsis in the esophageal body and no relaxation in the lower esophageal sphincter are present after swallowing *D*. *Arrows*, 0.5 cm cranial pull-through of the catheter

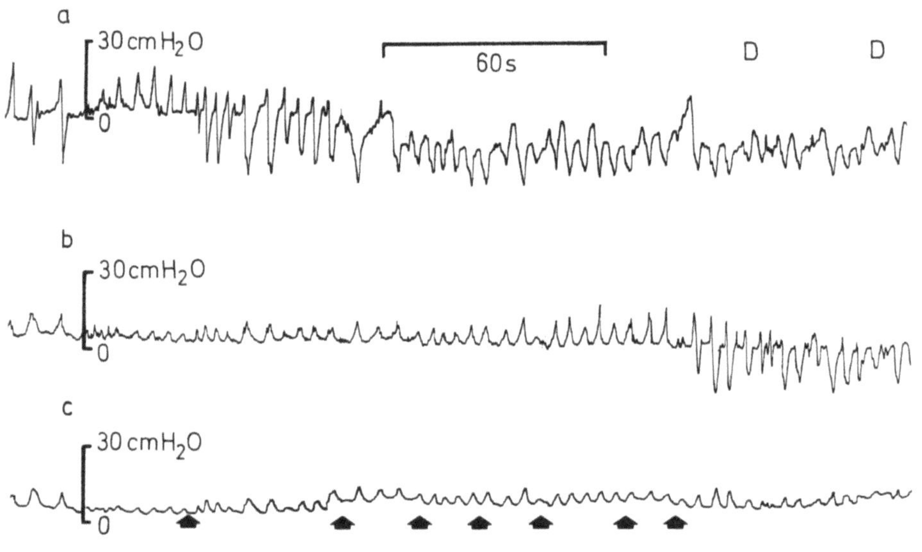

Fig. 7 a–c. Progressive systemic sclerosis. Intraluminal pressure profile of the lower esophageal sphincter (left-hand side of **a** and right-hand side of **b**) together with intragastric recording **c**. No zone of elevated pressure at the gastroesophageal junction is visible. Lack of peristaltic sequences in the esophageal body after swallowing *D*. *Arrows* indicate 0.5 cm cranial pull-through of the catheter

disorders or to evaluate esophageal motor alterations which may induce further damage to the esophagus. In progressive systemic sclerosis and in systemic lupus erythematosus, lesions, located mainly at the level of the smooth muscle, cause a decrease in lower esophageal sphincter pressure and lack of peristalsis in the distal segment of the esophageal body (Fig. 7). Normal inhibition of the lower esophageal sphincter and normal peristalsis in the upper part of the esophageal body are maintained (GARRETT et al. 1971; TATELMAN and KEECH 1966). In polymyositis and dermatomyositis, lesions, located mainly at the level of the striated muscle, are associated with normal motor behavior of the distal tract of the esophageal body with lack of peristalsis in the proximal tract. Not infrequentely however, these diseases induce alterations at all levels of the esophageal body so that differentiation of collagen disorders by means of manometry may be difficult or impossible (KILMAN and GOYAL 1976). Esophageal aperistalsis is a frequent finding in patients with Raynaud's phenomenon, even in the absence of systemic disease, but systemic sclerosis will develop in some of these patients (ATKINSON 1976).

B. The Stomach

I. Motor Activity

The main function of motor activity of the stomach is to receive and mix ingesta with gastric juice, to grind solid components finely, and to modulate emptying of contents into the duodenum. The different motor characteristics of the proximal and distal parts of the stomach and of the pylorus are integrated in order to perform these functions.

The *proximal stomach* is made up of the fundus and the proximal part of the body. In this area, changes in wall tension allow ingesta to be received without variation in intragastric pressure. Sustained and long-lasting contractions are present at this level (LIND et al. 1961). The motor activity of the proximal part of the stomach is mainly concerned with the regulation of gastric emptying of liquids.

The *distal stomach* is made up of the distal part of the body and of the antrum. It mixes ingesta with gastric juice and grinds and regulates emptying of solid components. Motor function of this area is characterized by annular contractions, originating in the body and propagating downwards along the antrum. Control electrical activity spreads away from a pacemaking area located in the upper part of greater curvature (KELLY and CODE 1971). It regulates frequency, velocity of propagation, and coordination of the contractions which are called peristaltic. In humans, control electrical activity has a frequency of 3 cycles/min, but the contractions are caused by the presence of spike potentials (KWONG et al. 1972; SARNA et al. 1972). Therefore the frequency varies from 0 to 3 contractions/min, depending upon whether or not all cycles of the control electrical activity are accompanied by spike potentials.

In the postprandial period, spike potentials and peristaltic contractions appear continuously and/or intermittentely; during fasting a change takes place with a cyclic pattern displaying absence, intermittent, and continuous presence of spike potentials (CODE and MARLETT 1975). This cyclic motor behavior, the so-called interdigestive myoelectric complex or migrating myoelectric complex, originates in the gastric pacemaker, and progresses distally to the duodenum, jejunum, and ileum (CODE and MARLETT 1975).

At the level of the *gastroduodenal junction* there is a sphincter in which low intraluminal pressures can be recorded. However, it has been claimed that the pylorus is open most of the time (ATKINSON et al. 1957a) and with the antrum forms a single motor function unit (THOMAS 1957). The motor activity of the pylorus is not fully understood, but it has been shown that this tract does not regulate gastric emptying of liquids (STEMPER and COOKE 1976), that it regulates transit of solid contents, and prevents duodenogastric reflux (FISHER and COHEN 1973).

1. Gastric Filling

Filling of the stomach is not a passive phenomenon. During swallowing the proximal stomach relaxes to receive the ingested food. This mechanism has been called receptive relaxation and is characterized by a decrease in intragastric pressure preceding the arrival of the bolus and lasting until swallowing ceases (CANNON and LIEB 1911). In the proximal stomach, wall tension varies according to the intraluminal distension in such a way that increments in intragastric volume cause only slight variations in initial pressure or have no effect. Receptive relaxation and adaptation to distension are the two mechanisms that allow filling of the stomach in the absence of rapid pressure increments and, therefore, prevent rapid gastric emptying.

2. Mixing and Grinding of Solid Contents

When ingesta arrive in the distal part of the stomach they are thoroughly mixed with gastric juice and solid contents are ground. Peristaltic contractions segment and propel the contents distally. Force and rate of propagation increae progressively as the contractions move distally; when the contractions reach the most distal part of the stomach the whole prepyloric antral segment contracts almost simultaneously "antral systole" (CARLSON et al. 1966). As peristalsis, in this sequence, ends with a systolic contraction of the distal antrum (and perhaps of the pylorus), the contents cannot progress distally and move backwards into the gastric body. This process of propulsion, segmentation, and retropulsion is repeated over and over until the contents are finely ground. In dogs, the stomach is able to discriminate and to prevent emptying of solid particles greater than 2 mm (MEYER et al. 1979).

3. Gastric Emptying

The modality of gastric emptying varies according to the osmolality (HUNT and PATHAK 1960), energy (HUNT and STUBBS 1975), lipids (HUNT and KNOX 1968), tryptophan (STEPHENS et al. 1976), and acid (HUNT and KNOX 1972) present in the gastric contents. Duodenal and jejunal receptors for acid, tryptophan, osmolality, and lipids inhibit gastric emptying via a neurohumoral pathway. In similar experimental conditions, the rate of emptying from the stomach to the duodenum is related to the gradient resulting from the interaction between the intragastric and the intraduodenal pressures and from the resistance to flow present at the antropyloric segment (NELSEN and KOHATSU 1971).

Gastric emptying of liquids is different and independent of solids; liquids empty rapidly, with an exponential pattern and according to the intragastric volume (HUNT and KNOX 1968); solids empty more gradually and independently of gastric volume (HEADING et al. 1976; MEYER et al. 1976; HINDER and KELLY 1977). Emptying of liquids is regulated mainly by pressure gradients secondary to wall tension and contractions of the proximal stomach. The emptying time of solid contents is regulated mainly by the antral peristaltic contractions which allow the passage of particles once ingesta are well ground (MEYER et al. 1979). However even solid substances that cannot be reduced in volume are nevertheless emptied into the duodenum, their transit through the pylorus occurring during the activity front of the migrating myoelectric complex (HINDER and KELLY 1977).

II. Gastric Manometry and Studies of Gastric Emptying in Clinical Practice

Owing to the anatomic configuration of the stomach, intragastric pressure cannot be accurately recorded. Fairly accurate recordings of intraluminal pressure in viscera with a virtual lumen can be obtained with open-tip catheters and small balloons, but they tend to understimate pressure in the wide gastric chamber. Large balloons transmit both intraluminal pressure variations and wall contractions and can even stimulate motor activity. Thus intragastric pressure studies are not used in clinical practice and alterations of gastric motor function, if any, remain to be described. However, gastric emptying can be easily and accurately evaluated. This aspect of gastric function has in fact been extensively investigated both from a physiologic and a clinical viewpoint.

Although the practical relevance of the measurement appear to be limited by the wide distribution of the results, studies performed in homogeneous populations of patients have shown alterations in gastric emptying in several conditions. Besides mechanical obstruction due to lesions in the antrum, pylorus, and duodenal bulb, slowing of gastric emptying may also occur in numerous conditions caused by nervous and metabolic alterations, infectious diseases, and drugs (RIMER 1966).

Slow gastric emptying has been reported in patients with atrophic gastritis (DAVIES et al. 1971), rapid emptying occurs in patients with duodenal ulcer (GRIFFITH et al. 1968; FORDTRAN and WALSH 1973), Zollinger–Ellison syndrome (DUBOIS et al. 1977), and pancreatic insufficiency (MALLINSON 1968; LONG and WEISS 1974). The characteristics of gastric emptying in patients with reflux esophagitis have not been fully clarified (LITTLE et al. 1977; CSENDES and HENRIQUEZ 1978; BEHAR and RAMSBY 1978). All vagotomies induce acceleration of liquid emptying and, except for proximal gastric vagotomy, slowing of solid emptying (COOKE 1975; KELLY 1976). After subtotal gastrectomy, emptying of both liquid and solid contents is accelerated; after vagotomy plus pyloroplasty emptying of liquids is faster, while emptying of solids is either faster or slower (MACGREGOR et al. 1977a, b).

C. The Small Intestine

I. Motor Activity

Motor activity of the small intestine is organized to mix chyme with digestive secretion, to allow ample contact between the contents and the mucosal surface and to propel the contents in an aboral direction. Contractions in the small intestine are regulated by the electrical characteristics of the smooth muscle cells. As in the

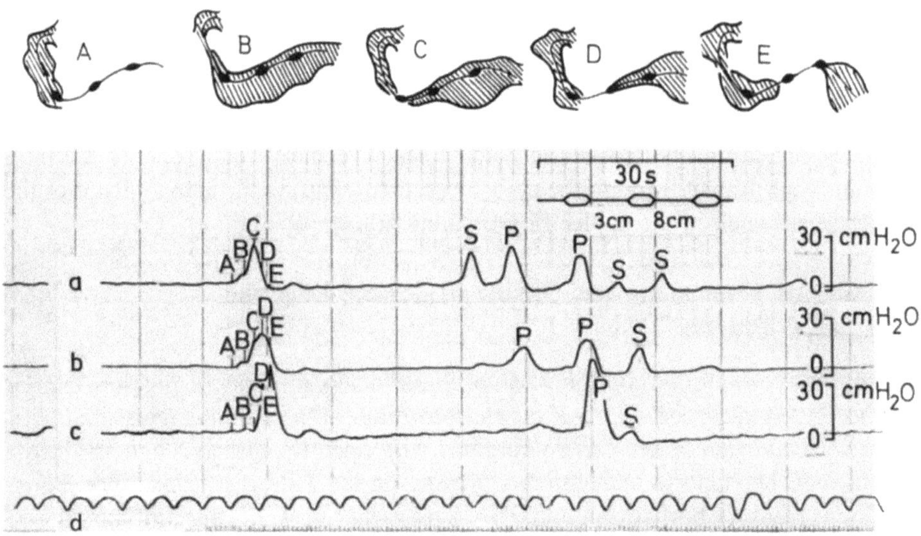

Fig. 8 a–d. Intraluminal pressure recordings obtained by three small balloons placed 3 cm apart in the duodenum. Tracings recorded by proximal **a**, middle **b**, and distal **c** balloons, respectively. Following the entrance of barium sulfate suspension into the duodenum, synchronized cinefluorography **d** is used to correlate movements of the wall and displacement of contents with intraluminal pressure variations. *S*, segmenting contractions; *P*, peristaltic contractions. Schematic drawings, corresponding to each point *(A–E)* marked on tracings, illustrate the sequence of motor events related to peristaltic contractions (TORSOLI et al. 1971 a)

stomach, control activity is invariably present. Slow wave frequency is constant at each level of the intestine, but is not the same at all levels. A decrease is in fact observed from the duodenum to the terminal ileum; in humans, the highest frequency is 11–12 cycles/min at the level of the duodenal loop; the lowest, 8–9 cycles/min, in the terminal ileum (CHRISTENSEN et al. 1966). The decrease in frequency is not uniform but shows a stepwise reduction from segment to segment (DIAMANT and BORTOFF 1969). In intestinal segments displaying the same frequency, the slow waves appear sequentially in an aboral direction, not synchronously. Electrical control activity does not stimulate motor contractions, which, as in the stomach, are caused by the occurrence of spike potentials (CHRISTENSEN 1971). The frequency of contractions for each small intestinal segment may therefore vary from zero to the maximal slow wave frequency of that segment.

Small intestinal motor activity is characterized, fundamentally, by two types of movements: segmenting contractions and peristalsis. Segmenting local activity appears as ring-like contractions of the wall which divide the lumen into segments. These annular contractions are about 1–2 cm long and occur at intervals of 3–4 cm. This motor aspect, on manometric recordings with small balloons, appears as monophasic pressure variations with amplitude ranging from 5 to 60 cmH_2O and duration from 2 to 5 s (Fig. 8). These appear either isolated or in groups, sometimes simultaneously at different levels, but in all instances without a propagating pattern. Segmenting activity, however, may give rise to pressure gradients determining displacement of contents in either direction (TORSOLI et al. 1971 a). Seg-

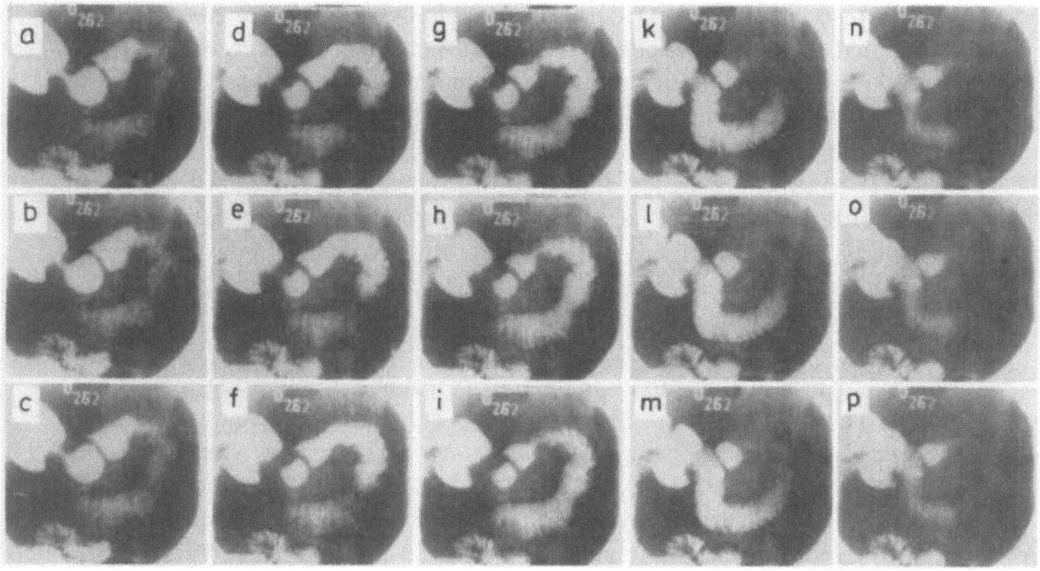

Fig. 9 a–p. Cinefluorographic sequence displaying a peristaltic motor event at duodenal loop level which displaces barium sulfate suspension beyond the duodenojejunal junction. Cinefluorography performed with subject in prone position (TORSOLI et al. 1971 a)

menting contractions are sometimes present for short periods in adjacent intestinal tracts displaying the maximal frequency allowed by the electrical control activity. This motor pattern, referred to as basic rhythm or rhythmic segmentation, causes bidirectional displacement of contents between the two adjacent areas (FAULK et al. 1954; CORAZZIARI et al. 1972). Similar movement of contents, observed during radiologic studies, have been described as pendular movements (HERTZ 1907).

Peristalsis is a complex motor activity characterized by relaxation of the wall preceding a ring-like contraction moving aborad. Peristaltic movement displaces contents in an aboral direction for short tracts of about 4–5 cm. In the first segment of the small intestine, however, it is not infrequent to find the contents moving from the duodenum beyond the angle of Treitz (TORSOLI et al. 1971 a; Fig. 9). Moreover, there is evidence that the activity front of the interdigestive myoelectric complex corresponds to a peristaltic sequence moving along the entire, or a part of, the small intestine (CODE and MARLETT 1975). On manometric recordings, peristaltic motor activity appears as monophasic waves, very similar to segmenting contractions, but arranged in a coordinated temporal and spatial sequence moving aborad (Fig. 8). The rate of peristaltic progression, in the upper part of the small intestine, is about 1–3.3 cm/s (TORSOLI et al. 1971 a).

In humans, retrograde displacement of contents for short distances has been observed during X-ray studies in both the jejunum and the ileum, but only in the duodenum have these movements been described as associated with a coordinated motor activity appearing as a sequential wall contraction moving in an oral direction (BORGSTRÖM and ARBORELIUS 1971; TORSOLI et al. 1971 a).

A difference in motor behaviour is observed in the small intestine between the postprandial and fasting periods. In the fasting state, manometric recordings from any level of the small intestine show a cyclic motor pattern of four phases corresponding to the migrating or interdigestive myoelectric complex (SZURSZEWSKI 1969; VANTRAPPEN et al. 1977). In phase I, contractions are absent or infrequent; in phase II, contractions are few and repetitive, appearing in short bursts at different levels either synchronously or in a sequential order, with a progressive increase in frequency; in phase III, there is a series of repetitive contractions lasting for several minutes with the same frequency as that of electrical control activity; phase IV, of short duration, is a transition period from the maximal activity of phase III to motor quiescence of phase I. Of the four phases, phase III has been most extensively investigated. It corresponds to the activity front of the migrating myoelectric complex. This front moves distally involving the entire small intestine and, as soon as it reaches the terminal ileum, a new front starts again from the stomach or the duodenum (SZURSZEWSKI 1969; SZURSZEWSKI et al. 1970; CODE and MARLETT 1975). Corresponding to the myoelectric activity front are wall contractions, apparently peristaltic, which move aborad for some 30–40 cm. These progressive sequences of motor contractions empty the entire small intestine of bacteria, cellular debris, food residue, and digestive secretion (CODE and SCHLEGEL 1974). Spike potentials moving for shorter distances in aboral progression have been observed during phase II of the migrating myoelectric complex only in the upper tract of the small intestine (FLECKENSTEIN and ÖIGAARD 1978). As myoelectric and mechanical activities vary cyclically, so does transit of contents through the small intestine. Progression is slow in phase I but gradually increases in phases II and III (SARR and KELLY 1979).

The absence or derangement of the migrating myoelectric complex has been considered a possible cause of the bacterial overgrowth syndrome following the modification in the emptying pattern in the jejunoileal loops (VANTRAPPEN et al. 1977). Motor variations of the migrating myoelecric complex are also time related with fluctuations in gastrointestinal secretory activity. It has been reported that the activity front at the level of the duodenum is preceded by an increase in the acid and pepsin gastric secretion and in bile flow and is followed by an increase in secretion of bicarbonate and enzymes from the pancreas (VANTRAPPEN et al. 1979b).

The myoelectric complex and the corresponding mechanical sequence are immediately interrupted with food ingestion. In the postprandial period, the four phases previously described are not identifiable. There are no phases of motor quiescence and periods alternating regular and irregulat spike potentials are observed (RAYNER et al. 1979). Similarly, progression of contents is no longer cyclical and resembles the pattern observed in phase II of the myoelectric complex (SARR and KELLY 1979), with aboral progression for short distances during periods of regular spike potentials (RAYNER et al. 1979).

II. Manometry of the Small Intestine in Clinical Practice

The relative inaccessibility of the small intestine to catheters, and the extreme variability of manometric recordings from subject to subject, and also in the same subject at different times, have so far discouraged pressure studies of the small intestine for clinical purposes. Investigations on the migrating myoelectric complex have led to a better understanding of the physiologic and pharmacologic aspects of small intestine motility, but are of no diagnostic value, except perhaps in the bacterial overgrowth syndrome (VANTRAPPEN et al. 1977). Moreover, motor disorders frequently present at the level of the small intestine (CONNELL 1974) are secondary to diseases and/or alterations in which no further practical information can be obtained from the study of motor behaviour.

The transit of barium sulfate suspension or radioopaque markers through the small intestine are easily observed with X-rays. Comparative studies of jejunoileal transit after administration of a barium meal, with and without the addition of lactose, have been suggested as a diagnostic tool in the identification of patients with disaccharidase deficiency (LAWS and NEALE 1966). Nevertheless, even this test appears to be of little use for diagnostic purposes except in cases of an exceedingly abnormal transit alteration, on account of the extreme variability in the flow rate of contents (THOMPSON and SANDERS 1972).

D. The Large Bowel

I. Motor Activity

Motor activity of the large bowel is responsible for the deposit, transportation, and periodic expulsion of the contents, with the various tracts of the viscus carrying out these functions in different degrees. The large bowel is separated from the small intestine by the ileocecal sphincter.

1. Ileocecal Sphincter

The ileocecal sphincter prevents reflux of the cecal contents into the ileum and, intermittently, allows transit from the ileum into the cecum. The sphincteric nature of the ileocecal junction is indicated by the finding of a high pressure zone at this level compared with adjacent tracts. Pressure rises and falls during intraluminal distension of the proximal colon and of the ileum, respectively (COHEN et al. 1968). In the cat, the frequency of electrical control activity in the terminal ileum is not coordinated with that present in the proximal colon; however coordinated action potentials propagate distally through the junction, especially in the postprandial period (WIENBECK et al. 1974). In humans, manometric recordings in an ileocolon transplant following esophagectomy showed a peristaltic pattern, moving from the ileum to the proximal colon following prostigmine administration (A. TORSOLI and E. CORAZZIARI unpublished work).

2. Colon

As in the small bowel, the timing of wall contractions in the various tracts of the large bowel are regulated by the electrical control activity. In contrast to the small bowel, controversy exists regarding the interpretation of the various characteristics of this electrical activity. It is not clear, for instance, whether control eletrical activity is constantly present (PROVENZALE and PISANO 1971; BARDAKAJIAN et al. 1976; SARNA et al. 1979) or appears intermittently (TAYLOR et al. 1975; SNAPE et

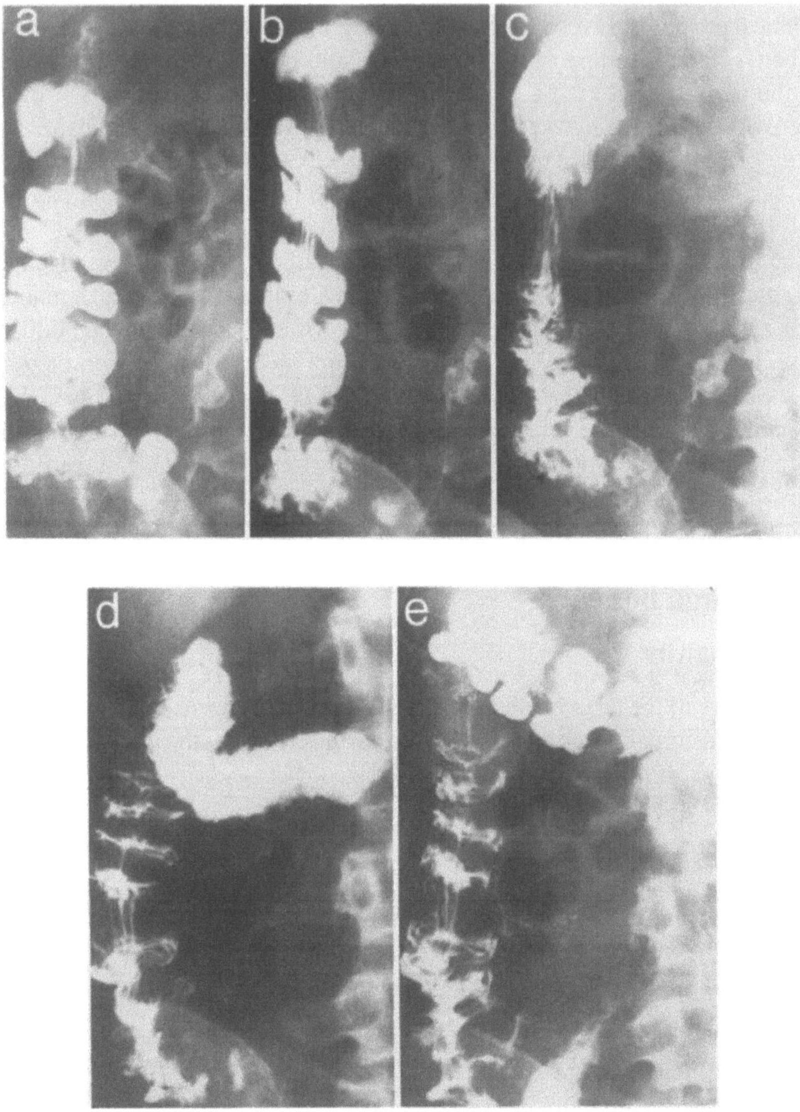

Fig. 10 a–e. Cinefluorographic sequence displaying a peristaltic **a**, motor event at the level of the right colon. Haustra modify orientation **b** and then disappear **c** as contents are displaced distally **c** and **d**; haustra are present again in the segment proximal to the displaced contents **d** and then at the level of contents **e** after termination of the motor event (Cassano and Torsoli 1966)

al. 1976). As for proximal, middle, and distal colon, corresponding to the cecum, ascending tract, transverse, descending tract, and sigmoid, respectively, it is generally agreed that a different myoelectric pattern probably determines their different motor behavior (Provenzale and Pisano 1971; Taylor et al. 1975; Caprilli et al. 1975; Sarna et al. 1979).

As in the small intestine, local segmenting contractions and peristalsis are the basic movements of colonic motor activity. Local segmenting activity is character-

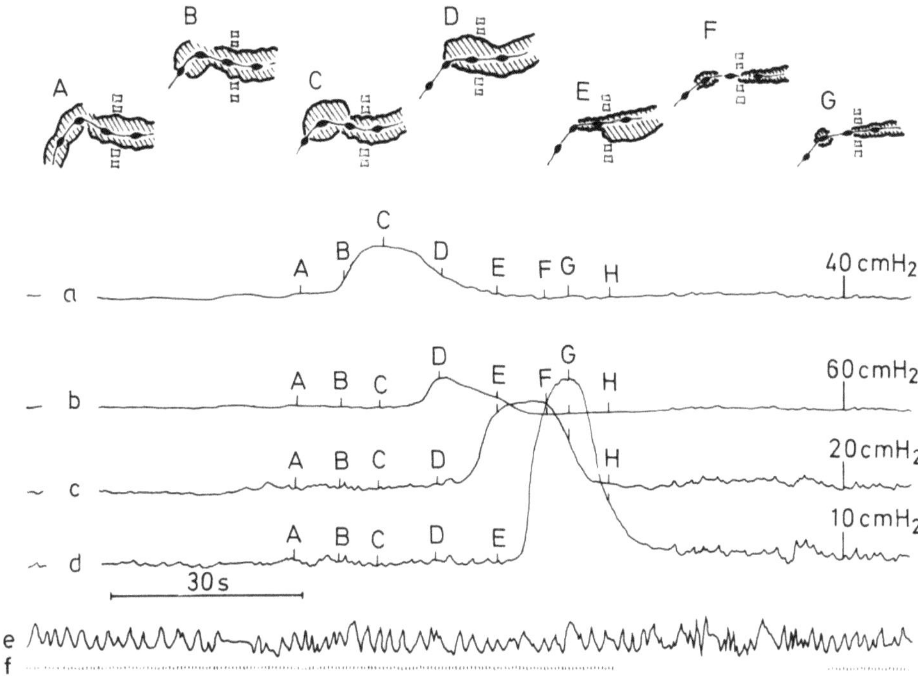

Fig. 11 a–f. Intraluminal pressure recordings obtained by four small balloons placed 5 cm apart in right flexure and transverse colon. Tracings recorded by proximal **a**, proximal intermediate **b**, distal intermediate **c**, and distal **d** balloons. Respiration **e** is also shown. Following arrival of barium sulfate suspension at the level of right flexure, synchronized cinefluorography **f** is used to correlate movements of the wall and displacement of contents with intraluminal pressure variations. Schematic drawings, corresponding to each point marked *(A–G)* on the tracings, display the sequence of motor events (Torsoli et al. 1971 b)

ized by wall contractions which, partly or completely, involve the circumference of the viscus. They do not show a propagating pattern, are sometimes synchronous at different levels, and frequently appear in an apparently irregular fashion (Ritchie 1968). On manometric tracings, segmenting activity corresponds to monophasic waves of various amplitude and duration that, in adjacent segments, appear either simultaneously or with no temporal relation (Connell 1968). Segmenting contractions are almost the only motor activity recorded in the various segments of the colon; their frequency during fasting is higher in the sigmoid than in the cecum, ascending tract (Misiewicz et al. 1966 b; Torsoli et al. 1968). Local activity does not usually cause any displacement of contents, but may sometimes give rise to intraluminal pressure gradients which induce retropulsion or propulsion of the contents (Cassano and Torsoli 1966).

Peristaltic activity is characterized by progressive coordinated movements, propagating in an aboral direction, causing displacement of the contents for short or even long distances. On radiology, these movements, which begin with a progressive change in the spatial orientation of colonic folds and finally disappear, consist of a progressive contraction of the wall preceded aborally by dilatation of the lumen (Fig. 10). On manometric tracings this motor activity appears as positive monophasic waves in temporal sequence moving in an aboral direction (Fig. 11;

HARDCASTLE and MANN 1968; TORSOLI et al. 1971 b). Compared with local activity, peristalsis in the colon is a fairly infrequent event, being more often observed at the level of the transverse and descending colon. Following administration of suitable stimuli, however, peristalsis has been described at the level of the more proximal parts of the colon (TORSOLI et al. 1971 a). Peristalsis is elicited every time intraluminal distension exceeds the threshold level (CHAUVE et al. 1976) which differs from subject to subject. This threshold level of intraluminal distension decreases in the presence of colonic contents with low pH (CORAZZIARI et al. 1977). In contrast to other species (ELLIOT and BARCLAY-SMITH 1904; CHRISTENSEN et al. 1974), no antiperistaltic motor activity has been described in humans, despite the frequent radiologic observations of retrograde displacement of the contents, especially at the level of the proximal and middle tracts of the colon.

Colonic motor activity is affected by psychic condition (ALMY et al. 1949), physical activity, and food ingestion (CONNELL 1968). Food ingestion, in particular, stimulates the segmenting activity in the cecum, ascending colon, and in the sigmoid; it has been reported that the increase in motor activity may be similar in the two tracts (MISIEWICZ et al. 1966) or relatively greater at the level of the proximal colon (WANGEL and DELLER 1965; CASSANO and TORSOLI 1966; TORSOLI et al. 1968). Likewise, after food ingestion, progression of contents is stimulated and peristaltic movements occur more frequently (HOLTZNECHT 1909; CASSANO and TORSOLI 1966).

3. Rectoanal Region

The motor behaviour in this tract differs greatly between resting conditions and during intraluminal distension of the rectal ampulla.

a) Resting Motor Activity

Electrical activity during resting conditions shows the same characteristics in the rectum, particularly the proximal part, as in the colon. Manometric recordings of the rectum display total inactivity, irregularly alternating with periods of monophasic pressure variations which appear with a higher average frequency than in the sigmoid (CONNELL 1961; CHIN KIM and BARBERO 1963). Myoelectric activity is constantly present at the level of the puborectalis muscle and the internal anal sphincter. The frequency increases temporarily in the erect position (TAVERNER and SMIDDY 1959) and is stimulated, independently of consciousness, by a spinal reflex starting in the muscle itself (MELZAK and PORTER 1964). Control electrical activity is constantly present at the level of the internal anal sphincter, at a higher frequency than in any other segment of the digestive tract (USTACH et al. 1970).

Intraluminal pressure in the anal canal is higher than in the rectal ampulla, the highest pressure being recorded about 2 cm from the anal verge in male subjects (HANCOCK 1976). Variations in intraluminal pressure have been recorded in the anal canal. Contraction waves are either of low amplitude with frequency progressively increasing in an aboral direction from 10 to 20 waves/min or of higher amplitude, synchronous at all levels of the canal and ranging in frequency from 0.6

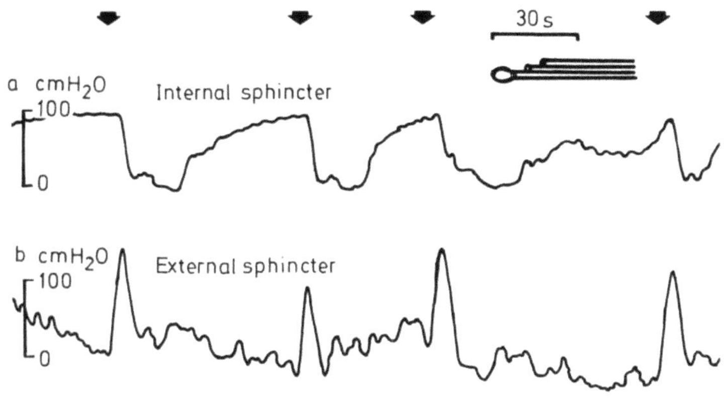

Fig. 12a, b. Intraluminal pressure recordings from the upper anal canal **a** and lower anal canal **b** in a normal subject. During rectal distension *(arrows)* inhibition of the upper anal canal and contraction of the lower anal canal occur

to 1.9 waves/min (HANCOCK 1976). Pressure variations showing an aboral increase in frequency are secondary to the motor activity of the internal anal sphincter (KERREMANS 1969). The high pressure zone of the anal canal is due to the internal anal sphincter and the puborectalis muscle (DICKINSON 1978), while the role of the external anal sphincter is still controversial (DUTHIE and WATTS 1965; VARMA and STEPHENS 1972; FRENCKNER and VON EULER 1975). The motor frequency gradients present at the level of the rectosigmoid tract and anal canal are usually considered to be the mechanism which ensures continence.

b) Motor Activity During Intraluminal Distension of the Rectal Ampulla

Within well-defined limits, prolonged and gradual distension of the rectal ampulla induces adaptation of the rectum to the intraluminal contents and is therefore not accompanied by the urge to evacuate; at times it may induce temporary contraction of the wall (ARHAN et al. 1976). This adaptive mechanism, together with the anatomic characteristics of the rectoanal tract (PHILLIPS and EDWARDS 1965), allows the deposit of fecal contents in the rectal ampulla. Rapid intraluminal distension and/or decrease in the adaptive mechanism of the wall are felt at a conscious level and facilitate the defecation reflex (FRENCKNER and VON EULER 1975; FARTHING and LENNARD-JONES 1978). Intrarectal distension, through a reflex mechanism, induces a decrease in pressure of the proximal part and, less frequently, an increase in pressure of the distal part of the anal canal (KERREMANS 1969; Fig. 12). The fall in pressure is secondary to the inhibition of the internal anal sphincter, where, at the same time, electrical control activity is interrupted (USTACH et al. 1970). The increase in pressure in the distal part of the anal canal parallels an "increment in myoelectrical activity at the level of the external anal sphincter" (MELZAK and PORTER 1964). Volume and/or pressure within the rectal ampulla affect the motor response at the level of the anal canal. During prolonged distension with small volumes, inhibition of the internal anal sphincter is only partial and temporary, but can become maximal and continuous by increasing the intrarectal volume

(IRHE 1974). The external anal sphincter also relaxes completely, after an initial contraction, if intrarectal distension is progressively increased (MELZAK and PORTER 1964). Maximal inhibition of the two sphincters induces the desire to defecate and the act of defecation itself.

4. Transit of Large Bowel Contents

Transit of large bowel contents is very slow compared with other segments of the digestive tract. Radioopaque markers usually take an average of 2–3 days to go through the large bowel, maximal times reported being 4 (ZAPPONI et al. 1979) and 7 days (MARTELLI et al. 1978). Although progression is the result of large bowel motor activity, transit undergoes interruptions and retropulsions to such an extent that mixing of food residues or markers ingested at time intervals of 24–48 h has been demonstrated (CASSANO and TORSOLI 1966; CASSANO et al. 1967; WIGGINS and CUMMINGS 1976). Radiologic observations suggest that the cecum, ascending colon serves as a reservoir for contents, however transit of radioopaque markers appears to indicate that their progression occurs in a fairly uniform fashion through the various segments of the large bowel (MARTELLI et al. 1978), and the proximal and distal parts of the colon as well as the rectum play a similar role in the progression of contents through the large bowel (ZAPPONI et al. 1979).

II. Large Bowel Manometry and Transit Time in Clinical Practice

Since the colonic segments are relatively inaccessible, the majority of manometric studies in clinical practice have been performed at the level of the rectosigmoid and rectoanal regions. Intraluminal pressure studies of the rectosigmoid tract have shown that motor activity is, on the average, increased in patients with symptomatic diverticulosis of the sigmoid (CASSANO and TORSOLI 1966; WEINREICH and ANDERSEN 1976b), but data show a considerable overlap with those obtained in a normal control group. Much controversy exists regarding motor activity in the rectosigmoid tract in patients with chronic constipation and with irritable colon syndrome (CONNELL 1962; RITCHIE and TUCKEY 1969; WALLER and MISIEWICZ 1972; MEUNIER et al. 1978; POZZESSERE et al. 1979). Some of these discrepancies may be due to the marked variability of motor activity in a given subject and from one subject to another (WEINREICH and ANDERSEN 1976a), and to the difficulties encountered in performing investigations on rather heterogeneous populations comprising patients with a variety of ill-defined, subjective, and variable symptoms. Intraluminal pressure studies of the rectosigmoid tract therefore provide no useful information for diagnostic purposes.

Conversely, evaluation of motor activity at the level of the anal canal has proved to be useful to differentiate Hirschsprung's disease from other conditions of megarectum and/or megacolon and chronic constipation. The manometric examination is particularly useful in infants (TOBON and SCHUSTER 1974; BOSTON et al. 1977) as it is easy to perform and safe; moreover, it is the only test that may help in the diagnosis of Hirschsprung's disease in the presence of a short aganglionic segment (DEVROEDE 1978). In intraluminal pressure studies on patients

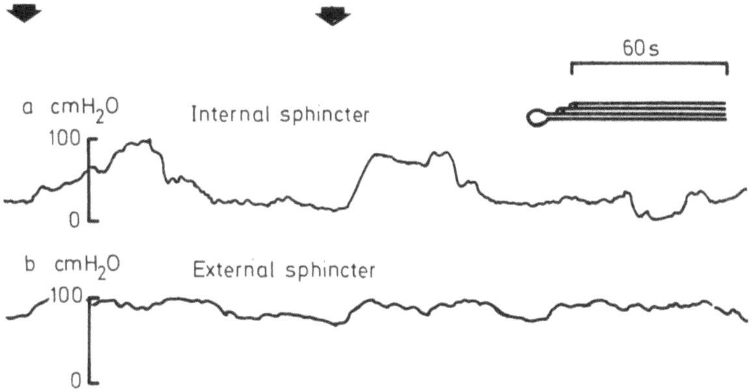

Fig. 13a, b. Intraluminal pressure recordings from the upper anal canal **a** and lower anal canal **b** in a patient with Hirschsprung's disease. During rectal distension *(arrows)* contractions of both upper and lower anal canals occur

with Hischsprung's disease, inhibition of the internal anal sphincter during intrarectal distension is lacking (HOWARD and NIXON 1968; AARONSON and NIXON 1972; Fig. 13). Motor behaviour similar to that occurring in Hirschsprung's disease has been described in cases of systemic sclerosis (SCHUSTER 1966), whole thickness sphincterotomy, chronic rectal ischemia (DEVROEDE 1978), and following transection of the rectum (SCHUSTER 1968). The rectoanal inhibitory reflex is instead present in all other cases of megacolon and/or chronic constipation. In the latter group, however, inhibition may be only partial and/or after distension of the rectal ampulla with abnormally large volumes (CLAYDEN and LAWSON 1976). In patients with chronic constipation and fecal incontinence, relaxation of the internal anal sphincter occurs with normal intrarectal distension, but the stimulus for defecation is felt at the conscious level with larger volumes (MEUNIER et al. 1976).

Finally, anorectal manometry has also proved to be useful in the treatment of fecal incontinence secondary to various disorders (CERULLI et al. 1979). It is in fact possible, during manometric monitoring of the anal canal, to train patients with fecal incontinence to increase their sensitivity to intrarectal stimuli. The patient is asked to contract the external anal sphincter during rectal distension with progressively decreasing volumes (Fig. 14). Learning to perform this voluntary act in the right time relationship with minimal rectal distension can rapidly be transformed into an automatic reflex act.

Measurement of oroanal transit time is of great importance in patients complaining of chronic constipation; it discriminates between those with a real slowing of contents and others who, although presenting the same disturbances, have a transit time within normal limits (HINTON et al. 1969; CORAZZIARI et al. 1979). The latter group cannot be differentiated from the former, on clinical grounds, and may represent as many as half the patients complaining of chronic constipation (CORAZZIARI et al. 1979). Futhermore, measurement of large bowel segmental transit times in patients with real slowing of transit indicates where progression of con-

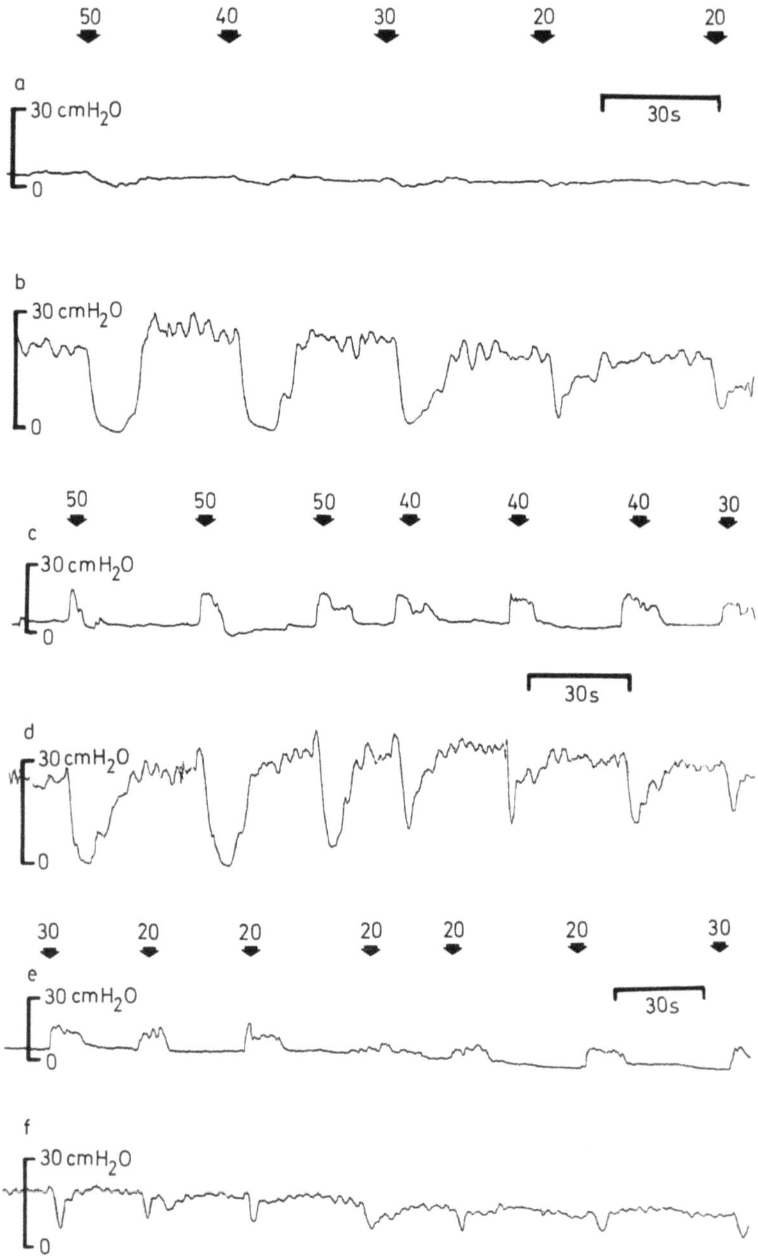

Fig. 14a–f. Intraluminal pressure recordings obtained by two small balloons placed at the level of the lower anal canal **a, c, e** and upper anal canal **b, d, f** in a patient with fecal incontinence. *Arrows*, inflation of a large ballon placed in the rectal ampulla with volumes of air indicated in ml. Tracings are from a single session. Recordings before biofeedback conditioning **a, b**; during rectal distension: inhibition of the upper anal canal and no response of the lower canal. Recordings during biofeedback conditioning **c, d**; patient observes tracing and, during rectal distension, is asked to contract the external anal sphincter; during distension with decreasing volumes of air: inhibition of the upper anal canal and contraction of the lower anal canal. Recordings after biofeedback conditioning **d, e**; during rectal distension, performed out of sight of the patient: inhibition of the upper canal and contraction of the lower anal canal

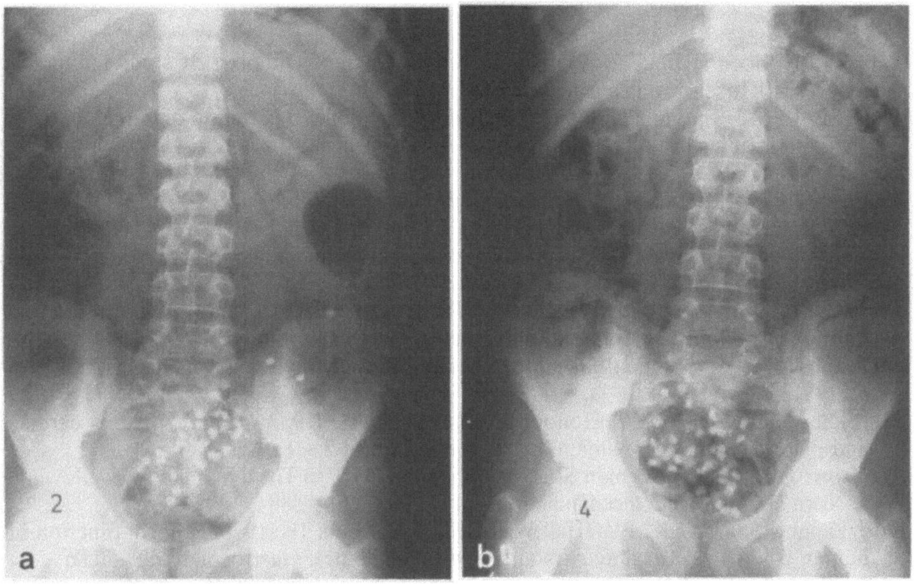

Fig. 15 a, b. Radioopaque markers retained in the rectal ampulla 2 days **a** and 4 days **b** after ingestion

tents is delayed (Fig. 15). Slowing of transit may occur only in the rectum, only in the distal colon, or in the entire large bowel (CASSANO and TORSOLI 1966; CORAZZIARI et al. 1975; MARTELLI et al. 1978). In patients with idiopathic muscular strictures, slowing of radioopaque markers occurs at the level of the distal colon (CASSANO and TORSOLI 1968).

E. Conclusions

Studies of gastrointestinal motility have developed considerably in the last 20 years. One of the most difficult problems in physiology, i.e., gastrointestinal movements (BAYLISS and STARLING 1899), has been to a large extent elucitated. However, clinical relevance of manometric investigations appears to be limited, except in the esophagus and the anorectal region. In these areas, intraluminal pressure studies are now part of the usual diagnostic tools.

Radiologic investigation of the gastroesophageal junction has, so far, not given satisfactory results and a pH–manometric study is useful whenever motor abnormality of the cardia is suspected. In the other tracts of the alimentary canal, however, radiologic studies still represent, in clinical practice, the major source of information on motor activity. Unfortunately, radiologic data cannot be quantified and no significant progress in the methodologic approach of radiologic studies has been made recently. The radiologic methods used to investigate gastrointestinal motility have not improved significantly over the long and dangerous fluoroscopic techniques developed by the pioneer radiologists. Efforts should be made to improve these radiologic methods.

References

Aaronson I, Nixon HH (1972) A clinical evaluation of anorectal pressure studies in the diagnosis of Hirschsprung's disease. Gut 13:138–146
Almy TP, Kern F Jr, Tulin M (1949) Alterations in colonic function in man under stress. II. Experimental production of sigmoid spasm in healthy persons. Gastroenterology 12:425–436
Anuras S (1978) Intestinal pseudoobstruction. Gastroenterology 74:1318–1324
Arhan P, Faverdin C, Persoz B, Devroede G, Dubois F, Dornic C, Pellerin D (1976) Relationship between viscoelastic properties of the rectum and anal pressure in man. J Appl Physiol 41:677–682
Arndorfer RC, Stef JJ, Dodds WJ, Linchon JH, Hogan WT (1977) Improved infusion system for intraluminal esophageal manometry. Gastroenterology 73:23–27
Atkinson M (1976) Oesophageal motor changes in systemic disease. Clin Gastroenterol 5:119–133
Atkinson M, Edwards DAW, Honour AJ, Rowlands EN (1957a) Comparison of cardiac and pyloric sphincters. A manometric study. Lancet 2:918–922
Atkinson M, Kramer P, Wyman SM, Ingelfinger FJ (1957b) The dynamics of swallowing. I. Normal pharyngeal mechanism. J Clin Invest 36:581–588
Bardakajian B, Sarna SK, Waterfall WE, Daniel EE, Lind JF (1976) Control function of human colonic electrical activity analysed by computer. Gastroenterology 70:86
Bayliss WM, Starling EH (1899) The movements and innervation of the small intestine. J Physiol (Lond) 24:99–143
Behar J, Ramsby G (1978) Gastric emptying and antral motility in reflux esophagitis. Effect of oral metoclopramide. Gastroenterology 74:253–256
Behar J, Biancani P, Spiro HM, Storer EH (1974) Effect of an anterior fundoplication on lower esophageal sphincter competence. Gastroenterology 67:209–215
Bennett JR (1973) The physician's problem. In: Symposium on gastroesophageal reflux and its complications. Sect 5. Gut 14:246–249
Berlin BP, Fienstein JI, Tedesco F, Ogure JH (1977) Manometric studies of the upper esophageal sphincter. Ann Otol Rhinol Laryngol 86:598–602
Bombeck CT, Battle WS, Nyhus LM (1972) Spasm in the differential diagnosis of gastroesophageal reflux. Arch Surg 104:477–483
Borgström S, Arborelius M Jr (1971) A technique for studying propulsion and the displacement of contents in the duodenum and proximal jejunum. Rend Gastroenterol 3:174–177
Boston VE, Cywes S, Davies MRQ (1977) Qualitative and quantitative evaluation of internal anal function in the newborn. Gut 18:1036–1044
Brand DL, Martin D, Pope CE II (1977) Esophageal manometrics in patients with angina-like chest pain. Am J Dig Dis 22:300–304
Cannon WB, Lieb CW (1911) The receptive relaxation of the stomach. Am J Physiol 29:267–273
Caprilli R, Vernia P, Frieri G, Melchiorri P (1975) Two electrical rhythms in the colon. Rend Gastroenterol 7:65–66
Carlson HC, Code CF, Nelson RA (1966) Motor action of the canine gastroduodenal junction: a cineradiographic pressure and electric study. Am J Dig Dis 11:155–172
Cassano C, Torsoli A (1966) Indirizzi moderni nello studio delle malattie croniche non neoplastiche del colon. In: Pozzi L (ed) Rel LXVII Congr Soc Ital Med Intern, Rome
Cassano C, Torsoli A (1968) Idiopathic muscular strictures of the sigmoid colon. Gut 9:325–331
Cassano CC, Amoruso M, Arullani P, Badalamenti G (1967) Ricerche sui tempi di transito gastrointestinale totali e parziali. Arch Ital Mal App Dig 34:290–293
Cerulli MA, Nikoomanesh P, Schuster MM (1979) Progress in biofeedback conditioning for fecal incontinence. Gastroenterology 76:742–746
Chattopadhyay DK, Pope CE II (1979) Lower esophageal sphincter pressure's variability destroys its usefulness. Gastroenterology 76:1111
Chauve A, Devroede G, Bastin E (1976) Intraluminal pressures during perfusion of the human colon in situ. Gastroenterology 70:336–340

Chin Kim I, Barbero GJ (1963) The pattern of rectosigmoid motility in children. Gastroenterology 45:57–66
Christensen J (1971) The controls of gastrointestinal movements: some old and new views. N Engl J Med 285:85–98
Christensen J, Schedl HP, Clifton JA (1966) The small intestinal basic rhythm (slow wave) frequency gradient in normal and in patients with a variety of diseases. Gastroenterology 50:309–315
Christensen J, Anuras S, Hauser RL (1974) Migrating spike bursts and electrical slow waves in the cat colon: effect of sectioning. Gastroenterology 66:240–247
Clayden GS, Lawson JON (1976) Investigation and management of longstanding chronic constipation in childhood. Arch Dis Child 51:918–923
Code CF, Marlett JA (1975) The interdigestive myo-electric complex of the stomach and small bowel of dogs. J Physiol (Lond) 246:289–309
Code CF, Schlegel JF (1974) The gastrointestinal interdigestive housekeeper: motor correlates of the interdigestive myoelectric complex of the dog. In: Daniel EE et al. (eds) Proceedings of the Fourth International Symposium on Gastrointestinal Motility. Mitchell, Vancouver, pp 631–634
Cohen BR (1965) Cardiospasm in achalasia: demonstration of an abnormally elevated esophagogastric sphincter pressure with partial relaxation on swallowing. Gastroenterology 48:864
Cohen BR, Wolf BS (1968) Cineradiographic and intraluminal pressure correlations in the pharynx and esophagus. In: Alimentary canal. American Physiological Society, Washington DC (Handbook of physiology, vol IV, sect 6, pp 1814–1860)
Cohen S, Harris LD (1972) The lower esophageal sphincter. Gastroenterology 63:1066–1073
Cohen S, Harris LD, Levitan R (1968) Manometric characteristics of the human ileocecal junctional zone. Gastroenterology 54:72–75
Connell AM (1961) The motility of the pelvic colon. I. Motility in normals and in patients with asymptomatic duodenal ulcer. Gut 2:175–186
Connell AM (1962) The motility of the pelvic colon. II. Paradoxical motility in diarrhea and constipation. Gut 3:342–348
Connell AM (1968) Motor action of the large bowel. In: Alimentary canal. American Physiological Society, Washington DC (Handbook of physiology, vol IV, sect 6, pp 2075–2091)
Connell AM (1974) Clinical aspects of motility. Med Clin N Am 58/6:1201–1216
Cooke AR (1975) Control of gastric emptyng and motility. Gastroenterology 68:804–816
Cooper JD, Gill SS, Nelems JM, Pearson FG (1977) Intraoperative and postoperative esophageal findings with Collis gastroplasty and Belsey hiatal hernia repair for gastroesophageal reflux. J Thor Cardiovasc Surg 74:744–751
Corazziari E, Capurso P, Anzini F, Torsoli A (1972) Rhythmic mechanical activity of the duodenum. Digestion 5:344
Corazziari E, Dani S, Pozzessere C, Anzini F, Torsoli A (1975) Colonic segmental transit times in chronic non organic constipation. Rend Gastroenterol 7:67–69
Corazziari E, Mineo TC, Anzini F, Torsoli A, Ricci C (1977) Functional evaluation of colon transplants used in esophageal reconstruction. Am J Dig Dis 22:7–12
Corazziari E, Pozzessere C, Dani S, Anzini F, Torsoli A (1978) Intraluminal pH and esophageal motility. Gastroenterology 75:275–277
Corazziari E, Pozzessere C, Bausano G et al. (1979) Cooperative study on chronic constipation. Preliminary data. Ital J Gastroenterol 11:142
Creamer B, Olsen AM, Code CF (1957) The esophageal sphincters in achalasia of the cardia (cardiospasm). Gastroenterology 33:293–301
Csendes A, Heriquez A (1978) Gastric emptying in patients with reflux esophagitis or benign stricture of the esophagus secondary to gastroesophageal reflux compared to controls. Scand J Gastroenterol 13:205–207
Davies WT, Kirkpatrick JR, Owen GM, Shields R (1971) Gastric emptying in atrophic gastritis and carcinoma of the stomach. Scand J Gastroenterol 6:297–301
Devroede G (1978) Constipation: mechanisms and management. In: Sleisenger MH, Fordtran JS (eds) Gastrointestinal disease. Saunders, Philadelphia London Toronto, pp 368–386

Diamant NE, Bortoff A (1969) Effects of transection on the intestinal slow wave frequency gradient. Am J Physiol 216:734–743
Dickinson VA (1978) Progress report. Maintenance of anal continence; a review of pelvic floor physiology. Gut 19:1163–1174
Dodds WJ, Stef JJ, Hogan WJ (1976) Factors determining pressure measurement accuracy by intraluminal esophageal manometry. Gastroenterology 70:117–123
Donner MW, Silbiger ML, Hookman P, Hendrix TR (1966) Acid barium swallows in the radiographic evaluation of clinical esophagitis. Radiology 87:220–225
Dubois A, Endewegh PV, Gardner JD (1977) Gastric emptying and secretion in Zollinger-Ellison syndrome. J Clin Invest 59:255–263
Duthie HL, Watts JM (1965) Contribution of the external anal sphincter to the pressure zone in the anal canal. Gut 6:64–68
Elliott TR, Barclay-Smith E (1904) Antiperistalsis and other activities of the colon. J Physiol (Lond) 31:272
Ellis FH, Schlegel JF, Lynch VP, Payne WS (1969) Cricopharyngeal myotomy for pharyngoesophageal diverticulum. Ann Surg 170:340–349
Farthing MJG, Lennard-Jones JE (1978) Sensibility of the rectum to distension and the anorectal distension reflex in ulcerative colitis. Gut 19:64–69
Faulk DL, Anuras S, Christensen J (1978) Chronic intestinal pseudoobstruction. Gastroenterology 74:922–931
Faulk WT, Code CP, Marlock CG, Bargen JA (1954) A study of the motility patterns and the basic rhythm in the duodenum and upper part of the jejunum of human beings. Gastroenterology 26:601–611
Fisher R, Cohen S (1973) Physiological characteristics of the human pyloric sphincter. Gastroenterology 64:67–75
Fleckenstein P, Öigaard A (1978) Electrical spike activity in the human small intestine: a multiple electrode study of fasting and diurnal variations. Am J Dig Dis 23:776–780
Fleshler B (1967) Diffuse esophageal spasm. Gastroenterology 52:559–564
Fordtran JS, Walsh JH (1973) Gastric acid secretion rate and buffer control of the stomach after eating: results in normal subjects and in patients with duodenal ulcer. J Clin Invest 52:645–657
Fox JE, Wideins EI, Beck IT (1973) Observer variation in esophageal pressure assessment. Gastroenterology 65:884–888
Frenckner B, Von Euler C (1975) Influence of pudendal block on the function of the anal sphincter. Gut 16:482–489
Fyke FE Jr, Code CF (1955) Resting and deglutition pressures in the pharyngoesophageal region. Gastroenterology 29:24–34
Garrett JM, Winkelmann RK, Schlegel JF, Code CF (1971) Esophageal deterioration in scleroderma. Mayo Clin Proc 46:92–96
Gerhardt DC, Schuck TJ, Bordeaux TA, Winship DH (1978) Human upper esophageal sphincter. Response to volume, osmotics, and acid stimuli. Gastroenterology 75:268–274
Griffith GH, Owen GM, Campbell H, Shields R (1968) Gastric emptying in health and gastroduodenal disease. Gastroenterology 54:1–7
Hancock BD (1976) Measurement of anal pressure and motility. Gut 17:645–651
Hardcastle JD, Mann CV (1968) Study of large bowel peristalsis. Gut 9:512–520
Hay DJ, Goodall RJ, Temple JG (1979) The reproducibility of the station pull-through technique for measuring LESP. Br J Surg 66:93–97
Heading RC, Tothill P, McLoughlin GP, Shearman DJG (1976) Gastric emptying rate measurement in man: a double isotope scanning technique for simultaneous study of liquid and solid components of a meal. Gastroenterology 71:45–50
Heitmann P (1971) The immediate effect of pneumatic dilatation on intraluminal yield pressures in achalasia of the esophagus. Rend Gastroenterol 3:141–142
Hertz AF (1907) The passage of food along the human alimentary canal. Guy Hosp Rep 61:389–427
Hinder PA, Kelly KA (1977) Canine gastric emptying of solids and liquids. Am J Physiol 233:E335–E340

Hinton JM, Lennard-Jones JE, Young AC (1969) A new method for studying gut transit times using radioopaque markers. Gut 10:842–847
Holtznecht G (1909) Die normale Peristalik des Kolons. MMW 56:2401–2403
Howard ER, Nixon HH (1968) Internal anal sphincter: observations on development and mechanism of inhibitory responses in premature infants and children with Hirschsprung's disease. Arch Dis Child 43:569–578
Hunt JN, Knox MT (1968) Regulation of gastric emptying. In: Alimentary canal. American Physiological Society, Washington DC (Handbook of physiology, vol IV, sect 6, pp 1917–1935)
Hunt JN, Knox MT (1972) The slowing of gastric emptying by four strong and three weak acids. J Physiol (Lond) 222:187–208
Hunt JN, Pathak JD (1960) The osmotic effects of some simple molecules and ions on gastric emptying. J Physiol (Lond) 154:254–269
Hunt JN, Stubbs DF (1975) The volume and energy content of meals as determinants of gastric emptying. J Physiol (Lond) 245:209–225
Irhe T (1974) Studies on anal function in continent and incontinent patients. Scand J Gastroenterol [Suppl 25] 9
Kelly KA (1976) Gastric motility in health and after gastric surgery. Viewpoints Dig Dis 8 (2)
Kelly KA, Code CF (1971) Canine gastric pacemaker. Am J Physiol 220:112–117
Kerremans R (1969) Morphological and physiological aspects of anal continence and defecation. Arscia Vitgaven, Brussels, pp 197–222
Kilman WJ, Goyal RK (1976) Disorders of pharyngeal and upper esophageal sphincter motor function. Arch Intern Med 136:592–601
Kramer P (1970) Diffuse esophageal spasm. In: Bayless TM (ed) Modern treatment. Management of esophageal disease. Harper & Row, New York, pp 1151–1162
Kwong NK, Brown BH, Whittaker GE, Duthie HL (1972) Effects of gastrin I, secretin, and cholecystokinin-pancreozymin on the electrical activity, motor activity, and acid output of the stomach in man. Scand J Gastroenterol 7:161–170
Laws JW, Neale G (1966) Radiological diagnosis of disaccharides deficiency. Lancet 2:139–142
Liebermann-Meffert D, Allgower M, Schmid P, Blum AL (1979) Muscular equivalent of the lower esophageal sphincter. Gastroenterology 76:31–38
Lind JF, Duthie HL, Schlegel JF, Code CF (1961) Motility of the gastric fundus. Am J Physiol 201:197–202
Lipshutz WH, Eckert RJ, Gaskins RD, Baluton DE, Lukash WM (1974) Lower esophageal sphincter after surgical treatment of gastroesophageal reflux. N Engl J Med 291:1107–1110
Little AG, DeMeester TR, Rezai-Zadeh K, Skinner DB (1977) Abnormal gastric emptying in patients with gastroesophageal reflux. Surg Forum 28:347–348
Long WB, Weiss JB (1974) Rapid gastric emptying of fatty meals in pancreatic insufficiency. Gastroenterology 67:920–925
MacGregor IL, Parent JA, Meyer JH (1977a) Gastric emptying of liquid meals and pancreatic and biliary secretion after subtotal and truncal vagotomy with pyloroplasty. Gastroenterology 72:195–205
MacGregor IL, Martin P, Meyer JH (1977b) Gastric emptying of solid food in normal man and after subtotal gastrectomy and truncal vagotomy with pyloroplasty. Gastroenterology 72:206–211
Mallinson CN (1968) Effect of pancreatic insufficiency and intestinal lactose deficiency on the gastric emptying of starch and lactose. Gut 9:737
Martelli H, Devroede G, Arhan P, Dugnay C, Dorric C, Faverdin C (1978) Some parameters of large bowel motility in normal man. Gatroenterology 75:612–618
McCallum RW, Kline HH, Curry N, Sturdevant RAL (1975) Comparative effects of metoclopramide and bethanecol on lower esophageal sphincter pressure in reflux patients. Gastroenterology 68:1114–1118
Melzak J, Porter NH (1964) Studies of the reflex activity of the external sphincter ani in spinal man. Paraplegia 1:277–296

Meunier P, Mollard P, Marechal J-M (1976) Physiopathology of megarectum: the association of megarectum with encopresis. Gut 17:224–227
Meunier P, Rochas A, Lambert R (1978) Sigmoid motility in constipation. Gastroenterology 74:1136
Meyer JH, McGregor IL, Gueller R, Martin P, Cavalieri R (1976) ^{99m}Tc-tagged chicken liver as a marker of solid food in the human stomach. Am J Dig Dis 21:296–304
Meyer JH, Thomson JB, Cohen MB, Scadchehr A, Mandiola SA (1979) Sieving of solid foods by the canine stomach and sieving after gastric emptying. Gastroenterology 76:804–813
Misiewicz JJ, Connell AM, Pontes FA (1966) Comparison of the effect of meals and prostigmine on the proximal and distal colon in patients with and without diarrhea. Gut 7:468–473
Monges H, Salducci J, Nandy B (1978) The upper esophageal sphincter during vomiting, eructation, and distension of the cardia: an electromyographic study in the unanesthesized dog. In: Duthie HL (ed) Gastrointestinal motility in health and disease. MTP Press, Lancaster, pp 575–584
Nelsen TS, Kohatsu S (1971) The stomach as a pump. Rend Gastroenterol 3:65–70
Pérez-Avila C, Irvor II (1975) Interpretation of LESP measurements. Br J Surg 62:663
Phillips SF, Edwards DAW (1965) Some aspects of anal continence and defecation. Gut 6:396–406
Pope CE II (1967) A dynamic test of sphincter strenght. Its implication to the lower esophageal sphincter. Gastroenterology 52:779–786
Pope CE II (1978) Esophageal motility. Who needs it? Gastroenterology 74:1337–1338
Pozzessere C, Corazziari E, Dani S, Anzini F, Torsoli A (1979) Basal and caerulein stimulated motor activity of sigmoid colon in chronic constipation. Ital J Gastroenterol 11:107–109
Provenzale L, Pisano M (1971) Methods for recording electrical activity of the human colon in vivo. Am J Dig Dis 16:712–722
Rayner V, Wenham G, Rhind SM, White F, Bruce JB (1979) Digesta transit by x-ray screening, glucose absorption, insulin secretion, and the migrating myoelectric complex in the pig. In: Abstracts of the 7 th International Symposium on Gastrointestinal Motility. The University of Iowa, Iowa City, p 42
Rimer DG (1966) Gastric retention without mechanical obstruction. Arch Intern Med 117:287–299
Rinaldo JA, Levey JF (1968) Correlation of several methods for recording esophageal sphincteral pressures. Am J Dig Dis 3:882–890
Ritchie JA (1968) Colonic motor activity and bowel function. Part I. Normal movement of contents. Gut 9:442–456
Ritchie JA, Tuckey MS (1969) Intraluminal pressure studies at different distances from the anus in normal subjects and in patients with the irritable colon syndrome. Am J Dig Dis 14:96–106
Sarna SK, Daniel EE, Kingma JE (1972) Stimulation of electrical control activity of the stomach by an array of relaxation oscillators. Am J Dig Dis 17:229–235
Sarna SK, Bardakjian BL, Waterfall WE, Lind JF, Daniel EE (1979) Human colonic electrical activity (ECA). In: Abstracts of the 7 th International Symposium on Gastrointestinal Motility. The University of Iowa, Iowa City, p 68
Sarr MG, Kelly KA (1979) Jejunal transit of liquids and solids during jejunal interdigestive and digestive motor activity. In: Abstracts of the 7 th International Symposium on Gastrointestinal Motility. The University of Iowa, Iowa City, p 52
Schuster MM (1966) Clinical significance of motor disturbances of the enterocolonic segment. Am J Dig Dis 11:320–335
Schuster MM (1968) Motor action of rectum and anal sphincters in continence and defecation. In: Alimentary canal. American Physiological Society, Washington DC (Handbook of physiology, vol IV, sect 6, pp 2121–2140)
Snape WJ, Carlson GM, Cohen S (1976) Colonic myoelectric activity in the irritable bowel syndrome. Gastroenterology 70:326–330

Sokol EM, Heitmann P, Wolf BS, Cohen BR (1966) Simultaneous cineradiographic and manometric study of the pharynx, hypopharynx, and cervical esophagus. Gastroenterology 51:960–974
Stef JJ, Dodds JW, Hogan WJ, Linehan JH, Stewart ET (1974) Intraluminal esophageal manometry: an analysis of variables affecting recording fidelity of peristaltic pressures. Gastroenterology 67:221–230
Stemper TJ, Cooke AR (1976) Effect of a fixed pyloric opening on gastric emptying in the cat and the dog. Am J Physiol 230:813–817
Stephens JR, Woolson RF, Cooke AR (1976) Osmolyte and tryptophan receptors controlling gastric emptying in the dog. Am J Physiol 231:848–853
Szurszewski JH (1969) A migrating electric complex of the canine smal intestine. Am J Physiol 217:1757–1763
Szurszewski JH, Elvebach LK, Code CF (1970) Configuration and frequency gradient of electric slow wave over canine small bowel. Am J Physiol 218:1468–1473
Tatelman M, Keech MK (1966) Esophageal motility in systemic erythematosus, rheumatoid arthritis and scleroderma. Radiology 86:1041–1046
Taverner D, Smiddy FG (1959) An electromyographic study of the normal function of the external anal sphincter and pelvic diaphragm. Dis Colon Rectum 2:153–160
Taylor I, Duthie HL, Smallwood R, Linkens D (1975) Large bowel myoelectrical activity in man. Gut 16:808–816
Thomas JE (1957) Mechanics and regulation of gastric emptying. Physiol Rev 37:453–474
Thompson JR, Sanders I (1972) Lactose barium small bowel study. Efficacy of a screening method. AJR 116:276–278
Tobon F, Schuster MM (1974) Megacolon: special diagnostic and therapeutic features. Johns Hopkins Med J 135:91–105
Torsoli A, Ramorino ML, Crucioli V (1968) The relationship between anatomy and motor activity of the colon. Am J Dig Dis 13:462–467
Torsoli A, Corazziari E, Waller LS, Anzini F (1971 a) Duodenal peristalsis in man. Rend Gastroenterol 3:168–173
Torsoli A, Ramorino ML, Ammaturo MV, Capurso L, Arcangeli G, Paoluzi P (1971 b) Mass movements and intracolonic pressures. Am J Dig Dis 16:693–696
Turano L (1957) Malattie non neoplastiche dell'esofago. In: Pozzi L (ed) Atti del Congr Ital Med Intern Rome, pp 1–72, September 1957
Ustach T, Tobon F, Hambrecht T, Bass D, Schuster MM (1970) Electrophysiological aspects of human sphincter function. J Clin Invest 49:41–48
Vantrappen G, Hellemans J Deloof W, Valembois P, Vandenbroucke J (1971) Treatment of achalasia with pneumatic dilatations. Gut 12:268–275
Vantrappen G, Janssens J, Hellemans J, Ghoos Y (1977) The interdigestive motor complex of normal subjects and patients with bacterial overgrowth of the small intestine. J Clin Invest 59:1158–1166
Vantrappen G, Janssens J, Hellemans J, Coremans G (1979 a) Achalasia, diffuse esophageal spasm, and related disorders. Gastroenterology 76:450–457
Vantrappen G, Peeters TL, Janssens J (1979 b) The secretory component of the interdigestive complex. In: Abstracts of the 7th International Symposium on Gastrointestinal Motility. The University of Iowa, Iowa City, p 51
Varma KK, Stephens D (1972) Neuromuscular reflexes of rectal continence. Aust NZ J Surg 41:263–272
Waller SL, Misiewicz JJ (1972) Colonic motility in constipation or diarrhea. Scand J Gastroenterol 7:93–96
Wangel AG, Deller DJ (1965) III Mechanisms of constipation and diarrhea with particular reference to the irritable colon syndrome. Gastroenterology 48:69–84
Weinreich J, Andersen D (1976 a) Intraluminal pressure in the sigmoid colon. I. Method and results in normal persons. Scand J Gastroenterol 11:577–580
Weinreich J, Andersen D (1976 b) Intraluminal pressures in the sigmoid colon. II. Patients with sigmoid diverticula and related conditions. Scand J Gastroenterol 11:581–586
Wienbeck M (1976) The present status of esophageal manometry. Acta Hepatogastroenterol 23:59–67

Wienbeck M, Holger J, Janssen H (1974) Electrical control mechanisms of the ileo-colic junction. In: Daniel EE (ed) Proceedings of the 4th International Symposium on Gastrointestinal Motility. Mitchell, Vancouver, pp 97–107
Wiggins HS, Cummings JH (1976) Evidence for the mixing of residue in the human gut. Gut 17:1007–1011
Winans CS (1972) The pharyngoesophageal closure mechanism: a manometric study. Gastroenterology 63:768–777
Zapponi GA, Bausano G, Corazziari E, Anzini F, Torsoli A (1979) Progressione del contenuto attraverso l'intestino crasso in soggetti con tempo di transito normale. Ital J Gastroenterol [Suppl 1] 11:132

Subject Index

Handbook of Experimental Pharmacology

Continuation of "Handbuch der experimentellen Pharmakologie"

Springer-Verlag
Berlin
Heidelberg
New York

Volume 17
Ions alcalino-terreux

Part 1
Systèmes isolés

Part 2
Organismes entiers

Volume 18
Histamine and Anti-Histaminics

Part 1
Histamine. Its Chemistry, Metabolism and Physiological and Pharmacological Actions

Part 2
Histamine II and Anti-Histaminics

Volume 19
5-Hydrocytryptamine and Related Indolealkylamines

Volume 20: Part 1
Pharmacology of Fluorides I

Part 2
Pharmacology of Fluorides II

Volume 21
Beryllium

Volume 22: Part 1
Die Gestagene I

Part 2
Die Gestagene II

Volume 23
Neurohypophysial Hormones and Similar Polypeptides

Volume 24
Diuretica

Volume 25
Bradykinin, Kallidin and Kallikrein

Volume 26
Vergleichende Pharmakologie von Überträgersubstanzen in tiersystematischer Darstellung

Volume 27
Anticoagulantien

Volume 28: Part 1
Concepts in Biochemical Pharmacology I

Part 3
Concepts in Biochemical Pharmacology III

Volume 29
Oral wirksame Antidiabetika

Volume 30
Modern Inhalation Anesthetics

Volume 32: Part 2
Insulin II

Volume 34
Secretin, Cholecystokinin, Pancreozymin and Gastrin

Volume 35: Part 1
Androgene I

Part 2
Androgens II and Antiandrogens/Androgene II und Antiandrogene

Volume 36
Uranium - Plutonium - Transplutonic Elements

Volume 37
Angiotensin

Volume 38: Part 1
Antineoplastic and Immunosuppressive Agents I

Handbook of Experimental Pharmacology

Continuation of "Handbuch der experimentellen Pharmakologie"

Part 2
Antineoplastic and Immunosuppressive Agents II

Volume 39
Antihypertensive Agents

Volume 40
Organic Nitrates

Volume 41
Hypolipidemic Agents

Volume 42
Neuromuscular Junction

Volume 43
Anabolic-Androgenic Steroids

Volume 44
Heme and Hemoproteins

Volume 45: Part 1
Drug Addiction I

Part 2
Drug Addiction II

Volume 46
Fibrinolytics and Antifibrinolytics

Volume 47
Kinetics of Drug Action

Volume 48
Arthropod Venoms

Volume 49
Ergot Alkaloids and Related Compounds

Volume 50: Part 1
Inflammation

Part 2
Anti-Inflammatory Drugs

Volume 51
Uric Acid

Volume 52
Snake Venoms

Volume 53
Pharmacology of Ganglionic Transmission

Volume 54: Part 1
Adrenergic Activators and Inhibitors I

Part 2
Adrenergic Activators and Inhibitors II

Volume 55: Part 1
Antipsychotics and Antidepressants I

Part 2
Antpsychotics and Antidepressants II

Part 3
Alcohol and Psychotomimetics, Psychotropic Effects of Central Acting Drugs

Volume 56, Part 1 + 2
Cardiac Glycosides

Volume 57
Tissue Growth Factors

Volume 58
Cyclic Nucleotides
Part 1: **Biochemistry**
Part 2: **Physiology and Pharmacology**

Volume 59
Mediators and Drugs in Gastrointestinal Motility
Part 1: **Morphological Basis and Neurophysiological Control**
Part 2: **Endogenis and Exogenis Agents**

Volume 60
Pyretics and Antipyretics

Springer-Verlag
Berlin
Heidelberg
New York

MIX
Papier aus verantwortungsvollen Quellen
Paper from responsible sources
FSC® C105338
FSC
www.fsc.org

If you have any concerns about our products,
you can contact us on
ProductSafety@springernature.com

In case Publisher is established outside the EU,
the EU authorized representative is:
Springer Nature Customer Service Center GmbH
Europaplatz 3, 69115 Heidelberg, Germany

Printed by Libri Plureos GmbH
in Hamburg, Germany